Handbook of Intensive Care Medicine

Handbook of Intensive Care Medicine

Edited by Damien Newman

AMERICAN
MEDICAL PUBLISHERS
www.americanmedicalpublishers.com

American Medical Publishers,
41 Flatbush Avenue,
1st Floor, New York,
NY 11217, USA

Visit us on the World Wide Web at:
www.americanmedicalpublishers.com

ISBN: 978-1-63927-102-3

Cataloging-in-Publication Data

Handbook of intensive care medicine / edited by Damien Newman.
p. cm.
Includes bibliographical references and index.
ISBN 978-1-63927-102-3
1. Critical care medicine. 2. Emergency medicine. 3. Intensive care units. I. Newman, Damien.
RC86.7 .H363 2022
616.028--dc23

Table of Contents

Preface

This book has been an outcome of determined endeavour from a group of educationists in the field. The primary objective was to involve a broad spectrum of professionals from diverse cultural background involved in the field for developing new researches. The book not only targets students but also scholars pursuing higher research for further enhancement of the theoretical and practical applications of the subject.

Intensive care medicine deals with the diagnosis and treatment of critically ill patients that need advanced monitoring and life saving support. Its diagnosis and treatment are carried out in special intensive care units within the hospital. Some of the equipment used in such units are ventricular assist devices, hemodynamic and cardiac monitoring systems, intra-aortic balloon pumps, extracorporeal membrane oxygenation circuits, continuous renal replacement equipment, etc. These equipment help in hemofiltration, mechanical ventilation, and invasive monitoring. There are many drugs that are used under intensive care. These include inotropes, sedatives, antibiotics and analgesics. This book explores all the important aspects of intensive care medicine in the present day scenario. It elucidates the concepts and innovative models around prospective developments with respect to intensive care medicine. This book will help the readers in keeping pace with the rapid changes in this field.

It was an honour to edit such a profound book and also a challenging task to compile and examine all the relevant data for accuracy and originality. I wish to acknowledge the efforts of the contributors for submitting such brilliant and diverse chapters in the field and for endlessly working for the completion of the book. Last, but not the least; I thank my family for being a constant source of support in all my research endeavours.

Editor

1

Involvement of ICU families in decisions: fine-tuning the partnership

Elie Azoulay*, Marine Chaize and Nancy Kentish-Barnes

Abstract

Families of patients are not simple visitors to the ICU. They have just been separated from a loved one, often someone they live with, either abruptly or, in nearly half the cases, because a chronic condition has suddenly worsened. They must cope with a serious illness of a loved one, while having to adapt to the unfamiliar and intimidating ICU environment. In many cases, the outcome of the critical illness is uncertain, a situation that causes considerable distress to the relatives. As shown by our research group and others, families exhibit symptoms of anxiety (70%) and depression (35%) in the first few days after admission, as well as symptoms of stress (33%) and difficulty understanding the information delivered by the healthcare staff (50%). Furthermore, relatives of patients who die in the ICU are at risk for psychiatric syndromes such as generalized anxiety, panic attacks, depression, and posttraumatic stress syndrome. In this setting of psychological distress, families are asked to consider sharing in healthcare decisions about their loved one in the ICU. This article aims to foster the debate about the shared decision-making process. We have three objectives: to transcend the overly simplistic position that opposes paternalism and autonomy, to build a view founded only on an evaluation of actual practice and experience in the field, and to keep the focus squarely on the patient. Families want information and communication time from the staff. Nurses and physicians need to understand that families can share in decisions only if the entire ICU staff actively promotes family involvement and, of course, if the family wants to participate in all or part of the decision-making process.

Keywords: Information; Communication; End of life; Bereavement; Randomized controlled trials

Review

Introduction

Advances in medicine have considerably improved life expectancy, in part by allowing patients to survive critical illnesses. In some countries, patients who want to participate actively in decisions about their healthcare are strongly encouraged to do so. In the ICU, however, and in many areas of acute care, patients often exhibit cognitive impairments that prevent them from providing informed consent or participating in decisions designed to avoid nonbeneficial interventions or to determine which treatment option provides the best risk-benefit trade-off [1,2]. Consequently, their families are often asked to speak for them when difficult decisions must be made. These decisions hinge around complex and potentially distressing issues such as the duty to preserve life, the right to a peaceful and dignified death, and the balance between length of life and quality of life [3].

When the patient cannot communicate, the private haven of the doctor-patient relationship is replaced by intercommunication between the entire medical staff and several of the patient's relatives. Involving the family in the decision-making process raises complex challenges. Not all patients discuss their wishes with their family. The family members may have difficulty shifting their perspective from what *they* want to what they believe the *patient* wants. Finally, some family members may consciously or subconsciously make decisions without a clear understanding of what is at stake [4] or defend their own best interests rather than the patient's [5-8], without making reference to possible interference from the information provided on the Internet [9].

Unfortunately, the debate about sharing decisions with families of the ICU patient was long confined to a confrontation between paternalism and autonomy [10]. These two models of the doctor-patient relationship are

* Correspondence: elie.azoulay@sls.aphp.fr
Medical Intensive Care Unit, Hôpital Saint-Louis, ECSTRA team, Biostatistics and clinical epidemiology, UMR 1153 (Center of Epidemiology and Biostatistic Sorbonne Paris Cité, CRESS), INSERM, Paris Diderot Sorbonne University, Paris, France

obsolete in our opinion, as are the reasons put forward to explain the differences in medical decisions that occur across countries [11-13].

Our objective with this review article is to strengthen the case for involving families in the decision-making process in the ICU. We will draw only from evidence supplied by epidemiological studies and practice evaluation surveys done in ICUs in France and elsewhere. Similarly, the concepts that we suggest are founded on clinical experience and on an analysis of complex situations.

The doctor-patient relationship: theoretical models

The doctor-patient relationship shifted from the paternalistic to the autonomy model in the 1970s [14]. According to the paternalistic model, the patient is passive and unable to make wise choices. The physician knows best and protects the patient (acting as a guardian) from making mistakes [15]. The patient trusts the doctor, who exercises control, makes all the decisions, and establishes priorities regarding the management plan, usually based on the scientific evidence. The paternalistic model was called into question when studies showed considerable variability in practice patterns within small geographic areas whose populations were similar in terms of health status and resources, as well as for health conditions whose management is laid out in clinical guidelines [16]. Subsequent studies established that this variability was due to the influence on decision-making of individual factors of such training [17] and cultural and religious values [13]. In addition, when several treatments are available, the best trade-off between benefits and risks depends in large part on the patient's perceptions and consequently cannot be determined by the physician alone. Similarly, whether treatment limitation decisions are appropriate depends in part on whether the quality of life that would be obtained should the patient survive with full-code treatment is acceptable to the patient. Studies establishing the role for subjective factors made a strong case for patients (or their families) playing an active role in choosing which types of healthcare they received. Thus, the autonomy model was developed as the antithesis of the paternalistic model.

The autonomy model gained popularity in the 1980s in North America and other English-speaking countries. In this model, the doctor is a consultant who informs the patients and families of the diagnosis and treatment options, describes the risks and advantages of each option, and listens to the patients to identify their preferences. Ultimately, the decision about which option to use lies with the patient or family. In this model, patients and families are assumed to have an objective understanding of scientific data that allows them to make informed choices without guidance. However, this model was rapidly recognized to have a number of shortcomings. Patients and families do not always gain a clear understanding of the scientific problems involved in decisions about healthcare [5,18-20]. They may be coping with severe pain, other symptoms of serious illness, or marked emotional distress, which may limit their ability to step back and gain an objective perspective on their health situation [20]. Family members acting as surrogates may experience difficulty in separating what they feel is best from what they believe the patient would think is best [21-24]. When a critical illness occurs, complex decisions must be made under considerable time pressure, placing an additional constraint on the patient and family. These obstacles to full patient autonomy prompted the development of a model in which decision-making is shared by the patient or family and by the physician.

In the shared decision model, patients or families and physicians work together as partners to make healthcare decisions [12,25]. Importantly, establishing a sound partnership requires careful attention to effective communication. The 2003 international consensus statement on managing ICU patients at the end of life strongly recommends the shared decision model as a dynamic strategy that allows adaptation to each specific situation [26]. The physicians' goal in the shared decision model is to empower families by helping them to understand what is at stake and, if they so wish, to share in the decision-making process. Conversations are held to allow the healthcare staff to supply scientific information and the families to explain the values and preferences of the patient, vent their emotions, and voice their concerns. During these conversations, the healthcare workers can provide emotional support to the patient and families, verify that the information supplied has been understood, indicate which course of action they deem best and why, and help families identify psychological and emotional barriers to objective decision-making. Furthermore, healthcare workers trained in using the shared decision model have learned to identify not only emotional and cognitive factors affecting the decision-making of patients and families but also their personal preferences and values, which may color their judgment in a way that differs from the patient's preferences and values [27-29].

In theory, the shared decision model combines the advantages of the paternalistic and autonomy models, by allowing patients or families to contribute to the extent that they can, while receiving guidance from the healthcare team. However, in everyday practice, sharing decisions has proved difficult to accomplish, particularly for ICU patients who are represented by their families. In a study from Seattle in the US, ten criteria defining shared decision-making were developed [30]. These criteria were then used to evaluate audiotapes of end-of-life family conferences in four ICUs. The results showed that only 1 of 51 decisions met all ten criteria, and the mean value on a

10-point shared decision-making scale (Table 1) was only 6.1 ± 1.8 [30]. These results establish the existence of obstacles to shared decision-making.

Obstacles to shared decision-making include difficulties experienced by patients and families in understanding the information they receive [18,19] and emotional distress of sufficient magnitude to impair the patient's or family's ability to make decisions that are in the patient's best interests [18-20]. In addition, because of organizational factors or of the rapid progression of a life-threatening illness, the healthcare team may not have enough time to hold the conversations required to build trust and to get to know the patient and family. The patient or family also needs time to form an opinion about the healthcare team. Furthermore, information about treatment options is usually available in terms of means for patient populations, whereas individual patients are interested only in the effects of the treatment on themselves. Shared decision-making requires that the healthcare workers tailor the information and discussion to the background, wishes, and experience of each patient or family. Shared decision-making assumes that the ICU staff can convey their knowledge in simple and readily understandable words that nevertheless allow the patient or family to grasp the nuances and consequences of each decision. There is a convincing evidence that the manner in which information is conveyed to patients strongly influences the nature of the decisions made [31]. For instance, in a study of patients with lung cancer, patients were asked to choose between surgery and radiation therapy, which were considered equivalent in terms of effectiveness and safety. When communicating the results of these two strategies to the patients, the statistics were framed in two different ways, with emphasis either on survival or on mortality. With the survival framing, 18% of patients chose radiation therapy, compared to 44% with the mortality framing [31]. Thus, there is no doubt that physicians consciously or subconsciously influence the choices made by their patients. This example illustrates the tight links between patient autonomy and the quality and objectivity of the information supplied to the patient. As

Table 1 Relationship between coded physician behaviors and shared decision-making (adapted from White [30] and Charles [25])

Dimension of shared decision-making	Coded physician behaviors	Practical example
Providing medical information	1. Discuss the nature of the decision. What is the essential clinical issue we are addressing?	1. Last week, we told you that he had severe cardiac insufficiency. But now, the stroke makes his/her odds of immediate survival very dismal
	2. Describe treatment alternatives What are the clinical reasonable choices?	2. Instead of performing the tracheostomy now, we could extubate him/her and see if it works
	3. Discuss the pro and cons of the choices	3. Each strategy has strengths and weaknesses, and it is important to balance each strategies
	4. Discuss uncertainty What is the likelihood of success of treatment?	4. We are beginning new antibiotics for this VAP, but his/her status may worsen
	5. Assess family understanding Is the family an informed participant with a working understanding of the decision	5. Check whether family has actually grasped which decision is being made and what are its consequences
Eliciting patient's values and preferences	6. Elicit patient's values and preferences What is known about patient's preferences and values?	6. As you know him/her well since a long time, could you please tell us what he would have said if he/she were sharing this discussion with us
Exploring the family's preferred role in decision-making	7. Discuss the family's role in decision-making	7. Family should be offered a role in decision-making even if some will decline
	8. Assess the need for input from others Is there anyone else the family would like to consult?	8. Is the primary physician, the general practitioner, or any close friend that the family would like to consult?
Deliberating and decision-making	9. Explore the context of the decision How will the decision affect the patient's life?	9. Terminal weaning with likely immediate death versus decision of no escalation of treatment
	10. Elicit the family's opinion about the treatment decision What does the family think is the most appropriate decision for the patient	10. The decision is that we are not going back to surgery as it is likely to fail and to prolong unnecessary suffering. What do you think of this decision?

emphasized further in this article, in addition to the information itself, a crucial point is communication with families, including a willingness to listen and to engage in meaningful conversations.

In most of the satisfaction scales developed for the ICU, participation in care, discussions, and decisions is listed among the factors that increase family satisfaction [32-34]. In Canada, where surrogates make decisions for the patients they represent, surrogate satisfaction with the decision-making process was found to increase with the quality of the information received [32]. On both sides of the Atlantic, participation of families in decisions is associated with greater satisfaction [32,33,35-37]. When 8,000 residents of France were surveyed, 90% of responses indicated a desire to have family members share in decisions about their care should they require ICU admission [38]. In France and in other countries, the overwhelming majority of healthcare providers are willing to have families share in medical decisions. However, an unwillingness of family members to share in decisions must be honored. The delegation of decisional authority is after all an autonomous decision. In a French study, more than half of the families did not want to share in medical decisions [7], and the number of relatives willing to share decisions was even lower among families that were satisfied with the quality of the information they received. Sharing in decisions can result in a substantial burden being placed on the families. Thus, in families of patients involved in end-of-life medical decisions, the risk of posttraumatic stress symptoms was increased 3 months after the death [39]. However, the staff should seek to determine whether the unwillingness to share in decisions is related to psychological distress, which may be amenable to alleviation, or to poor understanding of the situation, requiring additional information and communication efforts.

Specific challenges arise when patients die in the ICU. Families of patients who die in the ICU have higher rates of anxiety and depression symptoms [40,41], sleepiness [20], psychiatric syndromes (e.g., panic attacks, generalized anxiety, and pathological grief reaction) [42], and posttraumatic stress [39]. They report overwhelming guilt and regrets about the circumstances of their loved one's death in the ICU [6,43-46]. Clearly, the extreme vulnerability of these families warrants intensified communication efforts [47]. In a large cohort study, the death of a spouse led to severe distress in the surviving spouse, who had a nearly 20% increase in the risk of death [48]. These studies emphasize that families entering the grieving process need to be accompanied by communication strategies that combine empathy, compassion, listening, attending, and palliation. Similarly, ICU nurses and physicians can experience considerable distress when patients die in the ICU. Thus, the management of dying patients and their families are major determinants of conflicts in the ICU [49], as well as of burnout syndrome [50,51]. Clearly, all those involved in end-of-life situations need help and support. Preventing burnout syndrome and conflicts with families or within the staff are strong reasons to work actively on communication strategies that support families, with the primary goal of easing the grieving process and of diminishing the risk of pathological grieving. Clinicians should be aware of their duty when managing ICU conflicts and developing strategies aimed at reducing burnout.

Thus, although shared decision-making is clearly preferred today over other models, we are still learning about how to best respect the patient's autonomy (often via the family) while providing the appropriate level of guidance. Whereas the paternalism and autonomy models had fairly simple rules designed to confine the patient-physician interaction within narrow boundaries, shared decision-making is emerging as a spectrum of interaction patterns whose characteristics are specific to each patient or family. Shared decision-making must be fine-tuned to each case. If healthcare workers are to use the shared decision model, they must be highly skilled in communicating with the patient or family, as well as clearly aware of their personal sources of bias.

Fine-tuning shared decision-making

ICU teams must develop a staff-family relationship that is not only proactive but also context-sensitive [52-54]. It should also be reminded that the decision-making process is not a 'single shot decision'. Instead, most decisions require time to adapt, cope, and sometimes negotiate. For the sake of simplicity, we present the process of making a decision as a simplicity and binary event; however, we do recognize that this is not the reality.

The shared decision model has clear limitations but can be improved by directing attention to the needs of each specific situation [55]. In particular, the nature of healthcare decisions for ICU patients varies widely, and an important step is the identification of decisions for which offering a role to the family is not only an ethical obligation but also likely to benefit all those involved. These decisions are often characterized by either uncertainty regarding the outcome of an intervention [56] (e.g., the patient may survive with or without severe cognitive deficiencies) or the superiority of one intervention over another [57] (two interventions with similar effectiveness and safety profiles are available). In both situations, moral or religious beliefs and personal values play a major role in determining which is the best choice. There is a crucial need for shared decision-making, even when the outcome is easy to predict. When recovery of preexisting physical and cognitive function is almost certain to occur, or when a low-risk intervention is mandatory (e.g., insertion of a parenteral nutrition catheter), *information* during a conversation, with or without the help of a printed information sheet, helps to improve comprehension and to decrease anxiety and depression symptoms in the family members [56]. This strategy also empowers the relatives for an accurate decision-making process. When a high-risk intervention is mandatory on an emergency basis (e.g., blood transfusion in a patient with hemorrhagic shock due to stab wounds), the need for immediate treatment overrides the duty to provide information first. When death is almost certain to be the outcome regardless of whether life-supporting interventions are used, the focus of communication with the family should be on *palliative strategies* designed to maximize patient comfort and on negotiation with the family members to minimize any feelings of guilt [58,59]. Midway between these two situations, the outcome is difficult to predict and specific communication efforts are needed to help the family cope with this uncertainty (e.g., *n*th surgical procedure or additional chemotherapy course) [60]. The ICU staff must use a considerate and sensitive approach to help the family understand that death or disability is a distinct possibility but that there is hope for recovery with a good quality of life. Finally, when two interventions similar in terms of effectiveness and safety are available, the family's input about the patient's preferences and values is crucial.

The patient autonomy model was initially described as the physician providing impartial information then leaving decisional authority entirely to the patient or family. Because the patient and family may experience difficulties understanding the scientific issues involved or preventing their emotions from affecting their ability to make decisions that are in their best interest, a version of the autonomy model known as neopaternalism was developed [61]. Neopaternalism adjusts the concept of autonomy to the reality of patient and family capabilities by having the healthcare staff give a clear description of their personal opinions, based on their experience and on what they believe is in the patient's best interests [61]. In the shared decision model, such as description, can serve as a useful starting point for discussions with patients or families.

Families may be given the opportunity to exercise their right to autonomy (formal autonomy) yet be prevented by bounded cognition from making the decisions they deem in the best interests of the patient (effective autonomy). Bounded cognition is the set of cognitive, information, and time limitations that affect the rationality of decision-making by both families and healthcare workers. A systematic analysis of these limitations (debiasing [31]) may help to circumvent them. Specific efforts must be made to identify cognitive and emotional influences that may bias the decisions of both the family and the staff. For instance, a bias toward overconfidence in decisions can be counterbalanced by a description of alternative outcomes. Staff members must be aware of experiences and emotions that may affect the way they frame the information they give to families. Families can be helped to understand how their fears, past experiences, or current state of emotional distress may influence their decisions in a way that runs counter to the patient's values and wishes.

Regardless of the clinical, social, and psychological situation, families may decide to delegate their decisional authority to the ICU staff. This decision should be respected. After all, a decision to delegate is also an expression of autonomy. Families who delegate their decisional authority must be kept informed of changes in the patient's situation and offered the possibility of entering the decision-making process at any time if they so wish.

Thus, instead of a power-based description of the physician-patient (family) relationship as either paternalistic or autonomous, this relationship is best viewed as a complex partnership in which power has no place. In the shared decision-making model, the healthcare workers bring their scientific knowledge and experience to the partnership, whereas the family members bring their familiarity with the patient's values and wishes, symptoms, and quality of life. Both the staff and the family strive to gain awareness of factors that may bias their decisions. The staff presents the options with their expected outcomes and both the staff and family indicate which option they prefer and why. Careful attention is given to ensure that the family understands what is at stake and has a clear grasp of any uncertainty regarding the outcome. The staff must be aware that delivering fully objective information may be nearly impossible.

Clearly, the development of the family-staff partnership requires specific and intensive efforts. A prerequisite is good teamwork within the ICU. Actions likely to foster a healthy family-staff partnership are outlined below.

Conclusions

Ten key points to improve family care in the ICU (Table 2)

1) The nurse-physician liaison pair

We strongly recommend that the nurse and physician inform the family together, if at all possible. In addition to having didactic advantages, this approach ensures that the ICU team is perceived as united and that families do not receive contradictory information. It also highlights the valuable role for the nurse in the communication process and provides a written record of each conversation [62].

Along the same line, patient comfort should be evaluated by the liaison pair, to the extent possible, most notably at the end of life in the ICU. Having the physicians and nurses work together to evaluate pain at the end of life decreases the rate of associated conflicts [49,63,64].

Table 2 Ten key points to improve family care in the ICU

Ten key points
The nurse-physician liaison pair
Regular debriefing meetings attended by both physicians and nurses
Sharing decisions between physicians and nurses (decision-making meetings)
Moving from information to communication
Opening the ICU visiting hours
Informal and brief conversation with the family at ICU admission
Formal meeting on the third ICU day
The end-of-life conference
The ICU discharge visit
Evaluating information and communication practices and teaching communication skills to healthcare workers

2) Regular debriefing meetings attended by both physicians and nurses

Debriefing meetings provide physicians and nurses with a unique opportunity to exchange their points of view about a specific patient, a family member, or a complex medical case. Importantly, these meetings allow the participants to openly share their perhaps very personal perceptions of a person or situation and also to gain awareness of their own sources of bias. They are associated with greater satisfaction among families and nurses [35,51] and with lower within-team conflict rates [49]. Ideally, each team should meet once a week, and physicians on night duty should hold meaningful discussions with the night shift nurses.

3) Sharing decisions between physicians and nurses (decision-making meetings)

These meetings are also known as ethics meetings. They are considered as a prelude to possible treatment limitation decisions. The entire history of the patient is reviewed, and the irreversible nature of the current medical situation is confirmed. These meetings are the mark of a collegial decision-making process, which is far more common in France than in other countries [65]. When making decisions, physicians tend to rely on statistical data (to identify futility) and nurses on qualitative data (pain, anxiety, and quality of life). These differences underline the complementarity of input from nurses and physicians in the decision-making process [66].

4) Moving from information to communication

Among the key features of communication, listening alleviates distress in families [29,58,59,61,67]. In end-of-life conferences, families who spend more time describing their concerns and verbalizing their emotions and difficulties have higher levels of satisfaction and a lower risk of pathological grieving [58,67,68]. In addition, letting families choose the time of the conference so that they can arrange for a larger number of members to attend (i.e., parents or children) substantially improves the quality of communication.

5) Opening the ICU visiting hours

We will touch briefly on this topic, which would deserve an extensive review. We suggest that ICU teams keep an open mind and evaluate this issue in a nondogmatic manner. Five key points can be borne in mind when considering visiting hour policies [69]. (a) Suggesting and discussing new options works better than imposing a change. A good way to open the debate is to have a task force of physicians and nurses discuss the pros and cons of each option. (b) Evaluate openness to a change in policy among healthcare workers, families, and patients. (c) A 24-h visiting policy is not always the best option. For instance, in an ICU that allows visits during two 2-h periods, allowing visits from noon to 11 pm would constitute a major improvement. Further broadening of the visiting policy is likely to occur later on. (d) The visiting time is not the same as the information time. A more liberal visiting policy requires increased efforts to organize the delivery of information (i.e., start a round of the families at 2:30 pm). (e) Finally, the visiting policy and organization of information delivery should be explained clearly in the family information leaflet [18,70,71].

6) Informal and brief conversation with the family at ICU admission [5]

When a new patient arrives, the ICU staff is often busy settling the patient in, reading the medical chart, and performing life-supporting interventions. Nevertheless, a resident or senior physician should take a few minutes to *actively approach* the family and say a few words. Useful information at this stage is that the patient is being taken care of, that the symptoms are being analyzed although it is still too early for a diagnosis, that life-supporting measures (e.g., antibiotics, dialysis, ventilation) are being taken, and that more will be known about the situation on the next day. A team that knows how to gain the family's confidence at the time of admission is more likely to succeed in building a trust-based relationship that will persist throughout the ICU stay [72]. The impact of the information leaflet can also be enhanced by this brief information [70] that could definitely discourage the use of the Internet [9] and to patient-targeted googling [73].

7) Formal meeting on the third ICU day [74,75]

This meeting is crucial to the organization of information and to the development of the communication strategy. In our experience, the day 3 meeting is a powerful tool. On day 3, the ICU workers actively approach the family to organize a formal meeting for the next day or when the family can arrange for several members to attend. The format is formal, and the meeting must occur in a quiet place. Pagers and phones should be turned off. Staff members should identify themselves. The family members should then be asked to say, in their own words, what they know about the situation, and any errors in communication should be corrected. The family should be able to understand the prognosis and to detect the signs indicating that the treatment is working (e.g., awakening, resumption of urine output, discontinuation of vasopressors, and/or extubation). Importantly, the physicians and nurses must tell the family that they are available (together) to answer any subsequent questions and should arrange for another meeting 48 h later or earlier if needed.

8) The end-of-life conference [27,29,58,67,68]

The end-of-life conference applies the day 3 meeting concept to patients who die in the ICU. It was first described by Randall Curtis and the Seattle group then validated by the Famiréa group in France [27,29,58,67,68]. Major objectives for the team are to acknowledge the value of the family's input, to check that the family members understand the information they have received given so far, to spend much more time *listening* than speaking, to indicate clearly that the best interests of the patient are at the heart of everything that is being said (the focus is on the patient), and to invite the family to ask questions [63]. At completion of the end-of-life conference, we give the family a brochure derived from the SPARADRAP brochure developed by a multidisciplinary pediatric task force (www.sparadrap.fr).

9) The ICU discharge visit

Both patients and families are vulnerable at discharge from the ICU. The high intensity of care and numerous staff-family interactions in the ICU must be left behind, which may generate feelings of abandonment. Anxiety may result from the need to deal with an unknown department, new nurses, and new policies for patient management and information. A study by the Famiréa group is currently evaluating the ICU discharge visit. This visit is a valuable opportunity for reassuring the patient and family and providing information, for instance about the common occurrence of symptoms such as nightmares and the expectation that these symptoms will resolve within a few weeks. Handing the ICU discharge summary to the patient and suggesting a visit to the usual physician should the post-ICU symptoms persist are additional ways to provide support.

10) Evaluating information and communication practices and teaching communication skills to healthcare workers

This step must become a standard practice. Evaluating our communication practices allows us to make further progress. Teaching communication skills to nurses and physicians is the key to improve our practices [76]. Changes for patients and families in the short and medium terms must be measured.

Finally, if you remain unconvinced that families are more than simple visitors to the ICU, ask yourself these three questions [77]:

1. When a patient is unable to communicate, who is most likely to have the knowledge needed to ensure that the management strategy respects the patient's values, preferences, and choices: you or the family?

In all likelihood, the family is in the best position to defend the patient's *best interests*. Obviously, these considerations do not apply to patients who do not want their families to receive information about their health situation. Furthermore, if the various members of the healthcare team feel the family's description of the choices the patient would have made is biased by a conflict of interest, then the decisions must focus on the patient's best interests, and advice from an independent consultant must be obtained and recorded in the medical chart.

2. Who is most deeply affected on a personal level by the results of the medical decisions?

Family members experience severe distress when a loved one is suddenly admitted to the ICU. They often use terms such as 'cruel' or 'violent' to describe their suffering and feelings of emptiness. Although they are often unable to make decisions alone, and although clearly they must not be made to bear the burden of responsibility and guilt associated with major decisions, they must be involved in the process that will allow them to understand why a given decision is in the best interests of their loved one. In both curative care and palliative care, only daily information and effective communication can allow families to understand and accept that the decision made collegially by the ICU team is the best possible one. The decision remains based on medical considerations, except in the rare cases where the patient has repeatedly stated an unwillingness to become dependent on a life-supporting technique or to witness his or her own decline [78]. In this case, the decision belongs to the patient and is either taken by the patient or based on advance directives (very rarely) or statements made to the family, usual doctor, or referring physician.

3. If the patient dies, who will experience the most distress?

The burden is of course greatest for the family. Family members are at risk for pathological grieving, [45,79-82], depression [42], posttraumatic stress disorder, [39,83], and death [48].

Abbreviation
ICU: intensive care unit.

Competing interests
The authors declare that they have no competing interests.

Authors' contributions
EA has drafted the review article. MC and NKB have reviewed and made significant suggestions and changes in the manuscript. All authors read and approved the final manuscript.

References

1. Cassell EJ, Leon AC, Kaufman SG: **Preliminary evidence of impaired thinking in sick patients.** *Ann Intern Med* 2001, **134:**1120–1123.
2. Ferrand E, Bachoud-Levi AC, Rodrigues M, Maggiore S, Brun-Buisson C, Lemaire F: **Decision-making capacity and surrogate designation in French ICU patients.** *Intensive Care Med* 2001, **27:**1360–1364.
3. Long AC, Kross EK, Engelberg RA, Downey L, Nielsen EL, Back AL, Curtis JR: **Quality of dying in the ICU: is it worse for patients admitted from the hospital ward compared to those admitted from the emergency department?** *Intensive Care Med* 2014, **2014:**13.
4. Upadya A, Muralidharan V, Thorevska N, Amoateng-Adjepong Y, Manthous CA: **Patient, physician, and family member understanding of living wills.** *Am J Respir Crit Care Med* 2002, **166:**1430–1435.
5. Azoulay E, Cattaneo I, Ferrand E, Pochard F: **L'Information au patient de Réanimation et à ses proches: le point de vue de la SRLF.** *Reanimation* 2001, **10:**571–581.
6. Azoulay E, Pochard F: **Communication with family members of patients dying in the intensive care unit.** *Curr Opin Crit Care* 2003, **9:**545–550.
7. Azoulay E, Pochard F, Chevret S, Adrie C, Annane D, Bleichner G, Bornstain C, Bouffard Y, Cohen Y, Feissel M, Goldgran-Toledano D, Guitton C, Hayon J, Iglesias E, Joly LM, Jourdain M, Laplace C, Lebert C, Pingat J, Poisson C, Renault A, Sanchez O, Selcer D, Timsit JF, Le Gall JR: **Schlemmer B; FAMIREA Study Group: Half the family members of intensive care unit patients do not want to share in the decision-making process: a study in 78 French intensive care units.** *Crit Care Med* 2004, **32:**1832–1838.
8. Azoulay E, Pochard F, Chevret S, Arich C, Brivet F, Brun F, Charles PE, Desmettre T, Dubois D, Galliot R, Garrouste-Orgeas M, Goldgran-Toledano D, Herbecq P, Joly LM, Jourdain M, Kaidomar M, Lepape A, Letellier N, Marie O, Page B, Parrot A, Rodie-Talbere PA, Sermet A, Tenaillon A, Thuong M, Tulasne P, Le Gall JR, Schlemmer B, French Famirea Group: **Family participation in care to the critically ill: opinions of families and staff.** *Intensive Care Med* 2003, **29:**1498–1504. Epub 2003 Jul 1410.
9. Bouju P, Tadie JM, Uhel F, Letheulle J, Fillatre P, Lavoue S, Camus C, Le Tulzo Y, Gacouin A: **Internet use by family members of intensive care unit patients: a pilot study.** *Intensive Care Med* 2014, **40:**1175–1176.
10. Prendergast T: **Research agenda or (North) American cultural hegemony?** *Crit Care Med* 2001, **29:**2024–2025.
11. Sprung CL, Cohen SL, Sjokvist P, Baras M, Bulow HH, Hovilehto S, Ledoux D, Lippert A, Maia P, Phelan D, Schobersberger W, Wennberg E, Woodcock T, Ethicus Study Group: **End-of-life practices in European intensive care units: the Ethicus study.** *Jama* 2003, **290:**790–797.
12. Barnato AE, Tate JA, Rodriguez KL, Zickmund SL, Arnold RM: **Norms of decision making in the ICU: a case study of two academic medical centers at the extremes of end-of-life treatment intensity.** *Intensive Care Med* 2012, **38:**1886–1896.
13. Bulow HH, Sprung CL, Baras M, Carmel S, Svantesson M, Benbenishty J, Maia PA, Beishuizen A, Cohen S, Nalos D: **Are religion and religiosity important to end-of-life decisions and patient autonomy in the ICU? The Ethicatt study.** *Intensive Care Med* 2012, **38:**1126–1133.
14. Azoulay E, Sprung CL: **Family-physician interactions in the intensive care unit.** *Crit Care Med* 2004, **32:**2323–2328.
15. Cook D: **Patient autonomy versus parentalism.** *Crit Care Med* 2001, **29:**N24–N25.
16. Chassin MR, Brook RH, Park RE, Keesey J, Fink A, Kosecoff J, Kahn K, Merrick N, Solomon DH: **Variations in the use of medical and surgical services by the Medicare population.** *N Engl J Med* 1986, **314:**285–290.
17. Forte DN, Vincent JL, Velasco IT, Park M: **Association between education in EOL care and variability in EOL practice: a survey of ICU physicians.** *Intensive Care Med* 2012, **38:**404–412.
18. Azoulay E, Chevret S, Leleu G, Pochard F, Barboteu M, Adrie C, Canoui P, Le Gall JR, Schlemmer B: **Half the families of intensive care unit patients experience inadequate communication with physicians.** *Crit Care Med* 2000, **28:**3044–3049.
19. Rodriguez RM, Navarrete E, Schwaber J, McKleroy W, Clouse A, Kerrigan SF, Fortman J: **A prospective study of primary surrogate decision makers' knowledge of intensive care.** *Crit Care Med* 2008, **36:**1633–1636.
20. Verceles AC, Corwin DS, Afshar M, Friedman EB, McCurdy MT, Shanholtz C, Oakjones K, Zubrow MT, Titus J, Netzer G: **Half of the family members of critically ill patients experience excessive daytime sleepiness.** *Intensive Care Med* 2014, **40:**1124–1131.
21. Zier LS, Sottile PD, Hong SY, Weissfield LA, White DB: **Surrogate decision makers' interpretation of prognostic information: a mixed-methods study.** *Ann Intern Med* 2012, **156:**360–366.
22. White DB, Cua SM, Walk R, Pollice L, Weissfeld L, Hong S, Landefeld CS, Arnold RM: **Nurse-led intervention to improve surrogate decision making for patients with advanced critical illness.** *Am J Crit Care* 2012, **21:**396–409.
23. Scheunemann LP, Arnold RM, White DB: **The facilitated values history: helping surrogates make authentic decisions for incapacitated patients with advanced illness.** *Am J Respir Crit Care Med* 2012, **186:**480–486.
24. Schenker Y, Crowley-Matoka M, Dohan D, Tiver GA, Arnold RM, White DB: **I don't want to be the one saying 'we should just let him die': intrapersonal tensions experienced by surrogate decision makers in the ICU.** *J Gen Intern Med* 2012, **27**(12):1657–1665.
25. Murray E, Charles C, Gafni A: **Shared decision-making in primary care: tailoring the Charles et al. model to fit the context of general practice.** *Patient Educ Couns* 2006, **62:**205–211.
26. Carlet J, Thijs LG, Antonelli M, Cassell J, Cox P, Hill N, Hinds C, Pimentel JM, Reinhart K, Thompson BT: **Challenges in end-of-life care in the ICU. Statement of the 5th international consensus conference in critical care: Brussels, Belgium, April 2003.** *Intensive Care Med* 2004, **30:**770–784. Epub 2004 Apr 2020.
27. Curtis JR, Patrick DL, Shannon SE, Treece PD, Engelberg RA, Rubenfeld GD: **The family conference as a focus to improve communication about end-of-life care in the intensive care unit: opportunities for improvement.** *Crit Care Med* 2001, **29:**N26–N33.
28. Curtis JR, White DB: **Practical guidance for evidence-based ICU family conferences.** *Chest* 2008, **134:**835–843.
29. Lautrette A, Ciroldi M, Ksibi H, Azoulay E: **End-of-life family conferences: rooted in the evidence.** *Crit Care Med* 2006, **34:**S364–S372.
30. White DB, Braddock CH 3rd, Bereknyei S, Curtis JR: **Toward shared decision making at the end of life in intensive care units: opportunities for improvement.** *Arch Intern Med* 2007, **167:**461–467.
31. Schwab AP: **Formal and effective autonomy in healthcare.** *J Med Ethics* 2006, **32:**575–579.
32. Heyland DK, Rocker GM, Dodek PM, Kutsogiannis DJ, Konopad E, Cook DJ, Peters S, Tranmer JE, O'Callaghan CJ: **Family satisfaction with care in the intensive care unit: results of a multiple center study.** *Crit Care Med* 2002, **30:**1413–1418.
33. Heyland DK, Tranmer JE: **Measuring family satisfaction with care in the intensive care unit: the development of a questionnaire and preliminary results.** *J Crit Care* 2001, **16:**142–149.

34. Wasser T, Pasquale MA, Matchett SC, Bryan Y, Pasquale M: **Establishing reliability and validity of the critical care family satisfaction survey.** *Crit Care Med* 2001, **29:**192–196.
35. Azoulay E, Pochard F, Chevret S, Lemaire F, Mokhtari M, Le Gall JR, Dhainaut JF, Schlemmer B: **Meeting the needs of intensive care unit patient families: a multicenter study.** *Am J Respir Crit Care Med* 2001, **163:**135–139.
36. Schleyer AM, Curtis JR: **Family satisfaction in the ICU: why should ICU clinicians care?** *Intensive Care Med* 2013, **39:**1143–1145.
37. Jongerden IP, Slooter AJ, Peelen LM, Wessels H, Ram CM, Kesecioglu J, Schneider MM, van Dijk D: **Effect of intensive care environment on family and patient satisfaction: a before-after study.** *Intensive Care Med* 2013, **39:**1626–1634.
38. Azoulay E, Pochard F, Chevret S, Adrie C, Bollaert PE, Brun F, Dreyfuss D, Garrouste-Orgeas M, Goldgran-Toledano D, Jourdain M, Wolff M, Le Gall JR, Schlemmer B: **Opinions about surrogate designation: a population survey in France.** *Crit Care Med* 2003, **31:**1711–1714.
39. Azoulay E, Pochard F, Kentish-Barnes N, Chevret S, Aboab J, Adrie C, Annane D, Bleichner G, Bollaert PE, Darmon M, Fassier T, Galliot R, Garrouste-Orgeas M, Goulenok C, Goldgran-Toledano D, Hayon J, Jourdain M, Kaidomar M, Laplace C, Larché J, Liotier J, Papazian L, Poisson C, Reignier J, Saidi F, Schlemmer B, FAMIREA Study Group: **Risk of post-traumatic stress symptoms in family members of intensive care unit patients.** *Am J Respir Crit Care Med* 2005, **171:**987–994. Epub 2005 Jan 2021.
40. Pochard F, Azoulay E, Chevret S, Lemaire F, Hubert P, Canoui P, Grassin M, Zittoun R, le Gall JR, Dhainaut JF, Schlemmer B: **Symptoms of anxiety and depression in family members of intensive care unit patients: ethical hypothesis regarding decision-making capacity.** *Crit Care Med* 2001, **29:**1893–1897.
41. Pochard F, Darmon M, Fassier T, Bollaert PE, Cheval C, Coloigner M, Merouani A, Moulront S, Pigne E, Pingat J, Zahar JR, Schlemmer B, Azoulay E, French FAMIREA Study Group: **Symptoms of anxiety and depression in family members of intensive care unit patients before discharge or death. A prospective multicenter study.** *J Crit Care* 2005, **20:**90–96.
42. Siegel MD, Hayes E, Vanderwerker LC, Loseth DB, Prigerson HG: **Psychiatric illness in the next of kin of patients who die in the intensive care unit.** *Crit Care Med* 2008, **36:**1722–1728.
43. Abbott KH, Sago JG, Breen CM, Abernethy AP, Tulsky JA: **Families looking back: one year after discussion of withdrawal or withholding of life-sustaining support.** *Crit Care Med* 2001, **29:**197–201.
44. Curtis JR, Patrick DL, Engelberg RA, Norris K, Asp C, Byock I: **A measure of the quality of dying and death. Initial validation using after-death interviews with family members.** *J Pain Symptom Manage* 2002, **24:**17–31.
45. Cuthbertson SJ, Margetts MA, Streat SJ: **Bereavement follow-up after critical illness.** *Crit Care Med* 2000, **28:**1196–1201.
46. Malacrida R, Bettelini CM, Degrate A, Martinez M, Badia F, Piazza J, Vizzardi N, Wullschleger R, Rapin CH: **Reasons for dissatisfaction: a survey of relatives of intensive care patients who died.** *Crit Care Med* 1998, **26:**1187–1193.
47. Rabow MW, Hauser JM, Adams J: **Supporting family caregivers at the end of life: "they don't know what they don't know".** *Jama* 2004, **291:**483–491.
48. Christakis NA, Allison PD: **Mortality after the hospitalization of a spouse.** *N Engl J Med* 2006, **354:**719–730.
49. Azoulay E, Timsit JF, Sprung CL, Soares M, Rusinova K, Lafabrie A, Abizanda R, Svantesson M, Rubulotta F, Ricou B, Benoit D, Heyland D, Joynt G, Français A, Azeivedo-Maia P, Owczuk R, Benbenishty J, de Vita M, Valentin A, Ksomos A, Cohen S, Kompan L, Ho K, Abroug F, Kaarlola A, Gerlach H, Kyprianou T, Michalsen A, Chevret S, Schlemmer B: **Prevalence and factors of intensive care unit conflicts: the conflicus study.** *Am J Respir Crit Care Med* 2009, **180:**853–860.
50. Embriaco N, Azoulay E, Barrau K, Kentish N, Pochard F, Loundou A, Papazian L: **High level of burnout in intensivists: prevalence and associated factors.** *Am J Respir Crit Care Med* 2007, **175:**686–692. Epub 2007 Jan 2018.
51. Poncet MC, Toullic P, Papazian L, Kentish-Barnes N, Timsit JF, Pochard F, Chevret S, Schlemmer B, Azoulay E: **Burnout syndrome in critical care nursing staff.** *Am J Respir Crit Care Med* 2007, **175:**698–704. Epub 2006 Nov 2016.
52. Pochard F, Grassin M, Azoulay E: **Ethical principles for everyone.** *Ann Intern Med* 2001, **134:**1152. discussion 1152–1153.
53. Pochard F, Grassin M, Herve C: **Palliative options at the end of life.** *Jama* 1998, **279:**1065–1066. discussion 1066–1067.
54. Pochard F, Grassin M, Kentish-Barnes N, Azoulay E: **Patient autonomy and the end of life.** *Crit Care Med* 2003, **31:**662–663.
55. Whitney SN: **A new model of medical decisions: exploring the limits of shared decision making.** *Med Decis Making* 2003, **23:**275–280.
56. Goldstein NE, Back AL, Morrison RS: **Titrating guidance: a model to guide physicians assisting patients and families facing complex decisions.** *Arch Intern Med* 2008, **168:**1733–1739.
57. Whitney SN, McGuire AL, McCullough LB: **A typology of shared decision making, informed consent, and simple consent.** *Ann Intern Med* 2004, **140:**54–59.
58. Lautrette A, Darmon M, Megarbane B, Joly LM, Chevret S, Adrie C, Barnoud D, Bleichner G, Bruel C, Choukroun G, Curtis JR, Fieux F, Galliot R, Garrouste-Orgeas M, Georges H, Goldgran-Toledano D, Jourdain M, Loubert G, Reignier J, Saidi F, Souweine B, Vincent F, Barnes NK, Pochard F, Schlemmer B, Azoulay E: **A communication strategy and brochure for relatives of patients dying in the ICU.** *N Engl J Med* 2007, **356:**469–478.
59. Lilly CM, Daly BJ: **The healing power of listening in the ICU.** *N Engl J Med* 2007, **356:**513–515.
60. Azoulay E, Pochard F: **Meeting the needs of intensive care unit patients' family members: beyond satisfaction.** *Crit Care Med* 2002, **30:**2171.
61. Azoulay E: **The end-of-life family conference: communication empowers.** *Am J Respir Crit Care Med* 2005, **171:**803–804.
62. Jones C: **What's new on the post-ICU burden for patients and relatives?** *Intensive Care Med* 2013, **39:**1832–1835.
63. Puntillo K, Nelson JE, Weissman D, Curtis R, Weiss S, Frontera J, Gabriel M, Hays R, Lustbader D, Mosenthal A, Mulkerin C, Ray D, Bassett R, Boss R, Brasel K, Campbell M: **Palliative care in the ICU: relief of pain, dyspnea, and thirst—a report from the IPAL-ICU advisory board.** *Intensive Care Med* 2013, **40:**235–248.
64. Gelinas C, Chanques G, Puntillo K: **In pursuit of pain: recent advances and future directions in pain assessment in the ICU.** *Intensive Care Med* 2014, **40:**1009–1014.
65. Yaguchi A, Truog RD, Curtis JR, Luce JM, Levy MM, Melot C, Vincent JL: **International differences in end-of-life attitudes in the intensive care unit: results of a survey.** *Arch Intern Med* 2005, **165:**1970–1975.
66. Ferrand E, Lemaire F, Regnier B, Kuteifan K, Badet M, Asfar P, Jaber S, Chagnon JL, Renault A, Robert R, Pochard F, Herve C, Brun-Buisson C, Duvaldestin P, French RESSENTI Group: **Discrepancies between perceptions by physicians and nursing staff of intensive care unit end-of-life decisions.** *Am J Respir Crit Care Med* 2003, **167:**1310–1315. Epub 2003 Jan 1324.
67. McDonagh JR, Elliott TB, Engelberg RA, Treece PD, Shannon SE, Rubenfeld GD, Patrick DL, Curtis JR: **Family satisfaction with family conferences about end-of-life care in the intensive care unit: increased proportion of family speech is associated with increased satisfaction.** *Crit Care Med* 2004, **32:**1484–1488.
68. Curtis JR, Engelberg RA, Wenrich MD, Shannon SE, Treece PD, Rubenfeld GD: **Missed opportunities during family conferences about end-of-life care in the intensive care unit.** *Am J Respir Crit Care Med* 2005, **171:**844–849. Epub 2005 Jan 2007.
69. Levy MM, De Backer D: **Re-visiting visiting hours.** *Intensive Care Med* 2013, **39:**2223–2225.
70. Azoulay E, Pochard F, Chevret S, Jourdain M, Bornstain C, Wernet A, Cattaneo I, Annane D, Brun F, Bollaert PE, Zahar JR, Goldgran-Toledano D, Adrie C, Joly LM, Tayoro J, Desmettre T, Pigne E, Parrot A, Sanchez O, Poisson C, Le Gall JR, Schlemmer B, Lemaire F: **Impact of a family information leaflet on effectiveness of information provided to family members of intensive care unit patients: a multicenter, prospective, randomized, controlled trial.** *Am J Respir Crit Care Med* 2002, **165:**438–442.
71. Schnell D, Abadie S, Toullic P, Chaize M, Souppart V, Poncet MC, Schlemmer B, Azoulay E: **Open visitation policies in the ICU: experience from relatives and clinicians.** *Intensive Care Med* 2013, **39:**1873–1874.
72. McAdam JL, Arai S, Puntillo KA: **Unrecognized contributions of families in the intensive care unit.** *Intensive Care Med* 2008, **34:**1097–1101.
73. Clinton BK, Silverman BC, Brendel DH: **Patient-targeted googling: the ethics of searching online for patient information.** *Harv Rev Psychiatry* 2010, **18:**103–112.
74. Lilly CM, De Meo DL, Sonna LA, Haley KJ, Massaro AF, Wallace RF, Cody S: **An intensive communication intervention for the critically ill.** *Am J Med* 2000, **109:**469–475.
75. Lilly CM, Sonna LA, Haley KJ, Massaro AF: **Intensive communication: four-year follow-up from a clinical practice study.** *Crit Care Med* 2003, **31:**S394–S399.

76. Fallowfield L, Jenkins V, Farewell V, Saul J, Duffy A, Eves R: **Efficacy of a Cancer Research UK communication skills training model for oncologists: a randomised controlled trial.** *Lancet* 2002, **359:**650–656.
77. Arnold RM, Kellum J: **Moral justifications for surrogate decision making in the intensive care unit: implications and limitations.** *Crit Care Med* 2003, **31:**S347–S353.
78. Fried TR, Bradley EH, Towle VR, Allore H: **Understanding the treatment preferences of seriously ill patients.** *N Engl J Med* 2002, **346:**1061–1066.
79. Puntillo KA, Benner P, Drought T, Drew B, Stotts N, Stannard D, Rushton C, Scanlon C, White C: **End-of-life issues in intensive care units: a national random survey of nurses' knowledge and beliefs.** *Am J Crit Care* 2001, **10:**216–229.
80. Robinson SM, Mackenzie-Ross S, Campbell Hewson GL, Egleston CV, Prevost AT: **Psychological effect of witnessed resuscitation on bereaved relatives.** *Lancet* 1998, **352:**614–617.
81. Lundin T: **Long-term outcome of bereavement.** *Br J Psychiatry* 1984, **145:**424–428.
82. Maciejewski PK, Zhang B, Block SD, Prigerson HG: **An empirical examination of the stage theory of grief.** *Jama* 2007, **297:**716–723.
83. Jones C, Skirrow P, Griffiths RD, Humphris G, Ingleby S, Eddleston J, Waldmann C, Gager M: **Post-traumatic stress disorder-related symptoms in relatives of patients following intensive care.** *Intensive Care Med* 2004, **30:**456–460. Epub 2004 Feb 2004.

2

Sepsis-3 definitions predict ICU mortality in a low–middle-income country

Bruno Adler Maccagnan Pinheiro Besen[1,2*], Thiago Gomes Romano[3,4], Antonio Paulo Nassar Jr.[1,5], Leandro Utino Taniguchi[1,3], Luciano Cesar Pontes Azevedo[1,3], Pedro Vitale Mendes[1,3], Fernando Godinho Zampieri[6,7] and Marcelo Park[1]

Abstract

Background: Sepsis-3 definitions were published recently and validated only in high-income countries. The aim of this study was to assess the new criteria's accuracy in stratifying mortality as compared to its predecessor (Sepsis-2) in a Brazilian public intensive care unit (ICU) and to investigate whether the addition of lactate values would improve stratification.

Methods: Retrospective cohort study conducted between 2010 and 2015 in a public university's 19-bed ICU. Data from patients admitted to the ICU with sepsis were retrieved from a prospectively collected database. ICU mortality was compared across categories of both Sepsis-2 definitions (sepsis, severe sepsis and septic shock) and Sepsis-3 definitions (infection, sepsis and septic shock). Area under the receiving operator characteristic curves were constructed, and the net reclassification index and integrated discrimination index for the addition of lactate as a categorical variable to each stratum of definition were evaluated.

Results: The medical records of 957 patients were retrieved from a prospectively collected database. Mean age was 52 ± 19 years, median SAPS 3 was 65 [50,79], respiratory tract infection was the most common cause (42%, 402 patients), and 311 (32%) patients died in ICU. The ICU mortality rate was progressively higher across categories of sepsis as defined by the Sepsis-3 consensus: infection with no organ dysfunction—7/103 (7%); sepsis—106/419 (25%); and septic shock—198/435 (46%) ($P < 0.001$). For Sepsis-2 definitions, ICU mortality was different only across the categories of severe sepsis [43/252-(17%)] and septic shock [250/572-(44%)] ($P < 0.001$); sepsis had a mortality of 18/135-(13%) ($P = 0.430$ vs. severe sepsis). When combined with lactate, the definitions' accuracy in stratifying ICU mortality only improved with lactate levels above 4 mmol/L. This improvement occurred in the severe sepsis and septic shock groups (Sepsis-2) and the no-dysfunction and septic shock groups (Sepsis-3). Multivariate analysis demonstrated similar findings.

Conclusions: In a Brazilian ICU, the new Sepsis-3 definitions were accurate in stratifying mortality and were superior to the previous definitions. We also observed that the new definitions' accuracy improved progressively with severity. Serum lactate improved accuracy for values higher than 4 mmol/L in the no-dysfunction and septic shock groups.

Keywords: Infection, Intensive care unit, Sepsis, Septic shock, Lactate, Organ dysfunction

Background

Sepsis is a well-recognized worldwide healthcare issue, ultimately resulting in significant mortality [1], morbidity and resource utilization during and after critical illness [2]. Initial consensus definitions relied upon the systemic inflammatory response syndrome (SIRS) to infection as a fundamental aspect of sepsis definition, which was then stratified in severity according to the presence of organ dysfunction (severe sepsis) or vasopressor requirement despite adequate fluid resuscitation (septic shock) [3]. This had an important role in education and

*Correspondence: brunobesen@yahoo.com.br
[1] Intensive Care Unit, Emergency Department, Hospital das Clínicas, University of São Paulo Medical School, Rua Dr. Enéas Carvalho de Aguiar, 255, Room 6040, São Paulo ZIP 05403-000, Brazil
Full list of author information is available at the end of the article

the pathophysiological understanding of the transition between a homeostatic and a dys-homeostatic inflammatory response that results in organ dysfunctions.

In a second consensus conference, although a new panel of specialists agreed that SIRS was not necessary to the definition of sepsis, not much was changed. The panel recognized several factors that could be used to identify patients with severe sepsis and associated with increased mortality, ultimately leading to important efforts for the early recognition and treatment of severe sepsis and septic shock. This consensus also developed the PIRO concept (predisposition, infection, response, organ failure); however, this idea was not largely translated to clinical practice [4].

Sepsis definitions based on SIRS criteria have, though, been questioned as of late, as SIRS has been shown to be present in 93% of all patients admitted to intensive care (and therefore overly non-specific) [5]. Furthermore, up to 1 in every 8 patients with infection and organ dysfunction do not meet SIRS criteria [6]. Moreover, the methodology used to capture SIRS criteria may lead to substantial variability in defining sepsis cases [7, 8]. These and other concerns have led to the development and publication of new sepsis definitions (Sepsis-3), which were derived through a data-driven mortality risk stratification [9–11]. Although these new criteria have been validated in large databases, much controversy still surrounds them. Some criticisms include the new definitions' lack of validation in scenarios outside of high-income countries, and their non-utilization of lactate as a marker of organ dysfunction [12–16].

Therefore, in order to address these concerns, we aimed to evaluate whether the new Sepsis-3 definitions maintain their accuracy in a different setting from those in which the criteria were developed and whether they can discriminate intensive care unit (ICU) mortality better than the previous definitions (Sepsis-2). We also evaluated whether the addition of lactate to the definitions would improve upon the previous and new criteria's accuracy of ICU mortality discrimination.

Methods

Study design, population and ethical requirements

This was a retrospective cohort study of patients diagnosed with sepsis admitted to an ICU over a 6-year span, from January 2010 to December 2015. Data were retrieved from the prospectively collected database of a 19-bed ICU in a Brazilian, academic, tertiary medical center in São Paulo—Brazil (Hospital das Clínicas, University of São Paulo Medical School). The study protocol followed the tenets of the Declaration of Helsinki. The institutional review board (*Comissão para Análise de Projetos de* Pesquisa—CAPPesq) reviewed and approved this study (CAPPesq—protocol number 107.443). Since the study was retrospective in nature and did not involve patient identification, informed consent was waived as there was no intervention.

Setting and sepsis management

Our ICU is located in the Hospital das Clínicas, the largest healthcare complex in Latin America. At the time when the study was conducted, it consisted of seven specialized institutes, with a total of 2400 beds. In the Instituto Central, there are 7 ICUs, ours being mainly a Medical ICU, with patients from emergency surgery and trauma being admitted occasionally for logistical reasons.

The ICU is managed by staff as follows: one nursing assistant for every two beds; one nurse for every five beds; one respiratory therapist for every 10 beds; one staff physician for every 5–8 beds; and residents of internal medicine, critical care, physical therapy, nutrition and nursing. The studied ICU is classified as a strained unit as occupation rate has been above 95% since the beginning of the study period, and the mean SAPS 3 of the patients is 60 [17]. Neither quantitative resuscitation nor protocolized care is routinely used for sepsis management. Our approach to sepsis care is described in Additional file 1.

Data collection

Our database is an electronic health chart record fulfilled by physicians and respiratory therapists on a daily basis. Patients were selected using *sepsis, severe sepsis* or *septic shock* as an [All field] search term in the syndromic diagnosis fields of the database. Senior intensivists clinically adjudicated these diagnoses based on previous Sepsis-2 consensus. Patients with any acute organ failure were considered to have severe sepsis, while septic shock was defined when patients were on vasopressors despite fluid resuscitation. These were adjudicated independent of the presence of 2 SIRS criteria. The following clinical data were collected: age; gender; worst and best vital signs during the first ICU day; Simplified Acute Physiological Score (SAPS) 3; first day total Sequential Organ Failure Assessment (SOFA) score; syndromic diagnosis; etiological diagnosis; comorbidities; ICU length of stay (LOS); organ support measures; clinical ICU outcomes; and highest lactate level of the first day. Laboratory variables were retrieved from the electronic health database specific to laboratorial data.

Sepsis definitions

Sepsis-2 definitions were primarily used to classify our patients in the database. The categories (sepsis, severe sepsis and septic shock) were defined according to previously published consensus [4]. The new Sepsis-3 categories were defined as follows [9]:

- *Infection without acute organ dysfunction (no-dysfunction category)* infected patients with no significant additional organ dysfunction over the previous conditions, that is, a variation of total SOFA <2 over baseline (chronic organ dysfunction) during the first 24 h after ICU admission.
- *Sepsis (sepsis category)* infected patients with a total SOFA variation ≥2 over baseline clinical condition.
- *Septic shock (septic shock category)* infected patients with persistent hypotension [mean arterial blood pressure (MAP) <65 mmHg] after adequate fluid resuscitation needing vasopressors to keep MAP ≥65 mmHg. Additionally, the hypotension or need for vasopressors must be associated with lactate level >2 mmol/L measured during the first 24 h.

Baseline total SOFA score was considered to be 4 in patients undergoing chronic dialysis, and 2 or 3 in cirrhotic patients, depending on baseline bilirubin levels. For instance, according to the Sepsis-3 definition [9], a patient with chronic renal failure undergoing dialysis was considered to be in the sepsis group only when the total SOFA score was ≥6. Although the original validation of Sepsis-3 definitions did not include patients with ICU LOS <2 days [9], we included all patients in the period described, independently of LOS, in order to pragmatically test the definitions in our ICU.

Outcome

The primary outcome of interest was ICU mortality.

Statistical analysis

Continuous variables were assessed for normality using the Kolmogorov–Smirnov test. Parametric continuous variables were compared between groups using the *t* test; nonparametric variables were compared using the Mann–Whitney test. Categorical variables were compared between groups using the Chi-squared test.

We assessed the independent association between lactate and outcome regardless of definition (both Sepsis-2 and Sepsis-3) group using a logistic regression model. Six models were built, three for each definition considering three different cutoffs for lactate (as a continuous predictor, stratified at ≤2 or >2 mEq/L and at ≤4 and >4 mEq/L). Since serum lactate measurements were positively skewed, we used log transformation to fit it into the model as a continuous variable. We further assessed the independent association of Sepsis-3 category and lactate level after adjusting for age, severity at baseline (SAPS 3) and use of support measures (renal replacement therapy, mechanical ventilation). Demographic variables (age and sex) were selected based on univariate analysis, with p values < 0.2 used as cutoff. The other confounding variables were selected because of clinical relevance.

The effect of adding lactate (as a continuous variable or stratified at ≤2 or >2 mEq/L or at ≤4 or >4 mEq/L) on model performance was assessed through area under receiver operating characteristic curve (AUROC). AUROCs were compared using DeLong's test. Additionally, we assessed the impact of adding lactate to the model using continuous net reclassification improvement (NRI) and integrated discrimination index (IDI), as previously suggested [18]. NRI compares classifications from 2 models (in this case, with and without lactate) for changes by outcome for a net calculation of changes in the right correction. IDI integrates the NRI over all possible cutoffs and is equivalent to the difference in discrimination slopes. In this paper, based on the histograms of the probability of ICU mortality distributions, the cutoff values for reclassification were the following: <30; 30–60; and >60%. We do not report categorical NRI since no single probability cutoff has been defined for the decision-making process in caring for septic patients, as discussed in the Sepsis-3 consensus [10].

Missing values were handled as previously suggested for studies in critical care, when missing values are <5% [19]. There were 46 (<5%) missing lactate values of the first day, which were replaced by the first second day value, or by median imputation if there were not data available. All statistical analyses and graphs were done in R-free source software [20].

Results

The general characteristics of patients, as well as support measures, clinical outcomes, source of infection, and comorbidities are given in Table 1. For the whole group, mean age was 52 years, without gender differences. The most frequent infectious source was respiratory, followed by abdominal and urinary tract sources. The most frequent comorbidities were diabetes, heart failure and hypertension. Sixty percentage of patients used vasopressors; 44%, mechanical ventilation; and 24%, renal replacement therapy. ICU mortality was 32%. In univariate analysis, non-survivors had higher mean age, severity at admission (SAPS 3), more organ dysfunctions (SOFA) and higher worst lactate values. No infectious source was associated with mortality, neither comorbidities, except for hematological cancer. They also presented more frequently with septic shock when compared to other categories. Furthermore, invasive support measures were more frequently used in this population.

Figure 1 depicts that Sepsis-2 definitions show reasonable differentiation in mortality only between septic shock and severe sepsis patients, while Sepsis-3 definitions

Table 1 General characteristics, support measures and outcomes of patients

Variables	Whole group ($N = 957$)	Survivors ($N = 646$)	Non-survivors ($N = 311$)	P value[a]
General characteristics				
Age—yo	52 ± 19	50 ± 19	56 ± 18	<0.001
Gender (males/females)—*n*	504/453	331/315	173/138	0.291
SAPS 3	65 [50,79]	60 [48,72]	74 [59,90]	<0.001
Total SOFA (first day)	6 [3,9]	5 [3,8]	9 [6,12]	<0.001
Worst lactate (first day)—mmol/L	3.0 [2.0,4.0]	2.7 [1.9,3.7]	3.7 [2.2,5.8]	<0.001
Maximum SOFA (ICU stay)	7 [6,12]	6 [5,9]	12 [8,16]	<0.001
Support measures				
Vasopressors—*n* (%)	572 (60)	322 (50)	250 (80)	<0.001
Inotropes—*n* (%)	13 (1)	11 (2)	2 (1)	<0.001
Mechanical ventilation (first day)—*n* (%)	259 (27)	131 (20)	128 (41)	<0.001
(C)RRT (first day)—*n* (%)	102 (11)	51 (8)	51 (16)	<0.001
Mechanical ventilation (ICU stay)—*n* (%)	420 (44)	267 (41)	153 (49)	0.026
(C)RRT (ICU stay)—*n* (%)	233 (24)	137 (21)	96 (31)	0.001
Sepsis-2 classification				
Sepsis—*n* (%)	134 (14)	116 (18)	18 (6)	<0.001
Severe sepsis—*n* (%)	251 (26)	208 (32)	43 (14)	<0.001
Septic shock—*n* (%)	572 (60)	322 (50)	250 (80)	<0.001
Sepsis-3 classification				
No-dysfunction—*n* (%)	103 (11)	96 (15)	7 (2)	<0.001
Sepsis—*n* (%)	419 (44)	313 (48)	106 (34)	<0.001
Septic shock—*n* (%)	435 (45)	237 (37)	198 (64)	<0.001
Infection source				
Respiratory—*n* (%)	402 (42)	263 (41)	139 (45)	0.271
Abdominal—*n* (%)	107 (11)	75 (12)	32 (10)	0.619
Urinary tract—*n* (%)	84 (9)	63 (10)	21 (7)	0.157
Skin and soft tissue—*n* (%)	72 (8)	45 (7)	27 (9)	0.417
Febrile neutropenia syndrome—*n* (%)	32 (3)	19 (3)	13 (4)	0.420
Catheter related—*n* (%)	22 (2)	17 (3)	5 (2)	0.448
Primary bloodstream infection—*n* (%)	17 (2)	13 (2)	4 (1)	0.592
Osteoarticular—*n* (%)	17 (2)	10 (2)	7 (2)	0.610
Unidentifiable source—*n* (%)	167 (17)	117 (18)	50 (16)	0.493
Others[b]—*n* (%)	37 (4)	24 (4)	13 (4)	1.000
Comorbidities				
Diabetes mellitus—*n* (%)	196 (20)	124 (19)	72 (23)	0.174
Chronic heart failure—*n* (%)	107 (11)	71 (11)	36 (12)	0.860
Chronic arterial hypertension—*n* (%)	95 (10)	61 (9)	34 (11)	0.534
Dialysis dependent chronic renal failure—*n* (%)	66 (7)	48 (7)	18 (6)	0.429
Rheumatologic diseases—*n* (%)	59 (6)	37 (6)	22 (7)	0.497
Chronic obstructive pulmonary disease—*n* (%)	38 (4)	25 (4)	13 (4)	0.949
Hematologic cancer—*n* (%)	30 (3)	11 (2)	19 (6)	<0.001
Solid cancer—*n* (%)	26 (3)	17 (3)	9 (3)	0.977
Organ transplantation—*n* (%)	20 (2)	14 (2)	6 (2)	1.000
AIDS[c]—*n* (%)	19 (2)	12 (2)	7 (2)	0.867
Liver cirrhosis—*n* (%)	14 (1)	9 (1)	5 (2)	1.000
Outcomes				
Days on mechanical ventilation[d]	3 [1,6]	3 [1,6]	3 [1,4]	0.716
Days on (C)RRT[d]	3 [2,7]	3 [2,7]	3 [2,6]	0.181
Days on vasopressors[d]	2 [1,4]	2 [1,4]	2 [1,4]	0.991

Table 1 continued

Variables	Whole group ($N = 957$)	Survivors ($N = 646$)	Non-survivors ($N = 311$)	*P* value[a]
ICU Length of stay—days	5 [4,11]	5 [4,10]	6 [3,13]	0.994
ICU mortality—*n* (%)	311 (32)	0 (0)	311 (100)	na
Death within the first 48 h of ICU—*n* (%)	78 (8)	0 (0)	78 (25)	na
Discharge within the first 48 h of ICU—*n* (%)	85 (9)	85 (13)	0 (0)	na

[a] Comparison between survivors and non-survivors

[b] Others are endocarditis, meningitis, leptospirosis and mediastinitis

[c] AIDS denotes acquired immunodeficiency syndrome

[d] Results using only patients which needed the support. na denotes not applicable

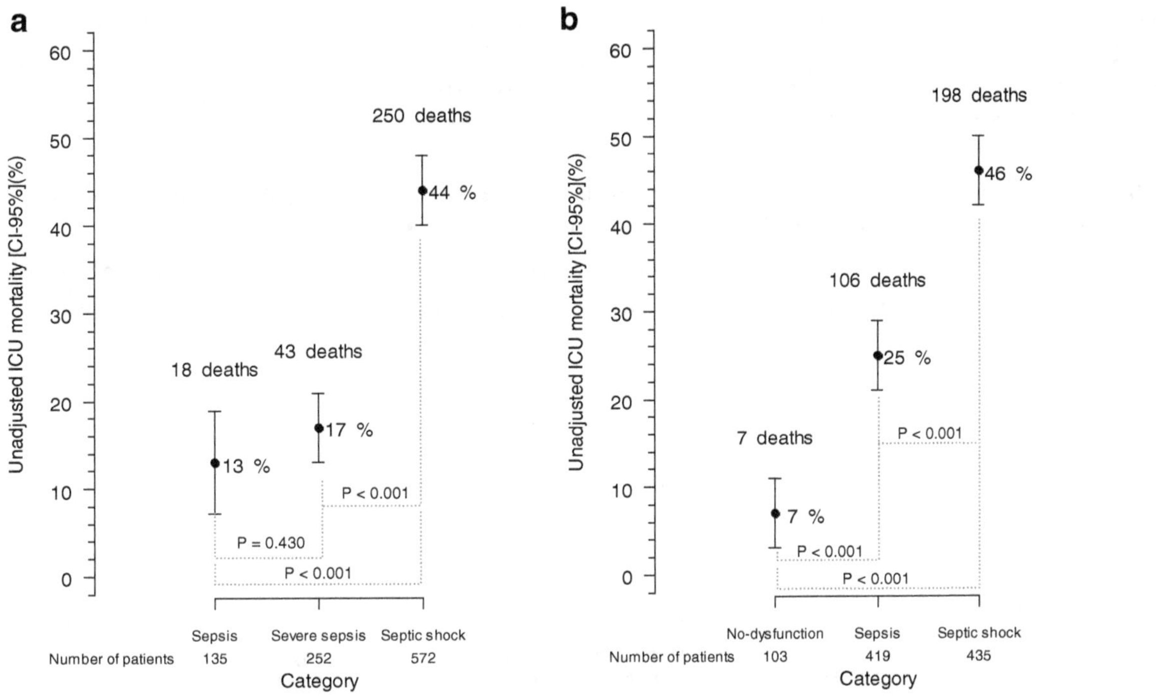

Fig. 1 Mortality stratified according to sepsis definition. **a** Mortality according to the Sepsis-2 definition (Pearson's Chi-squared test using the three categories $P < 0.001$. Pearson's Chi-squared post hoc analyses are shown in the figure). **b** Mortality according to the Sepsis-3 definition (Pearson's Chi-squared test using the three categories $P < 0.001$. Pearson's Chi-squared post hoc analyses are shown in the figure)

show clear stratification of mortality among the three categories (no-dysfunction, sepsis and septic shock). Additional file 2: Table 1s shows patients' re-allocation between both sepsis definitions. Sepsis-3 classification reduced the percentage of septic shock patients as compared to the previous definition.

Additional file 3: Figure 1s shows the median lactate levels of each sepsis category in both sepsis definitions. Significant differences between lactate levels occurred only in the septic shock categories for both definitions (Panels A and C) and between survivors and non-survivors in both septic shock definitions (Panels B and D). The mortality rates according to the sepsis definitions, sepsis categories and serum lactate concentrations are shown in Additional file 4: Fig. 2s. Lactate levels higher than 2 mmol/L were not clearly discriminative of mortality in the Sepsis-2 defined categories of severe sepsis or septic shock. In comparison, lactate levels >4 mmol/L clearly marked increased mortality in both the severe sepsis and septic shock categories of Sepsis-2 and in the no-dysfunction and septic shock categories of Sepsis-3.

Table 2 shows the associations of sepsis definitions with mortality and the additional impact of lactate inclusion in the multivariate model. Furthermore, Table 3 shows the association of Sepsis-3 definition with ICU mortality, after adjustment for lactate level, age, illness severity (assessed

Table 2 Multivariate models using ICU death as a dependent variable and sepsis definition and lactate as independent variables

	Lactate as a continuous variable		Lactate > 2 mmol/L		Lactate > 4 mmol/L	
	OR (CI 95%)	*P* value	OR (CI 95%)	*P* value	OR (CI 95%)	*P* value
Sepsis-2 model						
Sepsis	1	Reference	1	Reference	1	Reference
Severe sepsis	1.06 (0.97–1.16)	0.322	1.03 (1.01–1.19)	0.500	1.04 (0.95–1.19)	0.342
Septic shock	1.34 (1.22–1.44)	<0.001	1.33 (1.22–1.45)	0.001	1.32 (1.21–1.43)	0.001
Lactate	1.02 (1.02–1.03)	0.001	1.07 (1.00–1.14)	0.027	1.21 (1.14–1.30)	0.001
Sepsis-3 model						
No-dysfunction	1	Reference	1	Reference	1	Reference
Sepsis	1.21 (1.11–1.34)	<0.001	1.19 (1.08–1.32)	<0.001	1.21 (1.10–1.14)	<0.001
Septic shock	1.41 (1.28–1.56)	<0.001	1.49 (1.35–1.65)	<0.001	1.41 (1.28–1.56)	<0.001
Lactate	1.02 (1.01–1.03)	<0.001	0.97 (0.90–1.05)	0.466	1.19 (1.11–1.28)	<0.001

This analysis was performed using a binary logistic regression. The first model used lactate as a continuous variable (after logarithmic transformation in order to correct the positive skewness); the second and third models used lactate as a categorical variable

Lactate > 2 mmol/L represents all patients with lactate > 2 mmol/L, including those with lactate > 4 mmol/L

Table 3 Multivariate models using ICU death as a dependent variable and Sepsis-3 definition, lactate, age, SAPS 3 and requirement for RRT and mechanical ventilation as independent variables

	Lactate as a continuous variable		Lactate > 2 mmol/L		Lactate > 4 mmol/L	
	OR (CI 95%)	*P* value	OR (CI 95%)	*P* value	OR (CI 95%)	*P* value
Sepsis-3 model						
No-dysfunction	1	Reference	1	Reference	1	Reference
Sepsis	3.70 (1.75–9.12)	0.002	3.35 (1.57–8.27)	0.004	3.67 (1.73–9.07)	0.002
Septic shock	6.21 (2.94–15.27)	<0.001	7.31 (3.41–18.22)	<0.001	6.22 (2.94–15.31)	<0.001
Lactate	1.11 (1.06–1.16)	<0.001	0.94 (0.60–1.48)	0.811	2.28 (1.61–3.24)	<0.001
Age	1.01 (1.01–1.02)	<0.001	1.01 (1.01–1.02)	0.002	1.01 (1.00–1.02)	<0.001
SAPS 3	1.02 (1.01–1.03)	<0.001	1.02 (1.01–1.03)	<0.001	1.02 (1.01–1.03).	<0.001
RRT[a]	1.63 (1.15–2.31)	0.006	1.56 (1.11–2.21)	0.011	1.66 (1.17–2.36)	0.004
Mechanical ventilation[a]	1.29 (0.95–1.76)	0.107	1.26 (0.92–1.71)	0.146	1.27 (0.93–1.73)	0.131
	AUC[b] (CI 95%)	**Asymptotic *P* value**	**AUC[b] (CI 95%)**	**Asymptotic *P* value**	**AUC[b] (CI 95%)**	**Asymptotic *P* value**
Model accuracy	0.732 (0.698–0.766)	<0.001	0.725 (0.691–0.759)	<0.001	0.732 (0.698–0.766)	<0.001

[a] Support needed at any time of ICU stay; *RRT* renal replacement therapy; *SAPS* Simplified Acute Physiological Score

[b] AUC area under the curve

through SAPS 3), requirement for RRT and mechanical ventilation at any time of ICU stay.

Table 4 shows the accuracy of ICU death prediction of models using only the sepsis definitions and sepsis definitions added to lactate as a continuous and dichotomous variable. The accuracy significantly improved with the addition of lactate to the model.

Further evaluation of lactate's addition to the sepsis definitions model using the net reclassification index (NRI) and integrated discrimination increment (IDI) is presented in Additional file 2: Table 2s. In Sepsis-2 definitions, NRI as it relates to ICU mortality was 23.1 ($P < 0.001$) for lactate >2 mmol/L and 39.9 ($P < 0.001$) for lactate >4 mmol/L. For Sepsis-3 definitions, NRI was 39.9 ($P < 0.001$) for lactate levels >4 mmol/L. The discrimination slope of the updated model with lactate levels >4 mmol/L, as assessed by IDI, was 3.3 ($P < 0.001$) for Sepsis-2 and 2.7 ($P < 0.001$) for Sepsis-3. For lactate levels >2 mmol/L, IDI was 0.7 ($P = 0.021$) for Sepsis-2 criteria, while it was not significant for Sepsis-3.

Table 4 Predictive accuracy of mortality of sepsis definitions with or without lactate value

	Sepsis-2 definition		Sepsis-3 definition	
	AUC (CI 95%)	Asymptotic *P* value	AUC (CI 95%)	Asymptotic *P* value
Without lactate model	0.650 (0.619–0.680)	<0.001	0.615 (0.580–0.650)	<0.001
Lactate as a continuous variable[a]	0.704 (0.668–0.739)[b]	<0.001	0.649 (0.608–0.689)[b, d]	<0.001
Lactate > 2 mmol/L	0.664 (0.631–0.697)	<0.001	0.620 (0.584–0.656)	<0.001
Lactate > 4 mmol/L	0.686 (0.653–0.719)[b, c, d]	<0.001	0.636 (0.598–0.674)[b, c, d]	<0.001

The receiver operating curves (ROC) were constructed using the binary logistic regression probabilities of death using sepsis definitions and lactate categories. AUC area under the ROC curve

[a] Lactate as a continuous variable was logarithmically transformed in order to correct the positive skewness. Lactate > 2 mmol/L represents all patients with lactate > 2 mmol/L, including those with lactate > 4 mmol/L

[b] DeLong's test $P < 0.05$ versus without lactate model

[c] DeLong's test $P =$ ns versus lactate as a continuous variable

[d] DeLong's test $P < 0.05$ versus lactate > 2 mmol/L

Discussion

In this study, we demonstrate that Sepsis-3 is better than Sepsis-2 at stratifying mortality among septic patients admitted in a strained ICU of a developing country. Sepsis-3 criteria clearly categorized septic patients along a spectrum of severity, since mortality increased from 7% in no-dysfunction-infected patients to 25 and 46% for sepsis and septic shock patients, respectively. In contrast, in the Sepsis-2 definitions, only the septic shock criterion was associated with a significantly higher mortality when compared to the severe sepsis and sepsis categories (44, 17 and 13%, respectively). Moreover, a lactate level higher than 4 mmol/L improved the mortality prediction accuracy on both Sepsis-2 and Sepsis-3 definitions (Table 3).

The validity of sepsis definitions based on SIRS criteria has recently been called into question. This is because almost 90% of the patients admitted to an intensive care unit (ICU) meet the SIRS criteria, [5, 21]. Even SIRS criteria's high sensitivity has been questioned recently, as some patients with known infectious insult and new organ failures do not satisfy 2 SIRS criteria and therefore do not fulfill previous sepsis definitions [6]. Even more importantly, the categories of sepsis, severe sepsis and septic shock should indicate a real spectrum of severity to be considered as different outcome categories [14]. The present study reinforces a lack of accuracy of Sepsis-2 definitions of sepsis, severe sepsis and septic shock in stratifying patients' mortality risk. Additionally, our data demonstrate Sepsis-3 definitions of infection without organ dysfunction, sepsis and septic shock clearly represent progressive strata of mortality risk (Fig. 1).

High lactate values in sepsis may be the result of perfusion abnormalities or stress hyperlactatemia [22]. Regardless of the reason for its increase, early high lactate value is traditionally associated with worse outcomes in septic [23] and other critically ill patients [24, 25]. The fact that lactate was not maintained as a marker of organ dysfunction in the new sepsis definitions raised several concerns [26, 27], and the Surviving Sepsis Campaign suggested that lactate should continue to be measured to identify dysfunction [27]. In the original validation study of Sepsis-3 definitions, although high lactate levels were associated with higher mortality at different cutoffs regardless of hypotension or vasopressors, lactate was retained only for the characterization of septic shock [9]. In the present study, however, lactate was a prognostic factor for both definitions and reclassified some Sepsis-3-defined patients when its levels were above 4 mmol/L. In the assessment of the new septic shock definitions in the original validation study, lactate levels higher than 2 mmol/L were increasingly associated with higher odds of death [11]. In our study, cutoff levels above 2 mmol/L did not add any prognostic information in this stratum of severity, as expected, because it is included in the definition itself. However, in accordance with the validation paper, higher lactate levels (which we chose to add in the model as >4 mmol/L) were of prognostic significance.

In the validation of clinical criteria for sepsis, unfortunately, there was no clear mention to the added benefit of lactate for patients with SOFA scores <2, possibly because of lactate values missingness in the derivation (about 60%) and validation cohorts (about 90%) [10]. Interestingly, lactate was not retained in the novel qSOFA during model construction. However, the authors state that for a qSOFA score of 1, high lactate values characterized a population with similar risk to patients with a qSOFA score of 2 [10]. In our cohort, for patients without organ dysfunction, lactate levels higher than 4 mmol/L seem to categorize a population at higher risk of death (Table 2 and Additional file 4: Fig. 2s). Therefore, high lactate levels in patients without organ dysfunction as assessed by the SOFA score might improve risk stratification and change management of these patients, since they could be allocated to a higher level of care upfront in order to avoid further deterioration of their clinical status.

Sepsis-3 criteria for identifying septic patients have been extensively questioned since its publication [12, 15]. A possible decrease in awareness of sepsis and a need for massive educational programs to healthcare providers are among the main concerns. In this context, how Sepsis-3 criteria would perform for sepsis detection, especially in countries with high mortality rates, still needs validation. Our study was not designed to assess Sepsis-2 or Sepsis-3 as a screening tool, since only patients admitted to ICU were included. The role of Sepsis-2 criteria for identifying septic patients is undeniable, as was the case in a recent before–after study conducted in Brazil [28]. However, its accuracy to stratify severity can be called into question, as demonstrated by our data. Accordingly, our study clearly shows a better discriminative performance of Sepsis-3 in predicting ICU mortality.

Strengths of this study include the number of patients analyzed, the recent timeframe and the use of statistical methodologies such as net reclassification index, which allowed us to better evaluate the benefit of adding lactate to the new definition. Also, NRI was not used in the original validation study and our data missingness for lactate values was much lower (<5%), which could have yielded some of the above different results. Furthermore, this represents an external assessment of new criteria in a different setting than that of the original validation—an important step toward consistency for its findings.

There are, nevertheless, several limitations to be addressed, in light of which our findings should be interpreted. First, the retrospective nature of this study makes it difficult to elucidate known confounders that could have biased the outcome measures, such as differences in sepsis treatment. Second, this was a single-center study consisting mainly of medical patients and our results may not be generalizable to other centers, including from other developing countries, since there is wide variation in outcomes even within Brazil when comparing different settings [29, 30]. Third, we evaluated only patients admitted to the ICU and, therefore, our findings cannot be extrapolated to patients treated in wards and in the emergency room. This also threatens the generalizability of our results, since the original study captured a population with presumed infection not only in the ICU. Fourth, the validity of Sepsis-3 criteria in this study was assessed based on ICU mortality. Although ICU mortality is not the most appropriate endpoint to be evaluated, it reflects the pre-ICU and ICU care of septic patients, and in our scenario, identified a more specific point to improve the care of septic patients [31, 32].

Conclusions

The new clinical criteria of sepsis proposed by the third international consensus (Sepsis-3) could predict mortality in infected patients admitted to a strained ICU in a middle-income country. The prognostic value of the new definition of sepsis was progressive along all three categories, which denotes a spectrum of gravity of infectious process and could help in risk stratification for future studies in this area of research. This was not observed of the previous definitions (Sepsis-2) in our sample. Serum lactate improved accuracy for values higher than 4 mmol/L in the no-dysfunction and septic shock groups.

Additional files

Additional file 1: Appendix

Additional file 2: Tables

Additional file 3: Figure 1s Lactate levels according to the sepsis categories. **Panel A** shows lactate levels according to the Sepsis-2 definition. **Panel B** shows lactate levels according to the Sepsis-2 definition, stratified according to survival. **Panel C** shows lactate levels according to the Sepsis-3 definition. **Panel D** shows lactate levels according to the Sepsis-3 definition, stratified according to survival. * Kruskal-Wallis' test $P < 0.001$ among the three sepsis categories. Mann-Whitney's $P < 0.05$ *post-hoc* analysis vs. other categories. # Mann-Whitney's test $P < 0.05$ vs. survivors.

Additional file 4: Figure 2s Mortality according to the sepsis category and lactate concentration. Panel A shows the Sepsis-2 categories. Panel B shows the Sepsis-3 categories. Lactate > 2 mmol/L represents all patients with lactate > 2 mmol/L, including those with lactate > 4 mmol/L* Number of patients in the category. # Pearson's Chi-squared test $P < 0.001$ among the three sepsis categories (same lactate level). Pearson's Chi-squared test $P < 0.05$ *post-hoc* analysis vs. severe sepsis (same lactate level) category.$ Pearson's Chi-squared test $P < 0.001$ among the three sepsis categories (same lactate level). Pearson's Chi-squared test $P < 0.05$ *post-hoc* analysis vs. sepsis (same lactate level) category. % Pearson's Chi-squared test $P < 0.001$ among the three lactate categories (same sepsis category level). Pearson's Chi-squared test $P < 0.05$ *post-hoc* analysis vs. whole group and Lactate > 2 mmol/L (same sepsis category level) categories.

Abbreviations

ICU: intensive care unit; SOFA: Sequential Organ Failure Assessment; SAPS: Simplified Acute Physiological Score; SIRS: systemic inflammatory response syndrome; LOS: length of stay; IDI: integrated discrimination index; NRI: net reclassification improvement; AUROC: area under the receiving operational characteristics curve.

Authors' contributions

BAMPB, TGR and MP conceived of the study and acquired all data. MP and FGZ performed the statistical analysis. BAMPB, TGR and APNJ drafted the manuscript. LUT, LCPA, PVM, FGZ and MP revised the manuscript for important intellectual content. All authors read and approved the final manuscript.

Author details

[1] Intensive Care Unit, Emergency Department, Hospital das Clínicas, University of São Paulo Medical School, Rua Dr. Enéas Carvalho de Aguiar, 255, Room 6040, São Paulo ZIP 05403-000, Brazil. [2] Hospital da Luz, Amil, São Paulo, Brazil. [3] Research Institute, Hospital Sírio-Libanês, São Paulo, Brazil. [4] Nephrology Department, ABC Medical School, Santo Andre, Brazil. [5] A.C. Camargo Cancer Center, São Paulo, Brazil. [6] Research Institute, HCor-Hospital do Coração, São Paulo, Brazil. [7] Intensive Care Unit, Hospital Alemão Oswaldo Cruz, São Paulo, Brazil.

Competing interests
The authors declare that they have no competing interests.

References

1. Fleischmann C, Scherag A, Adhikari NK, Hartog CS, Tsaganos T, Schlattmann P, et al. Assessment of global incidence and mortality of hospital-treated sepsis. Current estimates and limitations. Am J Respir Crit Care Med. 2016;193(3):259–72.
2. Kahn JM, Benson NM, Appleby D, Carson SS, Iwashyna TJ. Long-term acute care hospital utilization after critical illness. JAMA. 2010;303(22):2253–9.
3. Bone RC, Balk RA, Cerra FB, Dellinger RP, Fein AM, Knaus WA, et al. Definitions for sepsis and organ failure and guidelines for the use of innovative therapies in sepsis. The ACCP/SCCM Consensus Conference Committee. American College of Chest Physicians/Society of Critical Care Medicine. Chest. 1992;101(6):1644–55.
4. Levy MM, Fink MP, Marshall JC, Abraham E, Angus D, Cook D, et al. 2001 SCCM/ESICM/ACCP/ATS/SIS international sepsis definitions conference. Intensive Care Med. 2003;29(4):530–8.
5. Sprung CL, Sakr Y, Vincent JL, Le Gall JR, Reinhart K, Ranieri VM, et al. An evaluation of systemic inflammatory response syndrome signs in the Sepsis Occurrence In Acutely Ill Patients (SOAP) study. Intensive Care Med. 2006;32(3):421–7.
6. Kaukonen KM, Bailey M, Pilcher D, Cooper DJ, Bellomo R. Systemic inflammatory response syndrome criteria in defining severe sepsis. N Engl J Med. 2015;372(17):1629–38.
7. Klein Klouwenberg PM, Ong DS, Bonten MJ, Cremer OL. Classification of sepsis, severe sepsis and septic shock: the impact of minor variations in data capture and definition of SIRS criteria. Intensive Care Med. 2012;38(5):811–9.
8. Gaieski DF, Edwards JM, Kallan MJ, Carr BG. Benchmarking the incidence and mortality of severe sepsis in the United States. Crit Care Med. 2013;41(5):1167–74.
9. Singer M, Deutschman CS, Seymour CW, Shankar-Hari M, Annane D, Bauer M, et al. The third international consensus definitions for sepsis and septic shock (sepsis-3). JAMA. 2016;315(8):801–10.
10. Seymour CW, Liu VX, Iwashyna TJ, Brunkhorst FM, Rea TD, Scherag A, et al. Assessment of clinical criteria for sepsis: for the third international consensus definitions for sepsis and septic Shock (sepsis-3). JAMA. 2016;315(8):762–74.
11. Shankar-Hari M, Phillips GS, Levy ML, Seymour CW, Liu VX, Deutschman CS, et al. Developing a new definition and assessing new clinical criteria for septic shock: for the third international consensus definitions for sepsis and septic shock (sepsis-3). JAMA. 2016;315(8):775–87.
12. Cortes-Puch I, Hartog CS. Change is not necessarily progress: revision of the sepsis definition should be based on new scientific insights. Am J Respir Crit Care Med. 2016;194(1):16–8.
13. Angus DC. Defining sepsis: A case of bounded rationality and fuzzy thinking? Am J Respir Crit Care Med. 2016;194(1):14–5.
14. Deutschman CS. Imprecise medicine: the limitations of sepsis-3. Crit Care Med. 2016;44(5):857–8.
15. Simpson SQ. New sepsis criteria: a change we should not make. Chest. 2016;149(5):1117–8.
16. Vincent JL, Mira JP, Antonelli M. Sepsis: older and newer concepts. Lancet Respir Med. 2016;4(3):237–40.
17. Gabler NB, Ratcliffe SJ, Wagner J, Asch DA, Rubenfeld GD, Angus DC, et al. Mortality among patients admitted to strained intensive care units. Am J Respir Crit Care Med. 2013;188(7):800–6.
18. Steyerberg EW, Vickers AJ, Cook NR, Gerds T, Gonen M, Obuchowski N, et al. Assessing the performance of prediction models: a framework for traditional and novel measures. Epidemiology. 2010;21(1):128–38.
19. Vesin A, Azoulay E, Ruckly S, Vignoud L, Rusinova K, Benoit D, et al. Reporting and handling missing values in clinical studies in intensive care units. Intensive Care Med. 2013;39(8):1396–404.
20. R Core Team. R: A language and environment for statistical computing. R Foundation for Statistical Computing, Vienna, Austria; 2014. http://www.R-project.org/. Accessed 25 May 2016.
21. Lai NA, Kruger P. The predictive ability of a weighted systemic inflammatory response syndrome score for microbiologically confirmed infection in hospitalized patients with suspected sepsis. Crit Care Resusc. 2011;13(3):146–50.
22. Van Lambalgen AA, Runge HC, van den Bos GC, Thijs LG. Regional lactate production in early canine endotoxin shock. Am J Physiol Endocrinol Metab. 1988;254(1):E45–51.
23. Noritomi DT, Soriano FG, Kellum JA, Cappi SB, Biselli PJ, Liborio AB, et al. Metabolic acidosis in patients with severe sepsis and septic shock: a longitudinal quantitative study. Crit Care Med. 2009;37(10):2733–9.
24. Shapiro NI, Howell MD, Talmor D, Nathanson LA, Lisbon A, Wolfe RE, et al. Serum lactate as a predictor of mortality in emergency department patients with infection. Ann Emerg Med. 2005;45(5):524–8.
25. Trzeciak S, Dellinger RP, Chansky ME, Arnold RC, Schorr C, Milcarek B, et al. Serum lactate as a predictor of mortality in patients with infection. Intensive Care Med. 2007;33(6):970–7.
26. Machado FR, Salomao R, Pontes de Acevedo LC, Lisboa T, Costa Filho R. Latin American Sepsis Institute (LASI). Why LASI did not endorse the new definitions of sepsis published today in JAMA; 2016. http://ilas.org.br/assets/arquivos/upload/declaracao%20sepse%203.0%20ILAS%20-%20English%20version.pdf. Accessed 25 May 2016.
27. Antonelli M, De Backer D, Dorman T, Kleinpell R, Levy M, Rhodes A. For the Surviving Sepsis Campaign Executive Committee. Surviving Sepsis Campaign Responds to Sepsis-3; 2016. http://www.survivingsepsis.org/SiteCollectionDocuments/SSC-Statements-Sepsis-Definitions-3-2016.pdf. Accessed 25 May 2016.
28. Noritomi DT, Ranzani OT, Monteiro MB, Ferreira EM, Santos SR, Leibel F, et al. Implementation of a multifaceted sepsis education program in an emerging country setting: clinical outcomes and cost-effectiveness in a long-term follow-up study. Intensive Care Med. 2014;40(2):182–91.
29. Silva E, Pedro Mde A, Sogayar AC, Mohovic T, Silva CL, Janiszewski M, et al. Brazilian Sepsis Epidemiological Study (BASES study). Crit Care. 2004;8(4):R251–60.
30. Conde KA, Silva E, Silva CO, Ferreira E, Freitas FG, Castro I, et al. Differences in sepsis treatment and outcomes between public and private hospitals in Brazil: a multicenter observational study. PLOS ONE. 2013;8(6):e64790.
31. Berenholtz SM, Pronovost PJ, Ngo K, Barie PS, Hitt J, Kuti JL, et al. Developing quality measures for sepsis care in the ICU. J Comm J Qual Patient Saf. 2007;33(9):559–68.
32. Berenholtz SM, Dorman T, Ngo K, Pronovost PJ. Qualitative review of intensive care unit quality indicators. J Crit Care. 2002;17(1):1–12.

3

A comparison of two insulin infusion protocols in the medical intensive care unit by continuous glucose monitoring

Christophe E. M. De Block[1*], Peter Rogiers[2], Philippe G. Jorens[3], Tom Schepens[3], Cosimo Scuffi[4] and Luc F. Van Gaal[1]

Abstract

Background: Achieving good glycemic control in intensive care units (ICU) requires a safe and efficient insulin infusion protocol (IIP). We aimed to compare the clinical performance of two IIPs (Leuven versus modified Yale protocol) in patients admitted to medical ICU, by using continuous glucose monitoring (CGM). This is a pooled data analysis of two published prospective randomized controlled trials. CGM monitoring was performed in 57 MICU patients (age 64 ± 12 years, APACHE-II score 28 ± 7, non-diabetic/diabetic: 36/21). The main outcome measures were percentage of time in normoglycemia (80–110 mg/dl) and in hypoglycemia (<60 mg/dl), and glycemic variability (standard deviation, coefficient of variation, mean amplitude of glucose excursions, mean of daily differences).

Results: Twenty-two subjects were treated using the Leuven protocol and 35 by the Yale protocol; >63,000 CGM measurements were available. The percentage of time in normoglycemia (80–110 mg/dl) was higher (37 ± 15 vs. 26 ± 11%, $p = 0.001$) and percentage of time spent in hypoglycemia was lower (0[0–2] vs. 5[1–8]%, $p = 0.001$) in the Yale group. Median glycemia did not differ between groups (118[108–128] vs. 128[106–154] mg/dl). Glycemic variability was less pronounced in the Yale group (median SD 28[21–37] vs. 47[31–71] mg/dl, $p = 0.001$; CV 23[19–31] vs. 36[26–50]%, $p = 0.001$; MODD 35[26–41] vs. 60[33–94] mg/dl, $p = 0.001$). However, logistic regression could not identify type of IIP, diabetes status, age, BMI, or APACHE-II score as independent parameters for strict glucose control.

Conclusions: The Yale protocol provided better average glycemia, more time spent in normoglycemia, less time in hypoglycemia, and less glycemic variability than the Leuven protocol, but was not independently associated with strict glycemic control.

Keywords: Intensive care unit, Continuous glucose monitoring, Insulin infusion protocol, Hypoglycemia

Background

Consensus exists that overt hyperglycemia (>150 mg/dl) in patients admitted to the intensive care unit (ICU) should be treated to improve morbidity and survival [1]. However, there is little agreement on the ideal target range of glycemia [2]. Strict glycemic control (80–110 mg/dl) is no longer recommended for most ICUs, but in highly standardized ICUs a strict target may be feasible without increasing hypoglycemia. Achieving strict glycemic control is a complex task since during ICU stay severity of illness and degree of insulin resistance may fluctuate, nutritional delivery may change, and interventions (e.g., administration of corticosteroids) may produce frequent changes in insulin needs [2]. Therefore, multiple insulin infusion protocols (IIPs) were created, all meant to balance efficacy with safety (avoid hypoglycemia), and attainability (nursing workload).

So far, no single IIP has been established as the most effective for obtaining tight glycemic control. Earlier observational studies and randomized controlled trials

*Correspondence: christophe.deblock@uantwerpen.be; christophe.deblock@uza.be
[1] Department of Endocrinology, Diabetology and Metabolism, Faculty of Medicine, Antwerp University Hospital and University of Antwerp, Wilrijkstraat 10, 2650 Edegem, Belgium
Full list of author information is available at the end of the article

(RCTs) in medical ICU (MICU) or mixed ICU settings, and targeting a glycemia between 80 and 110 mg/dl, reported that 22–60% of all blood glucose values were in target for paper-based IIPs [3–14], compared to 42–69% for computerized decision-supported algorithms [4, 10, 11, 14, 15]. The efficacy and safety of different IIPs on glycemic control have recently been investigated using computer simulation models [16, 17] and in RCTs in cardiac surgery patients [18, 19]. However, to the best of our knowledge, comparing the effect of different IIPs on glucose control has never been investigated in MICU patients. With this pooled data analysis of two published prospective RCTs [5, 6], we assessed the clinical performance of two IIPs (Leuven versus modified Yale protocol) in patients admitted to MICU, by means of continuous glucose monitoring (CGM), allowing a complete picture of glucometrics.

Methods

This is a pooled data analysis of two prospective RCTs conducted at the medical ICUs of the Antwerp University Hospital (45 beds, including 14 MICU beds) and Middelheim Hospital, a university-affiliated tertiary care center (36 beds, including 13 MICU beds) [5, 6]. Patients were recruited between 04/2004 and 03/2005 for the first study and between 07/2007 and 09/2009 for the second study. Both MICUs applied the same standards of care, with a nurse-to-patient ratio between 1:2.5 and 1:3.0. Each patient or the closest family member gave written informed consent. Patients were included if they were between 18 and 75 years, treated by IV insulin, and expected to stay in MICU for ≥3 days. Patients were not enrolled if pregnant, if surgery was the reason for admission, or if a do not reanimate code was present. The studies were approved by the ethics committees of both hospitals (Middelheim approval no. 2345 and UZA 6/43/211) and conducted in accordance with the amended Declaration of Helsinki.

Severity of illness was scored using the Acute Physiology And Chronic Health Evaluation II (APACHE-II) and the Sequential Organ Failure Assessment (SOFA) score [20, 21]. The neurologic score was zero when patients were sedated. Enteral nutrition was started as soon as possible, at 25 kcal/kg body weight per day.

Glucose monitoring

Forty-eight-hour CGM was initiated within the first 48 h after admission using a microdialysis-based device that is not equipped with alarms (GlucoDay® in the first study and GlucoDay®S in the second study, A. Menarini Diagnostics, Florence, Italy). The methodology has been described before [5, 6]. Briefly, a microdialysis fiber (Medica, Medolla, Italy) was inserted subcutaneously into the periumbilical region using an 18-gauge Teflon® (DuPont, Wilmington, DE) catheter as a guide. The device does not use any coagulant. The device uses a glucose oxidase-based amperometric biosensor to measure glucose concentrations in the interstitial dialysate every 3 min over a 48 h period.

Data analysis for accuracy and glucometrics was performed by applying, in silico to the CGM signal, a two-point calibration according to the manufacturer's requirements (one calibration every 24 h). This was performed in order to avoid an overestimation of the system's accuracy if one uses a higher number of calibration points. In the RT-CGM group, however, to be as safe as possible and to account for possible changes in subcutaneous glucose recovery due to hemodynamic alterations (e.g., hypotension, shock, vasoactive drugs), for each sensor, a six-point calibration was performed (after 2, 6, 12, 18, 24, and 36 h) using arterial BG values, but these data were not used for statistical analysis [6]. This was done to assure that the glucose readings and trends shown by RT-CGM would be clinically reliable. At present, RT-CGM is becoming more common practice, but at the time of the study, a real-time CGM device was not approved to make clinical adjustments of insulin therapy, and our ethical committee would not approve clinical decisions to be made solely on the basis of RT-CGM at that time. In order to avoid clinical decisions being made on potentially inaccurate CGM data, nurses had to take an additional arterial blood glucose sample. Thus, direct corroboration of the data was explicitly needed. The RT-CGM system was thus used only as a prompt to take an extra blood glucose sample if the rate of change in glucose exceeded 25 mg/dl per 30 min. Since no differences in glucometrics were observed in the REGIMEN trial between in patients randomized to RT-CGM versus blinded CGM, we pooled the data. For all patients, adjustments of insulin therapy were made on the basis of arterial blood glucose values [6].

Insulin infusion protocols

Twenty-two patients received continuous IV insulin (regular insulin Actrapid; Novo Nordisk, Bagsvaerd, Denmark) according to the Leuven protocol, targeting a blood glucose between 80 and 110 mg/dl [5, 13]. Thirty-five subjects were treated with IV insulin (insulin aspart, Novo Nordisk, Bagsvaerd, Denmark) according to a modified Yale protocol, targeting a blood glucose level between 80 and 120 mg/dl [6].

In both groups, arterial blood glucose levels were measured using an on-site blood gas analyzer (Rapidlab® 1265, Siemens, München, Germany) and they were used to adjust the insulin infusion rate. Insulin in a concentration of 50 units in 50 cc 0.9% NaCl was infused using the Injectomat Agilia® syringe infusion system (flow rate change: range 0.1–200 ml/h, Fresenius Kabi, Bad Homburg, Germany). In both groups, the arterial blood glucose sampling interval varied between 1 and 4 h. For more details on the insulin infusion protocols, the reader is referred to the original publications [5, 6].

Outcome parameters

The percentage of time spent in the target range of glycemia (80–110 mg/dl) was the primary outcome parameter. Secondary outcome variables were percentages of time spent in hypoglycemia (<60 mg/dl), in hyperglycemia (>150 and >200 mg/dl), and parameters of glycemic fluctuations (SD: standard deviation [22], CV: coefficient of variation [22], MAGE: mean amplitude of glucose excursions [23], CONGA: continuous overlapping net glycemic action [24], and MODD: mean of daily differences [25]. We also calculated the low blood glucose index (LBGI) and the high blood glucose index (HBGI) as measures of risk of hypo- and hyperglycemia [26]. All glucometric data reported are those calculated using CGM data. A CGM reading <60 mg/dl, confirmed by an arterial blood glucose sample <60 mg/dl, lasting for >6 min (6 min being the time of two CGM measurements) was defined as a hypoglycemic event. We rigorously followed the recommendations on measurement of blood glucose and reporting glycemic control in critically ill adults [27].

Statistical analysis

Results were analyzed using SPSS (SPSS Inc., Chicago, USA). Distributions of continuous data were tested for normality by Kolmogorov–Smirnov test. The unpaired *t* test or Mann–Whitney *U* test were used to determine differences between groups, with Bonferroni adjustments for multiple comparisons. Data are expressed as mean ± SD or median [25th–75th percentile]. Differences in distributions of categorical data were evaluated by χ^2 or Fisher's exact test. Stepwise forward logistic or linear regression analysis was performed to assess the strength and independency of associations. A two-tailed $p < 0.05$ was considered significant.

Results

Over 63,000 CGM data points were analyzed from 57 adults (men/women: 30/27, non-diabetic/diabetic: 36/21) admitted to the MICU. Mean age was 64 ± 12 years. They were severely ill as demonstrated by a mean APACHE-II score of 28 ± 7 and SOFA score of 10 ± 4. Table 1 shows reasons for admission and interventions used.

Comparison of Leuven versus Yale protocol

Twenty-two subjects were treated using the Leuven protocol and 35 by the Yale protocol. The distribution of diabetic subjects differed between groups (13/22 Leuven vs. 8/35 Yale; $p = 0.0016$). Patients in the Yale group tended to be older. Reasons for admission were comparable between groups with exception of neurologic disease/coma. Feeding habits were different in the two groups ($p = 0.003$) with enteral feeding being less frequently used in the Leuven group (3/22 vs. 20/35). The APACHE-II score was similar, whereas the SOFA score tended to be higher in the Yale group.

Patients in the Leuven group required much more IV insulin compared to those treated by the Yale protocol (Table 1). Despite a similar number of arterial blood glucose measurements, patients in the Yale protocol had better glucometrics with a higher percentage of time in target glycemia (80–110 mg/dl) (37 ± 15 vs. 26 ± 11%, $p = 0.001$) and a lower percentage of time spent in hypoglycemia (0[0–2] vs. 5[1–8]%, $p = 0.001$). Also percentage of time spent between 60 and 150 mg/dl (81 ± 7 vs. 66 ± 24%, $p < 0.0001$), 80–125 mg/dl (57 ± 18 vs. 36 ± 21%, $p < 0.0001$), between 80 and 145 mg/dl (74 ± 17 vs. 48 ± 23, $p < 0.0001$), and between 70 and 180 mg/dl (91 ± 10 vs. 69 ± 19%, $p < 0.0001$) was higher in the Yale group. Figure 1 shows the time-in-band for the different ranges of targets for both groups. Median glycemia, however, did not differ between groups (118[108–128] (log: 114[105–125]) vs. 128[106–154] (log: 122[99–136]) mg/dl) (Table 1). Glycemic variability was less pronounced with the use of the Yale protocol (median[IQR] SD 28[21–37] vs. 47[31–71] mg/dl, $p = 0.001$; median CV 23[19–31] vs. 36[26–50]%, $p = 0.001$; median MODD 35[26–41] vs. 60[33–94] mg/dl, $p = 0.001$). Significant better LBGI and HBGI were observed in the Yale group (Table 1). Eight insulin/glucose plots comparing non-diabetic and diabetic patients treated according to the Leuven protocol versus according to the modified Yale protocol are shown in Fig. 2, providing the reader with a good visual image.

Characteristics of subjects achieving strict versus above-target glycemic control

Subjects achieving strict glycemic control ($n = 19$), defined as having an average glycemia ≤110 mg/dl, did not differ with regard to gender, diabetic status, age, BMI, reason for admission, severity of illness, and interventions used as compared to the ones not obtaining an average glycemia ≤110 mg/dl, with the exception of the use of glucocorticoids ($p = 0.001$) (Table 2). The distribution according to insulin infusion protocol used (Leuven vs. Yale) also did not differ between groups. Insulin doses infused and a number of arterial blood glucose measurements were similar as well. Most glucometrics (% of time within target) including glycemic variability (SD, MODD, LBGI and HBGI) were better in the group achieving

Table 1 Baseline characteristics, interventions used and glucometrics of patients treated by the Leuven versus Yale protocol

	Total cohort	Leuven	Yale	Statistics
Number of patients	57	22	35	*p* value
Patient demographics				
Men/women	30/27	13/9	17/18	NS
Diabetic status (no/type1/type2)	36/6/15	9/4/9	27/2/6	0.0016
Age (years)	64 ± 12	60 ± 13	66 ± 10	0.055
BMI (kg/m^2)	26.8 ± 5.4	27.5 ± 7.1	26.3 ± 4.0	NS
Admission reason				
Septic shock	22	13	9	NS
Neurologic disease/coma	9	0	9	0.004
Cardiopulmonary resuscitation	9	1	8	NS
Respiratory failure	6	1	5	NS
Cardiogenic shock	7	3	4	NS
Other	4	4	0	NS
Severity of illness				
APACHE-II score	28 ± 7	27 ± 7	28 ± 7	NS
SOFA score	10 ± 4	9 ± 4	11 ± 3	0.072
Clinical interventions				
Mechanical ventilation	44	16	28	NS
Vasopressor therapy	35	14	21	NS
Inotropic therapy	20	6	14	NS
Hemodialysis	14	9	5	NS
No/total parenteral/enteral feeding	17/17/23	9/10/3	8/7/20	0.003
Glucocorticoids	27	12	15	NS
Blood transfusion	15	4	11	NS
Antibiotics	46	19	27	NS
Outcome parameters				
LOS in ICU (days)	15 ± 9	11 ± 6	17 ± 10	0.019
In hospital mortality	20	7	11	NS
Insulin dose				
Day 1 (units)		138 (48–190)	50 (27–80)	0.001
Day 2 (units)		116 (54–116)	56 (28–81)	0.006
Glucose parameters				
HbA1c (%)		6.3 (5.8–7.0)	6.0 (5.7–6.6)	NS
HbA1c (mmol/mol)		45 (40–53)	42 (39–49)	NS
Median glycemia (mg/dl)		128 (106–154)	118 (108–128)	NS
% of time at glycemia				
<60 mg/dl		5 (1–8)	0 (0–2)	0.001
80–110 mg/dl		26 ± 11	37 ± 15	0.001
>150 mg/dl		29 ± 23	17 ± 13	<0.0001
>200 mg/dl		13 ± 19	3 ± 5	<0.0001
60–150 mg/dl		66 ± 24	81 ± 7	<0.0001
70–180 mg/dl		69 ± 19	91 ± 10	<0.0001
Nr of art blood glc measurements/day		10 ± 2	10 ± 4	NS
Glucose variability parameters				
SD (mg/dl)		47 (31–71)	28 (21–37)	0.001
Coefficient of variation (%)		36 (26–50)	23 (19–31)	0.001
IQR		66 (47–82)	37 (27–43)	<0.0001
MAGE (mg/dl)		73 (47–128)	52 (37–83)	0.061 (NS)

Table 1 continued

	Total cohort	Leuven	Yale	Statistics
MODD (mg/dl)		60 (33–94)	35 (26–41)	0.001
M-100		10 (4–25)	4 (2–5)	<0.0001
CONGA1 (mg/dl)		20 (14–39)	15 (13–24)	NS
CONGA2 (mg/dl)		30 (22–53)	23 (18–34)	0.036
CONGA4 (mg/dl)		38 (28–66)	29 (20–43)	0.012
LBGI		2.6 (1.0–3.7)	0.7 (0.4–1.4)	0.011
HBGI		2.5 (1.0–8.0)	1.3 (0.5–1.8)	0.018
Glucose variability		42 (29–67)	28 (20–34)	0.001

Data are presented as numbers, as mean ± SD or median (25–75th percentile)

LOS in ICU length of stay in ICU, *IQR* interquartile range, *MAGE* mean amplitude of glycemic excursions, *MODD* mean of daily differences, *LBGI* low blood glucose index, *HBGI* high BGI

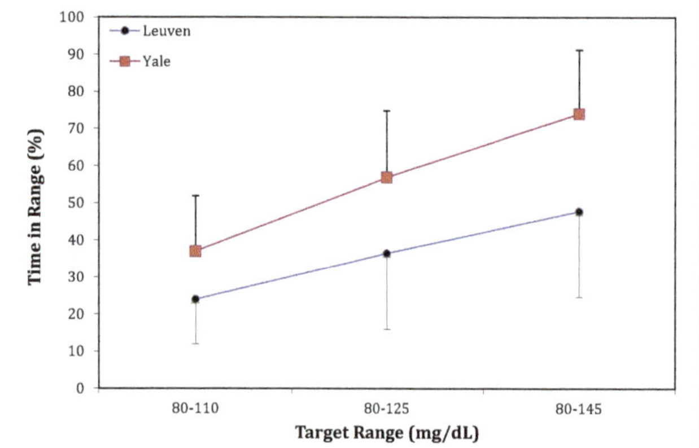

Fig. 1 Average percentage time in range and SD over the groups (Yale vs. Leuven) for the different glycemia target ranges. $P < 0.0001$ for all three ranges

strict glycemic control. Logistic regression analysis could not identify type of IIP, diabetes status, age, BMI, or APACHE-II score as independent parameters for strict glucose control. The only parameter which showed an independent association with strict glucose control was the administration of glucocorticoids ($p = 0.001$).

Characteristics of diabetic versus non-diabetic subjects

No differences in patient demographics except for BMI ($p = 0.02$), in reason for admission, severity of illness, and clinical interventions used, were present between diabetic ($n = 21$) and non-diabetic critically ill patients (Table 3). There were more diabetic patients in the Leuven protocol ($p = 0.009$). Diabetic subjects required more insulin, had a worse median glycemia (131[110–166] vs. 116[107–128] mg/dl, $p = 0.034$), spent less time in target glycemia (25 ± 12 vs. 36 ± 15%, $p = 0.006$), more time in hypoglycemia (4[1–10] vs. 0[0–1]%, $p = 0.001$) than non-diabetic subjects. All other glucometrics, including glycemic variability parameters, were worse as well in diabetic patients (see Table 3).

In the non-diabetic group, patients in the Yale protocol spent more time in target glycemia (40 ± 15 vs. 25 ± 10%, $p = 0.009$), less time in hypoglycemia (0[0–0] vs. 1[0–6]%, $p = 0.013$), and glycemic variability tended to be smaller (SD $p = 0.076$, CV $p = 0.057$, MODD $p = 0.021$) than those treated by the Leuven protocol. Median glycemia was similar (117[108–127] vs. 115[101–140]) in both groups (Additional file 1: Table S1). In the diabetic subjects, insulin needs were lower ($p = 0.044$) and patients spent less time at a glycemia >150 mg/dl (26 ± 21 vs. 35 ± 25%, $p = 0.003$) in the Yale compared to the Leuven group. However, median glycemia (120[108–140] vs. 136[111–169] mg/dl), time spent in hypoglycemia or at target range, and parameters of glycemic variability were similar between groups (Additional file 1: Table S1).

Discussion

Achieving strict glycemic control without risk of hypoglycemia in the ICU is difficult. It requires a comprehensive and safe insulin infusion protocol (IIP) that is both detailed enough and practical enough to be easily implemented by ICU nurses [2, 28]. Multiple IIPs have been developed, but to the best of our knowledge this is the first study comparing the clinical efficacy (% time in target glycemia) and safety (hypoglycemia, glycemic variability) of two IIPs in MICU patients by means of CGM. Overall, compared to existing data (see Table 4, [3–15, 29–38], both our IIPs were able to obtain reasonably strict glucose control without excessive risk of hypoglycemia. The percentage of time in normoglycemia was higher (37 vs. 26%), and percentage of time in hypoglycemia lower (0 vs. 5%) and glycemic variability was less pronounced in patients treated with the Yale IIP. Diabetes status can, however, be a confounding factor [34]. We

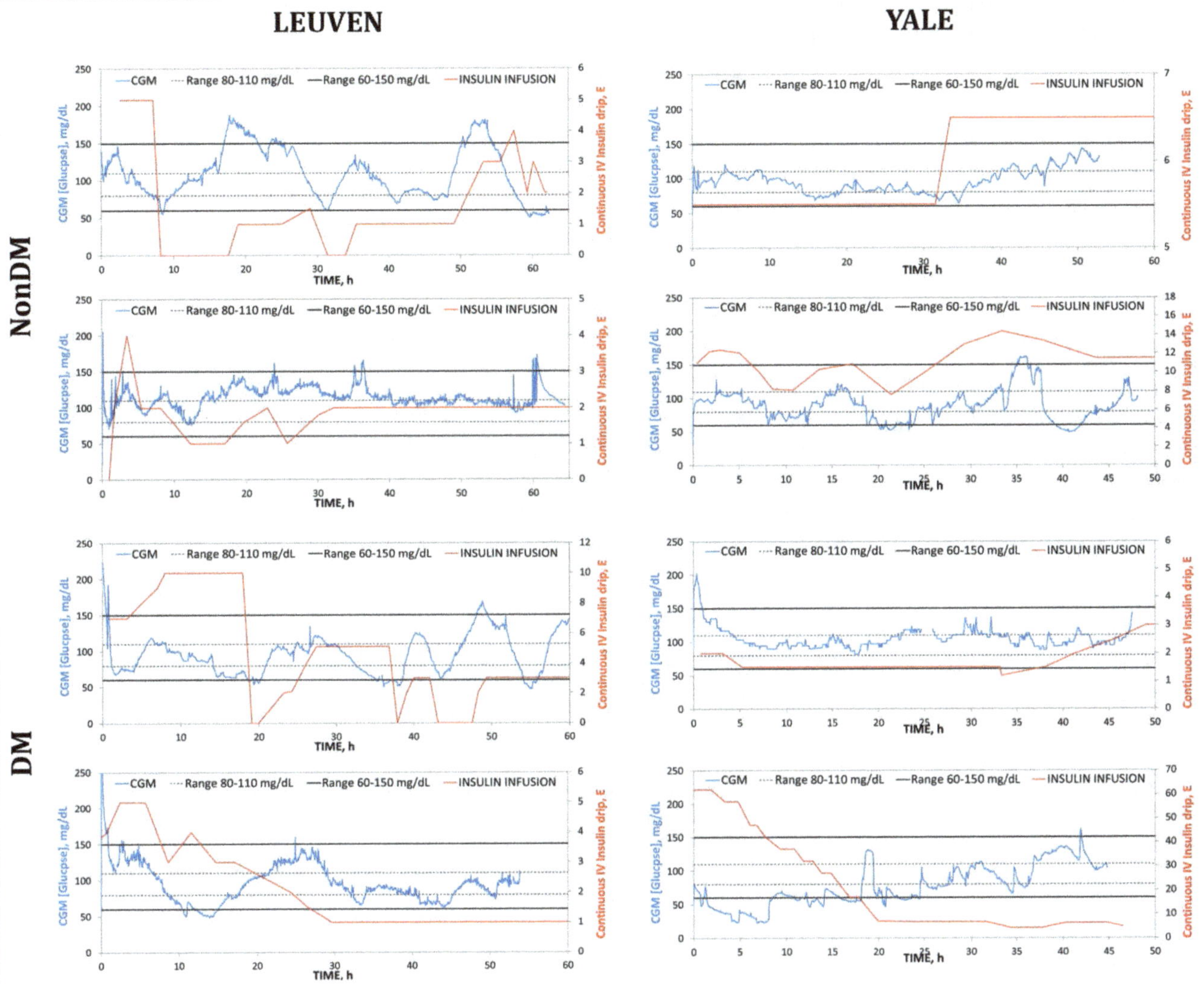

Fig. 2 Insulin glucose plots comparing 4 non-diabetic and 4 diabetic patients treated according to the Leuven protocol versus according to the modified Yale protocol. *CGM* continuous glucose monitoring

observed an imbalance in the number of diabetic subjects with more diabetic patients in the Leuven group. Diabetic as compared to non-diabetic subjects required more insulin, had worse glycemic control, and larger glycemic variability, thereby possibly blunting the effect of the IIP. However, logistic regression could not identify type of IIP, diabetes status, or severity of illness as independent parameters associated with strict glucose control. When comparing Yale versus Leuven protocol in non-diabetic subjects, patients in the Yale protocol had better glucometrics. This was evident, despite the low number of patients. In the diabetic subgroup, however, the advantages of the Yale protocol were less pronounced.

Up till now no single IIP has been established as the most effective for obtaining tight glycemic control [28, 39, 40]. The IIP should be tailored to the subset of patients being treated and to local resources, because an excellent validated IIP is no guarantee for optimal glucose control unless it is carefully implemented. Most IIPs show significant similarities, but differences relate to target glucose levels (80–110 mg/dl versus ranges varying between 90 and 180 mg/dl), initial glycemic threshold (>150–200 mg/dl), infusion rates, use of boluses, and frequency of monitoring. Changes in insulin infusion rate may relate to actual glycemia, direction and/or velocity of change in glycemia, degree of insulin resistance, and insulin dose. The population treated (surgical vs. medical ICU, diabetes status) may also affect the performance of the IIP [2, 28, 39, 40]. The competence of the nurses and clarity of instructions also influence outcome.

Table 2 Baseline characteristics, interventions used and glucometrics of patients reaching an average glycemia ≤110 mg/dl versus those with an average glycemia >110 mg/dl

	Avg glyc ≤ 110 mg/dl	Avg glyc >110 mg/dl	Statistics
Number of patients	19	38	
Patient demographics			
Men/women	8/11	22/16	NS
Diabetic status (no/type1/type2)	14/1/4	23/4/11	NS
Age (years)	65 ± 11	63 ± 12	NS
BMI (kg/m^2)	26.3 ± 3.8	27.1 ± 6.1	NS
Severity of illness			
APACHE-II score	27 ± 6	28 ± 7	NS
SOFA score	10 ± 4	10 ± 3	NS
Clinical interventions			
Mechanical ventilation	14	31	NS
Vasopressor therapy	12	23	NS
Hemodialysis	5	9	NS
No/total parenteral/enteral feeding	4/6/9	13/11/14	NS
Glucocorticoids	15	12	0.01
Antibiotics	17	29	NS
Protocol (Leuven/Yale)	7/12	15/23	NS
Insulin dose			
Day 1 (units)	62 (33–133)	63 (39–128)	NS
Day 2 (units)	67 (23–101)	70 (42–120)	NS
Glucose parameters			
HbA1c (%)	6.1 (5.6–6.7)	6.0 (5.8–6.9)	NS
HbA1c (mmol/mol)	43 (38–50)	70 (42–120)	NS
Median glycemia (mg/dl)	104 (100–108)	128 (119–141)	<0.0001
% of time at glycemia			
<60 mg/dl	5 (0–8)	0 (0–4)	0.067
80–110 mg/dl	41 ± 14	27 ± 13	0.001
>150 mg/dl	6 ± 6	28 ± 18	<0.0001
>200 mg/dl	1 ± 2	10 ± 16	0.017
60–150 mg/dl	89 ± 11	69 ± 19	<0.0001
70–180 mg/dl	86 ± 14	80 ± 19	NS
Nr of art blood glc measurements/day	10 ± 3	10 ± 4	NS
Glucose variability parameters			
SD (mg/dl)	25 (20–36)	38 (29–63)	0.003
Coefficient of variation (%)	25 (20–33)	29 (23–44)	NS
IQR	33 (27–55)	45 (35–76)	0.031
MAGE (mg/dl)	50 (34–72)	60 (43–100)	0.085
MODD (mg/dl)	29 (22–45)	42 (32–76)	0.005
M-100	2 (1–4)	6 (4–14)	0.001
CONGA1 (mg/dl)	15 (12–19)	21 (15–35)	0.008
CONGA2 (mg/dl)	22 (17–28)	32 (20–48)	0.010
CONGA4 (mg/dl)	29 (18–43)	42 (27–69)	0.011
LBGI	2.7 (0.9–3.8)	0.7 (0.2–1.9)	0.001
HBGI	0.3 (0.2–1.1)	2.0 (1.4–4.5)	<0.0001
Glucose variability	21 (17–28)	36 (29–53)	<0.0001

Data are presented as numbers, as mean ± SD or median (25–75th percentile)

LOS in ICU length of stay in ICU, *IQR* interquartile range, *MAGE* mean amplitude of glycemic excursions, *MODD* mean of daily differences, *LBGI* low blood glucose index, *HBGI* high BGI

Table 3 Baseline characteristics, interventions used and glucometrics of non-diabetic versus diabetic patients

	Non-DM	DM	Statistics
Number of patients	36	21	
Patient demographics			
Men/women	19/17	11/10	NS
Age (years)	65 ± 11	62 ± 12	NS
BMI (kg/m^2)	26 ± 4	29 ± 7	0.02
Severity of illness			
APACHE-II score	29 ± 6	26 ± 7	NS
SOFA score	11 ± 4	9 ± 3	NS (0.064)
Clinical interventions			
Mechanical ventilation	27	17	NS
Vasopressor therapy	23	12	NS
Hemodialysis	12	2	NS (0.06)
No/total parenteral/enteral feeding	7/13/16	10/4/7	NS (0.075)
Glucocorticoids	20	7	NS
Antibiotics	30	16	NS
Protocol (Leuven/Yale)	9/27	13/8	0.009
Insulin dose			
Day 1 (units)	48 (26–82)	127 (51–175)	0.001
Day 2 (units)	46 (25–85)	113 (67–168)	0.009
Glucose parameters			
HbA1c (%)	5.9 (5.6–6.3)	6.9 (6.1–7.3)	<0.0001
HbA1c (mmol/mol)	41 (38–45)	52 (43–56)	<0.0001
Median glycemia (mg/dl)	116 (107–128)	131 (110–166)	0.034
% of time at glycemia			
<60 mg/dl	0 (0–1)	4 (1–10)	0.001
80–110 mg/dl	36 ± 15	25 ± 12	0.006
>150 mg/dl	32 ± 15	24 ± 11	0.001
>200 mg/dl	3 ± 15	15 ± 20	0.001
60–150 mg/dl	83 ± 12	63 ± 23	<0.0001
70–180 mg/dl	90 ± 11	69 ± 19	<0.0001
Nr of art blood glc measurements/day	10 ± 4	10 ± 3	NS
Glucose variability parameters			
SD (mg/dl)	28 (21–35)	53 (40–75)	<0.0001
Coefficient of variation (%)	23 (19–30)	38 (29–51)	<0.0001
IQR	38 (28–45)	66 (41–108)	<0.0001
MAGE (mg/dl)	49 (35–66)	87 (56–127)	0.002
MODD (mg/dl)	35 (26–42)	59 (35–116)	<0.0001
M-100	4 (2–5)	12 (6–29)	<0.0001
CONGA1 (mg/dl)	15 (13–20)	30 (19–41)	<0.0001
CONGA2 (mg/dl)	22 (17–30)	44 (26–59)	<0.0001
CONGA4 (mg/dl)	30 (21–43)	60 (37–86)	<0.0001
LBGI	0.7 (0.3–1.8)	2.3 (0.9–3.7)	0.013
HBGI	1.2 (0.4–1.8)	3.0 (1.4–10.3)	0.002
Glucose variability	28 (20–34)	44 (34–79)	<0.0001

Data are presented as numbers, as mean ± SD or median (25–75th percentile)

LOS in ICU length of stay in ICU, *IQR* interquartile range, *MAGE* mean amplitude of glycemic excursions, *MODD* mean of daily differences, *LBGI* low blood glucose index, *HBGI* high BGI

Computerized decision-supported algorithms might provide superior glucose control compared to paper-based IIPs because of reduced errors by enabling the use of complex mathematical calculations and better protocol consistency. In MICUs and mixed ICUs where a glycemia between 80 and 110 mg/dl was targeted, 22–60% of all blood glucose values were reported to be in target for paper-based IIPs [3–14], compared to a higher percentage (42–69%) for computerized IIPs [4, 10, 11, 14, 15] (Additional file 1: Digital Content–Table S1). In contrast, in a before–after study in 192 surgical ICU patients, Barletta et al. [29] could not observe significant glucometric differences between the computer-assisted versus paper-based IIP. It is probably not the paper or computer that makes the largest difference; but the IIP algorithm itself and the competence of the staff.

A head-to-head comparison of different IIPs on glycemic control has only been performed in RCTs in cardiac surgery. Blaha et al. [18] compared two paper protocols with a computerized IIP in 120 patients, showing that the computerized IIP provided better average glucose control, but with a longer time in hypoglycemia risk range than the paper protocols. Dumont and Bourguignon [19] compared the effect of a computerized (EndoTool) versus a paper IIP (modified Portland protocol) in 300 ICU patients, showing better glucose control and nurses' satisfaction with the EndoTool IIP. In both studies, however, it was not only the protocol that differed but also the way it was implemented (paper vs. computerized), making it difficult to assess the true value of the protocol itself.

Measurement frequency is an inherent part of an IIP and will affect glucometrics. Recently, the effect of the IIP (Yale vs. University of Washington), frequency of glucose measurements (hourly vs. every 5 min), and measurement imprecision on glycemic control efficacy was studied using a simulation model [16]. In both IIPs, the rates of hypo- and hyperglycemia and of glycemic variability increased with increasing measurement imprecision. Others investigated the performance of the IIP versus methodology of glucose measurements (blood glucose meter vs. CGM) at different levels of measurement accuracy [17]. The protocol itself proved to have a greater effect on glycemic control efficacy than the glucose measurement method, with the Yale protocol showing the best performance. However, hypoglycemia risk was lower in CGM-informed IIPs [17]. Thus, efficacy of the IIP together with performance and accuracy of the CGM device used both contribute to the success of tight glucose control. In the future, validated computerized IIPs can be guided by real-time CGM in a semi-closed loop, thereby improving efficacy, safety and reducing nursing workload.

Comparison of glucometrics between studies using different IIPs is difficult due to differences in population,

Table 4 Summary of several insulin infusion protocols in different ICU settings

Authors	ICU type	Study	*n*	% Diabetic patients	Protocol	Target glycemia (mg/dl)	Method of glucose measurements
Goldberg et al. (2004)	MICU	Observational	52	56	Yale	100–139	Hospital glucose meter: near hourly measurements
Van den Berghe et al. (2006)	MICU	RCT	1200	17	Paper: Leuven	80–110	ABG: q1-4 h
Kulnik et al. (2008)	MICU	Observational	10	20	eMPC (computer)	80–110	Variable sampling rate: q20 min-4 h
Shetty et al. (2012)	MICU	Observational	90	66	Yale	120–160	POC meter: hourly measurements
Holzinger et al. (2010)	MICU	RCT	124	19	Leuven	80–110	CGM
De Block et al. (2015)	MICU	RCT	35	23	Yale	80–110	CGM
Finney et al. (2003)	Mixed	Observational	523	16	Paper	90–145	ABG
Juneja et al. (2007)	Mixed	Observational	2398	NR	Clarian Gluco Stabilizer	80–110	POC: q1-2 h
Chase et al. (2008)	Mixed	Observational	371	17	SPRINT	80–110	Sampling rate: q1-2 h
Morris et al. (2008)	Mixed	Before–after	755	NR	eProtocol-insulin versus paper	80–110	POC: q1-4 h
Preiser et al. GLU-CONTROL (2009)	Mixed	RCT	1078	21	Paper: glucontrol	80–110	POC: q1-4 h
NICE SUGAR (2009)	Mixed	RCT	6104	20	Paper: Leuven	81–108	ABG
Marvin et al. (2013)	Mixed	Retrospective	1657	NR	Computerized Yale	100–140	POC: variable time interval
Van Herpe et al. (2013)	Mixed	RCT	300	21	LOGIC-insulin computerized	80–110	ABG: variable time interval: q1-4 h
Krinsley et al. (2015)	Mixed	Retrospective	3297	23	Paper: Stamford	70–140	POC: q3 h
Vogelzang et al. (2005)	SICU	Observational	179	15	GRIP	72–135	POC blood gas analyzer: variable
Plank et al. (2006)	SICU: cardiothoracic surgery	RCT	60	23	eMPC versus paper	80–110	POC: variable sampling rate: q1 h-4 h
Hovorka et al. (2007)	SICU: cardiac surgery	RCT	60	45	eMPC	80–110	Variable sampling rate: q1 h-4 h
Saager et al. (2008)	SICU: cardiothoracic ICU	RCT	40	100	EndoTool (computer) versus paper	90–150	POC: hourly
Dortch et al. (2008)	SICU: trauma ICU	RCT	552		Computer versus paper	80–110	POC q1-4 h
Blaha et al. (2009)	SICU: cardiac surgery	RCT	120	14	eMPC versus paper (Matias versus Bath)	80–110	ABG: protocol dependent: q1-4 h
Barletta et al. (2011)	SICU	Before–after	192	28	Computer versus paper	80–110	POC: variable sampling rate: q30 min-2 h versus q2 h
Dumont et al. (2012)	SICU: cardiovascular ICU	RCT	300	43	Computer (EndoTool) versus paper (modified Portland)	80–150	NA

Table 4 continued

Authors	Duration of glucose monitoring	Glucometric to measure target	% of time at target glycemia: intervention versus control group	Mean glycemia (mg/dl): intervention versus control group	Hypoglycemia: intervention versus control group	Glycemic variability	References
Goldberg et al. (2004)	61 h	Percent of hourly BG values in target range	52%	124 ± 15	% of data at glc <60 mg/dl: 0.3%	NA	[8]
Van den Berghe et al. (2006)	NR	Mean morning BG	NA	111 ± 29 versus 153 ± 31	% of patients: glc <40 mg/dl: 18.7 versus 3.1%	NA	[13]
Kulnik et al. (2008)	72 h	Percent of BG values in target	47 ± 13%	109 ± 13	% data at glc <40 mg/dl: 0%	NA	[15]
Shetty et al. (2012)	59 h	Percent of BG values in target range	42%	156 ± 23	% of data <70 mg/dl: 0.3%	NA	[37]
Holzinger et al. (2010)	72 h	CGM data: percent of data in target range	59 ± 20 versus 55 ± 18	106 ± 18 versus 111 ± 10	Rate: 1.9% versus 11.5%	NA	[9]
De Block et al. (2015)	96 h	CGM data: percent of data in target range	37 ± 12 versus 34 ± 10	119 ± 17 versus 122 ± 11	% of time at glc <60 mg/dl: 0.6 ± 1.6 versus 2.4 ± 4.3%	No differences between groups in SD, MAGE, MODD, CV	[6]
Finney et al. (2003)	22–89 h	Time spent in glucose band 80–110 mg/dl	4 (0–20)%	NR	0 ± 1%	NA	[31]
Juneja et al. (2007)	NR	Percent of data in target range	52 versus 32%	107 ± 39	% data at glc <50 mg/dl: 0.4 versus 0.5%	NA	[10]
Chase et al. (2008)	53 h	Percent of BG values in target	54%	108 ± 27	% of data at glc <72 mg/dl: 3.8%	SD: 27 mg/dl	[4]
Morris et al. (2008)	4–22 days	Percent of BG values in target	42 versus 28%	116 versus 134	% data at glc <40 mg/dl: 11.1 versus 5.1%	NA	[11]
Preiser et al. GLUCONTROL (2009)	48–216 h (=2–9 days)	Proportion of time of BG values in range	43%	117 (IQR: 108–130) mg/dl	Proportion of time at glc <40 mg/dl: 5.9 ± 27%	SD: 36 mg/dl	[12]
NICE SUGAR (2009)	4.2 days (1.9–9.0 days)	Time-weighted mean BG	NR	115 ± 18 versus 144 ± 23	% of patients: glc <40 mg/dl: 6.8 versus 0.5%	NA	[7]
Marvin et al. (2013)	NR	Percent of hourly BG values in target range	92%	124	% of data 40–70 mg/dl: 1.1% and in 17.6% of patients	NA	[34]
Van Herpe et al. (2013)	26–113 h	Percent of BG values in target range	69 ± 17 versus 60 ± 19	106 ± 9 versus 107 ± 11	% data at glc <60 mg/dl: 0.6 versus 1.2%	Max change in glc/24 h: 31 versus 37 mg/dl	[14]
Krinsley et al. (2015)	36–120 h	Percent of time of BG values in target range	Non-DM versus DM: 81 (61–94) versus 55 (35–71)%	Non-DM versus DM: 121 (112–133) versus 140 (128–155) mg/dl	% of patients: glc <70 mg/dl: non-DM versus DM: 18 versus 31%	CV: non-DM versus DM: 18 versus 27%	[33]
Vogelzang et al. (2005)	1.6 (0.8–4.7) days	Percent of time of BG values in target	78 (66–88)%	121 (108–135)	% of patients: glc <40: 0.6%; glc <63: 11.2%	NA	[38]

Table 4 continued

Authors	Duration of glucose monitoring	Glucometric to measure target	% of time at target glycemia: intervention versus control group	Mean glycemia (mg/dl): intervention versus control group	Hypoglycemia: intervention versus control group	Glycemic variability	References
Plank et al. (2006)	48 h	Percent of time in target range	52 (17–92) versus 19 (0–71)%	117 (102–144) versus 131 (97–237)	Number of hypo episodes (<54 mg/dl) over 48 h: 0 versus 2	NA	[35]
Hovorka et al. (2007)	24 h	Percent of time in target range	60 ± 23 versus 28 ± 16	112 ± 20 versus 130 ± 20	% of data at glc <52 mg/dl: 0% versus 0%	NA	[32]
Saager et al. (2008)	9 h	Percent of BG values in target	84 versus 60%	126 ± 18 versus 147 ± 27	Episodes of hypo (<60 mg/dl) during ICU: 4 versus 1	NA	[36]
Dortch et al. (2008)	NR	Percent of BG values in target	42 versus 34%	116 ± 37 versus 120 ± 37	% data at glc <40 mg/dl: 0.2 versus 0.5%	NA	[30]
Blaha et al. (2009)	45–48 h	Time in target range	46 ± 3 versus 38 ± 3 versus 40 ± 3%	106 ± 4 versus 121 ± 4 versus 117 ± 4	Time in hypo (<52 mg/dl): 0 ± 0 versus 0.4 ± 0.2 versus 0.4 ± 0.3%	NA	[18]
Barletta et al. (2011)	67 versus 98 h	Percent of BG values in target	49 ± 14 versus 40 ± 12	113 ± 11 versus 116 ± 11	% data at glc <40 mg/dl: 2.1 versus 4.1%	SD: 25 ± 9 versus 31 ± 11 mg/dl	[29]
Dumont et al. (2012)	NA	Percent of BG values in target range	70 ± 15 versus 62 ± 18	138 ± 16 versus 141 ± 20	Number of hypo events <60 mg/dl: 7 (5%) versus 18 (11%)	SD:36 ± 18 versus 42 ± 21	[19]

MICU medical intensive care unit, *SICU* surgical ICU, *RCT* randomized controlled trial, *NR* not reported, *NA* not assessed, *ABG* arterial blood glucose, *POC* point of care, *SD* standard deviation

target glycemia, and frequency of glucose monitoring. In addition, many different glucometrics are reported in different studies, including metrics of central tendency (mean or median glycemia, time-averaged glucose, admission glycemia, proportion of glucose values in target), metrics of extremes (percentages or episodes of hypo- or hyperglycemia), and metrics of dispersion (SD, coefficient of variation, MAGE). The robustness of glucometrics depends largely on the number of measurements per time unit used for its calculation. Accurate assessment of time in target glycemia, or in hypo- or hyperglycemia, and of glucose variability can only be done by using validated CGM methodology.

Our study has some limitations and strengths. This is a pooled data analysis of two prospective RCTs conducted at the medical ICUs, using relatively old data. Indeed, patients were recruited between 04/2004 and 03/2005 for the first study and between 07/2007 and 09/2009 for the second study. However, pooling the CGM data is justifiable in our opinion because the same CGM sensor was used in both studies and the study population and standards of care in both services were comparable. However, our results might not be applicable to a mixed or surgical ICU setting. Despite more than 63,000 CGM glucose measurements being available for analysis, due to the small number of patients and heterogeneity of groups, statistical superiority of the Yale protocol could not be proven.

A major strength, in our opinion, when comparing IIPs, is the use of CGM data which provides a complete picture of glucometrics. We did not make use of study nurses particularly focused on glucose control, but implemented our study in a routine clinical setting, allowing a more clinically relevant picture.

In summary, the use of a safe and efficient IIP is a prerequisite to correctly implement strict glycemic targets. Both IIPs have proven to balance efficacy with safety (avoid hypoglycemia and glycemic variability) and attainability (nursing workload). Overall, the modified Yale protocol provided better glucose control with more time spent in normoglycemia, less time spent in hypoglycemia, and less glycemic variability as compared to the Leuven protocol.

Abbreviations

BMI: body mass index; CGM: continuous glucose monitoring; CONGA: continuous overlapping net glycemic; HBGI: high blood glucose index; ICU: intensive care unit; IIP: insulin infusion protocol; IV: intravenous; LBGI: low blood glucose index; MAGE: mean amplitude of glucose excursions; MICU: medical intensive care unit; MODD: mean of daily differences; RCT: randomized controlled trial(s); SD: standard deviation; UZA: Universitair Ziekenhuis Antwerpen (Antwerp University Hospital).

Authors' contributions

All authors made important intellectual contributions to the conception and analysis of the study. Every author reviewed and provided comments on manuscript drafts and gave final approval of this version to be published. CEMDB was responsible for the final design of the study. CEMDB, PR, and PGJ recruited patients, implemented the study protocol, and acquired data. CS, who was masked for clinical data and treatment arm, analyzed the CGM profiles with patients being coded. CEMDB and TS performed the statistical analysis. CEMDB drafted the manuscript. All authors read and approved the final manuscript.

Author details

[1] Department of Endocrinology, Diabetology and Metabolism, Faculty of Medicine, Antwerp University Hospital and University of Antwerp, Wilrijkstraat 10, 2650 Edegem, Belgium. [2] Intensive Care Unit, ZNA, General Hospital Middelheim, Antwerp, Belgium. [3] Intensive Care Unit, Antwerp University Hospital, University of Antwerp, Edegem, Belgium. [4] A. Menarini Diagnostics, Scientific and Technology Affairs, Florence, Italy.

Acknowledgements

We thank Dr. W. Verbrugghe, Dr. J. Gios, Dr. N. Verheyen (Antwerp University Hospital), and Dr. K. Bervoets (Middelheim Hospital) who contributed to patient recruitment. We gratefully acknowledge the nursing staff of the ICU wards in both hospitals, and all patients. The CGM devices (GlucoDayS) and fibers were provided at no charge by A. Menarini Diagnostics (Florence, Italy). The company had no influence on trial design, analysis, or preparation of the manuscript.

Part of this study was accepted for oral presentation at the 9th International Conference on Advanced Technologies and Treatments for Diabetes (ATTD 2016, Milan, Italy).

Competing interests

The authors declare that they have no competing interests.

References

1. Jacobi J, Bircher N, Krinsley J, Agus M, Braithwaite SS, Deutschman C, et al. Guidelines for the use of an insulin infusion for the management of hyperglycemia in critically ill patients. Crit Care Med. 2012;40(12):3251–76.
2. De Block C, Manuel-y-Keenoy B, Rogiers P, Jorens P, Van Gaal L. Glucose control and use of continuous glucose monitoring in the intensive care unit: a critical review. Curr Diabetes Rev. 2008;4(3):234–44.
3. Brunkhorst FM, Engel C, Bloos F, Meier-Hellmann A, Ragaller M, Weiler N, et al. Intensive insulin therapy and pentastarch resuscitation in severe sepsis. N Engl J Med. 2008;358(2):125–39.
4. Chase JG, Shaw G, Le Compte A, Lonergan T, Willacy M, Wong XW, et al. Implementation and evaluation of the SPRINT protocol for tight glycaemic control in critically ill patients: a clinical practice change. Crit Care. 2008;12(2):R49.
5. De Block C, Manuel-Y-Keenoy B, Van Gaal L, Rogiers P. Intensive insulin therapy in the intensive care unit: assessment by continuous glucose monitoring. Diabetes Care. 2006;29(8):1750–6.
6. De Block CE, Gios J, Verheyen N, Manuel-y-Keenoy B, Rogiers P, Jorens PG, et al. Randomized evaluation of glycemic control in the medical intensive care unit using real-time continuous glucose monitoring (REGIMEN Trial). Diabetes Technol Ther. 2015;17(12):889–98.
7. Finfer S, Chittock DR, Su SY, Blair D, Foster D, Dhingra V, et al. Intensive versus conventional glucose control in critically ill patients. N Engl J Med. 2009;360(13):1283–97.
8. Goldberg PA, Siegel MD, Sherwin RS, Halickman JI, Lee M, Bailey VA, et al. Implementation of a safe and effective insulin infusion protocol in a medical intensive care unit. Diabetes Care. 2004;27(2):461–7.
9. Holzinger U, Warszawska J, Kitzberger R, Wewalka M, Miehsler W, Herkner H, et al. Real-time continuous glucose monitoring in critically ill patients: a prospective randomized trial. Diabetes Care. 2010;33(3):467–72.
10. Juneja R, Roudebush C, Kumar N, Macy A, Golas A, Wall D, et al. Utilization of a computerized intravenous insulin infusion program to control blood glucose in the intensive care unit. Diabetes Technol Ther. 2007;9(3):232–40.
11. Morris AH, Orme J Jr, Truwit JD, Steingrub J, Grissom C, Lee KH, et al. A replicable method for blood glucose control in critically ill patients. Crit Care Med. 2008;36(6):1787–95.
12. Preiser JC, Devos P, Ruiz-Santana S, Melot C, Annane D, Groeneveld J, et al. A prospective randomised multi-centre controlled trial on tight glucose control by intensive insulin therapy in adult intensive care units: the Glucontrol study. Intensive Care Med. 2009;35(10):1738–48.
13. Van den Berghe G, Wilmer A, Hermans G, Meersseman W, Wouters PJ, Milants I, et al. Intensive insulin therapy in the medical ICU. N Engl J Med. 2006;354(5):449–61.
14. Van Herpe T, Mesotten D, Wouters PJ, Herbots J, Voets E, Buyens J, et al. LOGIC-insulin algorithm-guided versus nurse-directed blood glucose control during critical illness: the LOGIC-1 single-center, randomized, controlled clinical trial. Diabetes Care. 2013;36(2):188–94.
15. Kulnik R, Plank J, Pachler C, Wilinska ME, Groselj-Strele A, Rothlein D, et al. Evaluation of implementation of a fully automated algorithm (enhanced model predictive control) in an interacting infusion pump system for establishment of tight glycemic control in medical intensive care unit patients. J Diabetes Sci Technol. 2008;2(6):963–70.
16. Boyd JC, Bruns DE. Effects of measurement frequency on analytical quality required for glucose measurements in intensive care units: assessments by simulation models. Clin Chem. 2014;60(4):644–50.
17. Wilinska ME, Hovorka R. Glucose control in the intensive care unit by use of continuous glucose monitoring: what level of measurement error is acceptable? Clin Chem. 2014;60(12):1500–9.
18. Blaha J, Kopecky P, Matias M, Hovorka R, Kunstyr J, Kotulak T, et al. Comparison of three protocols for tight glycemic control in cardiac surgery patients. Diabetes Care. 2009;32(5):757–61.
19. Dumont C, Bourguignon C. Effect of a computerized insulin dose calculator on the process of glycemic control. Am J Crit Care. 2012;21(2):106–15.
20. Knaus WA, Draper EA, Wagner DP, Zimmerman JE. APACHE II: a severity of disease classification system. Crit Care Med. 1985;13(10):818–29.
21. Vincent JL, Moreno R, Takala J, Willatts S, De Mendonca A, Bruining H, et al. The SOFA (Sepsis-related Organ Failure Assessment) score to describe organ dysfunction/failure. On behalf of the Working Group on Sepsis-Related Problems of the European Society of Intensive Care Medicine. Intensive Care Med. 1996;22(7):707–10.
22. Rodbard D. The challenges of measuring glycemic variability. J Diabetes Sci Technol. 2012;6(3):712–5.
23. Service FJ, Molnar GD, Rosevear JW, Ackerman E, Gatewood LC, Taylor WF. Mean amplitude of glycemic excursions, a measure of diabetic instability. Diabetes. 1970;19(9):644–55.
24. McDonnell CM, Donath SM, Vidmar SI, Werther GA, Cameron FJ. A novel approach to continuous glucose analysis utilizing glycemic variation. Diabetes Technol Ther. 2005;7(2):253–63.
25. Molnar GD, Taylor WF, Ho MM. Day-to-day variation of continuously monitored glycaemia: a further measure of diabetic instability. Diabetologia. 1972;8(5):342–8.
26. Kovatchev BP, Cox DJ, Gonder-Frederick LA, Young-Hyman D, Schlundt D, Clarke W. Assessment of risk for severe hypoglycemia among adults with IDDM: validation of the low blood glucose index. Diabetes Care. 1998;21(11):1870–5.
27. Finfer S, Wernerman J, Preiser JC, Cass T, Desaive T, Hovorka R, et al. Clinical review: consensus recommendations on measurement of blood glucose and reporting glycemic control in critically ill adults. Crit Care. 2013;17(3):229.

28. Boutin JM, Gauthier L. Insulin infusion therapy in critically ill patients. Can J Diabetes. 2014;38(2):144–50.
29. Barletta JF, McAllen KJ, Eriksson EA, Deines G, Blau SA, Thayer SC, et al. The effect of a computer-assisted insulin protocol on glycemic control in a surgical intensive care unit. Diabetes Technol Ther. 2011;13(4):495–500.
30. Dortch MJ, Mowery NT, Ozdas A, Dossett L, Cao H, Collier B, et al. A computerized insulin infusion titration protocol improves glucose control with less hypoglycemia compared to a manual titration protocol in a trauma intensive care unit. JPEN J Parenter Enteral Nutr. 2008;32(1):18–27.
31. Finney SJ, Zekveld C, Elia A, Evans TW. Glucose control and mortality in critically ill patients. JAMA. 2003;290(15):2041–7.
32. Hovorka R, Kremen J, Blaha J, Matias M, Anderlova K, Bosanska L, et al. Blood glucose control by a model predictive control algorithm with variable sampling rate versus a routine glucose management protocol in cardiac surgery patients: a randomized controlled trial. J Clin Endocrinol Metab. 2007;92(8):2960–4.
33. Krinsley JS, Preiser JC. Time in blood glucose range 70 to 140 mg/dl >80% is strongly associated with increased survival in non-diabetic critically ill adults. Crit Care. 2015;19:179.
34. Marvin MR, Inzucchi SE, Besterman BJ. Computerization of the Yale insulin infusion protocol and potential insights into causes of hypoglycemia with intravenous insulin. Diabetes Technol Ther. 2013;15(3):246–52.
35. Plank J, Blaha J, Cordingley J, Wilinska ME, Chassin LJ, Morgan C, et al. Multicentric, randomized, controlled trial to evaluate blood glucose control by the model predictive control algorithm versus routine glucose management protocols in intensive care unit patients. Diabetes Care. 2006;29(2):271–6.
36. Saager L, Collins GL, Burnside B, Tymkew H, Zhang L, Jacobsohn E, et al. A randomized study in diabetic patients undergoing cardiac surgery comparing computer-guided glucose management with a standard sliding scale protocol. J Cardiothorac Vasc Anesth. 2008;22(3):377–82.
37. Shetty S, Inzucchi SE, Goldberg PA, Cooper D, Siegel MD, Honiden S. Adapting to the new consensus guidelines for managing hyperglycemia during critical illness: the updated Yale insulin infusion protocol. Endocr Pract. 2012;18(3):363–70.
38. Vogelzang M, Zijlstra F, Nijsten MW. Design and implementation of GRIP: a computerized glucose control system at a surgical intensive care unit. BMC Med Inform Decis Mak. 2005;5:38.
39. Steil GM, Deiss D, Shih J, Buckingham B, Weinzimer S, Agus MS. Intensive care unit insulin delivery algorithms: why so many? How to choose? J Diabetes Sci Technol. 2009;3(1):125–40.
40. Wilson M, Weinreb J, Hoo GW. Intensive insulin therapy in critical care: a review of 12 protocols. Diabetes Care. 2007;30(4):1005–11.

4

Patients with ANCA-associated vasculitis admitted to the intensive care unit with acute vasculitis manifestations: a retrospective and comparative multicentric study

Julien Demiselle[1,2], Johann Auchabie[1], François Beloncle[1], Philippe Gatault[3], Steven Grangé[4], Damien Du Cheyron[5], Jean Dellamonica[6], Sonia Boyer[6], Dimitri Titeca Beauport[7], Lise Piquilloud[1,8], Julien Letheulle[9], Christophe Guitton[10,11], Nicolas Chudeau[12], Guillaume Geri[13], François Fourrier[14], René Robert[15], Emmanuel Guérot[16], Julie Boisramé-Helms[17,18], Pierre Galichon[19], Pierre-François Dequin[20], Alexandre Lautrette[21], Pierre-Edouard Bollaert[22], Ferhat Meziani[17,18], Loïc Guillevin[23], Nicolas Lerolle[1*] and Jean-François Augusto[2]

Abstract

Purpose: Data for ANCA-associated vasculitis (AAV) patients requiring intensive care are scarce.

Methods: We included 97 consecutive patients with acute AAV manifestations (new onset or relapsing disease), admitted to 18 intensive care units (ICUs) over a 10-year period (2002–2012). A group of 95 consecutive AAV patients with new onset or relapsing disease, admitted to two nephrology departments with acute vasculitis manifestations, constituted the control group.

Results: In the ICU group, patients predominantly showed granulomatosis with polyangiitis and proteinase-3 ANCAs. Compared with the non-ICU group, the ICU group showed comparable Birmingham vasculitis activity score and a higher frequency of heart, central nervous system and lungs involvements. Respiratory assistance, renal replacement therapy and vasopressors were required in 68.0, 56.7 and 26.8% of ICU patients, respectively. All but one patient (99%) received glucocorticoids, 85.6% received cyclophosphamide, and 49.5% had plasma exchanges as remission induction regimens. Fifteen (15.5%) patients died during the ICU stay. The following were significantly associated with ICU mortality in the univariate analysis: the need for respiratory assistance, the use of vasopressors, the occurrence of at least one infection event in ICU, cyclophosphamide treatment, sequential organ failure assessment at admission and simplified acute physiology score II. After adjustment on sequential organ failure assessment or infection, cyclophosphamide was no longer a risk factor for mortality. Despite a higher initial mortality rate of ICU patients within the first hospital stay ($p < 0.0001$), the long-term mortality of hospital survivors did not differ between ICU and non-ICU groups (18.6 and 20.4%, respectively, $p = 0.36$). Moreover, we observed no renal survival difference between groups after a 1-year follow-up (82.1 and 80.5%, $p = 0.94$).

Conclusion: This study supports the idea that experiencing an ICU challenge does not impact the long-term prognosis of AAV patients.

Keywords: Anti-neutrophil cytoplasmic antibody, ANCA-associated vasculitis, Intensive care unit, Mortality

*Correspondence: nicolas.lerolle@univ-angers.fr
[1] Département de Réanimation Médicale et de Médecine Hyperbare, Centre Hospitalier Universitaire, 4 rue Larrey, 49933 Angers Cedex 9, France
Full list of author information is available at the end of the article

Background

Anti-neutrophil cytoplasmic antibodies (ANCAs)-associated vasculitis (AAV) are life-threatening multisystem autoimmune diseases characterized by necrotizing inflammation of small- to medium-sized vessels [1, 2]. There are three differentiated entities based on clinical and pathological criteria: microscopic polyangiitis (MPA), granulomatosis with polyangiitis (GPA) and eosinophilic granulomatosis with polyangiitis (EGPA) [3]. Their clinical spectrum partially overlaps. Indeed, rapidly progressive glomerulonephritis is the typical renal presentation of MPA and GPA, but is rarely present in EGPA [1]. Diffuse alveolar hemorrhage (DAH) is the most critical lung injury observed with all entities, but more frequently with MPA and GPA [4, 5]. Other respiratory presentations include pulmonary infiltrates and nodules, the latter being observed predominantly in GPA [6]. Even though ANCA negativity does not exclude AAV diagnosis, diffuse forms of AAV are usually associated with serum positivity for ANCAs [1, 7]. Given their high level of specificity, ANCA detection is critical for AAV diagnosis, and ANCA positivity with a compatible clinical diagnosis usually allows the initiation of immunosuppressive treatments [8, 9].

The prompt initiation of immunosuppressive drugs to induce remission is critical for AAV patient prognosis. In generalized and severe forms, conventional induction treatment combines high doses of glucocorticoids and cyclophosphamide [10]. In addition, plasma exchange (PE) may be used in severe forms with DAH and/or severe renal involvement [11, 12]. Based on recent clinical trials, rituximab, the anti-CD20 monoclonal antibody, can be used as an alternative to cyclophosphamide. Under these regimens, AAV remission is achieved in 60–80% of the patients [13–17]. However, despite being adequately treated, some patients experience resistance to therapy or disease relapse. Moreover, a high mortality rate is observed in AAV patients, with rates reaching 10–15% within the first year following treatment initiation, the main causes of early death being infection events and vasculitis manifestations [18, 19]. Mortality rates of up to 20% after 5 years have been observed, and mortality has been shown to be higher with MPA than with EGPA and GPA [18].

To date, patients with the most severe forms of AAV—those requiring intensive care—have not been extensively and adequately analyzed. Indeed, most previous studies were small size studies, uncontrolled and monocentric. Moreover, they mingled AAV patients with manifestations related to vasculitis activity, and those with manifestations not related to it. Finally, data for AAV patients admitted to the intensive care unit (ICU) for AAV manifestations [20–24] are scarce and the prognosis of this specific population remains poorly determined.

We conducted this retrospective multicentric study to analyze disease presentation and outcome in AAV patients admitted to the ICU with acute vasculitis manifestations. Specifically, we intended to explore whether ICU admission was associated with adverse long-term outcomes. To this end, ICU-AAV patients were compared with a group of AAV patients admitted to two nephrology departments with an active disease but with no requirement of ICU care (non-ICU-AAV patients).

Methods

Population and inclusion criteria

We conducted a multicentric retrospective study in seventeen ICUs from French University and General Hospitals, and from Lausanne's University Hospital in Switzerland. Inclusion criteria included: over 18 years of age, ICU admission between January 2002 and December 2012, and newly diagnosed or relapsing AAV. Only patients with acute vasculitis manifestations were included in the study. To be included, AAV initial or relapse diagnosis had to be done during the ICU stay or within the thirty days immediately prior to ICU admission.

A number of non-ICU-AAV patients were used as a control group. This group included all consecutive AAV patients of two nephrology centers (Angers and Tours University Hospitals), who were diagnosed between January 2002 and December 2012. To be included in the control group, patients had to show active newly diagnosed or relapsing AAV. Patients who required further ICU admission within the month following admission to the nephrology department were excluded from the control group.

ANCA positivity by indirect immunofluorescence (cytoplasmic or perinuclear pattern) and ELISA (proteinase-3 (PR-3) or myeloperoxidase (MPO)) was required for inclusion in both groups (ICU and non-ICU groups).

The Institutional Ethics Committees of the Angers University Hospital and Lausanne Hospital approved the study protocol (N°2013/21 and N°164/14, respectively).

AAV diagnosis

Patients' medical files were analyzed, and the AAV subtype (GPA, MPA and EGPA) was determined according to the European Medicines Agency vasculitis classification algorithm [25]. For newly diagnosed patients, the date of AAV diagnosis was defined as the date of ANCA determination and the date of relapse for relapsing patients was defined as the date of hospital admission. The diagnosis of new onset AAV relied on ANCA positivity and presence of vasculitis manifestations. The diagnosis of relapsing AAV was retained when it was suspected by the physician, and when the retrospective analysis of the patient's medical history was consistent (i.e., typical clinical manifestation, increase in ANCA titer or biopsy-proven vasculitis activity).

For conflicting cases, the hospitalization report and the medical records were analyzed by 2 expert investigators (JFA and NL). If AAV activity remained doubtful, the patient was excluded from the study.

Data collection

Patients were identified from the ICU database of each hospital. All the data were collected retrospectively by a systematic screening of patients' medical records. The following data were collected: age, gender, height and weight, and significant aspects of past medical history. Organs affected by vasculitis were listed upon the presentation of newly diagnosed and relapsing patients. The ANCA type was recorded, and pathology data of biopsied organs were analyzed (when available) to confirm the diagnosis of vasculitis. Birmingham Vasculitis Activity Score (BVAS) 2003 was used to determine AAV activity [26].

ICU ANCA-associated vasculitis

For ICU-AAV patients, causes of ICU admission with simplified acute physiology score II (SAPS II) and sequential organ failure assessment (SOFA) score upon admission [27, 28] were recorded. The ratio of partial pressure of arterial oxygen over inspired-fraction of oxygen (PaO_2/FiO_2) with ventilation initiation, the serum creatinine level and the Acute Kidney Injury Network (AKIN) score [29] upon ICU admission were used to characterize the severity of respiratory and renal injuries. Supporting therapies used during the ICU stay and their duration (mechanical ventilation, renal replacement therapy, vasopressors), septic events (as documented in the ICU hospitalization report) and death were registered. Cause of death was classified by two authors (NL and JD) after patient's files review.

AAV treatment

In both groups, all specific AAV induction regimens and their timing were recorded, including steroid treatment, cyclophosphamide, rituximab and plasmapheresis treatments. The use of steroid boluses, and the dosages and the number of cyclophosphamide and rituximab boluses were analyzed, as well as the number of plasma exchanges.

Outcomes definition

For both groups, survival was analyzed until death, loss of follow-up or end of follow-up (December 2012). Survival free of end-stage renal disease of the ICU and non-ICU groups was also analyzed. Renal death was defined as the need for long-term (>3 months) renal replacement therapy.

Statistical analysis

Quantitative parameters were presented as median (interquartile range (IQR)) and qualitative parameters as absolute number and/or percentage. Categorical and continuous data were analyzed with Chi-square (or Fisher's exact test) and Mann–Whitney U tests, respectively. Results were presented as odd ratio (OR) with 95% confidence intervals (95 CIs); the Kaplan–Meyer method was used to analyze the survival rates of ICU and non-ICU groups. A log-rank test was used to compare the survival curves. All statistical tests were performed with a two-sided 0.05 level of significance applied. Statistical analysis was performed using SPSS software® 23.0 for Macintosh and Graphpad Prism®.

Results

Baseline characteristics of the ICU and non-ICU-AAV populations

Ninety-seven and ninety-five AAV patients with a median follow-up of 2.28 [IQR 0.2–4.7] and 4.18 [IQR 1.7–7.0] years were included in the ICU group and the non-ICU control group, respectively. Characteristics of the ICU and the non-ICU groups and the main AAV manifestations upon admission are detailed in Table 1. Groups were similar regarding gender and AAV subtype, but patients of the ICU group were significantly younger. Newly diagnosed AAV was significantly more common in the non-ICU group (93%) compared with the ICU group (79%). In the ICU group, 39 patients were diagnosed during the ICU stay and 58 were diagnosed before their admission to ICU. Disease activity assessed by BVAS showed no statistical difference between groups. Heart, lung and central neurological injuries were more frequent in ICU patients than in non-ICU patients. A notably high rate of alveolar hemorrhage was observed in ICU patients (64 vs. 10% in non-ICU patients), but the renal involvement rate was comparable. ANCA subtypes by immunofluorescence and ELISA were significantly different between groups. Indeed, 62% of ICU patients had PR3-ANCAs, and 68% of non-ICU patients had MPO-ANCAs.

Parameters specific to AAV-ICU group and assessment of organ support

The median ICU length of stay was 7 [IQR 4.5–17.5] days. Acute respiratory failure (alone or in combination with renal failure) was the main cause for ICU admission and accounted for 80% of ICU admissions. Approximately 70% of patients required respiratory assistance, which was initiated within 48 h following ICU admission in the large

Table 1 Baseline characteristics of the ICU and non-ICU ANCA-associated vasculitis groups

	ICU-AAV ($n = 97$)	Non-ICU-AAV ($n = 95$)	p
Baseline characteristics			
Sex (M/F)	45/52	54/41	0.147
Age (years)	62.0 (48.0–71.0)	68.0 (55.8–75.1)	0.016
Weight (kg)	71.5 (58.0–80.0)	70.0 (60.0–82.0)	0.877
Hypertension, *n* (%)	35 (36.1)	47 (49.5)	0.061
Diabetes mellitus, *n* (%)	11 (11.3)	9 (9.5)	0.672
AAV characteristics			
Diagnosis, *n* (%)			
GPA	58 (59.8)	45 (47.4)	0.084
MPA	37 (38.1)	48 (50.5)	0.084
EGPA	2 (2.1)	2 (2.1)	0.983
ANCA type			
By immunofluorescence			
cANCA, *n* (%)	61 (62.9)	33 (34.7)	<0.001
pANCA, *n* (%)	36 (37.1)	62 (65.3)	<0.001
By ELISA			
PR3-ANCA, *n* (%)	60 (61.9)	30 (31.6)	<0.001
MPO-ANCA, *n* (%)	37 (38.1)	65 (68.4)	<0.001
Disease status, *n* (%)			
Newly diagnosed AAV, *n* (%)	77 (79.4)	88 (92.6)	0.008
Relapsing AAV, *n* (%)	20 (20.6)	7 (7.4)	0.008
BVAS	23.0 (18.0–27.5)	19.5 (15.0–31.0)	0.273
Organ involvement, *n* (%) when specified			
Cutaneous signs	25 (25.8)	19 (20.0)	0.341
Ear, nose, throat	36 (37.1)	34 (35.8)	0.849
Heart	17 (17.5)	3 (3.2)	0.001
Digestive	9 (9.3)	3 (3.2)	0.134
Lung	85 (87.6)	30 (31.6)	<0.001
Alveolar hemorrhage	62 (63.9)	9 (9.5)	<0.001
Others	23 (23.7)	21 (22.1)	0.791
Renal	83 (85.6)	87 (91.6)	0.191
Serum creatinine	256.5 (115.3–527.8)	244.0 (132.0–377.5)	0.666
Renal replacement therapy	55 (56.7)	19 (20.0)	<0.001
Neurological	25 (25.8)	12 (12.6)	0.020
Central	8 (8.2)	0 (0)	0.007
Peripheral	17 (17.5)	12 (12.6)	0.343

majority of the patients. Acute kidney injury was highly prevalent, with AKIN score ≥1 in more than 90% of patients at the time of admission, and more than half of the patients required renal replacement therapy (RRT) during their ICU stay. RRT was initiated within 48 h after admission in 35% of patients. Vasopressors were required for 25% of the patients. Infection events were reported in 40% of the patients during the ICU stay, with an identified pathogen in 82% of them. These data are summarized in Table 2.

Site and nature of infectious events are detailed in Additional file 1: Table 1.

Immunosuppressive regimens

Ninety-nine percent of patients of the ICU and 98% of non-ICU groups received glucocorticoids for remission induction. Steroid pulses were given to 95 of the 97 (98%) patients in the ICU group, and to 80 of the 95 (84%) patients in the non-ICU group ($p < 0.001$). Glucocorticoids were combined with cyclophosphamide in 83 (85.6%) ICU patients and in 78 (82.1%) non-ICU patients ($p = 0.514$). PE was more frequently used in the ICU group than in the non-ICU group ($n = 48$, 54% vs. $n = 23$, 24%, respectively, $p < 0.001$).

Table 2 Characteristics and supportive therapies used with ICU-AAV patients

Length of stay (days)	7.0 (4.5–17.5)
Reasons for ICU admission, *n* (%)	
Respiratory failure	44 (45.4)
And renal failure	23 (23.7)
And neurological failure	1 (1.0)
Acute renal failure	17 (17.5)
And neurological failure	4 (4.1)
Neurological failure	4 (4.1)
Heart failure	3 (3.1)
Hemorrhagic shock	1 (1.0)
SOFA (at admission)	6 (4.0–9.0)
SAPS II	39.0 (31.0–51.0)
Respiratory assistance, *n* (%)	
Mechanical ventilation	
Invasive or/and noninvasive	66 (68.0)
Within 48 h of admission	58 (59.8)
Noninvasive ventilation only	19 (19.6)
Invasive ventilation only	36 (37.1)
Noninvasive and invasive ventilation	11 (11.3)
Length of respiratory assistance (days)	10.0 (5.5–18.5)
PaO_2/FiO_2	92.0 (58.8–182.0)
Kidney involvement	
Serum creatinine at admission, (μmol/L)	256.5 (115.3–527.8)
Maximum serum creatinine in ICU, (μmol/L)	348.0 (160.0–673.0)
AKIN score ≥1, *n* (%)	89 (91.8)
Renal replacement therapy, *n* (%)	55 (56.7)
Within 48 h of admission	34 (35.1)
Hemodynamic assistance	
Vasopressive amines, *n* (%)	26 (26.8)
Within 48 h	25 (25.8)
Length of treatment (days)	6.0 (3–11.5)
Infectious events	
Early/late*	29/10
Lung infection, *n* (%)	29 (74.4)**
Other sites, *n* (%)	10 (25.6)**
Patients with pathogen identified, *n* (%)	32 (82.1)**

* Diagnosed < or >48 h after ICU admission

**Among patients that experienced infection

The most common induction immunosuppressive regimen administered to the ICU group was a combination of glucocorticoids and cyclophosphamide used in 41 patients (42.3%) and a combination of glucocorticoids, cyclophosphamide and PE used in 42 patients (43.3%). In the non-ICU group, glucocorticoids and cyclophosphamide were the most frequent induction regimen (58.9% of patients). Data detailing immunosuppressive regimen used in ICU and non-ICU-AAV patients, and their timing according to ICU admission, are outlined in Additional file 2: Table 2.

Mortality and predictors of ICU mortality

Fifteen patients (15.5%) died during the ICU stay. SAPS II and ICU SOFA scores were significantly higher in non-survivors compared to survivors. The need for mechanical ventilation (invasive or not) and vasopressors was more frequent in the non-survivor group. The requirement of RRT tended to be higher in the non-survivor group, but remained statistically not significant. Moreover, infectious events during ICU stays were significantly more prevalent in non-survivors. Non-surviving patients received cyclophosphamide more frequently than surviving patients. We did not observe any difference between survivors and non-survivors according to the timing of immunosuppressive treatment, including cyclophosphamide, with respect to ICU admission (data not shown). These data are summarized in Table 3. In a multivariate logistic analysis, cyclophosphamide was no longer associated with mortality after adjustment on SAPS II or occurrence of infection events (Additional file 3: Table 3).

The cause of ICU death was attributed to refractory vasculitis manifestations in 6 (40%) patients (DAH in 5 patients, digestive involvement in 1), to multiple organ failure likely due to sepsis in 5 (33%) patients and to neurologic causes in 4 (27%) patients, including 3 cerebral hemorrhage while receiving anticoagulation for extracorporeal membrane oxygenation.

Long-term outcomes of ICU-AAV patients

Whether ICU stay can impact the prognosis of AAV patients had not been yet analyzed. Regarding hospital mortality, we observed that ICU-AAV patients had a poorer survival rate compared to non-ICU-AAV patients (Fig. 1a). Given that most deaths in the ICU group occurred soon after ICU admission, we next analyzed the long-term mortality of patients that survived to the first hospital stay (ICU or non-ICU patients). By this way, we were able to observe that the long-term mortality of AAV patients who survived to the first hospital stay was no longer different between the ICU and the non-ICU group (Fig. 1b). We also analyzed the renal outcome of groups. Long-term renal outcome was available for 67 ICU-AAV patients out of 82 and for all non-ICU-AAV patients. Survival analysis showed that renal survival was not significantly different between ICU and non-ICU patients after 1 year of follow-up (Fig. 1c).

Discussion

In the present work, we described 97 patients who required ICU admission at AAV diagnosis or relapse. Lung involvement (notably, DAH) was the prominent cause for ICU admission, 70% of the patients requiring mechanical ventilation. Fifty percent needed RRT and 25% needed vasopressors. Comparison with a

Table 3 Comparison between survivor and non-survivor ICU-AAV patients and univariate logistic regression analysis for ICU mortality

	Survivors ($n = 82$)	Non-survivors ($n = 15$)	p value	Univariate logistic regression		
				OR	95% CI	p
Baseline characteristics						
Gender (female), n (%)	41 (50)	4 (26.7)	0.158	0.36	0.11–1.24	0.105
Age (years), median [IQR]	61.0 [47.0–70.3]	67.0 [65.0–75.0]	0.212	0.98	0.94–1.02	0.311
Hypertension, n (%)	32 (39.0)	3 (20.0)	0.158	0.39	0.10–1.49	0.169
ANCA						
c-ANCA type, n (%)	54 (65.9)	7 (46.7)	0.157	0.45	0.15–1.38	0.164
AAV relapse, n (%)	19 (23.2)	1 (6.7)	0.185	0.24	0.03–1.92	0.177
AAV involvement						
Heart, n (%)	14 (17.1)	3 (20.0)	0.723	1.21	0.30–4.87	0.784
CNS, n (%)	5 (6.1)	3 (20.0)	0.104	3.85	0.81–18.2	0.089
Digestive, n (%)	7 (8.5)	2 (13.3)	0.626	1.64	0.31–8.83	0.559
ENT, n (%)	33 (40.2)	3 (21.4)	0.159	0.37	0.10–1.41	0.147
Kidney						
Serum creatinine (μmol/L), median [IQR]	364.0 [117.5–503.0]	229.0 [104.0–682.0]	0.824	1.00	0.99–1.00	0.878
AKIN > 1, n (%)	74 (90.2)	15 (100)	0.351	1.51	0.17–13.1	0.706
RRT, n (%)	43 (52.4)	12 (80.0)	0.086	3.53	0.93–13.5	0.064
Lung, n (%)	71 (86.6)	14 (93.3)	0.685	2.17	0.26–18.2	0.475
DAH, n (%)	51 (62.2)	11 (73.3)	0.562	1.67	0.49–5.71	0.412
Respiratory assistance, n (%)	52 (63.4)	14 (93.3)	0.032	8.51	1.07–67.9	0.043
Infectious event, n (%)	26 (31.7)	13 (86.7)	<0.001	14.0	2.94–66.6	0.001
Vasopressors, n (%)	17 (20.7)	9 (60.0)	0.002	5.73	1.79–18.4	0.003
Plasma exchange*, n (%)	39 (47.6)	7 (46.7)	0.949	0.96	0.32–2.91	0.949
Cyclophosphamide*, n (%)	52 (63.4)	14 (93.3)	0.032	8.51	1.07–67.9	0.043
SAPS II, median [IQR]	37.5 [28.8–49.3]	52.0 [33.0–66.0]	0.006	1.06	1.02–1.10	0.003
SOFA, median [IQR]	6.0 [4.0–9.0]	8.0 [6.0–13.0]	0.040	1.21	1.04–1.41	0.013
BVAS, median [IQR]	23.0 [18.0–28.0]	21.0 [20.0–27.0]	0.916	1.01	0.94–1.08	0.899

OR odd ratio, *CI* confidence interval, *ANCA* anti-neutrophil cytoplasmic antibodies, *c-ANCA* cytoplasmic ANCA, *AAV* ANCA-associated vasculitis, *CNS* central nervous system, *ENT* ear nose throat, *AKIN* acute kidney injury network score, *RRT* renal replacement therapy, *DAH* diffuse alveolar hemorrhage

* Started before or during the ICU stay

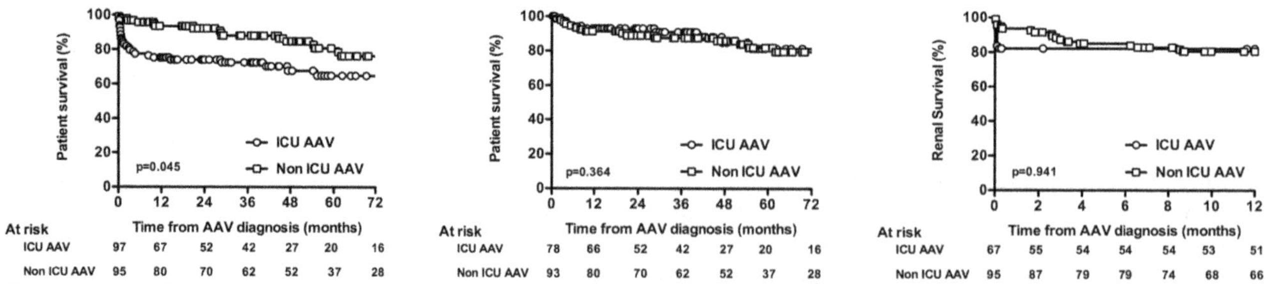

Fig. 1 **a** Survival of ICU and non-ICU-AAV patients and **b** survival of patients who survived to the first hospital stay. **c** Renal survival of ICU and non-ICU patients. Survivals were compared using the log-rank test

control group of AAV patients admitted to the nephrology department showed no difference in overall score of disease activity (BVAS), but ICU patients were younger and more likely to have PR3-ANCAs and GPA. A vast majority of ICU patients and non-ICU patients received an induction regimen with corticosteroid and cyclophosphamide, and ICU patients received PE more frequently. One-year mortality rate was higher in ICU patients due to high in-ICU fatality (15.5%) but, interestingly, in ICU survivors, 1-year survival after initial hospital admission was no different from non-ICU patients.

Several studies have already reported AAV patients admitted to ICU. Most included AAV patients admitted to ICU for reasons related to vasculitis manifestations and reasons unrelated to the same—such as our results cannot be readily compared. However, some of our results are in line with these reports, showing a majority of GPA among ICU-AAVs [20, 21, 30], and a high prevalence of DAH [20, 21, 24]. Previous studies have reported very variable rates of respiratory assistance (31–57%) [20, 23, 24, 31] and of RRT use (20–80%) [20, 23, 24], and variable mortality rates from 0 to 33% probably related to the heterogeneity of included patients [20, 23].

However, this study is the first to report on any long-term outcome of AAV patients with active disease after an ICU stay or to assess the impact of ICU stay in comparison with AAV patients initially admitted to non-ICU wards. Indeed, besides observing that ICU admission for acute organ dysfunction requiring organ support is associated with poor outcome, we thought that the main question was to determine the association between initial disease severity, invasive therapeutic procedures, and long-term outcome. Given that kidney involvement is a major prognostic factor in AAV [11], we estimated that AAV patients with kidney involvement constituted a pertinent control group. Unsurprisingly, a high death rate was observed with ICU patients at the early phase of the disease, but the observation that long-term outcome (both mortality and renal survival) in ICU survivors is no different from non-ICU patients is a key observation and deserves discussion. First, it can be noted that ICU patients were younger and more frequently had GPA compared with MPA, two factors related to better outcome in previous studies outside the ICU [32, 33]. The fact that GPA onset is usually earlier than MPA onset may explain the lower age and the greater frequency of patients with relapsing in the ICU group [33]. Due to the low death rate after the initial stay, no multivariate analysis to determine the association between ICU admission or not, AAV type and age with outcome was attempted. Beyond these limitations, our observation tends to show that initial disease severity, once adequately controlled by the induction regimen, is not associated with adverse long-term outcome and does not indicate a more severe disease. From an ICU point of view, it should be noted that this observation is at stake with several reports showing prolonged excess risk of death in ICU survivors in comparison with non-ICU patients [34]. Although the number of patients in our study limits the interpretation of this result, it favors the hypothesis that prolonged mortality in ICU patients is related to baseline conditions (here: the AAV disease) rather than to acute episodes [35].

Notwithstanding the relatively good prognosis with ICU survivors, ICU mortality is a concern that should be addressed. Intensity of acute organ dysfunction assessed through acute severity scores (SOFA, SAPS II and hence organ support requirement), cyclophosphamide and infection were associated with ICU death. In contrast, BVAS did not appear suitable for predicting short-term mortality of ICU-AAV patients [20]. Despite limitation of statistical analysis, cyclophosphamide did not appear as a risk factor for mortality after adjustment on SAPS II and infection occurrence. Although association between organ dysfunction and mortality is trivial in the ICU setting, the association between cyclophosphamide, infection and mortality is certainly not straightforward. Indeed, most infections were nosocomial infections in patients receiving mechanical ventilation, and the attributable mortality of such infections has been debated [36, 37]. Rather, it may represent an indicator of overall severity associated with an immunosuppressive state related to the condition which led to ICU admission (DAH and AAV), consequences of ICU care (tracheal intubation), and immunosuppressive treatments. Analysis of cause of death brings up additional relevant information, as infection causes and disease activity both represent the two major conditions associated with death. Finally, from our dataset, no straightforward message can be established for the purpose of determining whether ICU patients with AAV require a higher or lower level of immunosuppression, if this concept has any meaning.

Improved ICU outcome may come from more refined and individualized induction regimen. It has been proven that PE has benefited AAV patients with severe renal involvement (i.e., creatinine >500 μmol/L) when used in replacement of methylprednisolone boluses in AAV induction treatment, allowing the achievement of higher rates of renal recovery [11]. Moreover, evidence from clinical practice and retrospective studies also supports PE effectiveness in patients with DAH-related AAV [5, 12, 38]. However, our study does not show a clear-cut impact of PE on survival, this observation being clearly limited by the design of this study and the dataset. It should be noted that rituximab, which appeared as a novel option in both induction and maintenance regimens [14, 15] of AAV [39], was rarely used in our study. This may be explained by the date range of the study which ended in 2012, whereby rituximab was not able to pass into clinical practice. Given the limited data related to the use of rituximab in patients with severe forms of AAV including patient with DHA, The French Vasculitis Study Group recommended to use cyclophosphamide as a first-line treatment to induce remission [40]. However, recently, Cartin-Ceba et al. [41] suggested in a retrospective analysis that rituximab may be superior to cyclophosphamide to achieve remission at 6 months in AAV patients with DHA. We observed a high rate of infectious events, a majority of deaths related to DAH or sepsis in our study and an increased rate of cyclophosphamide use in non-survivors. Whether using rituximab in replacement of cyclophosphamide in this specific population may improve prognosis merits to be considered.

Our study undeniably has several limitations, starting with its retrospective design and restriction to AAV patients with ANCA positivity. Despite all efforts to be as exhaustive as possible, some data may have been missed. Given the very low prevalence of ICU admission for active AAV, a prospective study does not seem easily conceivable. We believe that the multicentric and controlled design of our study has contributed to limitation of center-dependent bias and to significant expansion of ICU-AAV-related knowledge, especially with regard to long-term prognosis of these patients.

Conclusion

Acute respiratory failure due to DAH is the most common vasculitis manifestation which puts AAV patients in the ICU. Despite a high early ICU mortality rate, patients who survive to ICU show comparable long-term mortality and renal prognosis compared to non-ICU-AAV patients.

Abbreviations

AAV: anti-neutrophil cytoplasmic antibodies-associated vasculitis; ANCA: anti-neutrophil cytoplasmic antibodies; AKIN: acute kidney injury network score; BVAS: Birmingham vasculitis activity score; DAH: diffuse alveolar hemorrhage; EGPA: eosinophilic granulomatosis with polyangiitis; ELISA: enzyme-linked immunosorbent assay; GPA: granulomatosis with polyangiitis; ICU: intensive care unit; MPA: microscopic polyangiitis; MPO: myeloperoxidase; PaO_2/FiO_2: ratio of partial pressure of arterial oxygen over inspired-fraction of oxygen; PE: plasma exchange; PR-3: proteinase-3; RRT: renal replacement therapy; SAPS II: simplified acute physiology score II; SOFA: sequential organ failure assessment.

Authors' contributions

JD and JA participated in conducting the study, collecting the data for the study and writing the manuscript. FB participated in the formulation of the study and conducting it, and collecting the data and revision of the manuscript. PG, SG, DDC, JD, SB, DT, LP, JL, CG, NC, GG, FF, RR, JLD, JBH, PG, PFD, AL, PEB and FM participated in collecting the data for the study and revision of the manuscript. LG participated in the formulation of the study and collecting data for it, and revision of the manuscript. NL and JFA participated in the formulation of the study and conducting it, and collecting the data for it, and in the writing of the manuscript. All authors read and approved the final manuscript.

Author details

[1] Département de Réanimation Médicale et de Médecine Hyperbare, Centre Hospitalier Universitaire, 4 rue Larrey, 49933 Angers Cedex 9, France. [2] Néphrologie-Dialyse-Transplantation, CHU Angers, 4 rue Larrey, 49933 Angers Cedex 9, France. [3] Service de Néphrologie et Immunologie Clinique, CHRU Tours, Tours, France. [4] Medical Intensive Care Unit, Rouen University Hospital, Rouen, France. [5] Service de Réanimation Médicale, CHU de Caen, Avenue de la Côte de Nacre, CS 30001, 14033 Caen Cedex 9, France. [6] Medical Intensive Care Unit, Archet 1 University Hospital, Route de St Antoine, CS 23079, 06202 Nice, France. [7] Medical Intensive Care Unit, Amiens University Medical Center, 80054 Amiens, Cedex 1, France. [8] Service de Médecine Intensive Adulte et Centre des Brûlés, Centre Hospitalier Universitaire Vaudois, Lausanne, Switzerland. [9] Service de Réanimation Médicale, Hôpital Pontchaillou, CHU Rennes, 2 rue Henri Le Guilloux, 35033 Rennes Cedex, France. [10] Medical Intensive Care Unit, Hôtel-Dieu, University Hospital of Nantes, 30 bd Jean Monnet, 44093 Nantes, France. [11] UMR 1064, Inserm, 30 bd Jean Monnet, 44093 Nantes, France. [12] Service de Reanimation Medico-Chirurgicale, Centre Hospitalier du Mans, 194 Avenue Rubillard, 72037 Le Mans, France. [13] Service de Réanimation Médicale, Hôpital Cochin, Paris, France. [14] Réanimation, Centre de Réanimation Polyvalente, Hôpital Roger Salengro, CHRU de Lille, Lille, France. [15] Service de Réanimation Médicale, CHU de Poitiers, Poitiers, France. [16] Service de Réanimation Médicale, Hôpital Européen Georges Pompidou, Paris, France. [17] Service de Réanimation Médicale, Nouvel Hôpital Civil, Hôpitaux Universitaires de Strasbourg, Strasbourg, France. [18] EA 7293, Fédération de Médecine Translationnelle de Strasbourg (FMTS), Faculté de Médecine, Université de Strasbourg, Strasbourg, France. [19] APHP, Hôpital Tenon, Urgences Néphrologiques et Transplantation Rénale, Paris, France. [20] Service de Réanimation Polyvalente, Hôpital Bretonneau, Tours, France. [21] Service de Réanimation Médicale Polyvalente, CHU Gabriel Montpied, 58 rue Montalembert, 63000 Clermont-Ferrand, France. [22] Service de Réanimation Médicale, CHU de Nancy Hôpital Central, 29 Avenue de Lattre de Tassigny, 54035 Nancy Cedex, France. [23] Département de Médecine Interne, Assistance Public des Hôpitaux de Paris, Hôpital Cochin, Paris, France.

Competing interests

The authors declare that they have no competing interests.

References

1. Jennette JC, Falk RJ. Small-vessel vasculitis. N Engl J Med. 1997;337:1512–23. doi:10.1056/NEJM199711203372106.
2. Jennette JC, Falk RJ, Hu P, Xiao H. Pathogenesis of antineutrophil cytoplasmic autoantibody-associated small-vessel vasculitis. Annu Rev Pathol. 2013;8:139–60. doi:10.1146/annurev-pathol-011811-132453.
3. Jennette JC, Falk RJ, Bacon PA, et al. 2012 revised International Chapel Hill consensus conference nomenclature of vasculitides. Arthritis Rheum. 2013;65:1–11. doi:10.1002/art.37715.
4. Rabe C, Appenrodt B, Hoff C, et al. Severe respiratory failure due to diffuse alveolar hemorrhage: clinical characteristics and outcome of intensive care. J Crit Care. 2010;25:230–5. doi:10.1016/j.jcrc.2009.04.009.
5. West S, Arulkumaran N, Ind PW, Pusey CD. Diffuse alveolar haemorrhage in ANCA-associated vasculitis. Intern Med Tokyo Jpn. 2013;52:5–13.
6. Thickett DR, Richter AG, Nathani N, et al. Pulmonary manifestations of anti-neutrophil cytoplasmic antibody (ANCA)-positive vasculitis. Rheumatol Oxf Engl. 2006;45:261–8. doi:10.1093/rheumatology/kei217.
7. Basu N, Watts R, Bajema I, et al. EULAR points to consider in the development of classification and diagnostic criteria in systemic vasculitis. Ann Rheum Dis. 2010;69:1744–50. doi:10.1136/ard.2009.119032.
8. Lionaki S, Blyth ER, Hogan SL, et al. Classification of antineutrophil cytoplasmic autoantibody vasculitides: the role of antineutrophil cytoplasmic autoantibody specificity for myeloperoxidase or proteinase 3 in disease recognition and prognosis. Arthritis Rheum. 2012;64:3452–62. doi:10.1002/art.34562.
9. Kallenberg CGM, Heeringa P, Stegeman CA. Mechanisms of disease: pathogenesis and treatment of ANCA-associated vasculitides. Nat Clin Pract Rheumatol. 2006;2:661–70. doi:10.1038/ncprheum0355.
10. Yates M, Watts RA, Bajema IM, et al. EULAR/ERA-EDTA recommendations for the management of ANCA-associated vasculitis. Ann Rheum Dis. 2016;75:1583–94. doi:10.1136/annrheumdis-2016-209133.
11. Jayne DRW, Gaskin G, Rasmussen N, et al. Randomized trial of plasma exchange or high-dosage methylprednisolone as adjunctive therapy for severe renal vasculitis. J Am Soc Nephrol. 2007;18:2180–8. doi:10.1681/ASN.2007010090.
12. Klemmer PJ, Chalermskulrat W, Reif MS, et al. Plasmapheresis therapy for diffuse alveolar hemorrhage in patients with small-vessel vasculitis. Am J Kidney Dis Off J Natl Kidney Found. 2003;42:1149–53.

13. Specks U, Merkel PA, Seo P, et al. Efficacy of remission-induction regimens for ANCA-associated vasculitis. N Engl J Med. 2013;369:417–27. doi:10.1056/NEJMoa1213277.
14. Stone JH, Merkel PA, Spiera R, et al. Rituximab versus cyclophosphamide for ANCA-associated vasculitis. N Engl J Med. 2010;363:221–32. doi:10.1056/NEJMoa0909905.
15. Jones RB, Tervaert JWC, Hauser T, et al. Rituximab versus cyclophosphamide in ANCA-associated renal vasculitis. N Engl J Med. 2010;363:211–20. doi:10.1056/NEJMoa0909169.
16. Hogan SL, Falk RJ, Chin H, et al. Predictors of relapse and treatment resistance in antineutrophil cytoplasmic antibody-associated small-vessel vasculitis. Ann Intern Med. 2005;143:621–31.
17. Pagnoux C, Hogan SL, Chin H, et al. Predictors of treatment resistance and relapse in antineutrophil cytoplasmic antibody-associated small-vessel vasculitis: comparison of two independent cohorts. Arthritis Rheum. 2008;58:2908–18. doi:10.1002/art.23800.
18. Flossmann O, Berden A, de Groot K, et al. Long-term patient survival in ANCA-associated vasculitis. Ann Rheum Dis. 2011;70:488–94. doi:10.1136/ard.2010.137778.
19. Guillevin L, Pagnoux C, Seror R, et al. The five-factor Score revisited: assessment of prognoses of systemic necrotizing vasculitides based on the French Vasculitis Study Group (FVSG) cohort. Medicine (Baltimore). 2011;90:19–27. doi:10.1097/MD.0b013e318205a4c6.
20. Frausova D, Brejnikova M, Hruskova Z, et al. Outcome of thirty patients with ANCA-associated renal vasculitis admitted to the intensive care unit. Ren Fail. 2008;30:890–5. doi:10.1080/08860220802353892.
21. Khan SA. Outcome of patients with small-vessel vasculitis admitted to a medical ICU. Chest. 2007;131:972. doi:10.1378/chest.06-2464.
22. Cruz BA. Prognosis and outcome of 26 patients with systemic necrotizing vasculitis admitted to the intensive care unit. Rheumatology. 2003;42:1183–8. doi:10.1093/rheumatology/keg322.
23. Monti S, Montecucco C, Pieropan S, et al. Life-threatening onset of systemic vasculitis requiring intensive care unit admission: a case series. Clin Exp Rheumatol. 2015;33:S126–31.
24. Burkhardt O, Köhnlein T, Wrenger E, et al. Predicting outcome and survival in patients with Wegener's granulomatosis treated on the intensive care unit. Scand J Rheumatol. 2007;36:119–24. doi:10.1080/03009740600958611.
25. Watts R, Lane S, Hanslik T, et al. Development and validation of a consensus methodology for the classification of the ANCA-associated vasculitides and polyarteritis nodosa for epidemiological studies. Ann Rheum Dis. 2007;66:222–7. doi:10.1136/ard.2006.054593.
26. Luqmani RA, Bacon PA, Moots RJ, et al. Birmingham vasculitis activity score (BVAS) in systemic necrotizing vasculitis. QJM Mon J Assoc Physicians. 1994;87:671–8.
27. Vincent JL, Moreno R, Takala J, et al. The SOFA (Sepsis-related Organ Failure Assessment) score to describe organ dysfunction/failure. On behalf of the Working Group on Sepsis-Related Problems of the European Society of Intensive Care Medicine. Intensive Care Med. 1996;22:707–10.
28. Le Gall JR, Lemeshow S, Saulnier F. A new simplified acute physiology score (SAPS II) based on a European/North American multicenter study. JAMA. 1993;270:2957–63.
29. Mehta RL, Kellum JA, Shah SV, et al. Acute kidney injury network: report of an initiative to improve outcomes in acute kidney injury. Crit Care Lond Engl. 2007;11:R31. doi:10.1186/cc5713.
30. Kimmoun A, Baux E, Das V, et al. Outcomes of patients admitted to intensive care units for acute manifestation of small-vessel vasculitis: a multicenter, retrospective study. Crit Care. 2015. doi:10.1186/s13054-016-1189-5.
31. Dumas G, Géri G, Montlahuc C, et al. Outcomes in critically Ill patients with systemic rheumatic disease: a multicenter study. Chest J. 2015;148:927. doi:10.1378/chest.14-3098.
32. Hilhorst M, van Paassen P, Tervaert JWC, Limburg Renal Registry. Proteinase 3-ANCA vasculitis versus myeloperoxidase-ANCA vasculitis. J Am Soc Nephrol JASN. 2015;26:2314–27. doi:10.1681/ASN.2014090903.
33. Franssen C, Gans R, Kallenberg C, et al. Disease spectrum of patients with antineutrophil cytoplasmic autoantibodies of defined specificity: distinct differences between patients with anti-proteinase 3 and anti-myeloperoxidase autoantibodies. J Intern Med. 1998;244:209–16.
34. Wunsch H, Guerra C, Barnato AE, et al. Three-year outcomes for Medicare beneficiaries who survive intensive care. JAMA. 2010;303:849–56. doi:10.1001/jama.2010.216.
35. Iwashyna TJ, Netzer G, Langa KM, Cigolle C. Spurious inferences about long-term outcomes: the case of severe sepsis and geriatric conditions. Am J Respir Crit Care Med. 2012;185:835–41. doi:10.1164/rccm.201109-1660OC.
36. Mitharwal SM, Yaddanapudi S, Bhardwaj N, et al. Intensive care unit-acquired infections in a tertiary care hospital: an epidemiologic survey and influence on patient outcomes. Am J Infect Control. 2016;. doi:10.1016/j.ajic.2016.01.021.
37. Van Vught LA, Klein Klouwenberg PMC, Spitoni C, et al. Incidence, risk factors, and attributable mortality of secondary infections in the intensive care unit after admission for sepsis. JAMA. 2016;315:1469. doi:10.1001/jama.2016.2691.
38. Beck L, Bomback AS, Choi MJ, et al. KDOQI US commentary on the 2012 KDIGO clinical practice guideline for glomerulonephritis. Am J Kidney Dis Off J Natl Kidney Found. 2013;62:403–41. doi:10.1053/j.ajkd.2013.06.002.
39. Pagnoux C, Guillevin L, French Vasculitis Study Group, MAINRITSAN investigators. Rituximab or azathioprine maintenance in ANCA-associated vasculitis. N Engl J Med. 2015;372:386–7. doi:10.1056/NEJMc1414728.
40. Charles P, Bienvenu B, Bonnotte B, et al. Rituximab: recommendations of the French Vasculitis Study Group (FVSG) for induction and maintenance treatments of adult, antineutrophil cytoplasm antibody-associated necrotizing vasculitides. Presse Medicale. 1983;42:1317–30. doi:10.1016/j.lpm.2013.08.003.
41. Cartin-Ceba R, Diaz-Caballero L, Al-Qadi MO, et al. Diffuse alveolar hemorrhage secondary to antineutrophil cytoplasmic antibody-associated vasculitis: predictors of respiratory failure and clinical outcomes. Arthritis Rheumatol. 2016;68:1467–76. doi:10.1002/art.39562.

5

External validation of SAPS 3 and MPM_0-III scores in 48,816 patients from 72 Brazilian ICUs

Giulliana Martines Moralez[1], Ligia Sarmet Cunha Farah Rabello[2,3], Thiago Costa Lisboa[4], Mariza da Fonte Andrade Lima[5], Rodrigo Marques Hatum[6], Fernando Vinicius Cesar De Marco[7], Alessandra Alves[8], Jorge Eduardo da Silva Soares Pinto[9], Hélia Beatriz Nunes de Araújo[10], Grazielle Viana Ramos[11], Aline Reis Silva[11], Guilherme Côrtes Fernandes[12], Guilherme Brenande Alves Faria[13], Ciro Leite Mendes[14], Roberto Álvaro Ramos Filho[15], Valdênia Pereira de Souza[16], Pedro Emmanuel Alvarenga Americano do Brasil[11,17], Fernando Augusto Bozza[11,17], Jorge Ibrain Figueira Salluh[2,18], Marcio Soares[2,18,19]* and On Behalf of the ORCHESTRA Study Investigators

Abstract

Background: The performance of severity-of-illness scores varies in different scenarios and must be validated prior of being used in a specific settings and geographic regions. Moreover, models' calibration may deteriorate overtime and performance of such instruments should be reassessed regularly. Therefore, we aimed at to validate the SAPS 3 in a large contemporary cohort of patients admitted to Brazilian ICUs. In addition, we also compared the performance of the SAPS 3 with the MPM_0-III.

Methods: This is a retrospective cohort study in which 48,816 (medical admissions = 67.9%) adult patients are admitted to 72 Brazilian ICUs during 2013. We evaluated models' discrimination using the area under the receiver operating characteristic curve (AUROC). We applied the calibration belt to evaluate the agreement between observed and expected mortality rates (calibration).

Results: Mean SAPS 3 score was 44.3 ± 15.4 points. ICU and hospital mortality rates were 11.0 and 16.5%. We estimated predicted mortality using both standard (SE) and Central and South American (CSA) customized equations. Predicted mortality rates were 16.4 ± 19.3% (SAPS 3-SE), 21.7 ± 23.2% (SAPS 3-CSA) and 14.3 ± 14.0% (MPM_0-III). Standardized mortality ratios (SMR) obtained for each model were: 1.00 (95% CI, 0.98–0.102) for the SAPS 3-SE, 0.75 (0.74–0.77) for the SAPS 3-CSA and 1.15 (1.13–1.18) for the MPM_0-III. Discrimination was better for SAPS 3 models (AUROC = 0.85) than for MPM_0-III (AUROC = 0.80) ($p < 0.001$). We applied the calibration belt to evaluate the agreement between observed and expected mortality rates (calibration): the SAPS 3-CSA overestimated mortality throughout all risk classes while the MPM_0-III underestimated it uniformly. The SAPS 3-SE did not show relevant deviations from ideal calibration.

Conclusions: In a large contemporary database, the SAPS 3-SE was accurate in predicting outcomes, supporting its use for performance evaluation and benchmarking in Brazilian ICUs.

Keywords: Severity-of-illness scores, Validation, Intensive care units, Outcomes, Standardized mortality rate

*Correspondence: marciosoaresms@gmail.com
[19] Department of Critical Care, D'Or Institute for Research and Education, Rua Diniz Cordeiro, 30. Botafogo, Rio de Janeiro 22281-100, Brazil
Full list of author information is available at the end of the article

Background

Severity-of-illness scores have broad applicability in intensive care setting. Although they should not be used on individual basis, they are useful to evaluate ICU performance, to monitor it overtime, to guide resource management and quality improvements, and for benchmarking purposes [1]. However, the performance of these models varies in different scenarios because of differences in case mix, clinical management patterns, admission policies as well as pre- and post-ICU care. Therefore, severity-of-illness scores must be validated prior to their use in a specific setting or geographic region.

The three most used severity-of-illness scores are the Acute Physiology and Chronic Health Evaluation (APACHE) [2], the Mortality Probability Models (MPM_0-III) [3] and the Simplified Acute Physiology Score (SAPS 3) [4, 5]. Among them, the only score developed using data from patients and intensive care units (ICU) worldwide (307 ICUs in 35 countries) was the SAPS 3 score. Besides a general standard equation, investigators also developed seven regional equations to estimate hospital mortality, thus allowing comparisons among ICUs on a more common level.

In 2009, the Brazilian Association of Intensive Care (Associação de Medicina Intensiva Brasileira, AMIB) chose the SAPS 3 score as the severity-of-illness score recommended for performance evaluation and benchmarking in Brazilian ICUs [6]. However, to our knowledge, validation studies reported conflicting results and were mostly single centered, involving specific patient populations [7–13] and with relatively small sample sizes [14–16]. Moreover, as the calibration of severity-of-illness scores is expected to deteriorate overtime, the performance of such instruments should be reassessed on a regular basis [17]. Therefore, in the present study, we aimed at to validate the SAPS 3 in a large contemporary cohort of patients admitted to Brazilian ICUs. In addition, we also compared the performance of the SAPS 3 with the MPM_0-III.

Methods

Design and setting

This was a secondary analysis of the ORCHESTRA study, a multicenter retrospective cohort study of critical care organization and outcomes in 59,693 patients admitted to 78 ICUs at 51 Brazilian hospitals during 2013 [18].

Selection of participants, data collection and definitions

Participating ICUs in the ORCHESTRA study were selected from the Brazilian Research in Intensive Care Network (BRICNet). For the purposes of the present study, we excluded ICUs exclusively admitting cardiac patients ($n = 6$) (Fig. 1) and a total of 72 ICUs at 50 hospitals were involved. We included all consecutive patients aged $\geq$16 years admitted to the participating ICUs during 2013. In the ORCHESTRA study, readmissions and patients with missing core data [age, location before ICU admission, main ICU admission diagnosis, SAPS 3 score, ICU and hospital length of stay (LOS) and vital status at hospital discharge] were excluded. In the present study, besides the patients admitted to cardiac units ($n = 3951$), we also excluded those who did not meet both the SAPS 3 and MPM_0-III eligibility criteria [patients aged <18 years ($n = 358$), who underwent cardiac surgeries ($n = 2971$), with acute myocardial infarction ($n = 3568$) and burns ($n = 29$)]. Therefore, a total of 48,816 patients constituted the study population.

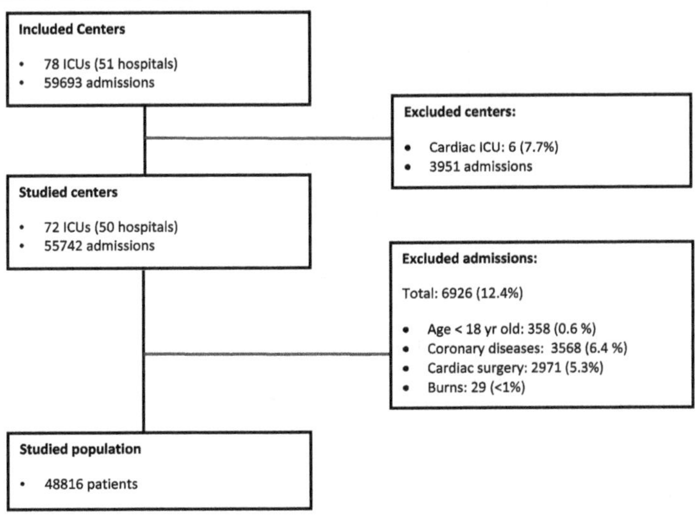

Fig. 1 Study flowchart

We obtained de-identified patient data from the Epimed Monitor System®, (Epimed Solutions®, Rio de Janeiro, Brazil), a commercial cloud-based registry for quality improvement, performance evaluation and benchmarking purposes. ICUs using the Epimed Monitor System® prospectively collect data in a structured electronic case report form, most typically using a trained case manager. Key data elements included demographics, admission diagnosis, location before ICU admission, comorbidities based on the Charlson Comorbidity Index [19], functional status one week before hospital admission [20], scores including the SAPS 3 score, MPM_0-III score and the Sequential Organ Failure Score (SOFA) [21], use of ICU support, ICU and hospital LOS and destination after hospital discharge. The SAPS 3 and MPM_0-III scores were calculated using data from the ICU admission (±1 h). As recommended, missing values were coded as the reference or "normal" category for each variable. Estimated mortality rates using both the standard equation (SAPS 3-SE) and the one customized for Central and South American countries (SAPS 3-CSA) are provided in the system. In the present study, the primary outcome of interest was in-hospital mortality at the patient level.

Statistical analysis

We described ICU and patient characteristics using standard descriptive statistics and reported continuous variables as mean ± standard deviation or median (25–75% interquartile range, IQR), as appropriate. We reported categorical variables as absolute numbers (frequency percentages).

We assessed models' discrimination (ability of each model to discriminate between patients who lived from those who died) by estimating the area under the receiver operating characteristic curve (AUROC). Comparisons between AUROCs by a pairwise evaluation of the three scores discrimination power were performed by Delong method [22]. We used the calibration belt, proposed by the GiViTI group [23, 24], to investigate the relationship between the observed and expected outcomes. Using this approach, a generalized polynomial logistic function between the outcome and the logit transformation of the predicted probability was fitted, with the respective 95 and 80% confidence intervals (CI) boundaries. A statistically significant deviation from the bisector (the line of perfect calibration) occurs when the 95% CI boundaries of the calibration belt do not include the bisector [23]. Calibration curves were constructed by plotting predicted mortality rates (x-axis) against observed mortality rates (y-axis). Standardized mortality rates (SMR) with respective 95% confidence intervals (CI) were calculated for each model by dividing observed by predicted mortality rates. A two-tailed p value <0.05 was considered statistically significant. We performed the statistical analyses using R (http://www.r-project.org) and SPSS 21 (IBM Corp., Armonk, NY).

Results

Our final sample consisted of 48,816 patients admitted by 72 ICUs in the study period (Fig. 1). Table 1 gives the main hospital and ICU characteristics. Most of ICUs were medical–surgical ($n = 62$, 86.1%) located at private hospitals ($n = 45$, 90.0%). Median number of patients per ICU was 517 (361–817).

Table 2 reports the main patients' characteristics. The main reasons for ICU admission were postoperative care (26.3%), followed by sepsis (22.3%), cardiovascular complications (11.3%) and neurological complications (11.4%). At ICU admission, invasive mechanical ventilation was used in 7550 (15.5%) and noninvasive ventilation was used in 4875 (10.0%) of patients. Vasopressors were required by 6158 (12.6%) and renal replacement therapy by 1578 (3.2%).

Table 1 Hospital and ICU characteristics

Characteristics	
Hospitals	**($n = 50$)**
Type of hospital	
Private, for profit	31 (62.0%)
Private, philanthropic	14 (28.0%)
Public	5 (10.0%)
Hospital beds (n)	
<150	19 (38.0%)
150–300	20 (40.0%)
≥301	11 (22.0%)
Intermediate/step-down unit	
No	25 (50.0%)
Yes	25 (50.0%)
Training programs in critical care	
No	28 (56.0%)
Yes	22 (44.0%)
ICUs	**($n = 72$)**
Medical–surgical ICU	
Yes	62 (86.1%)
No	10 (13.9%)
Active ICU beds (n)	22 (11–34)
≤10	23 (31.9%)
10–20	27 (37.5%)
>20	22 (30.6%)
ICU bed occupancy rate (%)	73 (62–83)

Results for continuous variables are reported as mean ± SD and median (IQR)
ICU intensive care unit, *IQR* interquartile range, *SD* standard deviation

Table 2 Main patients' characteristics and outcomes

Characteristics	
Patients (*n*)	**48,816**
Age (years)	65 (48–79)
<45	10,354 (21.2%)
45–64	13,555 (27.8%)
65–74	8661 (17.7%)
75–84	9666 (19.8%)
≥85	6580 (13.5%)
Gender	
Female	25,400 (52.0%)
Male	23,416 (48.0%)
Health insurance coverage	
Public health insurance	5779 (11.8%)
Private health insurance	36,821 (75.4%)
Admission costs paid with patient's own resources	6216 (13.7%)
Comorbidities	
Diabetes mellitus	11,037 (22.6%)
Cancer	9647 (19.8%)
Chronic renal failure	4469 (9.2%)
Coronary artery disease	2993 (6.1%)
Cardiac failure	2468 (5.1%)
Chronic pulmonary disease	2551 (5.2%)
Charlson Comorbidity Index (points)	1 (0–2)
Characteristics	***n* = 48,816**
Functional status before hospital admission	
Ambulant	36,835 (75.5%)
Minor assistance	8556 (17.5%)
Major assistance or bedridden	3425 (7.0%)
Source of ICU admission	
Emergency department	25,738 (52.7%)
Operating room	14,979 (30.7%)
Ward/floor	4212 (8.6%)
Transfer from other hospitals	1876 (3.8%)
Other	2011 (4.1%)
Hospital days prior to ICU admission (*n*)	0 (0–1)
Admission diagnostic category	
Scheduled surgery	12,825 (26.3%)
Emergency surgery	2854 (5.8%)
Cardiovascular**	5511 (11.3%)
Sepsis**	10,876 (22.3%)
Neurological**	5588 (11.4%)
Respiratory**	2542 (5.2%)
Gastrointestinal**	2263 (4.6%)
Other medical admissions**	6357 (13.0%)
SAPS 3 (points)	43 (34–53)
SOFA score on Day 1 (points)	1 (0–4)
Support on Day 1	
Mechanical ventilation	7550 (15.5%)
Noninvasive ventilation	4875 (10.0%)
Vasopressors	6158 (12.6%)
Renal replacement therapy	1578 (3.2%)
ICU LOS (days)	3 (1–5)
Hospital LOS (days)	8 (4–18)
ICU mortality	5385 (11.0%)
Hospital mortality	8031 (16.5%)
Destination at hospital discharge	
Home	37,683 (77.2%)
Other hospital	556 (1.1%)
Hospice/home care	355 (0.7%)
Other/unknown	2191 (4.5%)
Died	8031 (16.5%)

Results for continuous variables are reported as mean ± SD and median (IQR)

IQR interquartile range, *ICU* intensive care unit, *SAPS* Simplified Acute Physiology Score, *SOFA* Sequential Organ Failure Score, *LOS* length of stay, *SD* standard deviation

** These admission categories refer to medical diagnosis only

Median ICU and hospital LOS were 3 (1–5) and 8 (4–18) days, respectively. Mean SAPS 3 was 44.3 ± 15.4 points. A total of 5385 (11.0%) died in the ICUs; 2646 died in the hospital after the ICUs discharge and the hospital mortality rate was 16.5%. Table 2 reports the main patients' characteristics and outcomes.

Predicted mortality rates were 16.4 ± 19.3% (SAPS 3-SE), 21.7 ± 23.2% (SAPS 3-CSA) and 14.3 ± 14.0% (MPM_0-III). Table 3 gives the performance analyses for the studied scores. In summary, the SMR was appropriate using the SAPS 3-SE, while the SAPS 3-CSA overestimated and the MPM_0-III underestimated the hospital mortality. Overall, discrimination was good, but higher for the SAPS 3 score (Table 3). Calibration was acceptable for the SAPS 3-SE only. In the calibration belt analysis, there was only minimal over- (below the first percentile) and underprediction (between the 8th and 14th percentiles) in the first two risk deciles. Conversely, the SAPS 3-CSA uniformly overestimated mortality in all risk range and the MPM_0-III tended in general to underestimation (Figs. 2, 3).

As most of the included ICUs were located at private hospitals, we performed subgroup analyses according to the type of hospital and specific subgroups of patients (Additional file 1: eTable 1 and eFigures 1–8). In patients admitted to private hospitals, we found results comparable to the ones observed for all the studied population and the SAPS 3-SE was the only model with a good performance. However, in patients admitted to public hospitals, none of the models was accurate in predicting hospital mortality. Finally, we performed additional analyses of the SAPS 3 performance in all patients ($n = 55,742$) fulfilling only the eligibility criteria reported

Table 3 Scores performances comparison

	Mortality		Discrimination		Calibration*		Precision
	Predicted mortality (±SD)	SMR (95% CI)	AUROC	95% CI	Over the bisector 95% CI	Under the bisector 95% CI	Brier score
SAPS 3-SE	16.4 ± 19.3%	1.00 (0.98–1.02)	0.850	0.84–0.85	0.00–0.01	0.08–0.12	0.098
SAPS 3-CSA	21.7 ± 23.2%	0.75 (0.74–0.77)	0.850	0.84–0.85	Never	Always	0.103
MPMO-III	14.3 ± 14.0%	1.15 (1.13–1.18)	0.800	0.79–0.80	0.07–0.97	0.01–0.03	0.111

SAPS 3-SE Simplified Acute Physiology Score 3-Standard Equation, *SAPS 3-CSA* Simplified Acute Physiology Score 3-Customized equation for Central and South American Countries, *MPMO-III* Mortality Probability Models III, SMR Standardized mortality rates, *AUROC* area under the curve

* Calibration described as bisector deviation intervals, as proposed by GiViTI, (Italian Group for the Evaluation of Intervention in Intensive Care Medicine)

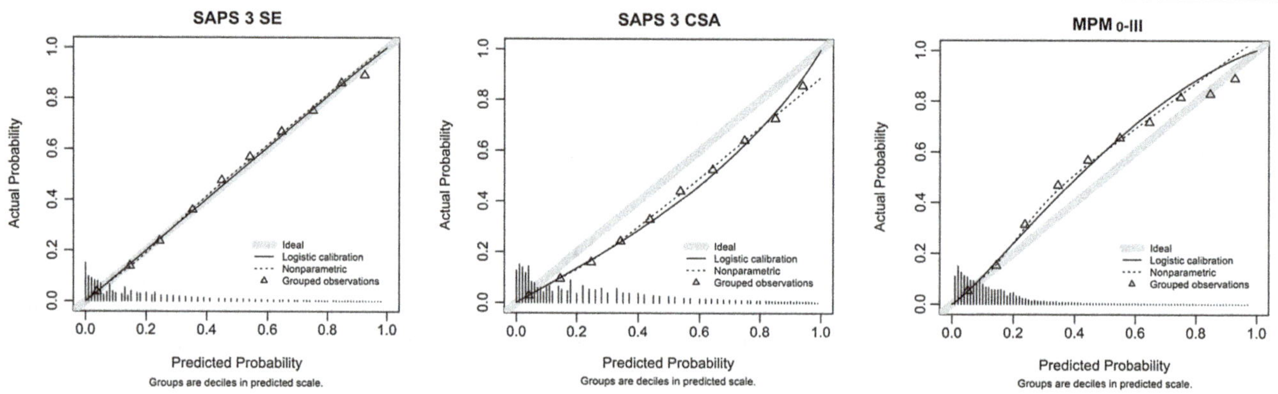

Fig. 2 Calibration plots for SAPS 3-SE, SAPS 3-CSA and MPM_0-III, with predicted mortality rates stratified by 10% intervals of mortality risk (*x*-axis) against observed mortality rates (*y*-axis)

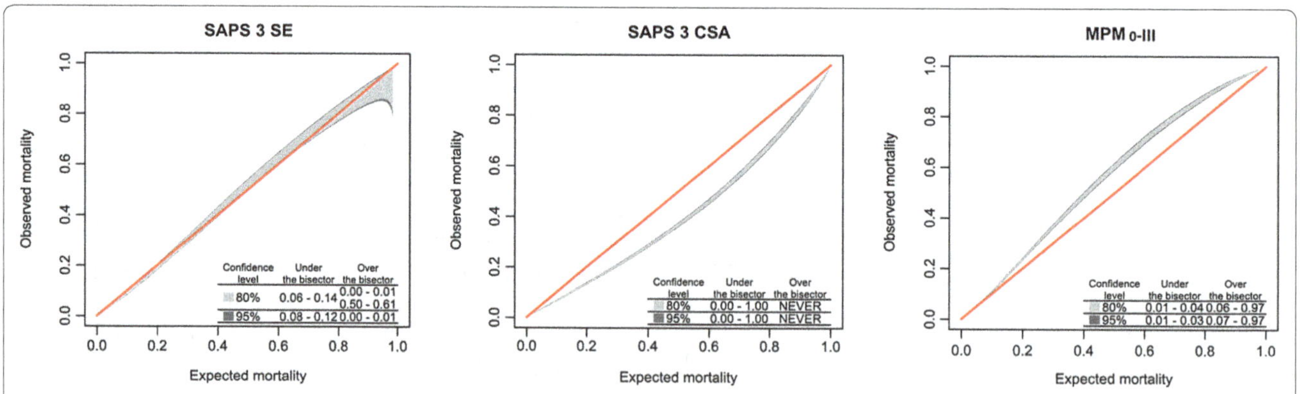

Fig. 3 Calibration Belt for SAPS 3-SE, SAPS 3-CSA and MPM_0-III, described as bisector deviation intervals, as proposed by GiViTI, (Italian Group for the Evaluation of Intervention in Intensive Care Medicine). The times the calibration belt significantly deviates from the bisector using 80 and 95% confidence levels are described in the lower right part of the *plots*

the original publication of the model [4]. Models' discrimination (AUROC = 0.855) for both the SAPS 3-SE and SAPS 3-CSA and calibration (Additional file 1: eFigure 3) were also appropriate. In Additional file 1: eTable 2, we provided information on patients' characteristics and outcomes for our cohort of patients and the one reported in the SAPS 3 study.

Discussion

In the present study, we demonstrated that the SAPS 3-SE was able to accurately predict outcomes in a large contemporary cohort of Brazilian ICU patients. Conversely, the MPM_0-III score had a relatively worse calibration and tended to significantly underestimate mortality, while the SAPS 3-CSA overestimated mortality despite a reasonable discrimination. Moreover, the SAPS 3-SE provided more precise estimations, resulting in a SMR closer to 1.0. In the calibration curves, the lines of observed mortality of the SAPS 3-SE were uniformly closer to the line of ideal prediction across all risk classes.

In the last years, mostly driven by official recommendations provided by AMIB, the SAPS 3 became the severity-of-illness score used in the vast majority of Brazilian ICUs to evaluate ICU performance as well as for benchmarking. However, validation studies of SAPS 3 were performed in specific subgroup of patients or in single-center studies involving a general ICU population [7–16]. In general, both the SAPS 3-SE and SAPS 3-CSA equations were evaluated in the studies. Overall, discrimination was usually good, but calibration results varied among the studies.

In these previous studies, the SAPS 3-SE had a poor calibration and tended usually to underestimate mortality [7–10, 12]. The SAPS 3-SE tended to overestimate mortality in only two studies (one of them comprising patients with acute coronary syndromes), both with a relatively low mortality rate [11, 16]. On the other hand, the SAPS 3-CSA accurately predicted mortality in five studies involving patients with cancer [8, 9], acute kidney injury [10, 12] and those who underwent surgical procedures [15]. Our results confirm that the MPM_0-III, however, was inaccurate in predicting mortality. These results are in line with almost all previous studies performed in Brazil [9, 10, 12, 16].

There is a known phenomenon with traditional calibration statistics (such as Hosmer–Lemeshow goodness of fit) in prediction models validation/calibration studies with many thousands included subjects, in which often p values are highly significant despite visually good calibration curves, very small absolute errors, and acceptable calibration slope and intercept. This occurs because with a large sample size the power is big enough to detect, as statistically significant, irrelevant small differences. At the other extreme, one must be cautious in the interpretation of calibration results with small cohorts, because, even when the calibration curve, the calibration intercept and slope points to a miscalibration, the p values of traditional calibration statistics may not be significant, raising concern about the study low power [25]. Therefore, in small cohorts, the lack of correspondence between expected and observed probabilities can also result in misaligned calibration curves, when sample size cannot be enough to achieve statistical significance [26]. In addition, specific subgroups of patients were included in these studies, whose results may not be fully transposed to general populations of critical care patients in different scenarios.

It is a well-known phenomenon that the performance of prognostic scores (chiefly the calibration) tends to deteriorate overtime. Zimmerman et al. [2] when reporting the development of the APACHE IV elegantly demonstrated this. Soares et al. [8] also documented the temporal compromising of calibration studying the SAPS 3 score in a cohort of patients with cancer admitted to the ICU over a 3-year period in Brazil. This is why the performance of prognostic scores should be reassessed periodically.

The cohort composition could also interfere with the score performance. Comparing our cohort and original SAPS 3 development cohort, we had comparable median age, but clinical patients predominated (67.9 vs. 43.5% in the SAPS 3 cohort), with lower median SAPS 3 scores (43 points vs. 48 points) and lower hospital mortality (16.5 vs. 23.5%) (Additional file 1: eTable 2). Despite these case mix differences, currently the SAPS 3-SE model was well fitted to our population, which might reflect changes in the provision of health care resulting in lower risk-adjusted mortality. In this sense, our results have potential implications for ICU performance evaluation and more importantly for benchmarking purposes in Brazilian ICUs. On the one hand, we provide robust evidence that although the SAPS 3 remains useful in our country, the customized equation for Latin American countries should be no longer used.

Our study has many strengths including being, to our knowledge, the largest validation study of severity-of-illness scores in Brazil and using more contemporary data from several centers countrywide. Moreover, we consider there is a negligible potential for discharge bias, [27] once our percentage of patients discharged to other hospitals and hospice care facilities was minimal.

Our study has also several limitations that should be considered in the interpretation of our results. First, although we have evaluated a large number of Brazilian ICUs, we used a convenience sample, predominantly composed by private hospitals and they may not be representative of the entire country. Second, we have not audited data collection, as we used data recorded in a registry for performance evaluation and benchmarking. Therefore, we cannot estimate the effect of missing variables in the scores estimations. However, trained healthcare professionals that work as case managers register data in all ICUs. Third, we did not assess end-of-life decisions, as they are not regularly registered in the database, and therefore, we were unable to account for this factor in the analysis.

In conclusion, using a large contemporary database, we demonstrated that the SAPS 3-SE was accurate in predicting outcomes, supporting its use for performance evaluation and benchmarking in Brazilian ICUs.

Abbreviations

AMIB: Associação de Medicina Intensiva Brasileira; APACHE: Acute Physiology and Chronic Health Evaluation; AUROC: area under receiver operating characteristic; BRICNet: Brazilian Research in Intensive Care Network; CI: confidence interval; ESM: electronic supplementary material; ICU: intensive care unit; LOS: length of stay; MPM0-III: Mortality Probability Model III; SAPS: Simplified Acute Physiology Score; SAPS 3-CSA: SAPS 3, customized equation for Central and South American Countries; SAPS 3-SE: SAPS 3, standard equation; SMR: standardized mortality rates; SOFA: sequential organ failure assessment.

Authors' contributions

GMM participated in study conception, data analysis and interpretation and drafting of the manuscript. LSCFR participated in study conception, data acquisition, data analysis and interpretation and drafting of the manuscript. TCL participated in data acquisition, data interpretation and revising manuscript for important intellectual content. MFAL, RMH, FVCM, AA, JESSP, HBNA, GVR, ARS, GCF, GBAF, CLM, RARF and VPS participated in data acquisition and revising manuscript for important intellectual content. PEAAB participated in data analysis and interpretation and drafting of the manuscript. FAB participated in data acquisition, data interpretation and revising manuscript for important intellectual content. JIFS participated in study conception, data interpretation and drafting of the manuscript. MS participated in study conception, data analysis and interpretation and drafting of the manuscript. The complete list of investigators is reported in electronic supplementary material (ESM). All authors read and approved the final manuscript.

Author details

[1] Graduate Program in Translational Medicine, D'Or Institute for Research and Education (IDOR), Rio de Janeiro, Brazil. [2] PPG Internal Medicine, Federal University of Rio de Janeiro, Rio de Janeiro, Brazil. [3] ICU, Hospital Copa D'Or, Rio de Janeiro, Brazil. [4] Complexo Hospitalar, Santa Casa de Misericórdia de Porto Alegre, Porto Alegre, Brazil. [5] ICU, Hospital Esperança Recife, Recife, Brazil. [6] ICU, Hospital Total Cor, Rio de Janeiro, Brazil. [7] ICU, Hospital viValle, São José dos Campos, Brazil. [8] ICU, Hospital Rios D'Or, Rio de Janeiro, Brazil. [9] ICU, Hospital Norte D'Or, Rio de Janeiro, Brazil. [10] Hospital do Coração do Brasil, Brasília, Brazil. [11] Department of Critical Care, D'Or Institute for Research and Education (IDOR), Rio de Janeiro, Brazil. [12] ICU, Santa Casa de Misericórdia de Juiz de Fora, Juiz de Fora, Brazil. [13] ICU, Hospital Oeste D'Or, Rio de Janeiro, Brazil. [14] ICU, Hospital Universitário Lauro Wanderley, João Pessoa, Brazil. [15] ICU, Hospital São Luiz – Unidade Jabaquara, São Paulo, Brazil. [16] Complexo Hospitalar de Niterói, Niterói, Brazil. [17] Instituto Nacional de Infectologia Evandro Chagas, Fundação Oswaldo Cruz-Fiocruz, Rio de Janeiro, Brazil. [18] Department of Critical Care and Graduate Program in Translational Medicine, D'Or Institute for Research and Education (IDOR), Rio de Janeiro, Brazil. [19] Department of Critical Care, D'Or Institute for Research and Education, Rua Diniz Cordeiro, 30. Botafogo, Rio de Janeiro 22281-100, Brazil.

Competing interests

Dr. Soares and Dr. Salluh are founders and equity shareholders of Epimed Solutions®, which commercializes the Epimed Monitor System®, a cloud-based software for ICU management and benchmarking. The other authors declare that they have no competing interests.

Funding

This study was supported in part by the National Council for Scientific and Technological Development (CNPq) (Grant No. 304240/2014-1), Carlos Chagas Filho Foundation for Research Support of the State of Rio de Janeiro (FAPERJ) and departmental funds from the D'Or Institute for Research and Education.

References

1. Salluh JIF, Soares M. ICU severity of illness scores: APACHE, SAPS and MPM. Curr Opin Crit Care. 2014;20(5):557–65.
2. Zimmerman JE, Kramer AA, McNair DS, Malila FM. Acute Physiology and Chronic Health Evaluation (APACHE) IV: hospital mortality assessment for today's critically ill patients. Crit Care Med. 2006;34(5):1297–310.
3. Higgins TL, Teres D, Copes WS, Nathanson BH, Stark M, Kramer AA. Assessing contemporary intensive care unit outcome: an updated Mortality Probability Admission Model (MPM0-III). Crit Care Med. 2007;35(3):827–35.
4. Metnitz PGH, Moreno RP, Almeida E, Jordan B, Bauer P, Campos RA, et al. SAPS 3: from evaluation of the patient to evaluation of the intensive care unit. Part 1: objectives, methods and cohort description. Intensive Care Med. 2005;31(10):1336–44.
5. Moreno RP, Metnitz PGH, Almeida E, Jordan B, Bauer P, Campos RA, et al. SAPS 3: from evaluation of the patient to evaluation of the intensive care unit. Part 2: development of a prognostic model for hospital mortality at ICU admission. Intensive Care Med. 2005;31(10):1345–55.
6. Associação Brasileira de Terapia Intensiva (AMIB). Regulamento técnico para funcionamento de unidades de Terapia Intensiva—AMIB. http://www.amib.org.br/fileadmin/RecomendacoesAMIB.pdf. 2009 [cited 2016 Jun 6].
7. de Oliveira VM, Brauner JS, Rodrigues Filho E, Susin RGA, Draghetti V, Bolzan ST, et al. Is SAPS 3 better than APACHE II at predicting mortality in critically ill transplant patients? Clin Sao Paulo Braz. 2013;68(2):153–8.
8. Soares M, Salluh JIF. Validation of the SAPS 3 admission prognostic model in patients with cancer in need of intensive care. Intensive Care Med. 2006;32(11):1839–44.
9. Soares M, Silva UVA, Teles JMM, Silva E, Caruso P, Lobo SMA, et al. Validation of four prognostic scores in patients with cancer admitted to Brazilian intensive care units: results from a prospective multicenter study. Intensive Care Med. 2010;36(7):1188–95.
10. Costa e Silva VT, de Castro I, Liano F, Muriel A, Rodriguez-Palomares JR, Yu L. Performance of the third-generation models of severity scoring systems (APACHE IV, SAPS 3 and MPM-III) in acute kidney injury critically ill patients. Nephrol Dial Transplant. 2011;26(12):3894–901.
11. Nassar Junior AP, Mocelin AO, Andrade FM, Brauer L, Giannini FP, Nunes ALB, et al. SAPS 3, APACHE IV or GRACE: which score to choose for acute coronary syndrome patients in intensive care units? Sao Paulo Med J Rev Paul Med. 2013;131(3):173–8.
12. Maccariello ER, Valente C, Nogueira L, Ismael M, Valenca RVR, Machado JES, et al. Performance of six prognostic scores in critically ILL patients receiving renal replacement therapy. Rev Bras Ter Intensiva. 2008;20(2):115–23.
13. Alves CJ, Franco GPP, Nakata CT, Costa GLG, Costa GLG, Genaro MS, et al. Evaluation of prognostic indicators for elderly patients admitted in intensive care units. Rev Bras Ter Intensiva. 2009;21(1):1–8.
14. Serpa Neto A, de Assuncao MSC, Pardini A, Silva E. Feasibility of transitioning from APACHE II to SAPS III as prognostic model in a Brazilian general intensive care unit. A retrospective study. Sao Paulo Med. J Rev Paul Med. 2015;133(3):199–205.
15. Silva Junior JM, Malbouisson LMS, Nuevo HL, Barbosa LGT, Marubayashi LY, Teixeira IC, et al. Applicability of the simplified acute physiology score (SAPS 3) in Brazilian hospitals. Rev Bras Anestesiol. 2010;60(1):20–31.
16. Nassar APJ, Mocelin AO, Nunes ALB, Giannini FP, Brauer L, Andrade FM, et al. Caution when using prognostic models: a prospective comparison of 3 recent prognostic models. J Crit Care. 2012;27(4):423.e1–7.
17. Keegan MT, Gajic O, Afessa B. Severity of illness scoring systems in the intensive care unit. Crit Care Med. 2011;39(1):163–9.
18. Soares M, Bozza FA, Angus DC, Japiassu AM, Viana WN, Costa R, et al. Organizational characteristics, outcomes, and resource use in 78 Brazilian intensive care units: the ORCHESTRA study. Intensive Care Med. 2015;41(12):2149–60.
19. Charlson ME, Pompei P, Ales KL, MacKenzie CR. A new method of classifying prognostic comorbidity in longitudinal studies: development and validation. J Chronic Dis. 1987;40(5):373–83.
20. Oken MM, Creech RH, Tormey DC, Horton J, Davis TE, McFadden ET, et al. Toxicity and response criteria of the Eastern Cooperative Oncology Group. Am J Clin Oncol. 1982;5(6):649–55.
21. Vincent JL, Moreno R, Takala J, Willatts S, De Mendonca A, Bruining H, et al. The SOFA (Sepsis-related Organ Failure Assessment) score to describe organ dysfunction/failure. On behalf of the Working Group

on Sepsis-Related Problems of the European Society of Intensive Care Medicine. Intensive Care Med. 1996;22(7):707–10.
22. DeLong ER, DeLong DM, Clarke-Pearson DL. Comparing the areas under two or more correlated receiver operating characteristic curves: a non-parametric approach. Biometrics. 1988;44(3):837–45.
23. Finazzi S, Poole D, Luciani D, Cogo PE, Bertolini G. Calibration belt for quality-of-care assessment based on dichotomous outcomes. PLoS ONE. 2011;6(2):e16110.
24. Poole D, Rossi C, Latronico N, Rossi G, Finazzi S, Bertolini G. Comparison between SAPS II and SAPS 3 in predicting hospital mortality in a cohort of 103 Italian ICUs. Is new always better? Intensive Care Med. 2012;38(8):1280–8.
25. Kramer AA, Zimmerman JE. Assessing the calibration of mortality benchmarks in critical care: The Hosmer–Lemeshow test revisited. Crit Care Med. 2007;35(9):2052–6.
26. Peek N, Arts DGT, Bosman RJ, van der Voort PHJ, de Keizer NF. External validation of prognostic models for critically ill patients required substantial sample sizes. J Clin Epidemiol. 2007;60(5):491–501.
27. Reineck LA, Pike F, Le TQ, Cicero BD, Iwashyna TJ, Kahn JM. Hospital factors associated with discharge bias in ICU performance measurement. Crit Care Med. 2014;42(5):1055–64.

6

What's new in multidrug-resistant pathogens in the ICU?

Gabor Zilahi[1], Antonio Artigas[2,3] and Ignacio Martin-Loeches[1,3,4,5*]

Abstract

Over the last several decades, antibacterial drug use has become widespread with their misuse being an ever-increasing phenomenon. Consequently, antibacterial drugs have become less effective or even ineffective, resulting in a global health security emergency. The prevalence of multidrug-resistant organisms (MDROs) varies widely among regions and countries. The primary aim of antibiotic stewardship programs is to supervise the three most influential factors contributing to the development and transmission of MDROs, namely: (1) appropriate antibiotic prescribing; (2) early detection and prevention of cross-colonization of MDROs; and (3) elimination of reservoirs. In the future, it is expected that a number of countries will experience a rise in MDROs. These infections will be associated with a high consumption of healthcare resources manifested by a prolonged hospital stay and high mortality. As a counteractive strategy, minimization of broad-spectrum antibiotic use and prompt antibiotic administration will aid in reduction of antibiotic resistance. Innovative management approaches include development and implementation of rapid diagnostic tests that will help in both shortening the duration of therapy and allowing early targeted therapy. The institution of more accessible therapeutic drug monitoring will help to optimize drug administration and support a patient-specific approach. Areas where further research is required are investigation into the heterogeneity of critically ill patients and the need for new antibacterial drug development.

Background

International health organizations, including the European Centre for Disease Prevention and Control (ECDC) and the Centers for Disease Control and Prevention (CDC), have used terms such as "crisis," "catastrophic consequences" and "nightmare scenario" to highlight the rapid emergence and spread of antibiotic resistance [1–4]. The World Health Organization (WHO) has identified antimicrobial resistance as one of the most important problems for human health with significant adverse impacts on clinical outcomes and higher costs due to consumption of healthcare resources [5].

*Correspondence: drmartinloeches@gmail.com
[1] Department of Clinical Medicine, Trinity Centre for Health Sciences, Multidisciplinary Intensive Care Research Organization (MICRO), Wellcome Trust-HRB Clinical Research, St James's Hospital, St James's University Hospital, Dublin 8, Ireland
Full list of author information is available at the end of the article

Epidemiology of highly resistant bacteria

A number of studies have been performed to assess the burden of infection in critical illness. The Intensive Care Over Nations (ICON) audit showed that more than one-third of the patients develop an infection during their intensive care unit (ICU) stay [6]. The Extended Prevalence of Infection in Intensive Care (EPIC) II study showed that 51 % of patients were considered to be infected while in ICU. The infection was of respiratory origin in 64 % of cases. *S aureus* (20.5 %) was the most frequent organism isolated, despite the overall predominance of Gram-negative organisms as a group: 62.2 % (*E. coli*, *Enterobacter* spp., *Klebsiella* spp., *Pseudomonas* spp. and *Acinetobacter* spp.) [7].

Antibiotic resistance is a serious problem in all parts of the world including Asia–Pacific, Latin America, Middle East, Europe and North America regions. A particular concern is the misuse or overuse of antibiotics, which has lead to the development of resistant or super-resistant bacterial strains. Two regions of particular concern, with existing high levels of antimicrobial resistance, are

South-East Asia and the Middle East where antibiotics can be easily bought over the counter [8, 9]. Findings from a cross-sectional study from Saudi Arabia showed that antibiotics were dispensed without a medical prescription in 244 (77.6 %) of 327 pharmacies analyzed, of which 231 (95 %) were dispensed without a patient request [10].

In Europe, the European Antimicrobial Resistance Surveillance Network (EARS-Net) has provided European reference data on antimicrobial resistance for public health purposes since the program began in 1999. Over the last 4 years (2011–2014), the proportion of *K. pneumoniae* and *E. coli* with resistance to fluoroquinolones, third-generation cephalosporins, aminoglycosides and a combined resistance to all three antibiotic groups has increased significantly. Large inter-country variations in *Acinetobacter* spp. resistance exist in Europe with a high percentage of resistant isolates being found in southern and southeast Europe. Similar patterns are observed with methicillin-resistant Staphylococcus aureus (MRSA) with resistance levels varying from 0.9 to 56 % depending on the country studied [11]. The recent "European Antimicrobial Resistance One Health ministerial conference 2016" highlighted the substantial antimicrobial resistance problem in Europe. For several antimicrobial group–bacterium combinations, a north-to-south and west-to-east gradient is evident in Europe. In general, lower resistance percentages are reported by countries in the north and higher percentages by countries in the south and east of Europe [12].

A group of international experts brought together by a joint initiative between the ECDC and the CDC, was tasked with creating a standardized international terminology to describe acquired resistance profiles in multidrug-resistant organisms [13]. MDROs have been divided into three categories depending on their resistance profile: 1. MDROs—non-susceptible to at least 1 agent in 3 antimicrobial categories; 2. extensively drug-resistant (XDR) organisms—non-susceptible to at least 1 agent in all but 2 or fewer antimicrobial categories; and 3. pan-drug-resistant (PDR) organisms—non-susceptible to all agents in all antimicrobial categories (Fig. 1).

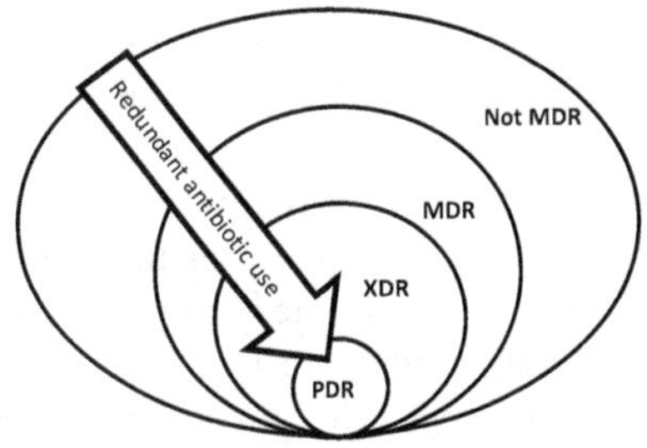

Fig. 1 Multidrug-resistant organisms (MDR) have been divided into three categories depending on their resistance profile: 1. MDR—non-susceptible to at least 1 agent in 3 antimicrobial categories; 2. extensively drug-resistant (XDR)—non-susceptible to at least 1 agent in all but 2 or fewer antimicrobial categories and 3. pan-drug-resistant (PDR)—non-susceptible to all agents in all antimicrobial categories

Over recent years, a new, comprehensive recommendation on classification of infections caused by Gram-positive and emerging Gram-negative multidrug-resistant pathogens has been launched. *E. faecium, S. aureus, K. pneumoniae, A. baumannii, P. aeruginosa* and *Enterobacter* spp. (ESKAPE) pathogens account for more than 80 % of infectious episodes in the ICU. As this acronym seems to help to highlight the problem of MDROs, some authors [14] claim a change to "ESCAPE" is warranted (*E. faecium, S. aureus, C. difficile, A. baumannii, P. aeruginosa* and *Enterobacteriaceae* spp.) in order to highlight the importance of *C.* difficile and incorporate not only *Enterobacter* spp. but also other *Enterobacteriaceae*spp. (namely, *Escherichia coli and Proteus* spp.) because of the increasing levels of antibiotic resistance (including extended-spectrum β-lactamases, carbapenemases and aminoglycoside resistance) and decreasing levels of fluoroquinolone susceptibility among these organisms. *E. coli* infections currently account for ~20 % of all cases of bacteremia in the UK and Ireland [15] with not just high rates of fluoroquinolone and amoxicillin–clavulanic acid (AMC) resistance, but also extended-spectrum beta-lactamase (ESBL) mechanisms with a possible link between high resistance and community antibiotic misuse [16]. In addition, ESBL *Enterobacteriaceae* spp. are responsible for outbreaks irrespective of location. Antibiotic selection of ESBL-producing Gram-negative pathogens is not just related to the total use of antimicrobial agents in hospitals, but also to the particular use of the fluoroquinolones and second- and third-generation cephalosporins [16]. *P. aeruginosa* has an extensive capability to become resistant to all type of antibiotics, create biofilms and demonstrate a high level of intrinsic resistance. These characteristics are caused by production of ESBL, overexpression of AmpC beta-lactamases and other drug-resistant mechanisms such as production of metallo-β-lactamases (MBLs) [17]. *Acinetobacter* spp., similar to *P. aeruginosa*, have an array of mechanisms by which they develop and horizontally transfer resistance. The most important of these is the production of beta-lactamases and aminoglycoside-modifying enzymes [18].

As a result of misuse of antibiotics, different pathogens are becoming increasingly resistant. The lack of regulatory policies regarding antibiotic prescription makes them easily accessible and cheap, which promotes overuse [19]. Gram-negative bacilli are often resistant to multiple antimicrobials. It is important to mention the newly emergence of the first plasmid-mediated polymyxin resistance mechanism, MCR-1, in Enterobacteriaceae in China [20]. This is especially worrisome because plasmid-mediated resistance can spread in an explosive manner and de-activate polymyxins, which are one of our last antibiotic options. On the other hand, carbapenems are another important last-line group of antibiotics for infections involving multidrug-resistant Gram-negative *Enterobacteriaceae* spp. The most important mechanism of carbapenem resistance in this group is the production of carbapenemases, although resistance can also result from the synergistic activity between AmpC-type and extended-spectrum beta-lactamases combined with decreased outer membrane permeability. Three major molecular classes of carbapenemases are recognized: A, B and D (Fig. 2). Although carbapenem resistance remains at relatively low levels in northern Europe, it does constitute a serious threat worldwide as a consequence of acquisition of carbapenemase genes with a higher prevalence in southern Europe and Asia. In South America, carbapenem-resistant *P. aeruginosa* and *A. baumannii* could be as high as 56 and 35 %, respectively [21]. Outbreaks of class A carbapenemases particularly plasmid encoded (*K. pneumoniae* carbapenemases [KPC]) producers also have been reported in several countries (Greece, Israel, China, Brazil, Argentina and USA) [22]. Some authors have proposed two concomitant epidemics of carbapenemase producers worldwide [23]: (1) community-acquired infections with carbapenemase-producing *E. coli* (New Delhi metallo-β-lactamase-1) (NDM-1 and OXA-48 types) and (2) nosocomial carbapenemase producers in *K. pneumoniae* of all types (KPC, IMP, VIM, NDM and OXA-48).

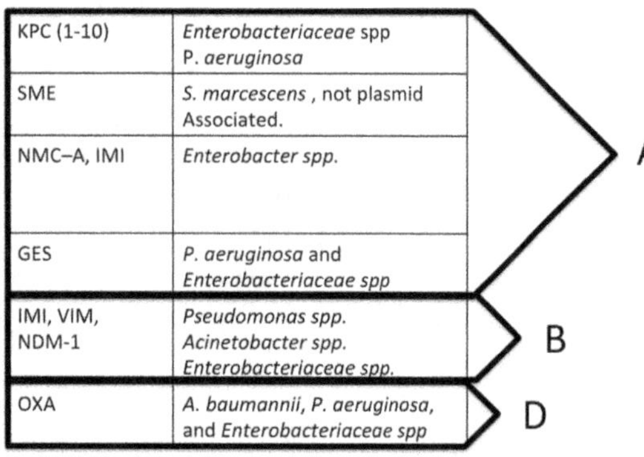

Fig. 2 Types of carbapenemases. *KPC Klebsiella pneumoniae* carbapenemase, *SME Serratia marcescens* enzyme, *MNC* not metallo-carbapenemase, *IMI* imipenem-hydrolyzing β-lactamase, *GES* Guiana extended spectrum, *IMI* imipenem-hydrolyzing β-lactamase, *VIM* Verona integron-encoded MBL, *NDM-1* New Delhi metallo-β-lactamase

There is an urgent need for development of new agents with activity against MDROs. The Infectious Diseases Society of America (IDSA) supported a program, so-called Bad Bugs, Need Drugs; 10 × '20 Initiative, with the aim of developing ten new systemic antibacterial drugs by 2020 [24]. In Europe, a recent report from the Economist Jim O'Neill in the UK expressed concern that the global financial cost of no action would be the loss of 10 million lives a year by 2050 and £69 tn ($100 tn) a year [25]. Infections by MDROs were associated with worse clinical outcomes compared with their susceptible counterparts [26]. While higher mortality associated with MDROs may be related to the virulence of the pathogen and a weak (comorbidity, age, etc.) or severely ill host (organ failure status, etc.) [27, 28], it is also important to highlight that delays in effective antimicrobial administration are also associated with high mortality [29].

Risk scoring/risk factors

There have been multiple attempts to identify patients at risk of MDROs with the implementation of risk scoring systems to initiate appropriate targeted antibiotic therapy. Unfortunately, the value of these scores is limited [30]. Most of the risk factors are shared among different MDRO species, and the same type of organism with various degrees of resistance might have distinct epidemiological characteristics. Martin-Loeches et al. [31] confirmed in a multicenter study that patients without risk factors listed in the 2005 ATS/IDSA guidelines admitted to ICU with hospital-acquired pneumonia (HAP) and/or ventilator-associated pneumonia (VAP) had a high prevalence of MDROs (50.7 %) confirming the difficulty of predicting MDROs based on risk stratification. Most clinicians use certain risk profiles (complex ICU stay, recent prior hospitalization or long-term care facility habitant, recent exposure to antimicrobials, etc.) to assess the need for broad-spectrum antibiotic therapy. This approach certainly improves adequate initial antibiotic choice, but again shares the same concerns with risk scores being non-specific and broad. If broad-spectrum antibiotics, based on risk scores or risk stratification, are prescribed, strict antibiotic stewardship programs should be also applied. This strategy, mainly based on de-escalation policies, will ultimately promote higher rates of appropriate antibiotic use. The recent launch of the IDSA/ATS guidelines for HAP/VAP will certainly help how to consider antibiotic treatment regarding the aforementioned concerns [32]. Strengths from these recently published guidelines are that VAP by MDR pathogens is significantly simplified and for the first time clinical parameters are included, namely septic shock on appearance of VAP and acute respiratory distress syndrome (ARDS) preceding VAP diagnosis.

Another approach is to perform regular surveillance. Based on previous observational studies MDROs colonization may precede bacteraemia in the ICU [33]. This early identification of MDROs—even before clinical infection—can guide the clinician toward appropriate empiric treatment. Brusselaers et al. [34] in a recent meta-analysis of tracheal aspirate surveillance concluded that such an approach has a high negative predictive value, i.e., if a recent surveillance culture does not contain MDROs, the newly symptomatic VAP is unlikely to be caused by MDROs (likelihood <10 %). However, the presence of MDROs only had a moderate positive predictive value with an overall 75 % sensitivity.

Rapid methods to diagnose multidrug resistance

One of the key aspects of avoiding the spread of resistant strains is early detection with the use rapid diagnostic tests. The methods currently used in hospitals for microbial detection tend to be labor-intensive, consume human resources and take more than a day to yield results. Newly developed rapid microbial detection tests, which biopharmaceutical industries have been slow to embrace, are precise, sensitive and generate results faster when compared with traditional culture-plate methods. There has been growing experience with rapid diagnostic techniques within the last decade, especially with MRSA. Harbarth et al. [35] using quick, multiplex immunocapture-coupled PCR (qMRSA) were able to decrease median time to notification from four days to one day which can help to identify previously unknown MRSA carriers rapidly. Experience with Gram-negative isolates such as carbapenemase-producing organisms (CROs), including the *Enterobacteriaceae* spp., is also evolving. Detection of patients carrying carbapenemase-producing microorganisms can significantly impact on infection control. Recently, Tato et al. assessed the performance of the Cepheid Xpert Carba-R assay (designed for the rapid detection and differentiation of the blaKPC, blaNDM, blaVIM, blaOXA-48 and blaIMP-1 genes) and found that sensitivity, specificity, positive and negative predictive values compared to reference culture and sequencing results were above 95 %. Worryingly, in addition to CROs, there has been an increase in reports of *Enterobacteriaceae* spp. resistant to polymyxins. Since conventional methods for detection of colistin-resistant isolates such as microdilution are time-consuming and methods like disk diffusion and the E-test are not reliable, Nordmann et al. [36] evaluated a new test: a chromogenic agar, shortening the results by 16 h compared to the reference broth dilution method, with a sensitivity and specificity of 99.3 and 95.4 %, respectively, compared to the standard microdilution method.

Shortening the turn-around time of positive blood culture identification and susceptibility results is essential to optimize antimicrobial treatment in patients with severe infections. One of the most widely used technologies nowadays that actually has revolutionized the process of care in microbiology laboratories is the matrix-assisted laser desorption ionization/time-of-flight mass spectrometry (MALDI-TOF MS) [37]. The introduction of mass spectrometry through MALDI-TOF in the diagnosis of bacteraemia and fungemia has represented a revolution due to the rapidity and reliability of the results that it can offer to microbiology services and laboratories through analysis of the mass spectrum of the bacterial protein directly from positive blood culture bottles [38]. Management of patients with bacteraemia has been optimized with the introduction of this methodology due to the rapid information.

Rapid diagnostic tests implemented in the current clinical practice should also consider an adequate workflow of information within a multidisciplinary working group approach that can process quickly and correctly the results from the microbiology laboratory to the bedside of the patient. An adequate process of care performance of rapid diagnostic tests such as MALDI-TOF will improve the quality of care, with the reduction of antibiotic expenditure and hospital stay and helping to infection control with the implementation of adequate and timing transmission-based precautions [39].

The basis for all infection control measures is the accurate and timely laboratory identification of MDROs. This will also deliver important information for regional and national containment strategies and hospitals. The implementation of rapid tests and the development of microbiology laboratory reference services is an urgent requirement.

Antibiotic stewardship (AMS) and infection control strategies

Antimicrobial stewardship (AMS) programs aim to provide assistance with optimal choice, dosage, pharmacokinetic–pharmacodynamic (PK/PD) characteristics and duration of antibiotics in order to reduce costs, adverse events and the development of resistance [40]. Even though the IDSA has published guidelines [41] about AMS programs, the ideal care bundle has yet to be identified as published articles vary greatly in their findings. A systematic review by Kaki et al. [42] assessing 24 mainly uncontrolled, before and after studies published in 2011 showed that marked heterogeneity exists with respect to interventions evaluated and no mortality benefit could be identified. Nevertheless, AMS was associated with an overall clinical benefit as evidenced by a reduction in antibiotic consumption, costs and antibiotic pressure that subsequently results in a decrease in resistance rates [42].

These measures are only effective if all stakeholders, supported by the relevant authorities, accept implementation and incorporate audits and feedback mechanisms. A recent example of such an initiative is the "Zero Resistance" program developed by The Spanish Society of Intensive Care Medicine and Coronary Care Units (SEMICYUC). The main objective of the "Zero Resistance" project is reduction in the cumulative incidence of patients with ICU-acquired MDR infections by 20 % with a bundle of 10 recommendations. The primary aim of the antibiotic program is to supervise the three most influential contributing factors to the development and transmission of MDROs, namely: (1) adequate prescription of antibiotics; (2) early detection and prevention of cross-colonization of MDR; and (3) elimination of reservoirs [43]. Results of this ambitious project will shed light on AMS programs in the near future.

De-escalation is defined as an AMS strategy of reducing the number of antibiotics or using narrower/targeted spectrum drugs. De-escalation has been found to be safe and associated with less antibiotic usage and shorter duration of therapy in observational studies. Theoretically, this will translate into a reduction of MDROs; nonetheless, it has yet to be clearly proven [44]. Two studies have recently been published looking at de-escalation in patients with severe sepsis. Leone et al. [45] conducted a multicenter non-blinded randomized non-inferiority trial of patients with severe sepsis and Garnacho-Montero et al. [46] a prospective observational study enrolling patients admitted to the ICU with severe sepsis or septic shock. While Leone et al. [45] found that de-escalation was inferior to continuation of the initial antibiotic therapy (length of stay as the primary outcome parameter), the study had important limitations (small numbers of patients and unbalanced groups at baseline; patients were younger and had lower disease severity). Garnacho-Montero et al. [46] demonstrated a protective effect of de-escalation in terms of mortality. In an observational, single-center study, Montravers et al. [47] prospectively analyzed the characteristics and outcomes of anti-infective de-escalation during healthcare-associated intra-abdominal infections and found that the presence of non-fermenting Gram-negative bacilli (NFGNB) and MDROs limited the implementation of a de-escalation program. De-escalation is a feasible option in patients with polymicrobial infections such as healthcare-associated intra-abdominal infections, but MDROs and NFGNB limit its implementation. Recently, De Bus [48] et al. analyzed the effect of de-escalation in 478 anti-pseudomonal antibiotic prescriptions and could not find lower rates of resistant organisms after exposure to anti-pseudomonal beta-lactam antibiotics. Interestingly, Carlier et al. [49] conducted a simulation study showing that the probability of achieving a PK/PD target was lower in the narrower-spectrum antibiotic group (amoxicillin–clavulanic acid, cefuroxime, flucloxacillin, cefazolin and cefepime) using conventional dosing as compared to broad-spectrum antibiotics like meropenem and piperacillin/tazobactam.

Combination antimicrobial therapy exploits the synergistic effect of some antibiotic groupings in addition to broadening the spectrum of activity against a suspected pathogen to ensure adequate coverage. The synergistic effect of combination therapy has been shown to be beneficial in vivo in invasive pneumococcal disease and toxic shock syndrome. Randomized controlled trials (RCTs), on the other hand, have failed to demonstrate a mortality benefit with B-lactam and aminoglycoside combinations, but renal damage was more frequent [50]. Treatment of infections caused by CROs using a combination of two or three active drugs has consistently been associated with improved outcomes, with carbapenems being included in the combination when the minimal inhibitory concentration (MIC) of the pathogen against meropenem does not exceed 8 mg/L [51, 52]. However, a survival benefit when using combination treatment for infections caused by multidrug-resistant Gram-negative bacteria is questionable [53–55]. As almost all these data originate from observational studies, the need for RCTs is clear.

There is an on-going debate about pharmacokinetic and pharmacodynamic (PK/PD) optimization. On the one hand, the critically ill patient has a higher than normal volume of distribution, impaired renal and hepatic clearance, altered plasma protein content and they also tend to be elderly with significant comorbidities. On the other hand, there is growing evidence that in selected patient populations renal clearance is actually augmented, which can lead to inadequate plasma concentrations for some of the important antibiotic groups like carbapenems, beta-lactams and cephalosporins. Yang et al. [56] published a systemic review showing that the extended or continuous infusion of beta-lactams (piperacillin/tazobactam) strategy was associated with a higher clinical cure rate and lower mortality than the conventional intermittent approach. In patients with multiorgan failure and renal replacement therapy, residual diuresis, type of membrane and body weight should be considered for beta-lactam dose titration [57, 58]. Another frequently used drug class to treat MDROs are the aminoglycosides. Recent studies have highlighted the need for dose adjustment in critically ill patients. De Montmollin et al. [59] found that one-third of the patients in ICU had an amikacin $C_{max} < 60$ mg/L with the recommended dose of 15 mg/kg of total body weight. This suggests the need for dose optimization based on creatinine clearance, total body weight and positive 24-h fluid balance in order to reach adequate therapeutic targets [60, 61]. Until drug assays are routinely available, a personalized approach to dosing should be considered for each patient based on local AMS.

Because of the increasing prevalence of Gram-negative MDROs worldwide, previously discarded antibiotics are being re-evaluated. Recent data suggest that the current dosage regimens of colistin are suboptimal in many critically ill patients [62]. To optimize the plasma level the administration of a loading dose has been proposed [63]. It has also recently been shown [64] that the dose of other "rescue" drugs such as fosfomycin should be increased for critically ill patients.

Infection control teams play a definitive role in antibiotic AMS programs by assisting with prompt detection of MDROs and promoting compliance with standard and transmission-based precautions. They also facilitate the use of other infection prevention strategies, such as implementing care bundles to prevent hospital-acquired infections, ensuring hand hygiene compliance and educating not only staff and patients, but also visitors about infection prevention topics. Therefore, infection control teams play a crucial part in AMS. Infection control and epidemiology professionals launched the concept of "synergy" to highlight the joint effort of infection prevention and AMS [65]. This initiative has three key aims: (1) minimize nosocomial infections, (2) decrease the use of additional antibiotics and (3) reduce MDROs.

Current and new treatment options

Two major organizations, the IDSA and ECDC, have analyzed the repertoire of drugs in the antibiotic R&D pipeline, and there are very few offering significant benefits over existing therapies (Table 1) [66].

MRSA is a major MDRO in ICU's around the globe. It is frequently treated with vancomycin, linezolid, daptomycin, ceftaroline or tigecycline. Linezolid was found to be superior for the treatment of HAP in the ZEPHyR trial [67] in terms of cure rate and nephrotoxicity. Daptomycin is a good alternative, but not licensed for pneumonia as the drug is inactivated by surfactant [68]. As a new alternative for MRSA, the novel tedizolid was found to be non-inferior to linezolid in early clinical response for an acute bacterial skin and skin structure infections (ABSSSI) [69]. Moreover, recent in vitro studies also confirmed activity against all Gram-positive isolates, which were inhibited by ≤ 1 µg/mL tedizolid in samples of patients with HAP. Antimicrobial susceptibility testing revealed that the MIC_{90} of tedizolid was 0.5 µg/mL for MRSA, which was fourfold lower than that of linezolid [70].

Enterococci are Gram-positive facultative anaerobes that live as commensals in the gastrointestinal tract, but they are not as virulent as *S. aureus* or *S. pneumoniae.* Donskey et al. [71] conducted a prospective study and found that vancomycin-resistant enterococci (VRE) in stool were associated with treatment with anti-anaerobic antimicrobials. More recently, an animal study found that in contrast to vancomycin, fidaxomicin (a new class of narrow spectrum macrocyclic antibiotic drugs) treatment caused minimal disruption of the intestinal flora and did not increase the rate of VRE and extended-spectrum β-lactamase-producing Klebsiella pneumoniae (ESBL-Kp) colonization [72]. Limiting the use of such agents may help decrease the spread of VRE. *Enterococci* spp. are likely to function as a reservoir of drug resistance determinants and can serve as the springboard for the spread of these genes to other Gram-positive pathogens [73]. It is important to highlight that there is a relatively high rate of VRE not susceptible to linezolid observed in ICU patients [31]. New agents like dalbavancin, oritavancin and telavancin seem promising [74].

Treatment of carbapenem-resistant *Enterobacteriaceae* spp. using monotherapy is often inadequate, and challenging cases may require the use of highly toxic agents. Aminoglycosides, polymyxins, tigecycline, fosfomycin and occasionally fluoroquinolones form the backbone of treatment. Recently, the US Food and Drug Administration (FDA) issued a warning regarding the risk of increased mortality in patients treated with tigecycline, observed in the clinical trials [75]. An observational study by Montravers et al. [76] found it can be used safely even in severe infections. However, a debate about the potential benefit of a high dosage regimen (200 mg daily) still needs to be resolved. Combination antimicrobial therapy has been shown to be superior in terms of cure rate when compared to monotherapy in multiple observational studies [77]. Emerging treatment options include ceftazidime–avibactam. Avibactam is a novel β-lactamase inhibitor with activity against class A, class C and some class D β-lactamases. It has activity against KPC-type carbapenemases and some OXA enzymes; however, it has no activity against metallo-β-lactamases (such as NDM-1) [78]. Ceftazidime–avibactam was approved by the Food and Drug Administration (FDA) in 2015 for the treatment of complicated intra-abdominal infections and complicated UTIs [79]. A newly released fifth-generation cephalosporin ceftolozane combined with a beta-lactamase inhibitor tazobactam has potent activity against *P. aeruginosa*, including various MDR types [80]. Another alternative for the treatment of MDR, XDR and PDR *Pseudomonas* ssp. is the use of intra-tracheal antibiotics (ITA), consisting mainly of aminoglycosides and polymyxins, with encouraging results seen to date. In

Table 1 Adapted from [66]

Company	Product	Class/structure	Mechanism of action	Lead indication
Actelion Ltd. (SIX:ATLN)	Cadazolid (179811)	Oxazolidinone–quinolone hybrid	Inhibit DNA replication and protein synthesis	*CDAD*
Affinium Pharmaceuticals Ltd.	AFN-1252	FabI enoyl-(acyl carrier protein) reductase inhibitor	Inhibit fabI	ABSSSI
CrystalGenomics Inc. (KOSDAQ:83790)	CG400549	FabI enoyl-(acyl carrier protein) reductase inhibitor	Inhibit fabI	Complicated ABSSSI
GlaxoSmithKline plc(LSE:GSK; NYSE:GSK)	GSK1322322	Peptide deformylase (PDF) inhibitor	Inhibit PDF	Bacterial infection
Furiex Pharmaceuticals Inc. (NASDAQ:FURX)/Johnson & Johnson (NYSE:JNJ)	JNJ-32729463 (JNJ-Q2)	Fluoroquinolone	Inhibit DNA replication	ABSSSI, CAP
Nabriva Therapeutics AG/ Forest Laboratories Inc. (NYSE:FRX)	BC-3781	Pleuromutilin	Inhibit protein synthesis	ABSSSI
Novartis AG (NYSE:NVS)	LFF571	Thiopeptide	Inhibit protein synthesis	*CDAD*
PolyMedix Inc. (OTCBB:PYMX)	Brilacidin (PMX-30063)	Defensin mimetics	Membrane lysis	ABSSSI
Rib-X Pharmaceuticals Inc.	Radezolid (RX-1741)	Oxazolidinone	Inhibit protein synthesis	CAP
Tetraphase Pharmaceuticals Inc.	Eravacycline (TP-434)	Tetracycline	Inhibit protein synthesis	cIAI
Theravance Inc. (NASDAQ:THRX)	TD-1792	Beta-lactam-glycopeptide hybrid	Inhibit cell wall synthesis	Gram-positive cSSSI
Wockhardt Ltd. (BSE:532300)	WCK 771	Fluoroquinolone	Inhibit DNA replication	*S. aureus*
Wockhardt Ltd. (BSE:532300)	WCK 2349	Fluoroquinolone	Inhibit DNA replication	Gram-positive cSSSI
Nanotherapeutics Inc.	Ramoplanin	Lipoglycodepsipeptide	Inhibit cell wall production	CDAD
2 M BioTech L.P.	CBR-2092	Rifamycin–quinolone hybrid	Inhibit DNA replication and RNA synthesis	*S. aureus*
Achaogen Inc.	ACHN-975	N-acetylglucosamine deacetylase (LpxC) inhibitor	Inhibit LpxC	Gram-negative
aRigen Pharmaceuticals Inc./ Green Cross Corp.	WAP-8294A2	Depsipeptide	Disrupt membrane	MRSA
Basilea Pharmaceutica AG (SIX:BSLN)	BAL30072	Beta-lactam (monocyclic)	Inhibit cell wall synthesis	Gram-negative
FAB Pharma S.A.S.	FAB001 (MUT056399)	FabI enoyl-(acyl carrier protein) reductase inhibitor	Inhibit fabI	*S. aureus*
Kalidex Pharmaceuticals Inc.	KPI-10	Fluoroquinolone	Inhibit DNA replication	Gram-negative and Gram-positive
Kyorin Pharmaceutical Co. Ltd. (Tokyo:4569)	KRP-AM1977X	Quinolone	Inhibit DNA replication	Gram-positive
MicuRx Pharmaceuticals Inc.	MRX-I	Oxazolidinone	Inhibit protein synthesis	Gram-positive
Novacta Biosystems Ltd.	NVB302	Lantibiotic	Inhibit cell wall synthesis	*CDAD*
Rempex Pharmaceuticals Inc.	Carbavance (RPX7009/biapenem)	Beta-lactamase inhibitor with boron core (RPX7009); beta-lactam (biapenem)	Inhibit cell wall synthesis	Gram-negative
Shionogi & Co. Ltd. (Tokyo:4507)/GlaxoSmithKline plc (LSE:GSK; NYSE:GSK)	S-649266	Beta-lactam	Inhibit cell wall synthesis	CAP
Tetraphase Pharmaceuticals Inc.	TP-2758	Tetracycline	Inhibit protein synthesis	cUTI

mechanically ventilated patients, the use of ITA for prevention or treatment of VAP has shown less toxicity as compared to systemic formulations [81]. A recent international survey reported that intra-tracheal antibiotic administration is a common therapeutic modality in ICUs; however, practice varies widely [82]. *Acinetobacter* spp. similar to *P. aeruginosa* have ample ways to develop and horizontally transfer resistance. Of greatest significance is the production of beta-lactamases and aminoglycoside-modifying enzymes [18]. Combination therapy including a polymyxin has commonly been the mainstay of treatment for *Acinetobacter spp*. However, a recent paper has highlighted the risk of nephrotoxicity when colistin and vancomycin are used in combination with no benefit to clinical outcome [83].

More recently, studies have been conducted revealing the benefits of treatment with "new" combination therapies for XDR or PDR organisms. In terms of PDR Gram-negative infections, Bulik et al. [84] found that double-carbapenem therapy (ertapenem and doripenem) for carbapenemase-producing *K. pneumoniae* had an enhanced efficacy over either agent alone both in vitro and in vivo in animal models. Giamarellou et al. [85] found that the use of ertapenem plus doripenem or meropenem resulted in treatment success without relapse at follow-up in patients with PDR *K. pneumoniae.*

As the vast majority of the antibiotic treatment is short term, many companies struggle to generate profit from the sales of anti-infective agents. The majority of products being approved are second-, third- or fourth-generation antibiotics, meaning they are follow-up compounds, without a novel mechanism of action. In addition to this, many novel antibiotics have struggled to reach the market due to difficulties in demonstrating efficacy or unacceptable side effects. Furthermore, for licensing purposes, new antibacterials must demonstrate non-inferiority against already marketed drugs. Finally, healthcare authorities are frequently reluctant to pay the high costs associated with clinical trials, hindering the development of novel antimicrobial agents.

As a result of the declining effectiveness of existing antibiotics and the steady decrease in new antibiotic development, alternative approaches to antibiotic therapy are appearing including immunotherapy and the use of bacteriophages. Immunotherapy initiated at the outset of an antibiotic course has the potential to result in beneficial effects; however, use is frequently limited by a narrow spectrum of action against specific target antigens. Another attractive approach to address the critical need for new antibiotics is the engineering of various components of the immune response such as monoclonal antibodies. For instance, a randomized, placebo-controlled phase I study found that IC43 (recombinant outer membrane protein-based vaccine against *P. aeruginosa*) could induce an antibody response in healthy volunteers [86]. Phase II and III studies are being conducted in mechanically ventilated patients (ClinicalTrials.gov Identifier: NCT01563263). Another cutting edge approach is the use of bacteriophages or phages. These are bacterial viruses that invade bacterial cells, disrupt metabolism, cause bacteriolysis and are highly specific and effective [87].

Future prospects

Infections with MDROs are already a threat in a number of countries. It is expected that in others with existing low level of MDROs, the number of infections due to MDR, XDR and even PDR organisms will rise. These infections are associated with an increased consumption of healthcare resources manifested by a prolonged hospital stay and an augmented mortality. In order to reduce antibiotic resistance rates, a strategy minimizing the use of broad-spectrum antibiotics and ensuring prompt antibiotic administration should be adopted. The development of rapid diagnostic tests will help by both shortening duration of therapy and allowing prompt-targeted therapy. The implementation of more accessible therapeutic drug monitoring will help to optimize drug administration and enable a more personalized approach to treatment. Some points require further investigation in clinical trials, such as the heterogeneity of patients admitted to ICU and the need for new drug development.

Since late 1980s, no new class of antibiotics has been discovered that is available for treatment of systemic bacterial infections. This discovery void is still impacting the therapeutic options to treat infections caused by multi-drug- or extensively drug-resistant bacteria. Recent findings regarding existing antibiotics combinations should also be mentioned. Combination therapy regimens with daptomycin with either oxacillin (enhancing in vivo efficacy to daptomycin monotherapy due to a daptomycin–oxacillin seesaw phenomenon in vitro) [88] or β-lactams [89] have been showed to enhance daptomycin efficacy against daptomycin-resistant strains. These examples just want to illustrate a "think outside of the box" model for existing drug combination for new research in the future. Certainly, it would need a deep remodel of the current drug regulation for new antibacterials and to adequately stimulate investment by the industry for new antimicrobial developments and ultimately to non-antibiotic approaches.

In summary, a steady resistance increase particularly to Gram-negatives, rising minimum inhibitory concentration in methicillin-resistant *Staphylococcus aureus* and the spread of multiresistant strains of pathogens in patients without classic risk factors in the ICU are key areas to delineate in future studies. Guidelines and recommendations will need to incorporate the ecology of the hospital setting and the severity of patient illness to provide a personalized patient approach to antimicrobial treatment in the future.

Authors' contributions

GZ, AA and IML contributed to draft the manuscript and approved the final version. All authors read and approved the final manuscript.

Author details

[1] Department of Clinical Medicine, Trinity Centre for Health Sciences, Multidisciplinary Intensive Care Research Organization (MICRO), Wellcome Trust-HRB Clinical Research, St James's Hospital, St James's University Hospital, Dublin 8, Ireland. [2] Critical Care Center, Parc Taulí Hospital-Sabadell, CIBERes, Parc Tauli s/n., Sabadell, Barcelona, Spain. [3] Centros de Investigación Biomédica en Red (CIBER), Madrid, Spain. [4] Wellcome Trust-HRB Clinical Research, Dublin, Ireland. [5] Department of Clinical Medicine, Trinity Centre for Health Sciences, Dublin, Ireland.

Acknowledgements

To Dr. Mary Aisling McMahon (Multidisciplinary Intensive Care Research Organization (MICRO), St James's University Hospital, Dublin, Ireland) for language edition.

Competing interests

IML, AA and GZ have no financial interest in any of the products mentioned in this paper.

References

1. Michael CA, Dominey-Howes D, Labbate M. The antimicrobial resistance crisis: causes, consequences, and management. Front Public Health. 2014;2:145.
2. Martin-Loeches I, Torres A, Rinaudo M, Terraneo S, de Rosa F, Ramirez P, et al. Resistance patterns and outcomes in intensive care unit (ICU)-acquired pneumonia. Validation of European Centre for Disease Prevention and Control (ECDC) and the Centers for Disease Control and Prevention (CDC) classification of multidrug resistant organism. J Infect. 2015;70:213–22.
3. Drinka P, Niederman MS, El-Solh AA, Crnich CJ. Assessment of risk factors for multi-drug resistant organisms to guide empiric antibiotic selection in long term care: a dilemma. J Am Med Dir Assoc. 2011;12:321–5.
4. Viswanathan VK. Off-label abuse of antibiotics by bacteria. Gut Microbes. 2014;5(1):3–4. doi:10.4161/gmic.28027.
5. http://www.who.int/drugresistance/documents/surveillancereport/en/. Accessed 20 Sept 2016.
6. Vincent JL, Marshall JC, Amendys-Silva SA, Francois B, Martin-Loeches I, Lipman J, et al. Assessment of the worldwide burden of critical illness: the Intensive Care Over Nations (ICON) audit. Lancet Respir Med. 2014;2:380–6.
7. Vincent J, Rello J, Marshall J, et al. International study of the prevalence and outcomes of infection in intensive care units. JAMA. 2009;302:2323–9.
8. Heddini A, Cars O, Qiang S, Tomson G. Antibiotic resistance in China—a major future challenge. Lancet. 2009;373(9657):30. doi:10.1016/S0140-6736(08)61956-X
9. Habibzadeh F. Lancet (London, England). 2013. http://www.thelancet.com/pb/assets/raw/Lancet/global-health/middle-east/Nov13_MiddleEastEd.pdf?elsca1=220713.
10. Bin Abdulhak AA, Altannir MA, Almansor MA, Almohaya MS, Onazi AS, Marei MA, et al. Non prescribed sale of antibiotics in Riyadh, Saudi Arabia: a cross sectional study. BMC Public Health. 2011;11:538.
11. http://ecdc.europa.eu/en/publications/Documents/antibiotic-resistance-in-EU-summary.pdf.
12. http://www.consilium.europa.eu/en/press/press-releases/2016/06/17-epsco-conclusions-antimicrobial-resistance/.
13. Magiorakos A-P, Srinivasan A, Carey RB, Carmeli Y, Falagas ME, Giske CG, et al. Multidrug-resistant, extensively drug-resistant and pandrug-resistant bacteria: an international expert proposal for interim standard definitions for acquired resistance. Clin Microbiol Infect. 2012;18:268–81.
14. Peterson LR. Bad bugs, no drugs: no escape revisited. Clin Infect Dis. 2009;49:992–3.
15. Livermore DM, Hope R, Brick G, Lillie M, Reynolds R. Non-susceptibility trends among *Enterobacteriaceae* from bacteraemias in the UK and Ireland, 2001-06. J Antimicrob Chemother. 2008;62(Suppl 2):ii41–54.
16. Knudsen JD, Andersen SE, Grp BI. A multidisciplinary intervention to reduce infections of ESBL-and AmpC-producing, gram-negative bacteria at a University Hospital. PLoS One. 2014;9(1):e86457. doi:10.1371/journal.pone.0086457.
17. Gupta R, Malik A, Rizvi M, Ahmed SM. Incidence of multidrug-resistant *Pseudomonas* spp. in ICU patients with special reference to ESBL, AMPC, MBL and biofilm production. J Glob Infect Dis. 2016;8:25–31.
18. Bonomo RA, Szabo D. Mechanisms of multidrug resistance in *Acinetobacter* species and *Pseudomonas aeruginosa*. Clin Infect Dis. 2006;43(Suppl 2):S49–56.
19. Ventola CL. The antibiotic resistance crisis: part 1: causes and threats. P T. 2015;40:277–83.
20. Liu Y-Y, Wang Y, Walsh TR, Yi L-X, Zhang R, Spencer J, et al. Emergence of plasmid-mediated colistin resistance mechanism MCR-1 in animals and human beings in China: a microbiological and molecular biological study. Lancet Infect Dis. 2016;16:161–8.
21. Marra AR, Camargo LFA, Pignatari ACC, Sukiennik T, Behar PRP, Medeiros EAS, et al. Nosocomial bloodstream infections in Brazilian hospitals: analysis of 2,563 cases from a prospective nationwide surveillance study. J Clin Microbiol. 2011;49:1866–71.
22. Nordmann P, Cuzon G, Naas T. The real threat of Klebsiella pneumoniae carbapenemase-producing bacteria. Lancet Infect Dis. 2009;9:228–36.
23. Nordmann P, Naas T, Poirel L. Global spread of carbapenemase-producing *Enterobacteriaceae*. Emerg Infect Dis. 2011;17:1791–8.
24. The 10 × '20 Initiative: pursuing a global commitment to develop 10 new antibacterial drugs by 2020. Clin Infect Dis. 2010;50:1081–3.
25. http://amr-review.org/sites/default/files/160518_Final%20paper_with%20cover.pdf.
26. Marchaim D, Gottesman T, Schwartz O, Korem M, Maor Y, Rahav G, et al. National multicenter study of predictors and outcomes of bacteremia upon hospital admission caused by *Enterobacteriaceae* producing extended-spectrum β-lactamases. Antimicrob Agents Chemother. 2010;54:5099–104.
27. Rello J, Rue M, Jubert P, Muses G, Sonora R, Valles J, et al. Survival in patients with nosocomial pneumonia: impact of the severity of illness and the etiologic agent. Crit Care Med. 1997;25:1862–7.
28. Rello J, Sole-Violan J, Sa-Borges M, Garnacho-Montero J, Munoz E, Sirgo G, et al. Pneumonia caused by oxacillin-resistant Staphylococcus aureus treated with glycopeptides. Crit Care Med. 2005;33:1983–7.
29. Kumar A, Ellis P, Arabi Y, Roberts D, Light B, Parrillo JE, et al. Initiation of inappropriate antimicrobial therapy results in a fivefold reduction of survival in human septic shock. Chest. 2009;136:1237–48.
30. Pogue JM, Kaye KS, Cohen DA, Marchaim D. Appropriate antimicrobial therapy in the era of multidrug-resistant human pathogens. Clin Microbiol Infect. 2015;21(4):302–12. doi:10.1016/j.cmi.2014.12.025.
31. Martin-Loeches I, Deja M, Koulenti D, Dimopoulos G, Marsh B, Torres A, et al. Potentially resistant microorganisms in intubated patients with hospital-acquired pneumonia: the interaction of ecology, shock and risk factors. Intensive Care Med. 2013;39(4):672–81. doi:10.1007/s00134-012-2808-5.
32. Kalil AC, Metersky ML, Klompas M, Muscedere J, Sweeney DA, Palmer LB, et al. Management of adults with hospital-acquired and ventilator-associated pneumonia: 2016 clinical practice guidelines by the Infectious Diseases Society of America and the American Thoracic Society. Clin Infect Dis. 2016;63:e61–111.
33. Oostdijk EAN, de Smet AMGA, Kesecioglu J, Bonten MJM. The role of intestinal colonization with gram-negative bacteria as a source for intensive care unit-acquired bacteremia. Crit Care Med. 2011;39:961–6.
34. Brusselaers N, Labeau S, Vogelaers D, Blot S. Value of lower respiratory tract surveillance cultures to predict bacterial pathogens in ventilator-associated pneumonia: systematic review and diagnostic test accuracy meta-analysis. Intensive Care Med. 2013;39(3):365–75. doi:10.1007/s00134-012-2759-x.
35. Harbarth S, Masuet-Aumatell C, Schrenzel J, Francois P, Akakpo C, Renzi G, et al. Evaluation of rapid screening and pre-emptive contact isolation for detecting and controlling methicillin-resistant Staphylococcus aureus in critical care: an interventional cohort study. Crit Care. 2006;10:25.

36. Nordmann P, Jayol A, Poirel L. Rapid detection of polymyxin resistance in *Enterobacteriaceae*. Emerg Infect Dis. 2016;22:1038–43.
37. Dixon P, Davies P, Hollingworth W, Stoddart M, MacGowan A. A systematic review of matrix-assisted laser desorption/ionisation time-of-flight mass spectrometry compared to routine microbiological methods for the time taken to identify microbial organisms from positive blood cultures. Eur J Clin Microbiol Infect Dis. 2015;34:863–76.
38. Huang AM, Newton D, Kunapuli A, Gandhi TN, Washer LL, Isip J, et al. Impact of rapid organism identification via matrix-assisted laser desorption/ionization time-of-flight combined with antimicrobial stewardship team intervention in adult patients with bacteremia and candidemia. Clin Infect Dis. 2013;57:1237–45.
39. Delport JA, Strikwerda A, Armstrong A, Schaus D, John M. Quality of care is improved by rapid short incubation MALDI-ToF identification from blood cultures as measured by reduced length of stay and patient outcomes as part of a multi-disciplinary approach to bacteremia in pediatric patients. PLoS One. 2016;11:618.
40. Bassetti M, De Waele JJ, Eggimann P, Garnacho-Montero J, Kahlmeter G, Menichetti F, et al. Preventive and therapeutic strategies in critically ill patients with highly resistant bacteria. Intensive Care Med. 2015;41(5):776–95. doi:10.1007/s00134-015-3719-z.
41. Dellit TH, Owens RC, Mcgowan JE, Gerding DN, Weinstein RA, Burke JP, et al. Guidelines for developing an institutional program to enhance antimicrobial stewardship. Clin Infect Dis Oxford J. 2007;44:159–77.
42. Kaki R, Elligsen M, Walker S, Simor A, Palmay L, Daneman N. Impact of antimicrobial stewardship in critical care: a systematic review. J Antimicrob Chemother. 2011;66:1223–30.
43. Montero JG, Lerma FÁ, Galleymore PR, Martínez MP, Rocha LÁ, Gaite FB, et al. Combatting resistance in intensive care: the multimodal approach of the Spanish ICU "Zero Resistance" program. Crit Care. 2015;19:114.
44. Blot S, Depuydt P, Vogelaers D, Decruyenaere J, De Waele J, Hoste E, et al. Colonization status and appropriate antibiotic therapy for nosocomial bacteremia caused by antibiotic-resistant gram-negative bacteria in an intensive care unit. Infect Control Hosp Epidemiol. 2005;26:575–9.
45. Leone M, Bechis C, Baumstarck K, Lefrant J-Y, Albanèse J, Jaber S, et al. De-escalation versus continuation of empirical antimicrobial treatment in severe sepsis: a multicenter non-blinded randomized noninferiority trial. Intensive Care Med. 2014;40:1399–408.
46. Garnacho-Montero J, Gutiérrez-Pizarraya A, Escoresca-Ortega A, Corcia-Palomo Y, Fernández-Delgado E, Herrera-Melero I, et al. De-escalation of empirical therapy is associated with lower mortality in patients with severe sepsis and septic shock. Intensive Care Med. 2014;40:32–40.
47. Montravers P, Augustin P, Grall N, Desmard M, Allou N, Marmuse J-P, et al. Characteristics and outcomes of anti-infective de-escalation during health care-associated intra-abdominal infections. London: Crit Care; 2016.
48. De Bus L, Denys W, Catteeuw J, Gadeyne B, Vermeulen K, Boelens J, et al. Impact of de-escalation of beta-lactam antibiotics on the emergence of antibiotic resistance in ICU patients: a retrospective observational study. Intensive Care Med United States. 2016;42:1029–39.
49. Carlier M, Roberts JA, Stove V, Verstraete AG, Lipman J, De Waele JJ. A simulation study reveals lack of pharmacokinetic/pharmacodynamic target attainment in de-escalated antibiotic therapy in critically Ill patients. Antimicrob Agents Chemother. 2015;59:4689–94.
50. Paul M, Grozinsky-Glasberg S, Soares-Weiser K, Leibovici L. Beta lactam antibiotic monotherapy versus beta lactam-aminoglycoside antibiotic combination therapy for sepsis. Cochrane Database Syst Rev. 2006;(1):CD003344. doi:10.1002/14651858.CD003344.pub2.
51. Tumbarello M, Viale P, Viscoli C, Trecarichi EM, Tumietto F, Marchese A, et al. Predictors of mortality in bloodstream infections caused by *Klebsiella pneumoniae* carbapenemase-producing *K. pneumoniae*: importance of combination therapy. Clin Infect Dis. 2012;55:943–50.
52. Daikos GL, Tsaousi S, Tzouvelekis LS, Anyfantis I, Psichogiou M, Argyropoulou A, et al. Carbapenemase-producing Klebsiella pneumoniae bloodstream infections: lowering mortality by antibiotic combination schemes and the role of carbapenems. Antimicrob Agents Chemother. 2014;58:2322–8.
53. Lopez-Cortes LE, Cisneros JM, Fernandez-Cuenca F, Bou G, Tomas M, Garnacho-Montero J, et al. Monotherapy versus combination therapy for sepsis due to multidrug-resistant *Acinetobacter baumannii*: analysis of a multicentre prospective cohort. J Antimicrob Chemother. 2014;69:3119–26.
54. Falagas ME, Rafailidis PI, Ioannidou E, Alexiou VG, Matthaiou DK, Karageorgopoulos DE, et al. Colistin therapy for microbiologically documented multidrug-resistant Gram-negative bacterial infections: a retrospective cohort study of 258 patients. Int J Antimicrob Agents. 2010;35:194–9.
55. Gu W-J, Wang F, Tang L, Bakker J, Liu J-C. Colistin for the treatment of ventilator-associated pneumonia caused by multidrug-resistant Gram-negative bacteria: a systematic review and meta-analysis. Int J Antimicrob Agents. 2014;44:477–85.
56. Yang H, Zhang C, Zhou Q, Wang Y, Chen L. Clinical outcomes with alternative dosing strategies for piperacillin/tazobactam: a systematic review and meta-analysis. PLoS One. 2015;10(1):e0116769. doi:10.1371/journal.pone.0116769.
57. Ulldemolins M, Martin-Loeches I, Llaurado-Serra M, Fernandez J, Vaquer S, Rodriguez A, et al. Piperacillin population pharmacokinetics in critically ill patients with multiple organ dysfunction syndrome receiving continuous venovenous haemodiafiltration: effect of type of dialysis membrane on dosing requirements. J Antimicrob Chemother. 2016;71:1651–9.
58. Ulldemolins M, Soy D, Llaurado-Serra M, Vaquer S, Castro P, Rodriguez AH, et al. Meropenem population pharmacokinetics in critically ill patients with septic shock and continuous renal replacement therapy: influence of residual diuresis on dose requirements. Antimicrob Agents Chemother. 2015;59:5520–8.
59. de Montmollin E, Bouadma L, Gault N, Mourvillier B, Mariotte E, Chemam S, et al. Predictors of insufficient amikacin peak concentration in critically ill patients receiving a 25 mg/kg total body weight regimen. Intensive Care Med. 2014;40:998–1005.
60. Marsot A, Guilhaumou R, Riff C, Blin O. Amikacin in critically ill patients: a review of population pharmacokinetic studies. Clin Pharmacokinet 2016. doi:10.1007/s40262-016-0428-x.
61. Burdet C, Pajot O, Couffignal C, Armand-Lefevre L, Foucrier A, Laouenan C, et al. Population pharmacokinetics of single-dose amikacin in critically ill patients with suspected ventilator-associated pneumonia. Eur J Clin Pharmacol. 2015;71:75–83.
62. Bergen PJ, Li J, Nation RL. Dosing of colistin-back to basic PK/PD. Curr Opin Pharmacol. 2011;11:464–9.
63. Plachouras D, Karvanen M, Friberg LE, Papadomichelakis E, Antoniadou A, Tsangaris I, et al. Population pharmacokinetic analysis of colistin methanesulfonate and colistin after intravenous administration in critically ill patients with infections caused by gram-negative bacteria. Antimicrob Agents Chemother. 2009;53:3430–6.
64. Parker SL, Frantzeskaki F, Wallis SC, Diakaki C, Giamarellou H, Koulenti D, et al. Population Pharmacokinetics of Fosfomycin in Critically Ill Patients. Antimicrob Agents Chemother. 2015;59:6471–6.
65. http://www.ahaphysicianforum.org/resources/appropriate-use/antimicrobial/content%20files%20pdf/APIC-synergy.pdf.
66. http://www.biocentury.com/antibioticsncepipeline.htm.
67. Chavanet P. The ZEPHyR study: a randomized comparison of linezolid and vancomycin for MRSA pneumonia. Med Mal Infect. 2013;43:451–5.
68. Henken S, Bohling J, Martens-Lobenhoffer J, Paton JC, Ogunniyi AD, Briles DE, et al. Efficacy profiles of daptomycin for treatment of invasive and noninvasive pulmonary infections with *Streptococcus pneumoniae*. Antimicrob Agents Chemother. 2010;54:707–17.
69. Prokocimer P. C DA, Fang E, Mehra P, Das A. Tedizolid phosphate vs linezolid for treatment of acute bacterial skin and skin structure infections: the establish-1 randomized trial. JAMA. 2013;309:559–69.
70. Lee Y, Hong SK, Choi S, Im W, Yong D, Lee K. In vitro activity of tedizolid against gram-positive bacteria in patients with skin and skin structure infections and hospital-acquired pneumonia: a Korean multicenter study. Ann Lab Med. 2015;35:523–30.
71. Donskey CJ, Chowdhry TK, Hecker MT, Hoyen CK, Hanrahan JA, Hujer AM, et al. Effect of antibiotic therapy on the density of vancomycin-resistant enterococci in the stool of colonized patients. N Engl J Med. 2000;343:1925–32.
72. Deshpande A, Hurless K, Cadnum JL, Chesnel L, Gao L, Chan L, et al. Effect of Fidaxomicin versus Vancomycin on Susceptibility to Intestinal Colonization with Vancomycin-Resistant Enterococci and Klebsiella pneumoniae in Mice. Antimicrob Agents Chemother. 2016;60:3988–93.
73. Miller WR, Munita JM, Arias CA. Mechanisms of antibiotic resistance in enterococci. Expert Rev Anti Infect Ther. 2014;12:1221–36.
74. Zhanel GG, Calic D, Schweizer F, Zelenitsky S, Adam H, Lagac-Wiens PRS, et al. New lipoglycopeptides: a comparative review of

dalbavancin, oritavancin and telavancin. Drugs. 2010;70(7):859–86. doi:10.2165/11534440-000000000-00000.
75. Bassetti M, Poulakou G, Giamarellou H. Is there a future for tigecycline? Intensive Care Med. 2014;40:1039–45.
76. Montravers P, Dupont H, Bedos JP, Bret P, Tigecycline Group. Tigecycline use in critically ill patients: a multicentre prospective observational study in the intensive care setting. Intensive Care Med. 2014;40(7):988–97. doi:10.1007/s00134-014-3323-7.
77. Qureshi ZA, Paterson DL, Potoski BA, Kilayko MC, Sandovsky G, Sordillo E, et al. Treatment outcome of bacteremia due to KPC-producing Klebsiella pneumoniae: superiority of combination antimicrobial regimens. Antimicrob Agents Chemother. 2012;56:2108–13.
78. Lucasti C, Popescu I, Ramesh MK, Lipka J, Sable C. Comparative study of the efficacy and safety of ceftazidime/avibactam plus metronidazole versus meropenem in the treatment of complicated intra-abdominal infections in hospitalized adults: results of a randomized, double-blind, Phase II trial. J Antimicrob Chemother. 2013;68:1183–92.
79. http://www.prnewswire.com/news-releases/actavis-receives-us-fda-approval-for-avycaz-ceftazidime-avibactam-300041592.html.
80. Zhanel GG, Chung P, Adam H, Zelenitsky S, Denisuik A, Schweizer F, et al. Ceftolozane/tazobactam: a novel cephalosporin/beta-lactamase inhibitor combination with activity against multidrug-resistant gram-negative bacilli. Drugs. 2014;74:31–51.
81. Michalopoulos AS, Falagas ME. Inhaled antibiotics in mechanically ventilated patients. Minerva Anestesiol. 2014;80:236–44.
82. Sole-Lleonart C, Rouby J-J, Chastre J, Poulakou G, Palmer LB, Blot S, et al. Intratracheal administration of antimicrobial agents in mechanically ventilated adults: an international survey on delivery practices and safety. Respir Care. 2016;61:1008–14.
83. Garnacho-Montero J, Amaya-Villar R, Gutirrez-Pizarraya A, Espejo-Gutirrez De Tena E, Artero-Gonzlez ML, Corcia-Palomo Y, et al. Clinical efficacy and safety of the combination of colistin plus vancomycin for the treatment of severe infections caused by carbapenem-resistant acinetobacter baumannii. Chemotherapy. 2014;59:225–31.
84. Bulik CC, Nicolau DP. Double-carbapenem therapy for carbapenemase-producing *Klebsiella pneumoniae*. Antimicrob Agents Chemother. 2011;55:3002–4.
85. Giamarellou H, Galani L, Baziaka F, Karaiskos I. Effectiveness of a double-carbapenem regimen for infections in humans due to carbapenemase-producing pandrug-resistant *Klebsiella pneumoniae*. Antimicrob Agents Chemother. 2013;57:2388–90.
86. Westritschnig K, Hochreiter R, Wallner G, Firbas C, Schwameis M, Jilma B. A randomized, placebo-controlled phase I study assessing the safety and immunogenicity of a *Pseudomonas aeruginosa* hybrid outer membrane protein OprF/I vaccine (IC43) in healthy volunteers. Hum Vaccin Immunother. 2014;10(1):170–83. doi:10.4161/hv.26565.
87. Sulakvelidze A, Alavidze Z, Morris JG. Bacteriophage therapy. Antimicrob Agents Chemother. 2001;45:649–59. doi:10.1128/AAC.45.3.649-659.2001.
88. Yang S-J, Xiong YQ, Boyle-Vavra S, Daum R, Jones T, Bayer AS. Daptomycin-oxacillin combinations in treatment of experimental endocarditis caused by daptomycin-nonsusceptible strains of methicillin-resistant Staphylococcus aureus with evolving oxacillin susceptibility (the "seesaw effect"). Antimicrob Agents Chemother. 2010;54:3161–9.
89. Mehta S, Singh C, Plata KB, Chanda PK, Paul A, Riosa S, et al. beta-Lactams increase the antibacterial activity of daptomycin against clinical methicillin-resistant Staphylococcus aureus strains and prevent selection of daptomycin-resistant derivatives. Antimicrob Agents Chemother. 2012;56:6192–200.

Epidemiology of extended-spectrum beta-lactamase-producing *Enterobacteriaceae* in an intensive care unit with no single rooms

Xavier Repessé[1], Margaux Artiguenave[1], Sophie Paktoris-Papine[1], Florence Espinasse[2], Aurélien Dinh[3], Cyril Charron[1], Faten El Sayed[4], Guillaume Geri[1,5,6] and Antoine Vieillard-Baron[1,5,6*]

Abstract

Background: The transmission of extended-spectrum beta-lactamase-producing *enterobacteriaceae* (ESBL) is prevented by additional contact precautions, mainly relying on isolation in a single room and hand hygiene. Contact isolation cannot be achieved in our 12-bed ICU, which has only double rooms. We report the epidemiology of ESBL imported, acquired and transmitted in an ICU with no single rooms.

Methods: We prospectively conducted an observational and non-interventional study in a French 12-bed ICU. Inclusion criteria were patients >18 years of age treated by at least two successive nursing teams. Patient characteristics at admission and clinical data during hospital stay were collected prospectively. ESBL carriage was monitored using rectal swabs collected at admission and once weekly during the ICU stay. Potential cross-transmission was studied (1) by identifying index patients defined as possible ESBL sources for transmission, (2) by classifying each ESBL strain according to the cefotaximase *München* (CTX_M) 1 and 9 groups and (3) by gene sequencing for remaining cases of possible transmission.

Results: From June 2014 to April 2015, of 550 patients admitted to the ICU, 470 met the inclusion criteria and 221 had at least two rectal swabs. The rate of ESBL colonization, mainly by *Escherichia coli*, at admission was 13.2%. The incidence of ESBL acquisition, mainly with *E. coli* too, was 4.1%. Mortality did not differ between ESBL carriers and non-carriers. In univariate analysis, ESBL acquisition was associated with male gender, SAPS II, SOFA, chronic kidney disease at admission, duration of mechanical ventilation, need for catecholamine and the ICU LOS. In multivariate analysis, SAPS II at admission was the only risk factor for ESBL acquisition. We confirmed cross-transmission, emanating from the same index patient, in two of the nine patients with ESBL acquisition (0.8%, 2/221). No case of cross-transmission in the same double room was observed.

Discussion and conclusion: Prevalence of ESBL colonization in our ICU was 13.2%. Despite the absence single rooms, the incidence of ESBL acquisition was 4.1% and cross-transmission was proven in only two cases, resulting from the same index patient who was not hospitalized in the same double room.

Background

Multidrug-resistant organisms (MDROs), and specifically third-generation cephalosporin-resistant *Enterobacteriaceae*, constitute a major problem in hospitals [1]. In the intensive care unit (ICU), Gram-negative resistant pathogens are responsible for longer hospitalizations and poorer outcomes [2, 3]. In the absence of new broad-spectrum antibiotics, there is a need to control antibiotic consumption and to prevent patient-to-patient cross-transmission. Recommended contact precautions, based on hand hygiene and the use of gowns, are considered as the cornerstone of preventive measures, along with isolation in a single room [4, 5],

*Correspondence: antoine.vieillard-baron@apr.aphp.fr; antoine.vieillard-baron@aphp.fr
[1] Intensive Care Unit, Section Thorax-Vascular Disease-Abdomen-Metabolism, Assistance Publique-Hôpitaux de Paris, University Hospital Ambroise Paré, 9, Avenue Charles-de-Gaulle, 92100 Boulogne-Billancourt, France
Full list of author information is available at the end of the article

especially for known carriers of resistant bacteria, defined as methicillin-resistant *Staphylococcus aureus*, extended-spectrum beta-lactamase (ESBL) and non-fermenting Gram-negative bacilli resistant to many antibiotics [6]. Moreover, ESBL-producing *Enterobacteriaceae* have the particularity of being part of the digestive flora, which means that specific precautions are required for the disposal of stools [6]. However, all these preventive precautions have mainly been evaluated in the context of hospital outbreaks of ESBL-producing *K. pneumoniae* or *E. cloacae* [7]. They have become debatable for very uncommon outbreaks of ESBL-producing *E. coli*, and it has been suggested that routine contact isolation in a single room could be challenged in a non-epidemic setting [8, 9].

We studied the analytic epidemiology of ESBL acquisition and transmission in an ICU without single rooms and the capacity for strict isolation of patients. Our hypothesis was that an ICU with double rooms is not associated with unexpected high acquisition and cross-transmission of ESBL, providing that contact precautions are strictly applied. Our secondary objectives were to report the incidences of and factors associated with ESBL acquisition and colonization at admission.

Methods

Study population and data collection

This non-interventional observational and usual care study was prospectively conducted in the 12-bed ICU of the tertiary university hospital Ambroise Paré (Boulogne-Billancourt, France). As for all our non-interventional studies, patients or their relatives were routinely informed that data recorded during hospitalization in the ICU may be used for observational research and scientific publications and that they may refuse at any time.

Consecutive patients were included if they met the following inclusion criteria:

- Patients >18 years old admitted to ICU.
- Taken in charge by at least two shifts of nurses during their stay in our ICU.

Our nurses operate 12-h shifts and each cares for between two and three patients, as recommended by French law. Patients given nursing care for a single shift, i.e., who were discharged or who died in the first 12 h following admission, were not included.

We recorded the main characteristics at admission, as age, gender, Simplified Acute Physiology Score (SAPS II) [10], SOFA [11], hospitalization within the 3 months before ICU admission, antibiotic exposure and travel within the 3 months before admission, transfer from another service or institution, as well as the main information concerning the ICU stay (mechanical ventilation and duration, ICU length of stay [LOS], antibiotic prescription, duration of antibiotic exposure, central venous and arterial catheters, dialysis, in-ICU mortality).

Hygiene and isolation protocol

Our 12-bed ICU has three units each of two double rooms, so that isolation of ESBL carriers in a single room cannot be achieved. Each double-room area is around 20 m^2. A rigid removable curtain (H 1.5 m, L 1.75 m) separates the two beds in each room. A preventive isolation protocol with contact precautions is routinely implemented in our unit at admission for patients expected to have high-risk factors for antibiotic resistance (age > 65 years, transfer from another ward or institution or already known ESBL carriage). We routinely used waterless alcohol-based hand rub and wore gowns before entering the room for such patients. These preventive measures were stopped when the first sample showed no MDRO. Moreover, our institution implemented measures for the elimination of *excreta* of MDRO carriers, in particular the widespread use of bedpan liners (Care-Bag, Cleanis, Paris, France) and a specific washbasin for the scrubbing of the bedpans. Finally, the manager of the infection control unit of the hospital (FE) conducts weekly checks that contact precautions are applied, in collaboration with the nursing officer of the ICU.

Consumption of alcohol-based hand rub (expressed in L/1000 patient-days or mL/patient-day) and of antibiotics (expressed in defined daily doses/1000 patient-days) is evaluated each year, and compliance with the hand hygiene protocol is assessed using blinded audits. These audits check compliance with the protocol by means of two care bundles each relating to three aspects of hand hygiene, one before the nurse provides healthcare and one after.

Microbiological analysis

Rectal swabs were sampled at admission and then weekly, every Monday, as recommended by our usual local protocol. They were sown on Drigalski medium (Biomérieux, Marcy l'Etoile, France) and then on ESBL selective medium, Chrom ID™ ESBL (Biomérieux, Marcy l'Etoile, France). After incubation at 35 °C, antimicrobial susceptibility was evaluated at 24 and 48 h for each colony that grew on the selective medium. The ESBL gene (*bla*) was amplified and analyzed by two polymerase chain reactions for a cefotaximase *München* (CTX_M) 1 and 9 groups. The gene *bla* was sequenced according to the Sanger method on the capillary sequencer ABI Prism 3130 (Applied Biosystems, Villebon-sur-Yvette, France) with the kit BigDye Terminator Cycle Sequencing (Thermo Fisher Scientific, Villebon-sur-Yvette, France). Comparison with already known sequences was made with the BLAST program (Basic Local Alignment Search Tool, blast.ncbi.nlm.nih.gov) from the National Center for Biotechnology Information.

ESBL acquisition was defined as a negative first screening at admission with a positive one during the ICU stay, at least 48 h after admission. ESBL colonization was defined as a positive ESBL screening at admission. All acquired carriers were considered as possible cases of patient-to-patient transmission. Patient-to-patient transmission was analyzed in three steps. The first step was the identification of potential index patients defined as known ESBL carriers hospitalized at the same time as the newly acquired carrier. The second step was the description and identification of ESBL as well as their comparison according to their CTX_M 1 or 9 groups. Transmission was excluded if the index's ESBL strains differed from the case's. Finally, the third step was the sequencing of the genes (*bla*) corresponding to the matched identified group. Transmission was excluded if the gene sequencing differed. Transmission was retained in the case of a matched ESBL group in two patients who had been hospitalized in the same period for at least one day if the gene sequencing was similar.

Statistical analysis

Categorical variables were described as *n* (%) and compared with Pearson's Chi-squared test or Fisher's exact test, as appropriate. Continuous variables were described as median [interquartile] and compared using a Mann–Whitney test.

Factors associated with ESBL acquisition were picked up using a univariate analysis. Then, clinically relevant factors significantly associated with ESBL acquisition in the univariate analysis were included in a multivariate logistic regression. ESBL acquisition was the dependent variable. Regarding the nonlinear relationship between ICU LOS, SAPS II and outcome, we used fractional polynomials (using the *mfp* Stata function) for a better fit between independent and dependent variables, as previously recommended [12]. We presented the results as the odds ratio of ESBL acquisition for the median of categories (named as reference), as previously reported [12]. The goodness of fit of the model was studied using the Hosmer–Lemeshow test. Statistical analysis was performed using MedCalc Software™, Ostend, Belgium. The multivariate logistic regression was performed using Stata 14.1 software (Stata Corp., College Station, TX, USA). A p value < 0.05 was considered as statistically significant.

Results

Settings and characteristics of the population

Of 550 patients admitted to the ICU between June 1, 2014, and April 30, 2015, 71 were not included because they were present in the ICU for only one 12-h nursing shift. Nine patients were excluded because no rectal swab was sampled at admission. Finally, 470 patients met the inclusion criteria (Fig. 1). Their mean age was 66.0 [54.0, 77.0] years, 60.2% ($n = 283$) were males, and their mean SAPS II was 46.0 [32.0, 62.0] (Table 1). The hospitalization LOS was 4.0 [2.0, 8.0] days, and duration of mechanical ventilation was 2.0 [0.0, 5.0] days. Two hundred and twenty-four patients (47.8%) received mechanical ventilation. Half of the patients received catecholamine and had at least one central venous catheter and/or an arterial catheter. In-ICU mortality was 13.2%.

The consumption of alcohol-based hand rub was 136.8 L/1000 patient-days in 2014 and 135.0 L/1000 patient-days in 2015. The consumption of antibiotics was 1453 DDD/1000 patient-days and 1331 DDD/1000 patient-days in 2014 and 2015, respectively. The blinded audits showed 63% compliance in 2014 and 77% in 2015.

ESBL-imported carriage

Of the 470 patients included, 62 (13.2%) carried an ESBL at ICU admission, with *Escherichia coli* in 77.9% of the strains (Table 2). The main characteristics of these patients are presented in Table 1. Four of these 62 patients were colonized with two strains of ESBL and one with three strains. As given in Table 1, no factor associated with ESBL-imported carriage, except a history of peripheral arterial disease ($p = 0.007$), was observed in univariate analysis, in particular age ($p = 0.8$), SAPS II ($p = 0.6$), hospitalization during the past three months ($p = 0.08$), transfer from another unit ($p = 0.8$) and antibiotic exposure during the past three months ($p = 0.5$).

ESBL acquisition

The incidence of ESBL acquisition was analyzed in 221 patients, whose characteristics are presented in Table 3. Nine patients acquired ESBL carriage, leading to an overall incidence of 4.1%. One of them acquired two different ESBL strains. The median time of acquisition was 8 [5–11] days. As reported in Table 3, in univariate analysis, those patients had higher SAPS II ($p = 0.007$) and SOFA ($p = 0.01$) scores, with a longer LOS (11 [9, 26] vs. 7 [5, 12] days, respectively, $p = 0.007$), than patients who did not acquire ESBL. All of them received mechanical ven-tilation ($p = 0.1$) and catecholamine infusion ($p = 0.001$). In multivariate analysis, only SAPS II at admission remained associated with ESBL acquisition (Table 4).

ESBL cross-transmission

All acquired ESBL carriers were considered as possible cases of transmission. The nine patients with ESBL acquisition were associated with 16 potential index patients for whom the chronological scale analysis is reported in

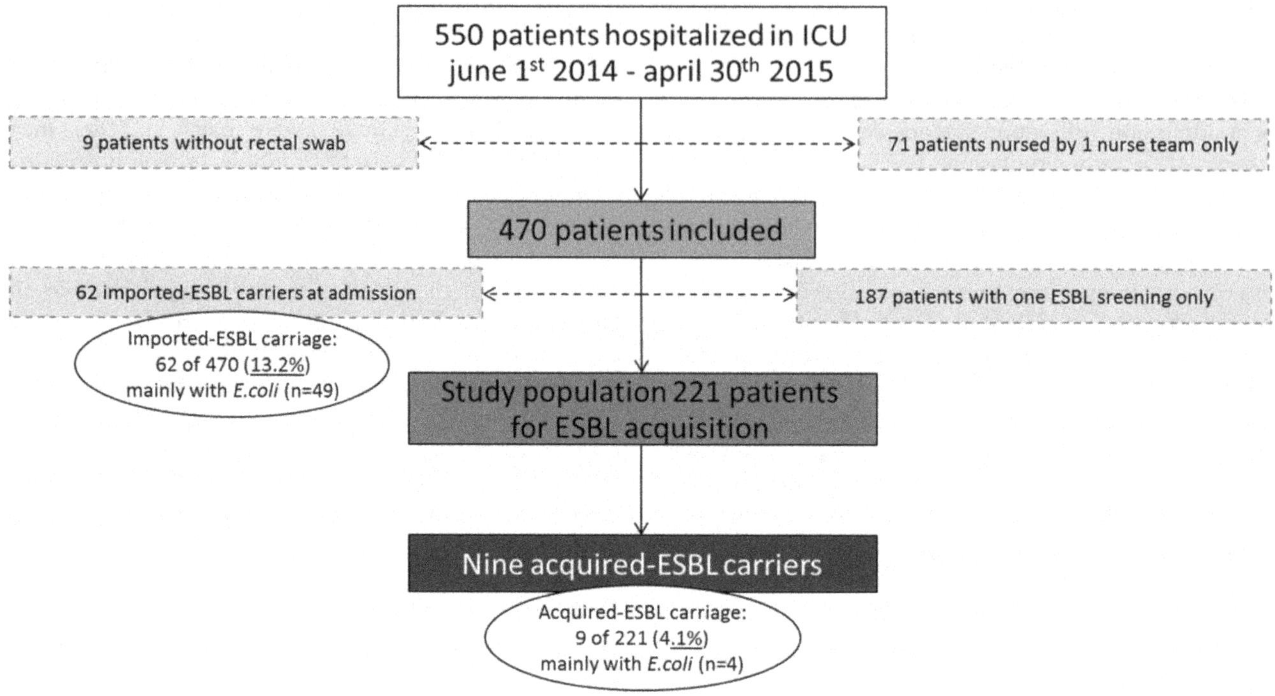

Fig. 1 Flowchart of the patients included in the study. *ESBL* extended-spectrum beta-lactamase, *ICU* intensive care unit

Additional file 1. Of five strains of *E. coli* isolated, three belonged to the group CTX_M 1 and 2 to the CTX_M 9 group (Table 2). The five other ESBL were mainly from the CTX_M 1 group ($n = 4$), and we were unable to identify the group in one case (*Citrobacter freundii*). The ESBL group excluded cross-transmission in four cases. For the five remaining acquired ESBL carriers, with the strain belonging to the same group as the potential index patient, gene sequencing identified the same gene for three patients (index P219 for two cases P203 and P220, Fig. 2). For these two cases of acquired ESBL (P203 and P220), patient-to-patient transmission was considered as proven. The acquired gene was observed in *E. coli* in one case (P203) and in *E. cloacae* in the other (P220). Both patients who acquired ESBL shared, respectively, one and two days with the index patient (Fig. 2). Neither was hospitalized in the same double room as the index patient: One patient was hospitalized in the same unit and the other in another one.

Discussion

In this prospective observational study in 470 consecutive patients admitted to a 12-bed medical and surgical ICU with no single rooms, the prevalence of imported ESBL carriage was 13.2% and the incidence of acquired carriage was 4.1%, mostly with *E. coli*. No factor was identified as associated with imported ESBL carriage, while the severity at admission (SAPS II) was independently associated with ESBL acquisition. Only two cases of cross-transmission from the same index patient were reported.

Imported carriage

The rate of imported ESBL carriage reported here is comparable to the 10–15% previously reported in three studies performed in French ICUs [13–15]. This prevalence is much higher than the 3.5% recently reported by Barbier et al. [16], but the latter study was performed in a historical cohort (1996–2016) of 16,734 patients admitted to 17 French ICUs and ESBL prevalence has changed dramatically in the last two decades. Although we noted no relation between severity at admission and imported ESBL, Alves et al. recently reported a lower rate of imported ESBL carriage of 8% in 308 patients with a much lower severity than in our population [17]. Finally, like Razazi et al. [13], we did not identify any impact of the ESBL-imported carriage on mortality, confirming the data of Barbier et al., who showed that ESBL infection was responsible for a 1.8-fold increase in mortality, while ESBL carriage had no impact on mortality [16].

Acquired carriage

Despite the unfavorable double-room configuration of our ICU, the 4.1% rate of ESBL acquisition was much lower than the 13% reported by Razazi et al. in a 24-bed ICU with eight single rooms but without any protocol of contact precautions for ESBL carriers [13]. It is close to

Table 1 Main characteristics of the population

Variable	All patients $n = 470$	No ESBL colonization $n = 408$	ESBL colonization $n = 62$	*p*
Age (years)	66.0 [54.0, 77.0]	66 [54, 77]	68 [57, 78]	0.5
Age > 65 years	256 (54.5)	218 (53.4)	38 (61.3)	0.3
Male gender	283 (60.2)	245 (60.0)	38 (61.3)	0.9
SAPS II	46.0 [32.0, 62.0]	45 [32, 62]	49 [37.3, 55.5]	0.5
SOFA score	7.0 [4.0, 9.0]	6 [4, 9]	7 [4.5, 8.5]	0.6
Preexisting conditions				
Heart failure	65 (13.9)	53 (13.0)	12 (19.3)	0.2
Peripheral arterial disease	60 (12.8)	45 (11.0)	15 (24.2)	0.007
Diabetes	110 (23.5)	91 (22.3)	19 (36.8)	0.2
Cirrhosis	21 (4.5)	18 (4.4)	3 (4.8)	0.8
Chronic obstructive pulmonary disease	69 (14.7)	59 (14.4)	10 (16.1)	0.9
Chronic kidney disease	61 (13.0)	52 (12.7)	9 (14.5)	0.8
Immunosuppression	75 (16.0)	62 (15.2)	12 (19.3)	0.5
Mechanical ventilation	283 (60.2)	248 (60.8)	35 (56.5)	0.6
Catecholamine use	224 (47.8)	190 (46.6)	34 (54.8)	0.3
Duration of mechanical ventilation (days)	2.0 [0.0, 5.0]	2.0 [0.0, 5.0]	1.0 [0.0, 4.0]	0.4
ICU length of stay (days)	4.0 [2.0, 8.0]	4 [2.0, 8.0]	4.0 [3.0, 8.0]	0.8
Transfer from another unit	239 (50.9)	206 (50.5)	33 (53.2)	0.8
Postoperative care	109 (23.2)	94 (23.0)	14 (22.6)	0.9
Hospitalization within the previous 3 months	243 (51.7)	204 (50)	39 (62.9)	0.08
Antibiotics within the previous 3 months	81 (17.2)	68 (16.7)	13 (20.1)	0.5
Antibiotics during ICU	346 (73.6)	303 (74.3)	43 (69.3)	0.5
Duration of antibiotic therapy	3.0 [0.0, 6.0]	3.0 [0.0, 6.0]	3.0 [0.0, 7.0]	0.8
Mortality	62 (13.2)	56 (13.7)	6 (9.7)	0.2

Categorical data are expressed as *n* (%)

Quantitative data are expressed as median [IQR]

Table 2 Summary of the 68 strains responsible for the 62 ESBL-imported carriages and of the ten strains responsible for the nine ESBL-acquired carriages

Strain	Imported ESBL				Acquired ESBL			
	n	CTX_M 1 group	CTX_M 9 group	Other group	*n*	CTX_M 1 group	CTX_M 9 group	Other group
E. coli	53	30	15	8	5	3	2	0
K. pneumoniae	10	8	0	2	1	1	0	0
E. cloacae	1	1	0	0	2	2	0	0
C. freundii	1	1	0	0	1	0	0	1
P. mirabilis	0	0	0	0	1	1	0	0
P. vulgaris	1	0	0	1	0	0	0	0
C. koseri	2	2	0	0	0	0	0	0
Total	68	43	15	11	10	7	2	1

that reported by Alves et al. in an ICU with only single rooms, in which contact precautions were also applied [17]. Unlike Barbier et al., who reported that half of the ESBL carriers acquired their ESBL during their ICU stay [16], and Gardam et al., who reported that ESBL acquisition accounted for two-thirds of ESBL carriage in the ICU [18], ESBL acquisition accounted for only 12.7% of all ESBL carriage in our study, confirming that ESBL carriage is mostly imported, whereas high-level cephalosporinase (HL-Case) is mostly acquired, in the ICU [19].

Table 3 Main characteristics of the study population for ESBL acquisition and factors associated with ESBL acquisition in univariate analysis

Variable	All patients $n = 221$	No ESBL acquisition $n = 212$	ESBL acquisition $n = 9$	*p*
Age (years)	67.0 [55.0, 77.0]	66.5 [55.0, 76.0]	82.0 [66.0, 82.0]	0.07
Age > 65 years	123 (55.6)	116 (54.7)	7 (78)	0.3
Male gender	144 (65.2)	137 (64.6)	7 (77.8)	0.5
SAPS II	49.0 [35.0, 66.0]	48.0 [35.0, 65.0]	72.0 [55.0, 77.0]	0.007
SOFA score	7.0 [4.0, 10.0]	7.0 [4.0, 10.0]	10.0 [9.0, 12.0]	0.01
Preexisting condition				
Heart failure	32 (14.5)	30 (14.1)	2 (28.6)	0.6
Peripheral arterial disease	25 (11.3)	22 (10.3)	3 (33.3)	0.07
Diabetes	54 (24.4)	51 (24)	3 (33.3)	0.5
Cirrhosis	10 (4.5)	9 (4.2)	1 (11.1)	0.4
Chronic obstructive pulmonary disease	39 (17.6)	37 (17.5)	2 (22.2)	0.7
Chronic kidney disease	36 (16.3)	32 (15.1)	4 (44.4)	0.04
Immunosuppression	38 (17.2)	36 (17.0)	2 (22.2)	0.7
Mechanical ventilation	166 (75.1)	157 (74.1)	9 (100)	0.1
Catecholamine use	132 (59.7)	123 (58.0)	9 (100)	0.01
Duration of mechanical ventilation (days)	4.0 [1.0, 10.0]	4.0 [0.0, 10.0]	9.0 [7.0, 11.0]	0.03
ICU length of stay (days)	8.0 [5.0, 12.0]	7.0 [5.0, 12.0]	11.0 [9.0, 26.0]	0.007
Transfer from another unit	124 (56.1)	117 (55.2)	7 (77.8)	0.3
Postoperative care	58 (26.2)	54 (25.5)	4 (44.4)	0.2
Hospitalization within the previous 3 months	123 (55.7)	117 (55.2)	6 (66.7)	0.7
Antibiotics within the previous 3 months	40 (18.1)	37 (17.5)	3 (33.3)	0.2
Antibiotics during ICU stay	193 (87.3)	184 (86.8)	9 (100)	0.6
Duration of antibiotic therapy	5.0 [3.0, 8.0]	5.0 [3.0, 8.0]	8.0 [5.0, 13.5]	0.1

Categorical data are expressed as *n* (%)

Quantitative data are expressed as median [IQR]

Table 4 Multivariate analysis of factors associated with ESBL acquisition

Variable	Reference	Odds ratio	95% Confidence interval
ICU length of stay (days)			
<4	3	0.92	0.82, 1.04
4–7	6	1.00	1.00, 1.00
7–10	9	1.08	0.96, 1.22
>10	15	1.28	0.89, 1.83
SAPS II			
<32	25	1.00	1.00, 1.00
33–45	40	1.89	1.11, 3.24
45–60	53	3.44	1.22, 9.68
>60	73	7.40	1.38, 39.59

Multivariate logistic regression including 218 complete observations

Hosmer–Lemeshow *p* value 0.6

SAPS II and ICU length of stay were included as continuous variables

SAPS II was not transformed

ICU length of stay was included using the following equation $x^2 - 1.96$ where $x = (\text{los})/10$

Covariates were included as continuous variables in the multivariable model

Presented odds ratios were calculated for the reference indicated in the table

In multivariate analysis, the severity (SAPS II) at admission was the only factor identified to be associated with the acquired carriage of ESBL, while some authors have reported that the duration of exposure to an ESBL carrier is independently associated with ESBL acquisition [13, 20]. Nevertheless, we found very short contact times for both cases of proven cross-transmission and ICU LOS was not independently associated with acquisition of ESBL in our study, which seems to temper the impact of the duration of contact in the mechanism of ESBL acquisition.

Our results confirm our hypothesis that a high level of infection control and a low rate of cross-transmission can be achieved despite the absence of isolation in single rooms, providing compliance with hand hygiene is high and antibiotic consumption is controlled. Consumption of alcohol-based hand rub for the study period was twice that usually reported in European ICUs [21], and the results of blinded audits of hand hygiene were considered very acceptable. Zahar et al. suggest that contact isolation is not needed to control the spread of ESBL-producing *E. coli* [9]. This was recently confirmed by Tschudin-Sutter

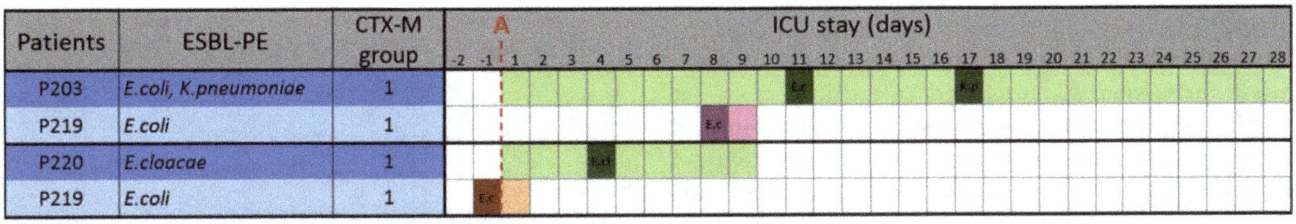

Fig. 2 Chronological scale of the two cases of ESBL cross-transmission in the ICU. The figure represents the timescale of ESBL cross-transmission. Patients are identified with their inclusion number. The two cases of cross-transmission (P203 and P220) are colored in *dark blue*, whereas the corresponding index patient (P219) is materialized in *light blue*. Index patient is defined as already known carriers of ESBL who shared at least one day of hospitalization with the case of ESBL acquisition. *Each line* represents the stay of one patient. A day of hospitalization is represented by *a square*. *Each block* separated by *bold lines* represents a case of cross-transmission. The ICU stays of the cross-transmitted ESBL patients are *green*, whereas the stay of the index patient is colored in *pink* if the index patient is hospitalized in a different unit, in *orange* for hospitalization in the same unit but not in the same room. The *dotted red line* indicates the arrival in the ICU of patients acquiring ESBL. *A* arrival, *Ec Escherichia coli*, *Ecl Enterobacter cloacae*, *Cf Citrobacter freundii*, *CTXm* cefotaximase München, *ESBL-PE* extended-spectrum beta-lactamase-producing *Enterobacteriaceae*, *ICU* intensive care unit, *Kp Klebsiella pneumoniae*, *P* patient, *Pm Proteus mirabilis*

et al. who showed no increase of transmission of ESBL-producing *E. coli* after contact precautions were discontinued, neither in an acute-care setting, nor in a geriatric hospital [20]. Moreover, Derde et al. demonstrated that 80% compliance with hand hygiene was associated with a decrease in *S. aureus* (MRSA) acquisition, even if it was not proven for vancomycin-resistant *Enterococci* (VRE) or highly resistant *Enterobacteriaceae* [22]. Guidelines concerning contact precautions and the recommended isolation rely on studies demonstrating their efficacy in controlling the spread of MRSA [23], VRE [24] and ESBL-producing *K. pneumoniae* [7], but such measures have not been fully validated for the now predominant CTX_M group of ESBL-producing *E. coli*. Isolation in single rooms could raise other issues since it has been shown to be associated with adverse outcomes, such as less patient–healthcare worker contact, delays in care provided, increased non-infectious adverse events and increased symptoms of depression and anxiety in patients [25].

Cross-transmission

Only two cases of proven cross-transmission were identified among the nine acquired ESBL carriers. Both transmissions emanated from the same index patient and did not occur in the same double room. These results are in accordance with former studies that showed that cross-transmission is quite a rare mechanism of ESBL acquisition. In a Swiss population including ICU and non-ICU patients, Tschudin-Sutter et al. [8] confirmed transmission by pulse-field gel electrophoresis in two (1.5%) of 133 contacts of ESBL carriers hospitalized in the same room at least 24 h before identification of ESBL carriage and then isolation in a single room. Among 19 acquired ESBL carriers, Alves et al. recently identified only one case of likely patient-to-patient cross-transmission [17]. In a study at the beginning of the 2000s in a transplantation unit of four rooms with four beds, eight double rooms and four single rooms, Gardam et al. reported possible patient-to-patient transmission in only six of 69 cases of ESBL acquisition [18]. In fact, the mechanism of acquisition of ESBL is not so obvious and the antibiotic exposure or the persistence of pathogens on inanimate surfaces could play an important role [26], even if the role of persistent environmental contamination as a reservoir for ESBL cross-transmission remains debatable. While *A. baumannii* is well known to survive in surface dust for months, other Gram-negative bacteria are not usually resilient to desiccation, while *E. coli*, *Klebsiella* spp. and *P. aeruginosa* are reportedly also able to survive more than a year on inert surfaces [26].

Limitations

We acknowledge that our study suffers from several limitations. First, the rate of acquisition could have been underestimated. Indeed, we did not perform a rectal swab at discharge and some patients may have acquired an ESBL between the last rectal swab and ICU discharge. Moreover, the number of patients could be considered as insufficient since 187/470 patients were not included in the analysis of the acquisition because they had only one rectal swab. Finally, it could be assumed that some cases of acquisition were not detected because of the lack of sensitivity of the rectal screening, in particular in patients with low levels of microorganisms, since we did not use enrichment before plating, which has been reported to improve sensitivity [27]. Nevertheless, several measures were applied to limit the number of false-negative screening results. First, nurses were trained to send for analysis only samples with a sufficient amount of stool on the swab. Second, the laboratory asked for a new sample if the standard cultures were sterile. Finally, swabs were seeded on a selective medium to improve the detection of ESBL. The second limitation is that our study does not allow understanding the mechanisms of acquisition when cross-transmission was excluded. We cannot rule out other hypotheses, such as transmission from unidentified carriers at admission, because of a lack of sensitivity of the rectal ESBL screening, and such as the impact of the selection pressure of antibiotics or the role of contamination by health care workers or inanimate surfaces.

Conclusion

We reported an ESBL colonization prevalence of 13.2% at ICU admission, mainly with *E. coli*, and an incidence of ESBL acquisition of 4.1%, among which we noted only two cases of ESBL cross-transmission. Our study demonstrates that, despite the lack of single rooms, it is possible to reach a high level of infection control and a low rate of cross-transmission. The impact of isolation in the prevention of ESBL cross-transmission in the absence of an epidemic setting and the mechanisms underlying ESBL acquisition remain to be elucidated.

Additional file

Additional file 1. The figure represents the timescale of ESBL acquisition. Patients are identified with their inclusion number. The nine patients who acquired ESBL during are colored in *dark blue*, whereas the 16 corresponding index patients are materialized in *light blue*. Index patients are defined as already known carriers of ESBL who shared at least one day of hospitalization with a case of acquisition. Among the 16 potential index patients, two were newly acquired ESBL carriers (P203 and P220). Eight index patients were hospitalized in the same unit and seven in a different one. Only one potential index patient was hospitalized in the same room. The median time of acquisition was 8 [5–11] days, while the median shared hospitalization with the index patients was 5 [3–9] days. *Each line* represents the stay of one patient. A day of hospitalization is represented by *a square*. *Each block* separated by *bold lines* represents a case of acquisition. The ICU stays of the patients who acquired ESBL are *green*, whereas the stay of the index patients is colored in *pink* if the index patient is hospitalized in a different unit, in *orange* for hospitalization in the same unit but not in the same room and in *yellow* for hospitalization in the same unit and the same room. The *dotted red line* indicates the arrival in the ICU of patients acquiring ESBL. The cases of transmission and their relatives' index patients are separated by a *horizontal black bold line*. *A* arrival, *Ec Escherichia coli*, *Ecl Enterobacter cloacae*, *Cf Citrobacter freundii*, *CTXm* cefotaximase München, *ESBL-PE* extended-spectrum beta-lactamase-producing *Enterobacteriaceae*, *ICU* intensive care unit, *Kp Klebsiella pneumoniae*, *P* patient, *Pm Proteus mirabilis*.

Abbreviations

ESBL: extended-spectrum beta-lactamase; CTX_M: cefotaximase *München*; ICU: intensive care unit; LOS: length of stay; MDRO: multidrug-resistant organism; SAPS II: Simplified Acute Physiology Score; SOFA: Sequential Organ Failure Assessment.

Authors' contributions

XR, CC, AD and AVB designed the study. XR, MA, SPP, FEL and FE collected data. XR, GG, AD and AVB analyzed the data. XR, GG and AVB wrote the manuscript. All authors read and approved the final manuscript.

Author details

[1] Intensive Care Unit, Section Thorax-Vascular Disease-Abdomen-Metabolism, Assistance Publique-Hôpitaux de Paris, University Hospital Ambroise Paré, 9, Avenue Charles-de-Gaulle, 92100 Boulogne-Billancourt, France. [2] Infection Control Unit, Section Biology Pathology and Health Products, Assistance Publique-Hôpitaux de Paris, University Hospital Ambroise Paré, 92100 Boulogne-Billancourt, France. [3] Infectious Diseases Department, Assistance Publique-Hôpitaux de Paris, University Hospital Ambroise Paré, 92100 Boulogne-Billancourt, France. [4] Microbiology Unit, Section Biology Pathology and Health Products, Assistance Publique-Hôpitaux de Paris, University Hospital Ambroise Paré, 92100 Boulogne-Billancourt, France. [5] Faculty of Medicine Paris Ile-de-France Ouest, University of Versailles Saint-Quentin en Yvelines, 78280 Saint-Quentin-en-Yvelines, France. [6] INSERM U-1018, CESP, Team 5 (EpReC, Renal and Cardiovascular Epidemiology), UVSQ, 94807 Villejuif, France.

Competing interests

The authors declare that they have no competing interests.

References

1. Peleg AY, Hooper DC. Hospital-acquired infections due to gram-negative bacteria. N Engl J Med. 2010;362:1804–13.
2. Vincent JL, Rello J, Marshall J, Silva E, Anzueto A, Martin CD, et al. International study of the prevalence and outcomes of infection in intensive care units. JAMA. 2009;302:2323–9.
3. Lautenbach E, Patel JB, Bilker WB, Edelstein PH, Fishman NO. Extended-spectrum beta-lactamase-producing *Escherichia coli* and Klebsiella pneumoniae: risk factors for infection and impact of resistance on outcomes. Clin Infect Dis. 2001;32:1162–71.
4. Siegel JD, Rhinehart E, Jackson M, Chiarello L. 2007 guideline for isolation precautions: preventing transmission of infectious agents in health care settings. Am J Infect Control. 2007;35:S65–164.
5. Tacconelli E, Cataldo MA, Dancer SJ, De Angelis G, Falcone M, Frank U, et al. ESCMID guidelines for the management of the infection control measures to reduce transmission of multidrug-resistant Gram-negative bacteria in hospitalized patients. Clin Microbiol Infect. 2014;20:1–55.
6. Société française d'hygiène hospitalière, Recommandations nationales. Prévention de la transmission croisée: précautions complémentaires contact. Consensus formalisé d'experts. Avril 2009.
7. Lucet JC, Decre D, Fichelle A, Joly-Guillou ML, Pernet M, Deblangy C, et al. Control of a prolonged outbreak of extended-spectrum beta-lactamase-producing enterobacteriaceae in a university hospital. Clin Infect Dis. 1999;29:1411–8.
8. Tschudin-Sutter S, Frei R, Dangel M, Stranden A, Widmer AF. Rate of transmission of extended-spectrum beta-lactamase-producing enterobacteriaceae without contact isolation. Clin Infect Dis. 2012;55:1505–11.
9. Zahar JR, Poirel L, Dupont C, Fortineau N, Nassif X, Nordmann P. About the usefulness of contact precautions for carriers of extended-spectrum beta-lactamase-producing *Escherichia coli*. BMC Infect Dis. 2015;15:512–9.
10. Le Gall JR, Lemeshow S, Saulnier F. A new simplified acute physiology score (SAPS II) based on a European/North American multicenter study. JAMA. 1993;270:2957–63.
11. Vincent JL, de Mendonca A, Cantraine F, Moreno R, Takala J, Suter PM, et al. Use of the SOFA score to assess the incidence of organ dysfunction/failure in intensive care units: results of a multicenter, prospective study. Working group on "sepsis-related problems" of the European Society of Intensive Care Medicine. Crit Care Med. 1998;26:1793–800.
12. Royston P, Ambler G, Sauerbrei W. The use of fractional polynomials to model continuous risk variables in epidemiology. Int J Epidemiol. 1999;28:964–74.
13. Razazi K, Derde LP, Verachten M, Legrand P, Lesprit P, Brun-Buisson C. Clinical impact and risk factors for colonization with extended-spectrum beta-lactamase-producing bacteria in the intensive care unit. Intensive Care Med. 2012;38:1769–78.
14. Thiebaut AC, Arlet G, Andremont A, Papy E, Sollet JP, Bernede-Bauduin C, et al. Variability of intestinal colonization with third-generation cephalosporin-resistant Enterobacteriaceae and antibiotic use in intensive care units. J Antimicrob Chemother. 2012;67:1525–36.

15. Carbonne H, Le Dorze M, Bourrel AS, Poupet H, Poyart C, Cambau E, et al. Relation between presence of extended-spectrum β-lactamase-producing Enterobacteriaceae in systematic rectal swabs and respiratory tract specimens in ICU patients. Ann Intensive Care. 2017;7:13–20.
16. Barbier F, Pommier C, Essaied W, Garrouste-Orgeas M, Schwebel C, Ruckly S, et al. Colonization and infection with extended-spectrum beta-lactamase-producing Enterobacteriaceae in ICU patients: What impact on outcomes and carbapenem exposure? J Antimicrob Chemother. 2016;71:1088–97.
17. Alves M, Lemire A, Decre D, Margetis D, Bige N, Pichereau C, et al. Extended-spectrum beta-lactamase—producing enterobacteriaceae in the intensive care unit: acquisition does not mean cross-transmission. BMC Infect Dis. 2016;16:147–55.
18. Gardam MA, Burrows LL, Kus JV, Brunton J, Low DE, Conly JM, et al. Is surveillance for multidrug-resistant enterobacteriaceae an effective infection control strategy in the absence of an outbreak? J Infect Dis. 2002;186:1754–60.
19. Grohs P, Podglajen I, Guerot E, Bellenfant F, Caumont-Prim A, Kac G, et al. Assessment of five screening strategies for optimal detection of carriers of third-generation cephalosporin-resistant Enterobacteriaceae in intensive care units using daily sampling. Clin Microbiol Infect. 2014;20:879–86.
20. Tschudin-Sutter S, Frei R, Schwahn F, Tomic M, Conzelmann M, Stranden A, et al. Prospective validation of cessation of contact precautions for extended-spectrum β-lactamase-producing *Escherichia coli*. Emerg Infect Dis. 2016;22:1094–7.
21. Hansen S, Schwab F, Gastmeier P, Pittet D, Zingg W, Sax H, et al. Provision and consumption of alcohol-based hand rubs in European hospitals. Clin Microbiol Infect. 2015;21:1047–51.
22. Derde LP, Cooper BS, Goossens H, Malhotra-Kumar S, Willems RJ, Gniadkowski M, et al. Interventions to reduce colonisation and transmission of antimicrobial-resistant bacteria in intensive care units: an interrupted time series study and cluster randomised trial. Lancet Infect Dis. 2014;14:31–9.
23. Jarlier V, Trystram D, Brun-Buisson C, Fournier S, Carbonne A, Marty L, et al. Curbing methicillin-resistant *Staphylococcus aureus* in 38 French hospitals through a 15-year institutional control program. Arch Intern Med. 2010;170:552–9.
24. Aumeran C, Baud O, Lesens O, Delmas J, Souweine B, Traore O. Successful control of a hospital-wide vancomycin-resistant *Enterococcus faecium* outbreak in France. Eur J Clin Microbiol Infect Dis. 2008;27:1061–4.
25. Morgan DJ, Diekema DJ, Sepkowitz K, Perencevich EN. Adverse outcomes associated with contact precautions: a review of the literature. Am J Infect Control. 2009;37:85–93.
26. Kramer A, Schwebke I, Kampf G. How long do nosocomial pathogens persist on inanimate surfaces? A systematic review. BMC Infect Dis. 2006;6:130–7.
27. Jazmati N, Hein R, Hamprecht A. Use of an enrichment broth improves detection of extended-spectrum-beta-lactamase-producing enterobacteriaceae in clinical stool samples. J Clin Microbiol. 2016;54:467–70.

8

Emergence of antimicrobial resistance to *Pseudomonas aeruginosa* in the intensive care unit: association with the duration of antibiotic exposure and mode of administration

Erlangga Yusuf[1*], Bruno Van Herendael[1,5], Walter Verbrugghe[2], Margareta Ieven[1], Emiel Goovaerts[3], Kristof Bergs[2], Kristien Wouters[4], Philippe G. Jorens[2] and Herman Goossens[1]

Abstract

Background: Antibiotics are frequently used in intensive care units (ICUs), and their use is associated with the emergence of bacterial resistance to antibiotics. The aim of this study was to investigate the association between the emergence of *Pseudomonas aeruginosa* resistance and the duration of antibiotic exposure or mode of administration in an ICU unit.

Methods: A 4-year cohort study of intensive care unit was performed in patients with *P. aeruginosa* isolates from clinical specimens, initially susceptible to the investigated antibiotics (piperacillin/tazobactam, ceftazidime, ciprofloxacin, meropenem and amikacin). Odds ratios (ORs) with 95% confidence interval (95% CI) of emergence of resistance were calculated using logistic regression analysis for various exposure periods to antibiotics (1–3, 4–7, 8–15 and >15 days) relative to no exposure with adjustment for age, sex, Simplified Acute Physiology Score 3 (SAPS 3) and length of stay. ORs on the emergence of *P. aeruginosa* resistance were also calculated for the various modes of administration.

Results: Included were 187 patients [mean age 61 years, 69% male, mean SAPS 3 score (SD): 59 (12.3)]. None of the antibiotics investigated showed the emergence of resistance within 1–3 days. Significant meropenem resistance emerged within 8–15 days [OR 79.1 (14.9–421.0)] after antibiotic exposure unlike other antibiotics (>15 days). No difference was observed between intermittent and extended administration of meropenem and between beta-lactam mono- or combined therapy.

Conclusions: Use of meropenem was associated with the emergence of resistance as soon as 8 days after exposure to the antibiotic.

Keywords: *Pseudomonas aeruginosa*, Antibiotic resistance, Extended infusion

Background

Pseudomonas aeruginosa is responsible for 9% of all healthcare-associated infections [1], and the resistance to *P. aeruginosa* is increasing [2]. Data from the European Centre for Disease Prevention and Control show that around 18% of *P. aeruginosa* strains are resistant to carbapenems, 15% resistant to at least three out of five antimicrobial classes with an antipseudomonal spectrum (piperacillin/tazobactam, ceftazidime, fluoroquinolones, carbapenems and aminoglycosides) and even 5% resistant to all five [3]. Antimicrobial resistance is of particular importance in the intensive care unit (ICU) because antibiotic use in this setting is extremely common [4]. Several studies have explored the risk factors for *P. aeruginosa* antimicrobial resistance in non-critically ill patients [5, 6]. These studies showed that among antipseudomonas antibiotics, meropenem was associated with the highest

*Correspondence: angga.yusuf@gmail.com
[1] Department of Microbiology, Antwerp University Hospital (UZA), University of Antwerp, Wilrijkstraat 10, 2650 Edegem, Belgium
Full list of author information is available at the end of the article

risk of resistance emergence [4, 7]. The risk factors for emerging antimicrobial-resistant *Pseudomonas aeruginosa* in the ICU are also worth investigating, especially to answer the question how quick the antibiotic resistance emerges after the exposure to antibiotics. Also, worthy of investigation is whether the use of extended infusion of meropenem and the combination of beta-lactam antibiotics with aminoglycosides are associated with less risk of the emergence of resistance. Extended infusion of meropenem (over 3–4 h) has been shown to improve microbiologic and clinical cure since it shows a time-dependent effect on bacterial eradication [8] but it is not clear whether extended infusion also reduces the emergence of resistance. Combination of beta-lactam antibiotics with aminoglycosides is often used in daily practice [9], for example in critically ill patients, because it increases the chance of treating the patients with one active antibiotic. Arguably, the risk of inappropriate antibiotic therapy (no active molecule) will increase in case of use of a beta-lactam alone, and inappropriate therapy is usually associated with a poor prognosis. Yet, the use of combination has not shown to have an added benefit, for example in neutropenic patients [10].

Therefore, the aim of this study was twofold: first to quantify the duration of antibiotic exposure and other risk factors for emergence of resistance and second to investigate whether the mode of administration of meropenem and combination beta-lactams and aminoglycosides were associated with lower emergence of resistance of previously susceptible *P. aeruginosa*.

Methods

Study setting and population

The cohort study was performed between June 2007 and June 2011 in adult patients admitted to the ICU of the Antwerp University Hospital (UZA) for at least 48 h. This ICU consists of 45 beds with approximately 2600 adult admissions yearly; it serves as tertiary care hospital in a city with the population of around 500,000 inhabitants. Included in the study were patients with >1 clinical (i.e., not screening) culture positive with *P. aeruginosa* from any site of the body (blood, upper (sputum) and lower respiratory tract (bronchoalveolar lavage), and wound, that were taken from a patient at least 2 days apart. Patients who were re-admitted after an initial stay in the ICU during the observed period as well as those on antibiotics prior to admission were excluded. On the included patients, we collected demographic data (age and sex), clinical characteristics (reason of ICU admission and Simplified Acute Physiology Score 3 ((SAPS 3), a validated marker of disease severity [11]), use of mechanical ventilation) and data on all antimicrobial drugs the patients received during the ICU stay (duration and mode of administration). The patients received standard dose of antibiotics or adjusted dose according to renal clearance. The standard intravenous doses were 4 g/2 g q.i.d. for piperacillin/tazobactam, 6 g o.d. for ceftazidime, 400 mg b.d. for ciprofloxacin, 1 g t.d. for meropenem and 15 mg/kg divided into three doses for amikacin. Amikacin was, apart from treatment of endocarditis with gentamicin, the only aminoglycoside used in our ICU.

Specimens

All cultures were analyzed according to standard hospital and laboratory protocol. Antibiotic susceptibility testing was performed using disk diffusion technique on Mueller–Hinton agar for piperacillin/tazobactam, ceftazidime, ciprofloxacin, meropenem and amikacin [12]. Zone diameters were interpreted according to CLSI (Clinical & Laboratory Standards Institute) guidelines (CLSI M100) as susceptible, intermediate or resistant. Intermediate isolates were considered in this present study as susceptible since the intermediate category also implies that a higher-than-normal dosage of a drug can be used [13].

Statistical analysis

All variables were assessed and described according to their distribution. Normally distributed variables were presented as mean with standard deviation (SD), and not normally distributed variables as median with range.

The outcome of the investigation was the emergence of resistance in *P. aeruginosa*, defined as phenotype switch of the relevant antibiotic from susceptible/intermediate at the initial culture to resistant at any follow-up culture. The determinant variable was the duration of the relevant antibiotic used by the patients. The patients were divided into groups according to the number of days of antibiotic exposure according to the literature [6, 14] as follows: not exposed, 1–3, 4–7, 8–15 and >15 days.

Goodman and Kruskal's gamma tests were first used to investigate an association between higher categories of exposure and higher numbers of the emergence of resistance. Associations were considered significant if p-values were <0.05. To further quantify the effect of antibiotic exposure on emergence of resistance per antibiotic, logistic regression analysis was performed to calculate odds ratios (ORs) with 95% confidence interval (95% CI) of emerging resistance to an antibiotic for patients in one of the exposed groups (1–3, 4–7, 8–15 and >15 days) compared to the group without exposure with adjustment for possible confounders age, sex and SAPS 3 scores. Further adjustment was made for the length of stay. The analyses were repeated using the emergence of resistance antibiotic on the phenotype switch of any antipseudomonal antibiotic as the outcome. Re-analyses were also performed after excluding possible cross-transmission. Arbitrarily, we defined possible cross-transmission as cases with phenotype switch to identical antibiogram with a potential source patient with overlapping time periods of 30 days. Due to the small number of the included study participants, the effect of interaction between antipseudomonal antibiotics was not investigated.

To investigate the effect of meropenem administration through extended or intermittent infusion and the effect of combination therapy versus monotherapy, the ORs (95% CI) were calculated using logistic regression analysis comparing the risk of emerging resistance in one regimen versus the risk in the comparator regimen. All analyses were performed using IBM SPSS Statistics for Windows version 23.0 (IBM Corp., Armonk, NY).

Results

Demographic of study participants

We identified 405 patients with at least one positive culture with *P. aeruginosa* during the study period. After exclusion of patients with only one isolate ($n = 168$), the length of stay <48 h ($n = 18$) and patients re-admitted to the ICU ($n = 32$), 187 patients (mean age of 61 years, 69% male) were included. The flowchart of included patients is presented in Fig. 1. The included patients had mean SAPS 3 score of 59 (12.3). Most of the patients had mechanical ventilation (84.0%) and vasopressors (88.8%) (Table 1).

During the ICU admission, 96% of the patients received at least one of the antipseudomonal antibiotics. The most common antibiotics used were piperacillin/tazobactam (61.0%) and meropenem (54.8%). The median length of stay was 29 days (range 2–145 days).

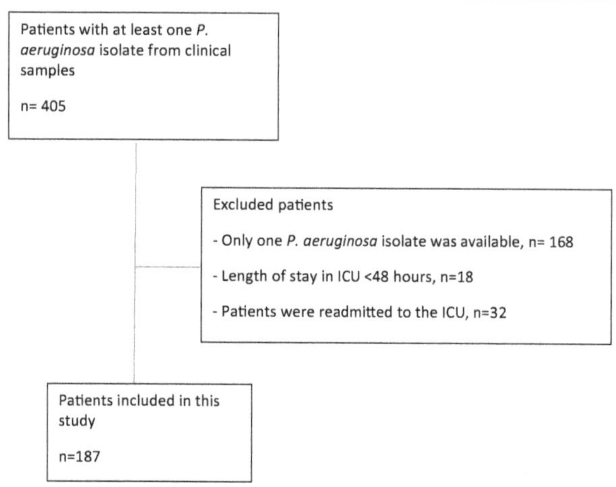

Fig. 1 Flowchart of included patients

Table 1 Demographic and clinical characteristics of the study cohort ($n = 187$)

Characteristics	Values
Mean age (SD), years	61 (14)
Male gender, *n* (%)	129 (69.0)
Mean Simplified Acute Physiology Score 3 score (SD)	59 (12)
Length of stay in intensive care unit, days, mean (range)	29 (2–145)
Previous non-antipseudomonal antibiotics, *n* (%)	79 (42.2)
Antibiotics during ICU stay	
Piperacillin/tazobactam, *n* (%)	114 (61.0)
Meropenem, *n* (%)	102 (54.8)
Ceftazidime, *n* (%)	73 (39.0)
Amikacin, *n* (%)	72 (38.5)
Ciprofloxacin, *n* (%)	69 (36.9)
Types of antibiotics received	
None	13 (7.4)
1	35 (19.9)
2–3	94 (53.5)
4–5	34 (19.2)
Reason for ICU admission, n (%)	
Cardiovascular/vascular	55 (29.4)
Respiratory	46 (24.6)
Neurological	32 (17.1)
Gastrointestinal	25 (13.4)
Sepsis/septic shock	15 (7.5)
Trauma	10 (5.3)
Others	5 (2.7)
Mechanical ventilation, *n* (%)	160 (83.8)
Therapy with one or more vasopressors, *n* (%)	169 (88.5)

SD standard deviation

From these patients, 1158 cultures were available (mean number cultures per patient 6, range 2–42). At baseline, the number of patients with an isolate susceptible to the antibiotic was 176 (94.1%) for piperacillin/tazobactam, 171 (91.4%) for ceftazidime, 133 for ciprofloxacin (71.1%), 124 (66.3%) for meropenem and 155 (82.9%) for amikacin. During the follow-up, phenotype switch from susceptible/intermediate to resistant for at least one antibiotic occurred in isolates from 38.1% of the patients during the ICU stay. During the ICU stay, 31.6% of *Pseudomonas* isolates became resistant to piperacillin/tazobactam, 27.5% to ceftazidime, 22.0% to meropenem, 13.3% to ciprofloxacin and 12.9% to amikacin.

Duration of antibiotics use and the emergence of resistance

Exposure to the relevant antibiotics was significantly associated with the emergence of resistance of *P. aeruginosa* for meropenem ($p < 0.001$), piperacillin/tazobactam ($p = 0.006$) and ceftazidime ($p = 0.006$). For ciprofloxacin, there was an association but did not reach statistic significant level ($p = 0.06$). There was no association with amikacin ($p = 0.33$). Other variables such as age, gender, SAPS 3 scores, previous antibiotic use, necessity use of mechanical ventilation or vasopressors and ICU length of stay were not associated with the emergence of *P. aeruginosa* resistance to any of the antipseudomonal antibiotics during ICU stay (data not shown).

Using antibiotics for less than 4 days was not significantly associated with emergence of resistance (Table 2). When the antibiotic was administered for longer than 15 days, we observed the emergence of resistance of *P. aeruginosa* to all antipseudomonal antibiotics, except to amikacin. The OR (95% CI) after adjusting for age, gender and SAPS 3 scores for the emergence of resistance for piperacillin–tazobactam was 4.7 (1.8–12.4) and for ciprofloxacin was 14.5 (2.8–75.0). Giving ceftazidime or meropenem between 8 and 15 days was associated with phenotypic switch of *P. aeruginosa* to these antibiotics. The ORs (95% CI) were 2.6 (1.1–6.0) and 10.0 (19.8–551.0), respectively. Further adjustment for length of stay changed the significant associations to not significant, except for meropenem (Table 2). The association between meropenem use and emergence of resistance remained even after adjustment for length of stay.

Among all antipseudomonal antibiotics, only meropenem use of 8–15 days and >15 days was associated with the emerging of resistance of any of antipseudomonal antibiotics. The ORs were 6.3 (2.4–16.8, $p = 0.0001$) and 2.6 (1.1–6.3, $p = 0.04$), respectively.

Eight patients (4.2%) were excluded due to possible cross-contamination. Re-analysis after excluding these patients did not significantly alter the results (data not shown).

Association between the mode of administration of meropenem and combination beta-lactams and aminoglycosides with emergence of resistance

Extended administration of meropenem was not associated with a lower risk of emerging *P. aeruginosa* resistance in comparison with intermittent administration (OR 1.1 (0.2–4.0). The proportion of patients who acquired resistance was 45.5% for extended administration ($n = 46$) and 43.5% for intermittent administration ($n = 11$).

The combination of piperacillin/tazobactam with amikacin was also not associated with a lower risk of acquiring *P. aeruginosa* resistance [OR 1.0 (0.4–2.5)]. The proportion of patients who acquired resistance was 37.5% for combination therapy ($n = 24$) and 37.2% for patients with monotherapy ($n = 86$).

Discussion

We observed in this study that exposure to meropenem, as short as 8 days, was already associated with emergence of resistance in *Pseudomonas aeruginosa*, even after adjustment for length of stay. We also found that extended infusion of meropenem and combination of beta-lactam antibiotics with amikacin did not reduce emergence of resistance. The present study used patient-based instead of surveillance-based approach. Instead of detecting the emergence of resistance in patients who endured regular screening cultures, the emergence of resistance was studied in clinical cultures. This approach is convenient in a clinical situation where surveillance cultures are not always routinely performed. The results of the present study are in line with those from surveillance-based approach studies that showed carbapenem as antibiotic class with the strongest potential for selection of resistance, for example from Carmeli et al. [15]. Unlike Carmeli and co-workers who used imipenem in their study, we used meropenem. Whether one type of carbapenem is more associated with emergence of resistance should be further explored. Earlier studies also showed that antipseudomonal antibiotics piperacillin/tazobactam, ceftazidime and ciprofloxacin were associated with the emergence of *P. aeruginosa* resistance in critically ill patients [7, 16, 17]. However, in our study, the significant effect disappeared after further adjustment with the length of stay, except for meropenem, which highlights meropenem as an antibiotic that selected for *P. aeruginosa* resistance.

Several studies have been published recently that investigated the molecular mechanisms of the resistance of *P. aeruginosa* to antipseudomonal antibiotics showing that mutated genes during the emergence of beta-lactam resistance differed for each antibiotic [18, 19]. Since we do not perform molecular analysis, our study does not allow the analysis of mechanisms involved in the emergence of resistance, either expression of intrinsic resistance mechanisms in response to antimicrobial exposure such as reduction in expression of the outer membrane proteins (porins) or increase production of an efflux pump to a variety of antibiotics.

To the best of our knowledge, the present study is the first to show that the emergence of resistance in initially susceptible *P. aeruginosa* isolates does not occur when the antibiotic was given for less than 4 days, even for meropenem. This is in line with results from Lodise et al. [6] that showed patients infected with a carbapenem-resistant *P. aeruginosa* were more likely to have been exposed to carbapenems for 3 days or more compared to patients infected with a carbapenem susceptible strain. The combination therapy beta-lactam and amikacin failed to decrease the emergence of resistance unlike in

Table 2 Odds ratios for the emergence of antipseudomonal antibiotic resistance by *Pseudomonas aeruginosa* in relation to antibiotic duration

Antibiotic duration	Number of patients	Events (%)	Odds ratio (95% confidence interval) adjusted for age, gender and SAPS 3 scores	Odds ratio (95% confidence interval) adjusted for age, gender, SAPS 3 scores and length of stay
Piperacillin–tazobactam ($n = 176$)				
Reference (i.e., use of other antibiotic than piperacillin–tazobactam or no antibiotic)	65	13 (21.2)	1	1
1–3 days	17	6 (35.3)	2.5 (0.8–8.0)	2.3 (0.7–8.2)
4–7 days	29	11 (37.9)	2.3 (0.8–6.1)	2.2 (0.7–6.4)
8–15 days	34	9 (26.5)	1.5 (0.6–4.1)	1.5 (0.5–4.3)
>15 days	29	16 (55.2)	4.7 (1.8–12.4)‡	1.7 (0.6–5.3)
Ceftazidime ($n = 171$)				
Reference (i.e., use of other antibiotic than ceftazidime or no antibiotic)	99	22 (22.2)	1	1
1–3 days	13	0	NA	NA
4–7 days	12	8 (66.7)	1.7 (0.4–6.6)	1.7 (0.4–7.4)
8–15 days	34	14 (41.2)	2.6 (1.1–6.0)‡	1.7 (0.7–4.3)
>15 days	13	7 (53.8)	3.4 (1.0–12.4)‡	0.7 (0.2–3.4)
Ciprofloxacin ($n = 128$)				
Reference (i.e., use of other antibiotic than ciprofloxacin or no antibiotic)	78	7 (9)	1	1
1–3 days	18	2 (5.6)	1.5 (0.3–7.9)	2.0 (0.3–11.7)
4–7 days	10	0	0	0
8–15 days	13	3 (23.1)	2.7 (0.5–13.3)	1.4 (0.2–850)
>15 days	9	5 (55.6)	14.5 (2.8–75.0)‡	1.9 (0.2–15.6)
Meropenem ($n = 123$)				
Reference (i.e., use of other antibiotic than meropenem or no antibiotic)	64	3 (4.7)	1	1
1–3 days	13	0 (0)	0.0	0.0
4–7 days	9	2 (5.6)	4.9 (0.7–37.2)	3.4 (0.4–30.2)
8–15 days	21	17 (81.0)	104.5 (19.8–551.0)‡	79.1 (14.9–421.0)‡
>15 days	16	5 (31.2)	10.0 (2.0–49.5)‡	4.6 (1.7–32.2)‡
Amikacin ($n = 148$)				
Reference (i.e., use of other antibiotic than amikacin or no antibiotic)	87	10 (11.5)	1	1
1–3 days	41	7 (17.1)	1.3 (0.4–4.2)	0.7 (0.2–2.6)
4–7 days	13	1 (7.7)	0.3 (0.03–3.0)	0.1 (0.01–2.2)
8–15 days	7	1 (14.3)	0.5 (0.05–5.1)	0.1 (0.01–2.9)
>15 days	0	0	0.0	0.0

‡ Statistically significant at $p < 0.05$

an in vitro study [20]. One of the possible explanations is that amikacin drug concentration may be suboptimal for *P. aeruginosa* in ICU patients. We did not always perform peak measurement of amikacin, and therefore, we do not know whether the pharmacokinetic/pharmacodynamic (PK/PD) target was achieved. In this study, the dose of 15 mg/kg divided into three doses was mostly used, yet some authors advised the use of 25 mg/kg/day [21].

Extended meropenem infusion was also not associated with less emergence of resistance compared with intermittent infusion. This effect may be true but alternative explanations such as optimal dosing are also possible and further study on this issue is needed.

This study has further limitations. Firstly, although using clinical specimens approach is convenient and mimic daily practice in many ICUs, this study cannot determine the exact date of phenotype switch because cultures were not regularly performed. Since the study was based on clinical specimens, the follow-up duration of the patients varied, i.e., the follow-up duration was the time frame between the first and the last positive culture for *P. aeruginosa*. A prospective study design with cultures taken at regular time frame will be a better study design despite in the routine practice *P. aeruginosa* could not always be re-isolated. Secondly, this study does not use genotyping to investigate the relatedness of the strains and to confirm the cross-transmission of resistant *P. aeruginosa*. However, cross-transmission estimated in this study (4.2%) is comparable with cross-transmission confirmed by genotyping (2.8%) as shown in a previous study [7], and the results of the analysis remain the same after excluding possible cross-transmission. It is also possible that several strains could be responsible for infection and this selection pressure cannot be differentiated from the emergence of resistance since no genotyping was performed. Thirdly, the results of this study might underestimate the effect since no minimum inhibitory concentration (MIC) values were available. Antipseudomonal antibiotics use might be associated with increasing MIC values that does not cause phenotypic switch on disk diffusion. Fourthly, the number of patients was relatively small and the study may be underpowered for several antibiotics that were used in low number, and lastly this study was performed in one center only.

Conclusions

The results of this study suggested that meropenem is associated with resistance of *P. aeruginosa* as soon after 8 days of use. This finding should be confirmed in other studies. All antipseudomonal antibiotics except amikacin are associated with the emergence of *P. aeruginosa* resistance. Physicians should weigh up the risk of resistance and the therapeutic benefit when meropenem or other antipseudomonal antibiotics are going to be used for a long period. Moreover, when physicians start empiric therapy with a carbapenem antibiotic, they should consider to de-escalate it within 48–72 h, once the culture results are known since the switch might be clinically beneficial for the patients.

Abbreviations

ICU: intensive care unit; SAPS 3: Simplified Acute Physiology Score 3; CLSI: Clinical & Laboratory Standards Institute; SD: standard deviation; OR: odds ratio; 95% CI: 95% confidence interval; MIC: minimum inhibitory concentration.

Authors' contributions

All authors contributed to the conception and design of the work. All authors performed the acquisition, analysis and interpretation of data. EY and BVH drafted the work. EY, BVH, WV, KW, PGJ and HG revised the work critically for important intellectual content. All authors gave final approval of the version to be published. All authors read and approved the final manuscript.

Author details

[1] Department of Microbiology, Antwerp University Hospital (UZA), University of Antwerp, Wilrijkstraat 10, 2650 Edegem, Belgium. [2] Department of Intensive Care Medicine, Antwerp University Hospital (UZA), University of Antwerp, Wilrijkstraat 10, 2650 Edegem, Belgium. [3] Department of Hospital Hygiene and Infection Control, Antwerp University Hospital (UZA), University of Antwerp, Wilrijkstraat 10, 2650 Edegem, Belgium. [4] Department of Biostatistics, Antwerp University Hospital (UZA), University of Antwerp, Wilrijkstraat 10, 2650 Edegem, Belgium. [5] Present Address: GZA Hospitals, Antwerp, Belgium.

Competing interests

The authors declare that they have no competing interests.

References

1. ECDC. European Centre for Disease Prevention and Control. Point prevalence survey of healthcareassociated infections and antimicrobial use in European acute care hospitals. Stockholm: ECDC; 2013.
2. ECDC. Antimicrobial resistance surveillance in Europe 2014. Annual Report of the European Antimicrobial Resistance Surveillance Network (EARS-Net). Stockholm: European Centre for Disease Prevention and Control; 2015.
3. European Centre for Disease Prevention and Control. Antimicrobial resistance surveillance in Europe 2013. Annual Report of the European Antimicrobial Resistance Surveillance Network (EARS-Net). [Internet]. Ecdc; 2014. p. 1–211.
4. Cobos-Trigueros N, Solé M, Castro P, Torres JL, Hernández C, Rinaudo M, et al. Acquisition of *Pseudomonas aeruginosa* and its resistance phenotypes in critically ill medical patients: role of colonization pressure and antibiotic exposure. Crit Care. 2015;19:218.
5. Peña C, Suarez C, Tubau F, Dominguez A, Sora M, Pujol M, et al. Carbapenem-resistant *Pseudomonas aeruginosa*: factors influencing multidrug-resistant acquisition in non-critically ill patients. Eur J Clin Microbiol Infect Dis. 2009;28(5):519–22.
6. Lodise TP, Miller C, Patel N, Graves J, McNutt LA. Identification of patients with *Pseudomonas aeruginosa* respiratory tract infections at greatest risk of infection with carbapenem-resistant isolates. Infect Control Hosp Epidemiol. 2007;28(8):959–65.
7. Ong DS, Jongerden IP, Buiting AG, Leverstein-van Hall MA, Speelberg B, Kesecioglu J, et al. Antibiotic exposure and resistance development in *Pseudomonas aeruginosa* and Enterobacter species in intensive care units. Crit Care Med. 2011;39(11):2458–63.
8. MacVane SH, Kuti JL, Nicolau DP. Prolonging β-lactam infusion: a review of the rationale and evidence, and guidance for implementation. Int J Antimicrob Agents. 2014;43(2):105–13
9. Vardakas KZ, Tansarli GS, Bliziotis IA, Falagas ME. β-Lactam plus aminoglycoside or fluoroquinolone combination versus β-lactam monotherapy for Pseudomonas aeruginosa infections: a meta-analysis. Int J Antimicrob Agents. 2013;41(4):301–10
10. Paul M, Dickstein Y, Schlesinger A, Grozinsky-Glasberg S, Soares-Weiser K, Leibovici L. Beta-lactam versus beta-lactam-aminoglycoside combination therapy in cancer patients with neutropenia. Cochrane database Syst Rev [Internet]. 2013;6(6):CD003038.
11. Moreno RP, Metnitz PGH, Almeida E, Jordan B, Bauer P, Campos RA, et al. SAPS 3–from evaluation of the patient to evaluation of the intensive care unit. Part 2: development of a prognostic model for hospital mortality at ICU admission. Intensive Care Med. 2005;31(10):1345–55.
12. CLSI. Performance standards for antimicrobial susceptibility testing; twentieth informational supplement. CLSI document M100-S20. 2010; p. 1–153.
13. Turnidge J, Paterson DL. Setting and revising antibacterial susceptibility breakpoints. Clin Microbiol Rev. 2007:20(3):391–408
14. Chastre J, Wolff M, Fagon JY, Chevret S, Thomas F, Wermert D, et al. Comparison of 8 vs 15 days of antibiotic therapy for ventilator-associated pneumonia in adults: a randomized trial. J Am Med Assoc. 2003;290(19):2588–98.
15. Carmeli Y, Troillet N, Eliopoulos GM, Samore MH. Emergence of antibiotic-resistant *Pseudomonas aeruginosa*: comparison of risks associated with different antipseudomonal agents. Antimicrob Agents Chemother. 1999;43(6):1379–82.
16. Georges B, Conil J-M, Dubouix A, Archambaud M, Bonnet E, Saivin S, et al. Risk of emergence of *Pseudomonas aeruginosa* resistance to beta-lactam antibiotics in intensive care units. Crit Care Med. 2006;34(6):1636–41.

17. Martínez JA, Delgado E, Martí S, Marco F, Vila J, Mensa J, et al. Influence of antipseudomonal agents on *Pseudomonas aeruginosa* colonization and acquisition of resistance in critically ill medical patients. Intensive Care Med. 2009;35(3):439–47.
18. Feng Y, Jonker MJ, Moustakas I, Brul S, ter Kuile BH. Dynamics of mutations during development of resistance by *Pseudomonas aeruginosa* against Five Antibiotics. Antimicrob Agents Chemother Internet. 2016;60(7):4229–36.
19. Solé M, Fàbrega A, Cobos-Trigueros N, Zamorano L, Ferrer-Navarro M, Ballesté-Delpierre C, et al. In vivo evolution of resistance of *Pseudomonas aeruginosa* strains isolated from patients admitted to an intensive care unit: mechanisms of resistance and antimicrobial exposure. J Antimicrob Chemother. 2015;70(11):3004–13.
20. Tam VH, Schilling AN, Neshat S, Poole K, Melnick DA, Coyle EA. Optimization of meropenem minimum concentration/MIC ratio to suppress in vitro resistance of *Pseudomonas aeruginosa*. Antimicrob Agents Chemother. 2005;49(12):4920–7.
21. De Montmollin E, Bouadma L, Gault N, Mourvillier B, Mariotte E, Chemam S, et al. Predictors of insufficient amikacin peak concentration in critically ill patients receiving a 25 mg/kg total body weight regimen. Intensive Care Med. 2014;40(7):998–1005.

9

Assessment of sepsis-induced immunosuppression at ICU discharge and 6 months after ICU discharge

Violette Zorio[1,2*], Fabienne Venet[2,3], Benjamin Delwarde[1,2], Bernard Floccard[1], Guillaume Marcotte[1], Julien Textoris[1,2], Guillaume Monneret[2,3] and Thomas Rimmelé[1,2]

Abstract

Background: Increase in mortality and in recurrent infections in the year following ICU discharge continues in survivors of septic shock, even after total clinical recovery from the initial septic event and its complications. This supports the hypothesis that sepsis could induce persistent long-term immune dysfunctions. To date, there is almost no data on ICU discharge and long-term evolution of sepsis-induced immunosuppression in septic shock survivors. The aim of this study was to assess the persistence of sepsis-induced immunosuppression by measuring expression of human leukocyte antigen DR on monocytes (mHLA-DR), CD4+ T cells, and regulatory T cells (Treg) at ICU discharge and 6 months after ICU discharge in patients admitted to the ICU for septic shock.

Methods: In this prospective observational study, septic shock survivors with no preexisting immune suppression or treatment interfering with the immune system were included. mHLA-DR, CD4+ T cells, and Treg expression were assessed on day 1–2, 3–4, and 6–8 after ICU admission, at ICU discharge, and 6 months after ICU discharge.

Results: A total of 40 patients were enrolled during their ICU stay: 21 males (52.5%) and 19 females, median age 68 years (IQR 58–77), median SOFA score on day 1–2 was 8 (IQR 7–9), and median ICU length of stay was 11 days (IQR 7–24). Among these 40 patients, 33 were studied at ICU discharge and 15 were disposed for blood sampling 6 months after ICU discharge. On day 1–2, mHLA-DR expression was abnormally low for all patients [median 4212 (IQR 2640–6047) AB/C] and remained abnormally low at ICU discharge for 75% of them [median 10,281 (IQR 7719–13,035) AB/C]. On day 3–4, 46% of patients presented CD4+ lymphopenia [median 515 (IQR 343–724) mm^{-3}] versus 34% at ICU discharge [median 642 (IQR 459–846) mm^{-3}]. Among patients with a 6-month blood sample, normal values of mHLA-DR were found for all patients [median 32,616 (IQR 24,918–38,738) AB/C] except for one and only another one presented CD4+ lymphopenia.

Conclusions: While immune alterations persist at ICU discharge, there is, at cellular level, no persistent immune alterations among septic shock survivors analyzed 6 months after ICU discharge.

Keywords: CD4+ T cells, HLA-DR, Immune system, Immunology, Immunosuppression, Regulatory T cells, Sepsis

Background

Despite progress in the therapeutic management of patients with sepsis and septic shock, hospital mortality of these patients has only slightly decreased in recent decades and remains around 20 and 40%, respectively [1]. While mortality in the first week has decreased, it has increased during subsequent weeks [2]. It is hypothesized that sepsis-induced immunosuppression occurring during this second phase of sepsis explains the "late" mortality, most likely due to increased risk of secondary infections [3].

Sepsis-induced immunosuppression is characterized by alterations affecting both innate and adaptive immunity.

*Correspondence: violette.zorio@gmail.com
[1] Department of Anesthesiology and Critical Care Medicine, Edouard Herriot hospital, Hospices Civils de Lyon, Lyon, France
Full list of author information is available at the end of the article

Among the biological parameters assessing the innate immune system, the level of the human leukocyte antigen DR expression on the surface of monocytes (mHLA-DR) is one of the best studied, and is recognized as an effective indicator of immunosuppression [4, 5]. Furthermore, a reduction in mHLA-DR is the only immune parameter shown to be an independent factor of nosocomial infection occurrence [6] and of mortality [7]. With regard to adaptive immunity, lymphopenia on the fourth day following the diagnosis of sepsis predicts mortality and may also serve as a biomarker for sepsis-induced immunosuppression [8]. Regulatory T cells (Treg) are less-well studied but present nevertheless well-defined and broad immunosuppressive properties [9–11]. Thus, in sepsis, the increase in the proportion of Treg cells among the total number of T CD4+ lymphocytes is correlated with poor prognosis [12].

Whereas the occurrence of immunosuppression during ICU stay is well documented, to date, there is almost no data on ICU discharge and on long-term evolution of sepsis-induced immunosuppression in survivors of septic shock. Some data support the hypothesis that sepsis could induce persistent long-term immune dysfunctions even long after the hospital discharge. Indeed, in the longer term, even after total clinical recovery in sepsis survivors, increase in mortality continues. It has been reported mortality of 43% after 1 year [13], 45% after 2 years [14], and 74% after 5 years [15] beyond hospital discharge. Furthermore, an increase of recurrent infections in the year following ICU discharge has also been reported in such patients [16, 17]. Taken together, persistent sepsis-induced immunosuppression at ICU discharge and in long term could be the underlying reason for this delayed mortality in sepsis survivors.

The aim of this study was to assess the persistence of sepsis-induced immunosuppression at the cellular level at ICU discharge and 6 months thereafter by measuring mHLA-DR, CD4+ T cells, and Treg expression in patients admitted for septic shock.

Methods

Study population

In this prospective cohort study, we included all patients who were admitted to the ICU for septic shock diagnosed for less than 48 h, and who were alive at the time of ICU discharge. The diagnosis of septic shock was retained in presence of sepsis associated with persistent hypotension despite adequate intravascular volume expansion and thus requiring initiation of vasopressors. We considered the diagnosis of septic shock when the required amount of vasopressors was greater than 0.25 μg/kg/min for at least 2 h. All patients under 18 years of age, pregnant women, as well as those with comorbidities related to the immune system or treatment interfering with the immune system were excluded (i.e., patients with hematological disease receiving or having received immunosuppressive drugs or immunomodulatory drugs within 5 years preceding inclusion, patients suffering from a solid tumor undergoing chemotherapy, from acquired aplasia, or from innate immune deficiency, patients who received extracorporeal life support (extracorporeal membrane oxygenation in context of acute respiratory distress syndrome or cardiogenic shock or extracorporeal circulation in relation to cardiac surgery) within 1 month prior to inclusion and patients treated with immunosuppressive drugs or corticosteroids at immunosuppressive doses.

Ethical requirements

Each analyzable patient—if clinical conditions allowed it—or every corresponding reliable person was informed orally about objectives and conduct of the study and received a note summarizing this information. Patients were included only when the non-opposition had been expressed. For this non-interventional study assessing clinical data and biological samples, oral informed consent from the patient or a relative was considered sufficient. Written informed consent is not required by French law for studies carried out in current care. The biological data collection is reported to the ministry of research (Registered Under the Number DC-2008-509).

Data collection

Patients were monitored clinically and biologically during their ICU stay. Blood samples were drawn: on day 1 or 2 (day 1–2), on day 3 or 4 (day 3–4), on day 6, 7, or 8 (day 6–8) of admission, and the day of ICU discharge (which could sometimes correspond to the day 6–8 sample, or more rarely to the day 3–4 sample for patients with rapid favorable outcome). Day 1 was the day of ICU admission. All survivors were asked to attend a consultation 6 months after ICU discharge, during which an additional blood sample was collected. Patients were contacted by telephone. Analyses included quantification of mHLA-DR at each time point and measurement of CD4+ T cells and Treg on day 3–4, at ICU discharge, and 6 months after ICU discharge. For each included patient, routine biological parameters and clinical data of ICU stay were collected. This 6-month post-ICU discharge consultation is usually offered to all patients admitted in our ICU irrespective of the reason for admission. During this medical consultation, we assess the psychological state of patients related to their ICU stay and we perform a medical examination.

mHLA-DR, CD4+ T cells and Treg measurement

At each time point, samples were collected using EDTA tubes. All blood samples were stained within 1 h after collection or were immediately stored at 4 °C, in accordance with the standardization recommendations for mHLA-DR measurement [18, 19]. For mHLA-DR measurement, staining and cell acquisition by flow cytometry (FC500, Beckman Coulter, Hialeah, FL, USA) were performed as described in the European standardized protocol and according to the manufacturer's recommendations (Quantibrite HLA-DR/Monocyte antibody cocktail, BD Bioscience, San Diego, CA, USA). Results were expressed as the number of anti-HLA-DR antibodies per cell (AB/C) (normal >15,000), which is correlated with the number of HLA-DR molecules expressed on each monocyte. CD4+ T cells were measured by flow cytometry based on expression of CD4; Treg cells were identified based on expression of CD4, CD25, and CD127, and results were expressed as the total number of Treg cells and as the proportion of the total number of CD4+ T cells.

Statistical analysis

Data are expressed as median (IQR). Comparison of baseline characteristics between patients with a blood sample at 6 months and those without was done using the Fisher's exact test or the Chi-square test, as appropriate. The Wilcoxon–Mann–Whitney's test was used to determine differences between immunological variables at each time point. Pearson's correlation coefficients were performed to study the correlation between immunological variables at ICU discharge and ICU length stay. Level of significance was set at 0.05. Calculations were performed using *R* statistical software [20].

Results

Study population

From March 2015 to May 2016, 40 patients with septic shock were enrolled, and from October 2015 to November 2016, they were contacted by telephone. A total of 15 patients (37.5%) came back to hospital 6 months after their ICU discharge and consented to give blood (Fig. 1). Twenty-five patients did not come back to the hospital 6 months after their ICU discharge: three patients died within 6 months, one patient was in a vegetative state in another health institution, six patients refused to come back, 11 patients were willing to come but unable to travel to the hospital, two patients moved to cities too far for them to travel back, and two patients could not be contacted by telephone. Among the 11 patients unable to travel to the hospital, one patient did not come back to the hospital because he suffered from a lung infection.

There were 21 (52.5%) male patients, and the median (IQR) age was 68 (58–77) years (Table 1). Most patients (82.5% of the total study population) needed surgery in addition to antibiotics (Table 1). Six patients (15%) experienced a secondary nosocomial infection during their ICU stay: three lung infections, two surgical site infection, and one urinary tract infection. The characteristics of those with a blood sample at 6 months were similar to those without, with two exceptions: diabetes mellitus was not a comorbidity of those with a sample at 6 months but present in 8 (32%) of those without ($p = 0.01$), and stomatological focus was not a source of septic shock among those without but present in 3 (20.0%) of those with a sample ($p = 0.04$; Table 1).

There was no statistically significant difference for all routine biological and immunological parameters performed during the first week after admission between the

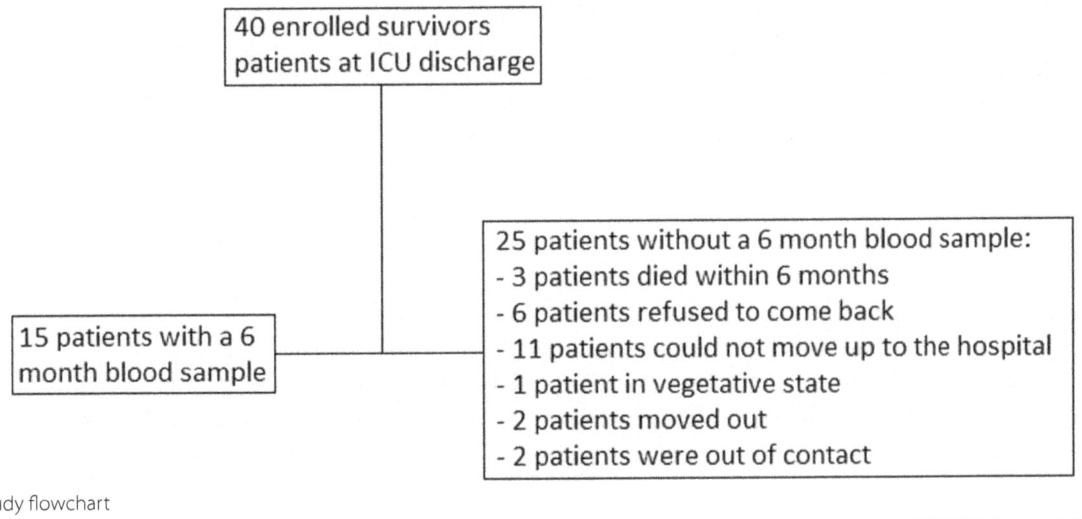

Fig. 1 Study flowchart

Table 1 Patient characteristics

	Total study population $n = 40$	Patients with a blood sample at 6 months $n = 15$	Patients without a blood sample at 6 months $n = 25$	*p* value
Age (years), median (IQR)	68 (58–77)	62 (48–72)	71 (62–78)	0.08
Male gender, *n* (%)	21 (52.5)	8 (53.3)	13 (52.0)	1
SOFA score on day 1–2, median (IQR)	8 (7–9)	9 (7–10)	7 (6–9)	0.38
SAPS II, median (IQR)	53 (43–66)	52 (48–62)	53 (42–69)	0.71
Maximum lactate (mmol/L), median (IQR)	2.7 (1.8–3.7)	3.5 (2.5–5.9)	2.4 (1.7–2.9)	0.37
Missing data, *n*	3		3	
Comorbidities, *n* (%)				
Chronic arterial hypertension	21 (52.5)	6 (40.0)	15 (60.0)	0.32
Chronic heart failure	6 (15.0)	1 (6.7)	5 (20.0)	0.38
Myocardial infarction	3 (7.5)	1 (6.7)	2 (8.0)	1
Stroke	2 (5.0)	1 (6.7)	1 (4.0)	1
Chronic obstructive pulmonary disease	9 (22.5)	2 (13.3)	7 (28.0)	0.44
Dialysis-dependent chronic kidney disease	1 (2.5)	0	1 (4.0)	1
Liver cirrhosis	0	0	0	1
Diabetes mellitus	8 (20.0)	0	8 (32.0)	0.01
Source of infection, *n* (%)				
Abdominal	20 (50.0)	6 (40.0)	14 (56.0)	0.51
Skin and soft tissue	7 (17.5)	1 (6.7)	6 (24.0)	0.22
Respiratory	5 (12.5)	2 (13.3)	3 (12.0)	1
Stomatological	3 (7.5)	3 (20.0)	0	0.04
Urinary tract	3 (7.5)	2 (13.3)	1 (4.0)	0.54
Osteoarticular	2 (5.0)	1 (6.7)	1 (4.0)	1
General management, *n* (%)				
Surgery	33 (82.5)	13 (86.7)	20 (80.0)	0.69
Medical only	7 (17.5)	2 (13.3)	5 (20.0)	0.69
Support measures, *n* (%)				
Norepinephrine	40 (100.0)	15 (100.0)	25 (100.0)	1
Dobutamine	5 (12.5)	1 (6.7)	4 (16.0)	0.63
Mechanical ventilation	31 (77.5)	11 (73.3)	20 (80.0)	0.70
Renal replacement therapy	12 (30.0)	4 (26.7)	8 (32.0)	1
Outcomes (days), median (IQR)				
Days on vasopressors	4 (3–5)	4 (3–10)	3 (2–5)	0.30
Days on mechanical ventilation	6 (3–8)	7 (4–9)	5 (2–7)	0.43
Patients involved, *n*	31	11	20	
Days on renal replacement therapy	8 (6–8)	10 (8–12)	7 (4–8)	0.05
Patients involved, *n*	12	4	8	
ICU length of stay	11 (7–24)	13 (6–25)	10 (7–24)	0.86
Hospital length of stay	37 (16–48)	37 (19–46)	37 (19–49)	0.75

IQR interquartile range, *SOFA* Sepsis-related Organ Failure Assessment, *SAPS II* Simplified Acute Physiology Score II, *ICU* intensive care unit

population with a 6 months blood sample and those without (Table 2). Seventy-four per cent of the total population had lymphopenia (lymphocytes <1.5 $mm^{-3} \times 10^3$) on day 1–2 and this persisted in 56% of patients on day 6–8.

mHLA-DR expression

At admission, the median (IQR) mHLA-DR was 4212 (2640–6047) AB/C and remained <10,000 AB/C at day 6–8 (Table 2). All patients had abnormal mHLA-DR (<15,000 AB/C) either on day 1–2 or day 3–4. Two

Table 2 Biological parameters

	Total study population $n = 40$	Patients with a blood sample at 6 months $n = 15$	Patients without a blood sample at 6 months $n = 25$	*p* value
Leukocytes ($mm^{-3} \times 10^3$), median (IQR)				
D1-2	16.6 (10.4–22.1)	15.3 (7.3–22.1)	16.6 (13.0–20.7)	0.41
Missing data, *n*	1	0	1	
D3-4	15.8 (10.1–21.3)	14.6 (10.6–21.5)	15.8 (9.7–19.7)	0.75
Missing data, *n*	9	1	8	
D6-8	14.2 (12.7–19.3)	13.8 (10.8–15.8)	15.4 (12.8–19.5)	0.88
Missing data, *n*	15	5	10	
Neutrophils ($mm^{-3} \times 10^3$), median (IQR)				
D1-2	13.7 (7.8–20.0)	13 (6.3–20.0)	13.9 (10.4–19.1)	0.47
Missing data, *n*	1	0	1	
D3-4	13 (8.8–18.5)	12.7 (9.5–18.9)	12.8 (8.4–16.3)	0.67
Missing data, *n*	9	1	8	
D6-8	11.8 (9.0–16.2)	11.6 (8.5–13.7)	12 (9.7–16.5)	0.76
Missing data, *n*	15	5	10	
Lymphocytes ($mm^{-3} \times 10^3$), median (IQR)				
D1-2	1 (0.5–1.5)	0.5 (0.3–0.9)	1.1 (0.7–1.8)	0.83
Missing data, *n*	1	0	1	
D3-4	1 (0.7–1.4)	1 (0.9–1.2)	1 (0.6–2.0)	0.99
Missing data, *n*	9	1	8	
D6-8	1.3 (1.0–2.2)	1.1 (1.0–1.3)	2 (1.0–2.2)	0.17
Missing data, *n*	15	5	10	
Monocytes ($mm^{-3} \times 10^3$), median (IQR)				
D1-2	0.5 (0.3–0.9)	0.4 (0.3–0.6)	0.6 (0.37–1.12)	0.78
Missing data, *n*	1	0	1	
D3-4	0.6 (0.4–0.9)	0.6 (0.4–0.7)	0.55 (0.42–1.0)	0.84
Missing data, *n*	9	1	8	
D6-8	0.7 (0.4–0.8)	0.4 (0.6–0.7)	0.7 (0.61–1.1)	0.35
Missing data, *n*	15	5	10	
mHLA-DR (AB/C), median (IQR)				
D1-2	4212 (2640–6047)	3321 (2246–6022)	4486 (2673–6047)	0.41
Missing data, *n*	4	3	1	
D3-4	4514 (3232–6497)	4989 (1484–7379)	4235 (3365–5555)	0.51
Missing data, *n*	1	1	0	
D6-8	7442 (4315–9724)	4817 (3059–9143)	7808 (5070–10,249)	0.13
Missing data, *n*	8	4	4	
ICU discharge	10,281 (7719–13,035)	10,228 (8719–11,826)	11,271 (7195–16,594)	0.54
Missing data, *n*	7	2	5	
6 months post-ICU discharge	32,616 (24,918–38,738)	32,616 (24,918–38,738)		
Missing data, *n*	25	0		
CD4+ T cells (mm^{-3}), median (IQR)				
D3-4	515 (343–724)	477 (356–670)	537 (344–963)	0.63
Missing data, *n*	1	1	0	
ICU discharge	642 (459–846)	765 (459–796)	628 (463–979)	0.85
Missing data, *n*	11	6	5	
6 months post-ICU discharge	797 (647–1057)	797 (647–1057)		
Missing data, *n*	26	1		
Treg percentage, median (IQR)				
D3-4	6.6 (5.0–9.3)	7 (5.1–10.8)	6.4 (4.9–9.0)	0.54

Table 2 continued

	Total study population $n = 40$	Patients with a blood sample at 6 months $n = 15$	Patients without a blood sample at 6 months $n = 25$	p value
Missing data, n	1	1	0	
ICU discharge	6.6 (5.2–7.9)	6.6 (5.0–8.3)	6.53 (5.5–7.6)	0.80
Missing data, n	11	6	5	
6 months post-ICU discharge	6.4 (4.7–8.0)	6.4 (4.7–8.0)		
Missing data, n	26	1		
Absolute Treg (mm^{-3}), median (IQR)				
D3-4	35 (22–45)	34 (22–43)	35 (23–47)	0.92
Missing data, n	1	1	0	
ICU discharge	39 (28–64)	39 (28–64)	38 (28–77)	0.85
Missing data, n	11	6	5	
6 months post-ICU discharge	44 (34–67)	44 (34–67)		
Missing data, n	26	1		

IQR interquartile range, *AB/C* anti-HLA-DR antibodies per cell, *ICU* intensive care unit

patients had normal mHLA-DR on day 6–8, whereas this was abnormal on day 3–4. At ICU discharge, eight patients (24%) had normal mHLA-DR. mHLA-DR was less than 5000 AB/C for 21 patients (58%) on day 1–2, for 22 patients (56%) on day 3–4, for 11 patients (34%) on day 6–8, and four patients (12%) at ICU discharge. For all patients, median mHLA-DR expression on day 1–2 was significantly lower to that at ICU discharge ($p < 0.0001$; Fig. 2). Three patients died within 6 months. One patient died from complications of incurable cytomegalovirus ileitis in a surgical unit 20 days after ICU discharge; for this patient mHLA-DR expression at ICU discharge was 9600 AB/C. Another patient died from an acute respiratory distress syndrome complicating lung infection in another critical care unit where he had been admitted 4 months after discharge from the study ICU; for this patient mHLA-DR expression at ICU discharge was 5555 AB/C. The last patient died at home 4 months after ICU discharge and the cause of death was cardiac arrest; for this patient mHLA-DR expression at ICU discharge was

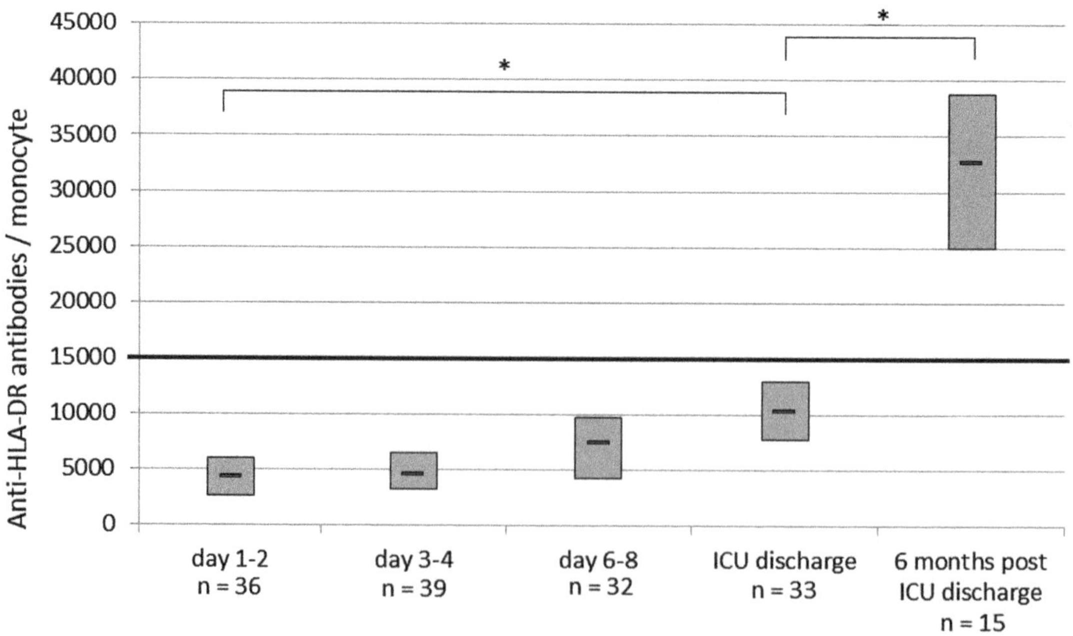

Fig. 2 mHLA-DR expression from day 1 after admission to ICU discharge. Box plot interpretation: box borders: 1st and 3rd quartile, central band in box: median value, *significantly different

28,447 AB/C. mHLA-DR expression on day 6–8 was not significantly different between those who had experienced a secondary nosocomial infection during ICU stay and those who had not done so ($p = 0.19$). mHLA-DR expression at ICU discharge was weakly correlated with the ICU length stay ($r = 0.44$, 95% CI 0.12–0.68, $p = 0.01$).

Among patients with a blood sample ($n = 15$), all but one patient had a normal level of mHLA-DR expression 6 months after ICU discharge (Fig. 2). The patient who had abnormal mHLA-DR expression suffered from recurrent abdominal sepsis requiring multiple surgical procedures since ICU discharge (29 days after his ICU admission) and was still hospitalized (in a surgical unit) 6 months after ICU discharge. For the 15 patients, median mHLA-DR expression on day 1–2 was significantly lower to that at ICU discharge ($p = 0.005$), and at 6 months after ICU discharge ($p < 0.0001$); median mHLA-DR expression 6 months after ICU discharge was significantly higher from median mHLA-DR at ICU discharge ($p = 0.0002$).

For the 11 patients who did not provide a blood sample at 6 months because they were unable to travel to the hospital, median mHLA-DR at ICU discharge was similar to those of the 15 with a blood sample at 6 months [median 11,497 (IQR 7195–21,032) AB/C vs. median 10,228 (IQR 8719–11,826) AB/C, respectively, $p = 0.32$].

CD4+ T cells

Eighteen patients (46%) had CD4+ lymphopenia (<500 mm^{-3}) on day 3–4 and 10 (34%) had CD4+ lymphopenia at discharge. The median (IQR) CD4+ T cells at ICU discharge was 642 (459–846) mm^{-3} (Table 2). Among the 15 patients with a blood sample at 6 months, only one patient presented CD4+ lymphopenia 6 months after ICU discharge (Fig. 3). This patient did not present a medical complication within this period. The number of CD4+ T cells at ICU discharge was not correlated with the ICU length of stay ($r = 0.23$, 95% CI −0.15 to 0.55, $p = 0.22$).

Treg expression

The median (IQR) percentage of Treg relative to total CD4+ T cells at ICU discharge was 6.6 (5.2–7.9)% (Table 2). Seven patients out of the 39 (18%) with data available had increased proportion of Treg among CD4+ T cells (>10%) on day 3–4, whereas only 3 out of 29 (10%) did so at ICU discharge; this difference did not reach statistical significance ($p = 0.49$). All patients who had an elevated proportion of Treg also had mHLA-DR <5000 AB/C either on day 1–2 or on day 3–4. Two patients had a proportion of Treg greater than 15% on day 3–4. These two patients also had the highest Sepsis-related Organ Failure Assessment score (SOFA score) at admission. Among the 15 patients with a blood sample at 6 months, none had an abnormal proportion of Treg 6 months after ICU discharge.

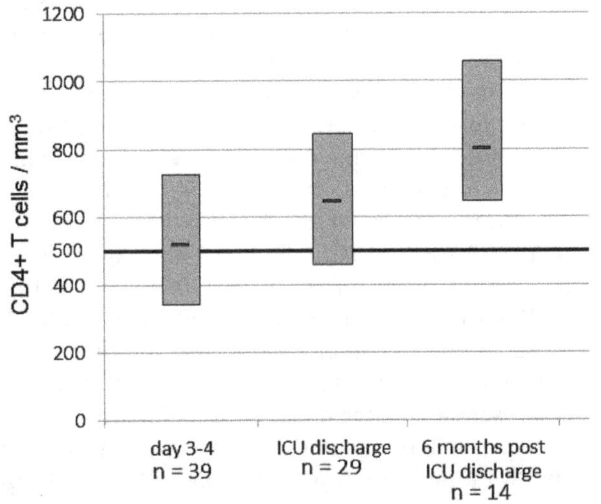

Fig. 3 CD4+ T cells from day 3 after ICU admission to 6 months after ICU discharge. Box plot interpretation: box borders: 1st and 3rd quartile, central band in box: median value

Discussion

This study found persistent cellular immune alterations in septic shock survivors at ICU discharge but no detectable long-term immune alterations 6 months after ICU discharge in some of them, as evidenced from mHLA-DR expression, CD4+ T cells, and relative proportion of Treg. Although unexpected, these data suggest that sepsis-induced immunosuppression at the cellular level based on these three markers is reversible after a period of time.

Among the biological parameters assessing the innate immune system, mHLA-DR seems to be an effective indicator of immune alterations [4, 5]. Its decreased expression represents one of the only immune marker shown to be an independent factor of occurrence of secondary nosocomial infections [6]. The interest of mHLA-DR expression assessment stands in the fact that this marker is a consequence of the effect of multiple mediators on the inflammatory response [21–23]. Its routine determination could be an important element of the immunological monitoring of septic patients [24, 25] or even of all patients undergoing an inflammatory injury and at risk of developing secondary infections. Usually, a patient is considered to be immunocompetent when mHLA-DR expression is above 15,000 AB/C. Values comprised between 10,000 and 15,000 AB/C may represent moderate immunosuppression, whereas values lower than 5000

AB/C may represent very deep immune alterations [18] which existed in 80% of patients in the present study, either on day 1–2 or on day 3–4. To our knowledge, there is no data in the medical literature assessing mHLA-DR expression at ICU discharge in patients admitted to the ICU for septic shock which would allow us to determine whether sepsis-induced immunosuppression persists. Herein, three-quarters of the patients have mHLA-DR below 15,000 AB/C at ICU discharge although they are usually free of organ failure at that moment. Furthermore, 12% of patients had mHLA-DR <5000 AB/C at ICU discharge, which represent a deep immune alteration. The immunological failure, not evaluated in routine, may represent a long-term persistent failure in the same way as renal failure in some patients. Among the three patients who died within 6 months post-ICU discharge, one died from cardiac arrest but two died from an infection and had abnormal mHLA-DR at ICU discharge. Interestingly, one of these infections was a CMV ileitis, which corresponds to a latent virus reactivation typically observed in context of deep immunosuppression.

With regard to adaptive immunity, CD4+ T lymphopenia occurring during sepsis is a major component of immunosuppression. It is also associated with higher risk of nosocomial infection and mortality [8, 26, 27]. Drewry et al. [8] reported that persistent lymphopenia on day 4 after the onset of sepsis predicted 28-mortality and 1-year survival. The medical literature on regulatory T cells is less abundant. Monneret et al. [12] reported in 2003 their relative increase in septic patients, which was later confirmed by others [28]. Their immunosuppressive properties affect both the antigen presenting cells of innate immunity and lymphocytes of adaptive immunity [29, 30]. Their presence correlates with a poor prognosis; in sepsis, their relative increase is observed early but persists only in patients dying later [12]. This negative association with survival was also reported in animal models [31]. We also recently reported that the increased proportion of Treg observed in sepsis was correlated with a decrease in lymphocyte proliferation [11]. Thus, Treg participates in the development of lymphocyte anergy described in sepsis which is significantly associated with increased mortality and the occurrence of secondary infections in septic patients [32]. In the present study, almost half of patients had CD4+ T lymphopenia on day 3–4 and this lymphopenia remained present for one-third of patients at ICU discharge although it was not correlated with the ICU length stay. The lack of correlation between immunological parameters and length of stay is probably caused by the small sample size resulting in a lack of power for correlation tests. Few patients (18%) had a percentage of Treg greater than 10%, but all of them had deep loss of mHLA-DR expression (i.e., mHLA-DR <5000 AB/C).

The study population was moderately old which may have affected immunological parameters. However, to our knowledge, modifications of mHLA-DR expression and CD4+ T cell count with age remain moderate [18, 33, 34]. Values found 6 months after ICU discharge were greater than the lower band of the normal range for all but one patient for mHLA-DR expression, and all but one for CD4+ T cell count. Thus, the immunosenescence does not seem to have an impact on the parameters measured.

With regard to immunological data at 6 months post-ICU discharge, the present results at the cellular level are in accordance with those from other investigators [35]. Arens et al. recently challenged the long-term persistence of sepsis-induced immunosuppression hypothesis in a retrospective cohort study composed of 8 sepsis survivors (without having studied immunological data during ICU stay, or at ICU discharge). They reported that immune alterations were minimal 26 months (range 9–52) after the septic event. There was no significant difference in lymphocyte profile (including Treg cell counts) and in expression of mHLA-DR between sepsis survivors and healthy volunteers. The expression of pattern recognition receptors (PRR) on leukocyte surface was not different between the two groups except for TLR-5, which was expressed at a lower level in the sepsis group. Finally, they only observed alterations regarding functional testing; after ex vivo stimulation of whole blood with potent activators, immune cells exhibited a decreased secretion of INF-γ, IL-10, IL-6, and TNF-α. Moreover, 62% of sepsis survivor patients had at least another episode of sepsis within the year prior to inclusion [35].

These findings raise the importance of functional tests, which must remain the reference to assess immune status as they directly measure the ability of cells to respond to pathogens. However, such tests are not always feasible in routine due to methodological difficulties such as a long incubation period, prolonged cellular purification procedures, and absence of standardization. Efforts are needed to facilitate practice of functional tests with the aim that their use becomes as common as that of static biomarkers.

The results presented herein complete two limitations of the study reported by Arens et al. [35]. Firstly, in the previous study, septic patients were not monitored during their ICU stay which means that sepsis-induced immunosuppression was not demonstrated in these patients. Secondly, the delay between septic event and mHLA-DR measurement was very long (median: 26 months), whereas herein it is demonstrated that mHLA-DR expression is already back to normal values as early as 6 months after ICU discharge. Additional studies with immunological monitoring within weeks following ICU discharge are needed to determine the timing of recovery of sepsis-induced immunosuppression.

Nevertheless, the present study has itself some limitations. For instance, only a small number of patients were studied at 6 months because a majority could not or refused to return to our hospital 6 months after the ICU discharge. Reasons for not coming back to the hospital were various. Most of these patients were elderly [median 71 (IQR 64–76) years (data not shown)], could not drive a car, could not take public transportation, and generally, they did not leave their home. This may have generated a selection bias in so far as participating patients were potentially in better clinical condition, which may have influenced results. We were not able to follow the immune status of patients with a bad outcome (those who died within 6 months or who suffered from new infections). This does not exclude the possibility that a sub-group of patients was not analyzed because of prolonged immune suppression. In other words, the analysis concerned only patients with a favorable outcome, whose immune functions returned to normal range. Data from the whole population are lacking, and these results need to be confirmed by a larger cohort. The small sample size also precludes a sub-analysis evaluating the immune status of patients suffering from complications in the long term in comparison with those who do not. However, these 15 patients were representative of the whole population, particularly for immunological parameters at ICU discharge. Thus, it should also be noted that 7.5% of patients alive at ICU discharge died within 6 months. Moreover, two other patients were out of contact and potentially also died. The total population had a favorable outcome because we included only patients who were alive at the time of ICU discharge, while mortality rate in septic shock is reported to reach up to 40% [1]. There is also a number of missing immunological data in particular at ICU discharge. This is due to the fact that measures could not be performed over the weekend or during the week outside the opening hours of the immunology laboratory. It would also have been interesting to have complete clinical data in particular the occurrence of infections since the ICU discharge for all patients who did not come back to the hospital 6 months after their ICU discharge. This could have allowed an exploration of a possible association with their immunological parameters at ICU discharge. Furthermore, we estimated only three immunological parameters, which also constitute a limit of the study.

If one hypothesizes that persisting long-term immune alterations may participate in increased risk for additional infections in septic patients, the present results are somehow unexpected. As opposed to mHLA-DR results, CD4+ T cells results and Treg results, the main result observed in the study reported by Arens et al. [35] is the ex vivo decreased whole blood cytokine secretion in long-term survivors. This is the confirmation that a single marker is likely to not be sufficient to fully monitor patient immune status. In addition, it supports the need to include functional testing in an immune monitoring panel which could detect some persistent immune alterations; additional research is needed to improve our understanding of long-term mortality in septic patients.

Conclusions

This study did not find any persistent immune alterations in septic shock survivors with good clinical outcome 6 months after ICU discharge as evidenced by mHLA-DR expression, CD4+ T cells and Treg count. This does not exclude that immune alterations are present in a sub-group of patients with a bad clinical outcome. Nevertheless, CD4+ lymphopenia and low mHLA-DR expression were still present at ICU discharge for most patients.

Abbreviations

mHLA-DR: expression of human leukocyte antigen DR on monocytes; Treg: regulatory T cells; ICU: intensive care unit; SOFA: Sepsis-related Organ Failure Assessment; IGS II: Simplified Index of Gravity II; AB/C: antibodies per cell.

Authors' contributions

Each author has participated sufficiently in the work to take public responsibility for the content. All authors read and approved the final manuscript.

Author details

[1] Department of Anesthesiology and Critical Care Medicine, Edouard Herriot hospital, Hospices Civils de Lyon, Lyon, France. [2] EA7426 Hospices Civils de Lyon – bioMérieux, University Claude Bernard Lyon 1 "Pathophysiology of Injury Induced Immunosuppression", Lyon, France. [3] Cellular Immunology Laboratory, Edouard Herriot hospital, Hospices Civils de Lyon, Lyon, France.

Competing interests

The authors declare that they have no competing interests.

References

1. SepNet Critical Care Trials Group. Incidence of severe sepsis and septic shock in German intensive care units: the prospective, multicentre INSEP study. Intensive Care Med. 2016;42:1980–9.
2. Delano MJ, Ward PA. Sepsis-induced immune dysfunction: can immune therapies reduce mortality? J Clin Investig. 2016;126:23–31.
3. Hotchkiss RS, Monneret G, Payen D. Immunosuppression in sepsis: a novel understanding of the disorder and a new therapeutic approach. Lancet Infect Dis. 2013;13:260–8.

4. Wolk K, Döcke WD, von Baehr V, Volk HD, Sabat R. Impaired antigen presentation by human monocytes during endotoxin tolerance. Blood. 2000;96:218–23.
5. Monneret G, Venet F. Sepsis-induced immune alterations monitoring by flow cytometry as a promising tool for individualized therapy. Cytom B Clin Cytom. 2016;90:376–86.
6. Landelle C, Lepape A, Voirin N, Tognet E, Venet F, Bohé J, et al. Low monocyte human leukocyte antigen-DR is independently associated with nosocomial infections after septic shock. Intensive Care Med. 2010;36:1859–66.
7. Monneret G, Lepape A, Voirin N, Bohé J, Venet F, Debard A-L, et al. Persisting low monocyte human leukocyte antigen-DR expression predicts mortality in septic shock. Intensive Care Med. 2006;32:1175–83.
8. Drewry AM, Samra N, Skrupky LP, Fuller BM, Compton SM, Hotchkiss RS. Persistent lymphopenia after diagnosis of sepsis predicts mortality. Shock. 2014;42:383–91.
9. Venet F, Pachot A, Debard A-L, Bohe J, Bienvenu J, Lepape A, et al. Human CD4+ CD25+ regulatory T lymphocytes inhibit lipopolysaccharide-induced monocyte survival through a Fas/Fas ligand-dependent mechanism. J Immunol. 2006;177:6540–7.
10. Lewkowicz P, Lewkowicz N, Sasiak A, Tchórzewski H. Lipopolysaccharide-activated CD4+ CD25+ T regulatory cells inhibit neutrophil function and promote their apoptosis and death. J Immunol. 2006;177:7155–63.
11. Venet F, Chung C-S, Kherouf H, Geeraert A, Malcus C, Poitevin F, et al. Increased circulating regulatory T cells (CD4(+)CD25 (+)CD127(−)) contribute to lymphocyte anergy in septic shock patients. Intensive Care Med. 2009;35:678–86.
12. Monneret G, Debard A-L, Venet F, Bohe J, Hequet O, Bienvenu J, et al. Marked elevation of human circulating CD4+ CD25+ regulatory T cells in sepsis-induced immunoparalysis. Crit Care Med. 2003;31:2068–71.
13. Winters BD, Eberlein M, Leung J, Needham DM, Pronovost PJ, Sevransky JE. Long-term mortality and quality of life in sepsis: a systematic review. Crit Care Med. 2010;38:1276–83.
14. Karlsson S, Ruokonen E, Varpula T, Ala-Kokko TI, Pettilä V. Finnsepsis Study Group. Long-term outcome and quality-adjusted life years after severe sepsis. Crit Care Med. 2009;37:1268–74.
15. Weycker D, Akhras KS, Edelsberg J, Angus DC, Oster G. Long-term mortality and medical care charges in patients with severe sepsis. Crit Care Med. 2003;31:2316–23.
16. Wang HE, Szychowski JM, Griffin R, Safford MM, Shapiro NI, Howard G. Long-term mortality after community-acquired sepsis: a longitudinal population-based cohort study. BMJ Open. 2014;4:e004283.
17. Linder A, Guh D, Boyd JH, Walley KR, Anis AH, Russell JA. Long-term (10-year) mortality of younger previously healthy patients with severe sepsis/septic shock is worse than that of patients with nonseptic critical illness and of the general population. Crit Care Med. 2014;42:2211–8.
18. Döcke W-D, Höflich C, Davis KA, Röttgers K, Meisel C, Kiefer P, et al. Monitoring temporary immunodepression by flow cytometric measurement of monocytic HLA-DR expression: a multicenter standardized study. Clin Chem. 2005;51:2341–7.
19. Monneret G, Elmenkouri N, Bohe J, Debard A-L, Gutowski M-C, Bienvenu J, et al. Analytical requirements for measuring monocytic human lymphocyte antigen DR by flow cytometry: application to the monitoring of patients with septic shock. Clin Chem. 2002;48:1589–92.
20. R Core Team. R: the R project for statistical computing [Internet]. 2013 [cited 2017 Jan 16]. https://www.r-project.org/.
21. Gonwa TA, Picker LJ, Raff HV, Goyert SM, Silver J, Stobo JD. Antigen-presenting capabilities of human monocytes correlates with their expression of HLA-DS, an Ia determinant distinct from HLA-DR. J Immunol. 1983;130:706–11.
22. Medzhitov R, Janeway C. Innate immunity. N Engl J Med. 2000;343:338–44.
23. Cheadle WG. The human leukocyte antigens and their relationship to infection. Am J Surg. 1993;165:75S–81S.
24. Volk HD, Reinke P, Döcke WD. Immunological monitoring of the inflammatory process: Which variables? When to assess? Eur J Surg Suppl. 1999;584:70–2.
25. Sáenz JJ, Izura JJ, Manrique A, Sala F, Gaminde I. Early prognosis in severe sepsis via analyzing the monocyte immunophenotype. Intensive Care Med. 2001;27:970–7.
26. Le Tulzo Y, Pangault C, Gacouin A, Guilloux V, Tribut O, Amiot L, et al. Early circulating lymphocyte apoptosis in human septic shock is associated with poor outcome. Shock. 2002;18:487–94.
27. Girardot T, Rimmelé T, Venet F, Monneret G. Apoptosis-induced lymphopenia in sepsis and other severe injuries. Apoptosis. 2017;22:295–305.
28. Leng FY, Liu JL, Liu ZJ, Yin JY, Qu HP. Increased proportion of CD4(+) CD25(+)Foxp3(+) regulatory T cells during early-stage sepsis in ICU patients. J Microbiol Immunol Infect. 2013;46:338–44.
29. Baecher-Allan C, Hafler DA. Human regulatory T cells and their role in autoimmune disease. Immunol Rev. 2006;212:203–16.
30. Belkaid Y. Regulatory T cells and infection: a dangerous necessity. Nat Rev Immunol. 2007;7:875–88.
31. Chen X, Bäumel M, Männel DN, Howard OMZ, Oppenheim JJ. Interaction of TNF with TNF receptor type 2 promotes expansion and function of mouse CD4+ CD25+ T regulatory cells. J Immunol. 2007;179:154–61.
32. Roth G, Moser B, Krenn C, Brunner M, Haisjackl M, Almer G, et al. Susceptibility to programmed cell death in T-lymphocytes from septic patients: a mechanism for lymphopenia and Th2 predominance. Biochem Biophys Res Commun. 2003;308:840–6.
33. Ferrando-Martínez S, Ruiz-Mateos E, Hernández A, Gutiérrez E, Rodríguez-Méndez Mdel M, Ordoñez A, et al. Age-related deregulation of naive T cell homeostasis in elderly humans. Age (Dordr). 2011;33:197–207.
34. Jentsch-Ullrich K, Koenigsmann M, Mohren M, Franke A. Lymphocyte subsets' reference ranges in an age- and gender-balanced population of 100 healthy adults—a monocentric German study. Clin Immunol. 2005;116:192–7.
35. Arens C, Bajwa SA, Koch C, Siegler BH, Schneck E, Hecker A, et al. Sepsis-induced long-term immune paralysis—results of a descriptive, explorative study. Crit Care Lond Engl. 2016;20:93.

10

Piperacillin–tazobactam as alternative to carbapenems for ICU patients

Benoit Pilmis[1,2], Vincent Jullien[3,4], Alexis Tabah[5,6], Jean-Ralph Zahar[7,8*] and Christian Brun-Buisson[9]

Abstract

Several studies suggest that alternatives to carbapenems, and particulary beta-lactam/beta-lactamase inhibitor combinations, can be used for therapy of extended-spectrum beta-lactamase-producing Enterobacteriaceae (ESBL-PE)-related infections in non-ICU patients. Little is known concerning ICU patients in whom achieving the desired plasmatic pharmacokinetic/pharmacodynamic (PK/PD) target may be difficult. Also, in vitro susceptibility to beta-lactamase inhibitors might not translate into clinical efficacy. We reviewed the recent clinical studies examining the use of BL/BLI as alternatives to carbapenems for therapy of bloodstream infection, PK/PD data and discuss potential ecological benefit from avoiding the use of carbapenems. With the lack of prospective randomized studies, treating ICU patients with ESBL-PE-related infections using piperacillin–tazobactam should be done with caution. Current data suggest that BL/BLI empirical use should be avoided for therapy of ESBL-PE-related infection. Also, definitive therapy should be reserved to patients in clinical stable condition, after microbial documentation and results of susceptibility tests. Optimization of administration and higher dosage should be used in order to reach pharmacological targets.

Keywords: Carbapenems, ESBL, Alternatives, Ecological consequences, Outcome

Introduction

Since the 1980s, extended-spectrum beta-lactamase (ESBL)-producing Enterobacteriaceae (ESBL-PE) have been spreading worldwide [1, 2]. Several reports underline the concomitant increasing use of carbapenems [3, 4]. Indeed, the recently published 2015 ESAC report noted a threefold increased use of carbapenems between 2010 and 2014 [5]. This induces a selective pressure for carbapenem-resistant isolates, and recent data suggest that even a brief exposure to carbapenems increases the risk of colonization with carbapenem-resistant bacteria (CRB) in intensive care unit patients [6].

To reduce the ecological risk associated with the increased consumption of last-line antibiotics, two main strategies are available: (1) searching for alternative treatments for ESBL-PE-related infections and (2) antimicrobial de-escalation (ADE). Therefore, the use of alternatives to carbapenems such as cephamycins, piperacillin–tazobactam and others for the treatment of ESBL-PE infections should be investigated. A recent systematic review, including two randomized controlled trials and 12 cohort studies, highlighted that the effects of ADE on antimicrobial resistance have not been properly studied [7]. However, this strategy is largely promoted by several scientific societies and specifically in critically ill patients [8, 9]. Indeed, for severely ill patients, international guidelines recommend the use of broad-spectrum antibiotics as first-line therapy to minimize the risk of inadequate initial antimicrobial treatment, and suggest streamlining initial antibiotic therapy and narrowing the spectrum whenever possible once the pathogen(s) are identified [10].

Until recently, the common rule is to treat infections caused by ESBL-producing organism with carbapenems. However, ESBLs are inhibited in vitro by beta-lactamase inhibitors and several studies have suggested the use of β-lactam/β-lactamase inhibitor combinations (BL/BLIs) such as piperacillin–tazobactam as a carbapenem-sparing strategy for the treatment of ESBL-PE-related infections [11–13]. The recent EUCAST and CLSI [14,

*Correspondence: jeanralph.zahar@aphp.fr
[7] Département de Microbiologie Clinique, Unité de Contrôle et de Prévention du risque Infectieux, Groupe Hospitalier Paris Seine Saint-Denis, AP-HP, CHU Avicenne, 125 rue de Stalingrad, 9300 Bobigny, France
Full list of author information is available at the end of the article

15] guidelines include BL/BLIs and other beta-lactams (cefepime, third generation cephalosporins, temocillin, cefoxitin) as treatment options for infections caused by ESBL-producing organisms. For a long time, AST categorization was based not only on MIC and zone diameter measurements but also on the detection of individual resistance mechanisms, i.e., interpretative reading. Even if in vitro results indicated susceptibility to a drug, the reported category was edited to "resistant" if the presence of a resistance mechanism was confirmed, e.g., in the case of extended-spectrum beta-lactamases (ESBLs). To limit the consumption of carbapenems, CLSI and EUCAST recently abandoned editing of AST reports based on the detection of ESBLs.

While several studies are conducted in ICU, data remain scarce concerning other beta-lactams in non-ICU- [16, 17] and ICU-infected [18–21] patients. Therefore, only BL/BLIs such as piperacillin–tazobactam (Pip–Taz) could be used in ICU patients, but there are concerns that: (1) no randomized controlled trials compared specifically carbapenems to Pip–Taz for the treatment of ESBL-PE-related infections [22]; (2) in vitro susceptibility to β-lactamase inhibitors might not predict clinical efficacy; and (3) the success of BL/BLIs depends on pharmacokinetic–pharmacodynamic target attainment, which current dosing recommendations may not guarantee. Therefore, alternatives are seldom used in clinical practice for treating serious infections caused by ESBL-PE.

In critically ill patients, pharmacokinetics of beta-lactam antibiotics differs from healthy volunteers. Lower than expected concentrations have been reported for meropenem, piperacillin, amoxicillin, as well as for cephalosporins [23–26]. Besides, the risk of treatment failure may be exacerbated when using antibiotics exposed to the inoculum effect [27], as are most beta-lactams.

This narrative review, based on microbiological, pharmacodynamics, clinical and ecological data, describes the available evidence for the use of Pip–Taz as an alternative to carbapenems in critically ill patients and to provide some guidance to prescribers for using these drugs when treating infections caused by ESBL-PE.

Methods

Literature search

A literature search was performed via PubMed, including all records from 1990 through April 2016. The following search pattern was applied: (ESBL OR extended-spectrum β-lactamases) AND (infection) AND (cefepime OR cefoxitine OR cephamycins OR flomoxef OR BL/BLI OR Piperacillin–tazobactam OR Carbapenems OR temocillin OR alternatives). Reference lists were cross-checked to identify further publications for possible inclusion. We restricted inclusion to studies published in the English, Spanish and French languages.

Selection criteria

We screened and included studies in three categories according to the following criteria: (1) pharmacokinetics and pharmacodynamics studies, where all studies investigating the PK/PD of the potential alternatives to carbapenems in ICU patients were included. (2) For clinical studies, we restricted inclusion to studies reporting mortality of patients receiving empirical or definitive treatment with a non-carbapenem therapy for an ESBL bacteremia in adult patients. Patients with community-, hospital- and healthcare-associated bacteremia were eligible for inclusion. (3) Finally, considering ecological studies, we included any published article reporting carbapenem-resistant Enterobacteriaceae (CRE). Among the eligible articles, studies were included if they reported on exposure to any previous antibiotic class as a risk factor associated with CRE acquisition.

Results

Microbiological susceptibility

Several studies suggested that ESBL-PE were susceptible to non-carbapenem beta-lactams. However, the prevalence of susceptibility depends on the species concerned, the antibiotic class and local epidemiology. ESBL-producing *E. coli* is usually regarded as more susceptible to all beta-lactams than ESBL-producing *K. pneumoniae*, piperacillin–tazobactam (Pip–Taz) being the most effective antibiotic [28]. North American data from the 2010–2014 SMART programs find that 4, 10 and 46% of ESBL-producing *E. coli* were susceptible to ceftriaxone, cefepime and ceftazidime, respectively [28], whereas 96–98 and 69% of ESBL-producing *E. coli* isolates from urinary tract [29] and from patients with pneumonia [30] were found susceptible in vitro to Pip–Taz, respectively. Conversely, only 26.9% of ESBL-producing *Klebsiella* spp. isolates from patients with pneumonia were susceptible to Pip–Taz [30]. Asian data on ESBL-producing *E. coli* find similar susceptibilities, with 1.6, 9.5, 33.4 and 84.5% isolates susceptible to cefotaxime, cefepime, ceftazidime and Pip–Taz, respectively [29]. It is noteworthy that in silico PK/PD studies aiming to evaluate the use of alternatives to carbapenems for treatment of ESBL-PE infections suggest that ESBL-Kp susceptibility is overestimated by conventional methods in comparison with E-test susceptibility testing.

Pharmacokinetics and pharmacodynamics studies

According to epidemiological data, two main antibiotics could be used as an alternative to carbapenems: piperacillin and cefoxitin. Others antibiotics suggested in the literature as temocillin, ceftolozane/tazobactam and/or ceftazidime/avibactam are less tested. Our goal was to define the optimal condition for using these antibiotics for ESBL-PE-related infections in ICU.

The pharmacokinetics of piperacillin in ICU patients was quite extensively investigated. There is, however, a lack of consensus on the pharmacokinetic/pharmacodynamic target to be achieved. Indeed targets as different as obtaining a free concentration > MIC (fT > MIC) or > 4 times the MIC (fT > 4xMIC) for 50 or 100% of a dose interval have been considered [31–36]. This is a crucial point as the dose to be administered will vary considerably according to the chosen target. There are, however, increasing data supporting a minimal efficacy criteria of fT > MIC = 100% in ICU patients, while a total trough concentration/MIC ratio of at least three was found to prevent the emergence of resistance in vitro [37–40]. Therefore, based on these more drastic PK/PD endpoints, it seems a dose of 4.5 g TID given as intermittent infusions should not be considered any more in ICU patients with normal renal functions [32, 36]. A 4.5-g × 4 daily dose appears more convenient, provided it is administered as prolonged infusion of at least 3 h [32, 34]. Indeed, for an intermittent bolus administration, a 4gx4 dose is associated with a very low probability of target attainment, even for the lowest PK/PD target of T > MIC = 50% [32]. However, even with a 4.5-g x 4 dose given by extended 3-h infusions, around one-third of the patients may not achieve a fT > MIC = 100%, which supports the need for an individual dose adjustment using therapeutic drug monitoring [35]. Such a result strongly supports the use of continuous infusion, and since this administration mode provides a better outcome than intermittent infusion [24], we believe a 16-g daily dose given as a continuous infusion, following a 4.5-g loading dose, should be considered as a starting point in ICU patients with normal renal function. Such an approach was found relevant for the treatment of ventilator-associated pneumonia, as it allowed the achievement of alveolar concentrations > 16 mg/L (i.e., the clinical breakpoint for gram-negative bacteria).

Slightly different results were observed in morbidly obese ICU patients, for whom the elimination half-life of piperacillin seems to be increased, compared to non-obese patients, resulting in an increased fT > MIC for equivalent doses [33]. Consequently, a 4.5-g × 4 daily dose given as a 4-h extended infusion should provide satisfying trough concentrations [33].

The pharmacokinetics of piperacillin in ICU patients undergoing continuous renal replacement therapy (CRRT) was also investigated, and similar results were found in case of venovenous hemofiltration or hemodiafiltration. A 4.5-g TID dose given as 30-min infusion should provide a free concentration > MIC for the entire dosing interval in almost all patients. Extending the infusion duration to 4 h should allow the attainment of several times the MIC. However, dose requirements seem to importantly depend on the membrane used and the effluent rate that are major aspects of CRRT poorly investigated to date [41, 42]. An interesting point is that piperacillin concentration in the dialysate effluent is equal to the free plasma concentration and can therefore be used for the individual adaptation of the dose via therapeutic drug monitoring (TDM) [43]. To our knowledge, the PK of piperacillin in the context of intermittent hemodialysis was not investigated to date in ICU patients. Based on the results obtained in sepsis-free volunteers with chronic renal failure [44], a dose of 4.5 g bid could be used as a starting point, with a subsequent TDM-guided individual adjustment of the dose. Conflicting results are available about the percentage of the dose that is eliminated by a 4-h session of hemodialysis (i.e., from 10 to 50%) [45, 46]. However, because a supplemental elimination is likely to occur during hemodialysis, it seems preferable to administrate the drug just after the end of the hemodialysis session.

Cefoxitin PK in ICU patients was not investigated to date. By using the PK parameters obtained in healthy subjects, it was shown that for a 8-g daily dose of cefoxitin, only an administration by continuous infusion provided a high probability to achieve targets of fT > MIC = 100% and fT > 4 × MIC = 100% for ESBL-PE [47]. However, since PK differences are expected in ICU subjects, PK data in this population are obviously needed [48].

Concerning temocillin, a 2-g TID dose given as intermittent 30-min infusion, provides a high probability to attain fT > MIC = 100% in ICU patients with normal renal function, provided the MIC is ≤ 4 mg/L. For higher MIC, administration of the same daily dose by continuous infusion is preferable [49]. In summary, among the different antibiotics suggested as alternatives to carbapenems, Pip–Tz is the one with the most frequent published PK/PD data in ICU. High daily doses and prolonged infusion should be promoted for ESBL-PE-related infections in ICU patients.

Clinical studies

The article selection process is shown in Fig. 1. Of the 54 articles selected initially, 23 provided data among patients treated with BL/BLIs for ESBL-producing Enterobacteriaceae-related infections (Table 1). Most of the published studies were retrospective (17/23; 73.9%), and all others were observational. Community-acquired, healthcare-associated and nosocomial infections were included without distinction. Among these 23 studies, 9 (39.1%), 6 (26%) and 7 (30.4%) evaluated antibiotic therapy as

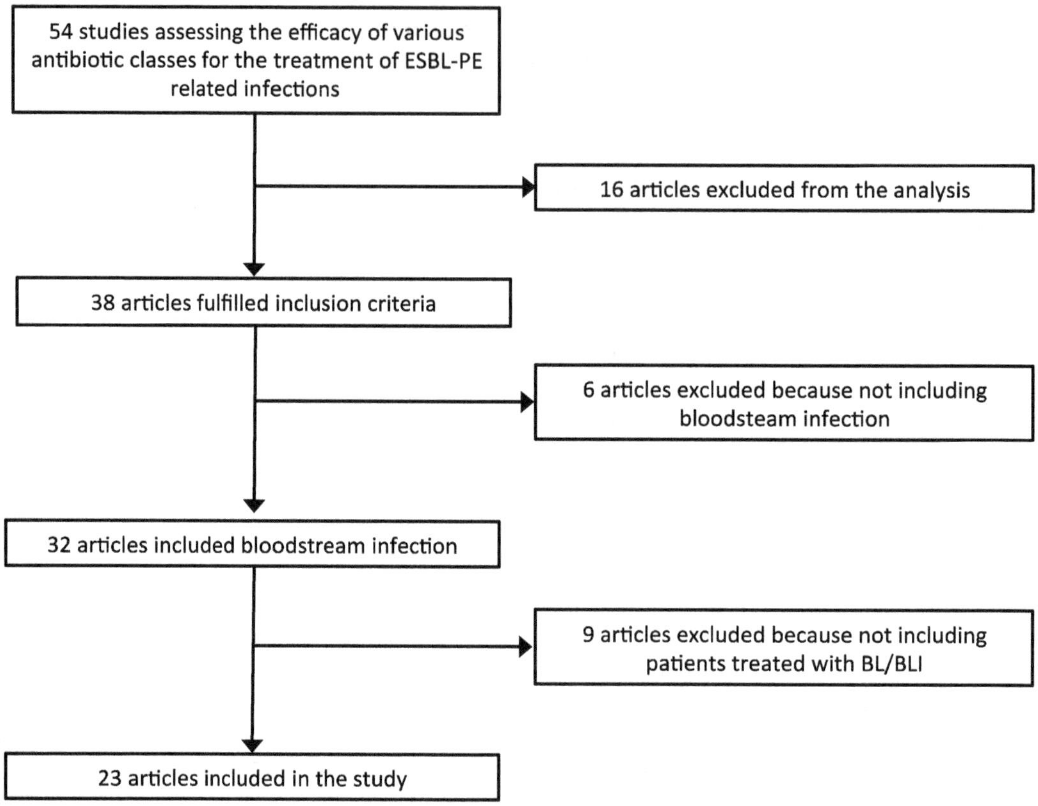

Fig. 1 Flow diagram of the selection process of the included studies

empirical therapy (ETC), definitive therapy or both, respectively. Among carbapenems, the selected molecule was available in 53% of included studies and imipenem–cilastatin was the most frequently used (45.7% of studies) followed by meropenem (35.2%) and ertapenem (19.1%).

Only 3 (13%) studies reported the doses of antibiotics [19, 20, 50] and none reported the modalities of antibiotic's administration. Indeed administered doses in patients without renal failure were variable; however, imipenem was used in most cases at an average dose of 0.5 g every 6 h, whereas 1 g every 8 h and 1 g every 24 h were used for meropenem and ertapenem, respectively. The two species most frequently involved were *E. coli* and *K. pneumoniae.* All patients included in these studies had bacteremia, and the two most frequent sites of infection were urinary tract and intra-abdominal infection. MIC was taken into account in adjusting antibiotic therapy in 11 (47.8%) of the 23 studies.

As mentioned above, 11 studies included between 6 and 131 ICU patients. In fact, some of the same patients were included in different cohorts [12, 51]. Only 4 studies [52–55] included patients with pneumonia caused by ESBL-PE, representing 8–50% of patients with ESBL-PE-related infections, indicating that less than 30 patients with ESBL-related pneumonia could be evaluated. Data regarding outcome for patients treated with carbapenems versus alternatives were available from 20 (86.9%) of the 23 studies including bacteremic patients. Surprisingly, potential confounding factors, such as severity of underlying diseases or of infection, were seldom reported.

Among studies including ICU patients, 6 (56%) compared BL/BLIs to carbapenems as empirical therapy. However, BL/BLIs was the only alternative compared to carbapenems in only 3 studies [12, 20, 51]. In these studies, *E. coli* and *K. pneumoniae* represented more than two-third of the isolates and MICs were taken into account in only one study [20]. The difference of mortality didn't reach statistical significance in two studies [12, 51]. However, Ofer-friedman et al. [20] conducted a multicenter observational study including non-urinary BSI and comparing BL/BLI to carbapenem for the treatment of ESBL. In contrast to other studies, E. *coli* accounted for only half of the bloodstream infections; the median piperacillin MIC was 8 mg/L, and approximately half of patients required ICU care. In this study, the mortality was significantly higher in the piperacillin–tazobactam group [OR 7.9 (1.2–53)]. Thus, BL/BLIs may lead a poorer outcome than carbapenem therapy for critically

Table 1 Studies characteristics

Author/year of publication	Study design, region	No. of patients, ESBL/total	Type of infection (*n*, %)	Bacteria (*n*, %)	ICU (*n*, %)	ETC/DTC	Treatment (*n*, %)	MIC	Administration (CI, PI or II)	Posology
Apisarnthanarak et al. [52]	SC case–control, 2003–2007, Thailand	36/146	UK (36, 100%)	*E. coli* *K. pneumoniae*	UK	ETC (36, 100%)	Cephalosporins (17, 47.2%) BL/BLI (10, 27.8%) Carbapenem (5, 13.9%) Fluoroquinolones (4, 11.1%)	N	UK	UK
Balakrishnan et al. [94]	MC retrospective cohort, 2008–2010, United Kingdom	42/42	UK	UK	UK	DTC (42, 100%)	Temocillin (42, 100%)	Y	II	Y
Bin et al. [95]	SC prospective cohort, 2002–2005, China	22/22	IIA (11, 50%) Primary bacteraemia (6, 27.2%) UTI (5, 22.7%)	*E. coli* (22, 100%)	UK	DTC (22, 100%)	Carbapenem (8, 36.4%) Cephalosporins (7, 31.8%) BL/BLI (7, 31.8%)	Y	Y	UK
Chaubey et al. [96]	MC prospective cohort, 2000–2007, Canada	79/79	Primary bacteraemia (39, 49.3%) UTI (38, 48.1%) Pneumonia (2, 2.5%) IIA (1, 1.3%)	*E. coli* (72, 91.1%) *K. pneumoniae* (7, 8.9%)	UK	ETC (74, 93.7%) DTC (79, 100%)	Carbapenem (16, 20.2%) BL/BLI (16, 20.2%) Aminoglycosides (16, 20.2%) Fluoroquinolones (16, 20.2%) Cephalosporins (16, 20.2%) Carbapenem (16, 20.2%) BL/BLI (16, 20.2%) Fluoroquinolones (16, 20.2%) Sulfamides (16, 20.2%) Aminoglycosides (16, 20.2%)	N	UK	UK
Chopra et al. [50]	MC retrospective cohort, 2005–2007, USA	145/145	UK	*E. coli* (24, 16.6%) *K. pneumoniae* (121, 83.4%)	Y (37, 25,5%)	ETC (128, 88.2%) DTC (110)	Cephalosporins (85, 58.6%) Carbapenem (50, 34.4%) Fluoroquinolones (6, 3.9%) Aminoglycosides (4, 3.1%) Carbapenem (103, 70.9%) Cephalosporins (41, 28.2%) BL/BLI (24, 16.4%) Fluoroquinolones (17, 11.8%) Amikacin (17, 11.8%) Tigecycline (12, 8.2%)	Y	UK	UK

Table 1 continued

Author/year of publication	Study design, region	No. of patients, ESBL/total	Type of infection (*n*, %)	Bacteria (*n*, %)	ICU (*n*, %)	ETC/DTC	Treatment (*n*, %)	MIC	Administration (CI, PI or II)	Posology
Chung et al. [97]	SC retrospective cohort, 2005–2010, Taiwan	122/122	UTI (47, 38.5%) Primary bacteraemia (21, 17.2%) IIA (22, 18%) Pneumonia (6, 4.9%) CVC (6, 4.9%) Skin and soft tissue (4, 3.3%) Surgical site infection (3, 2.5%) Other (13, 10.7%)	*E. coli* (122, 100%)	UK	DTC (107 87.7%)	Carbapenem (71, 57.9%) Non-BL/BLI (48, 39.3%) BL/BLI (3, 2.8%)	N	UK	UK
De Rosa et al. [98]	SC retrospective cohort, 2000–2007, Italy	128/128	Primary bacteraemia (61, 47.6%) IIA (55, 43%) UTI (12, 9.4%)	*E. coli* (80, 62.5%) *K. pneumoniae* (28, 21.9%) *P. mirabilis* (20, 15.6%)	Y (8, 6.3%)	ETC (97 75.8%)	Carbapenem (101, 79.3%) BL/BLI (10, 8.2%) Fluoroquinolone (8, 6.2%) Trimethoprim/sulfamethoxazole (1, 1%) Aminoglycosides (8, 6.2%)	N	UK	UK
Du et al. [16]	SC retrospective cohort, 1997–1999, China	23/85	Primary bacteraemia (9, 39.1%) IIA (5, 21.7%) Pneumonia (4, 17.4%) UTI (2, 8.7%) CVC (2, 8.7%) Other (1, 4.4%)	*E. coli* (16, 69.5%) *K. pneumoniae* (7, 30.5%)	N	DTC (23, 100%)	Carbapenem (13, 56.5%) Cephalosporins (7, 30.4%) Fluoroquinolone (2, 8.7%) Aminoglycosides (1, 4.4%)	N	UK	UK
Endimiani et al. [99]	SC retrospective cohort, 1997–2004, Italy	9/23	Primary bacteraemia (5, 55.6%) UTI (4, 44.4%)	*P. mirabilis* (9, 100%)	UK	ETC (9, 100%) DTC (9, 100%)	Cephalosporins (5, 55.6%) BL/BLI (4, 44.4%) Cephalosporins (4, 44.4%) BL/BLI (3, 33.3%) Carbapenem (2, 22.3%)	Y	Y	UK
Ferrandez et al. [100]	Retrospective cohort, 2000–2006, Spain	53/53	UK	*E. coli* *K. pneumoniae*	UK	–	Carbapenem (30, 56.6%) BL/BLI (5, 9.4%) Fluoroquinolone (4, 7.5%) Cephalosporins (2, 3.8%) Other (12, 22.7%)	Y	UK	UK
Gudiol et al. [101]	SC prospective observational study, 2006–2008, Spain	17/135	Primary bacteraemia (9, 52.9%) IIA (6, 35.3%) UTI (1, 5.9%) Other (1, 5.9%)	*E. coli* (17, 100%)	Y (2, 12%)	ETC (17, 100%) DTC (17, 100%)	BL/BLI (6, 35.3%) Carbapenem (5, 29.4%) Cephalosporins (5, 29.4%) Monobactam (1, 5.9%) Carbapenem (14, 82.3%) BL/BLI (2, 11.8%) Fluoroquinolone (1, 5.9%)	N	UK	UK

Table 1 continued

Author/year of publication	Study design, region	No. of patients, ESBL/total	Type of infection (*n*, %)	Bacteria (*n*, %)	ICU (*n*, %)	ETC/DTC	Treatment (*n*, %)	MIC	Administration (CI, PI or II)	Posology
Gutiérez-Gutiérez et al. [51]	MC, retrospective cohort study, 2004–2013, International	601/601	UTI (272, 45.2%) Other (258, 42.9%) IIA (71, 11.8%)	*E. coli* (439, 73%) *K. pneumoniae* (114, 19%) Other (48, 8%)	Y (64, 10.7%)	ETC (365, 60.7%) DTC (601, 100%)	Carbapenem (195, 53.5%) BL/BLI (169, 46.5%) Carbapenem (509, 84.7%) BL/BLI (92, 15.3%)	N	Y	II
Harris et al. [102]	SC retrospective cohort study, 2012–2013, China	92/92	UTI (43, 46.7%) Primary bacteramia (39, 42.2%) IIA (10, 11.1%)	*E. coli* (79, 85.9%) *K. pneumoniae* (13, 14.1%)	Y (11, 12.1%)	DTC (47, 51%)	Carbapenem (23, 48.9%) BL/BLI (24, 51.1%)	N	Y	II
Kang et al. [17]	SC retrospective cohort study, 1998–2002, South Korea	133/133	IIA (82, 61.6%) Primary bacteraemia (33, 24.8%) UTI (14, 10.5%) Pneumonia (4, 3.1%)	*E. coli* (67, 50.4%) *K. pneumoniae* (66, 49.6%)	N	ETC (133, 100%) DTC (133, 100%)	Non cephalosporins (29, 21.8%) Cephalosporins (104, 78.2%) Non cephalosporins (101, 75.9%) Cephalosporins (32, 24.1%)	Y	UK	UK
Kang et al. [69]	MC retrospective cohorts, 2008–2010, South Korea	114/114	UK	*E. coli* (78, 68.4%) *K. pneumonia* (36, 31.6%)	UK	ETC (114 100%)	Carbapenem (78, 68.4%) Piperacillin/tazobactam (36, 31.6%)	N	UK	UK
Lee et al. [53]	SC retrospective cohort, 2004–2005, Taiwan	27/27	Pneumonia (15, 55.5%) IIA (5, 18.5%) UTI (3, 11.1%) Primary bacteraemia (3, 11.1%) Other (1, 3.8%)	*K. pneumonia* (27, 100%)	Y (13, 48.1%)	DTC (27, 100%)	Carbapenem (20, 74%) Flomoxef (7, 26%)	Y	UK	UK
Lee and *al.* [21]	SC retrospective cohort, 2001–2008, Taiwan	121/206	CVC (48, 39.6%) Primary bacteraemia (32, 26.4%) Pneumonia (12, 9.9%) SSTI (9, 7.4%) UTI (9, 7.4%) IIA (6, 4.9%) Other (5, 4.3%)	*E. cloacae* (121, 100%)	Y (78, 64.4%)	ETC (114, 94.2%) DTC (114, 94.2%)	Cephalosporins (59, 49.1%) Carbapenem (26, 21%) BL/BLI (14, 11.4%) Other beta-lactam (13, 10.5%) Fluoroquinolones (3, 2.6%) Other Antibiotics (6, 5.4%) Carbapenem (53, 46.5%) Cephalosporins (38, 33.3%) Fluoroquinolones (16, 14%) BL/BLI (3, 2.6%) Other β-lactam (3, 2.6%) Other antibiotic therapy (1, 1%)	N	UK	UK

Table 1 continued

Author/year of publication	Study design, region	No. of patients, ESBL/total	Type of infection (*n*, %)	Bacteria (*n*, %)	ICU (*n*, %)	ETC/DTC	Treatment (*n*, %)	MIC	Administration (CI, PI or II)	Posology
Lee et al. [54]	MC retrospective cohort, 2002–2007, Taiwan	178/178	Pneumonia (43, 24.1%) UTI (39, 21.9%) CVC (37, 20.8%) IIA (28, 15.7%) Primary bacteraemia (25, 14%) SSTI (11, 6.3%)	ND	UK	DTC (178, 100%)	Carbapenem (161, 90,4%) Cefepime (17, 9.6%)	Y	Y	II
Lee et al. [103]	MC retrospective cohort, 2007–2012, Taiwan	389/389	UTI (88, 22.6%) CVC (86, 22.1%) Pneumonia (80, 20.5%) IIA (61, 15.7%) Primary bacteraemia (62, 16%) SSTI (12, 3.1%)	*E. coli* (156, 40.1%) *K. pneumoniae* (233, 59.9%)	UK	DTC (389, 100%)	Carbapenem (257, 66%) Flomoxef (132, 34%)	Y	UK	UK
Matsumura et al. [104]	MC retrospective cohort, 2005–2014, Japan	113/1440	UTI (57, 50.4%) IIA (32, 28.3%) Primary bacteraemia (19, 16.8%) Other (5, 4.5%)	*E. coli* (113, 100%)	UK	ETC (71, 62.8%) DTC (113, 100%)	Carbapenem (45, 63.7%) Cefmetazole/flomoxef (26, 36.6%) Carbapenem (54, 47.8%) Cefmetazole/flomoxef (59, 52.2%)	Y	UK	UK
Ofer-Friedman et al. [20]	MC retrospective cohort, 2008–2012, International	79/79	Pneumonia (27, 34.2%) SSTI (22, 27.8%) IIA (20, 25.3%) Primary bacteraemia (6, 7.6%) Undetermined (4, 5.1%)	*E. coli* (42, 53.1%) *K. pneumoniae* (22, 27.8%) *P. mirabilis* (15, 19.1%)	> 50%	ETC (33, 41.8%) DTC (79, 100%)	Carbapenem (24, 72.7%) Piperacillin/tazobactam (9, 27.3%) Carbapenem (69, 87.3%) Piperacillin/tazobactam (10, 12.7%)	Y	UK	UK
Qureshi et al. [105]	MC retrospective cohort, 2005–2008, USA	21/UK	UK	*E. cloacae* (21, 100%)	UK	ETC (21, 100%)	Cephalosporins (9, 42.8%) Carbapenem (8, 38%) BL/BLI (4, 19.2%)	Y	UK	UK
Paterson et al. [55]	Post hoc analysis MC prospective cohort, 1996–1997, International	85/455	UK	*K. pneumoniae* (85, 100%)	UK	ETC (71, 83.5%)	Monotherapy Carbapenem (27, 38%) Fluoroquinolones (11, 15.5%) Cephalosporins (5, 7%) BL/BLI (4, 5.6%) Aminoglycosides (2, 2.8%) Combination therapy (15, 21.1%) Sequential monotherapy (7, 10%)	N	UK	UK

Table 1 continued

Author/year of publication	Study design, region	No. of patients, ESBL/total	Type of infection (*n*, %)	Bacteria (*n*, %)	ICU (*n*, %)	ETC/DTC	Treatment (*n*, %)	MIC	Administration (CI, PI or II)	Posology
Pilmis et al. [106]	MC retrospective cohort, 2011, France	13/13	Primary bacteraemia (11, 84.6%) UTI (2, 15.4%)	*E. coli* (5, 38.4%) *K. pneumoniae* (7, 53.8%) *E. cloacae* (1, 7.8%)	UK	ETC (13, 100%) DTC (13, 100%)	Carbapenem (12, 92.3%) Cefoxitin (1, 7.7%) Carbapenem (11, 84.6%) Cefoxitin (2, 15.4%)	N	UK	UK
Retamar et al. [107]	Post hoc analysis MC prospective cohort, 2001–2007, Spain	39/39	UTI (11, 28.2%) Other source (28, 71.8%)	*E. coli* (39, 100%)	UK	ETC (39, 100%)	BL/BLI (39, 100%)	Y	UK	UK
Rodriguez-Bano et al. [12]	Post hoc analysis MC prospective cohorts, 2001–2007, Spain	192/192	UTI or IIA (121, 63%) Other sources (71, 37%)	*E. coli* (192, 100%)	Y (24, 12.6%)	ETC (103, 53.6%) DTC (174, 90.6%)	Carbapenem (31, 30%) BL/BLI (72, 70%) Carbapenem (120, 68.9%) BL/BLI (53, 31.1%)	N	UK	UK
Tamma et al. [19]	MC, Prospective cohort, 2008–2015, USA	213/331	CVC (97, 45.5%) IIA (55, 25.8%) UTI (44, 20.6%) Pneumonia (17, 8.1%)	*K. pneumoniae* (145, 68%) *E. coli* (66, 31%) *P. mirabilis* (2, 1%)	Y (71, 33.3%)	ETC (213, 100%)	Carbapenem (110, 51.6%) BL/BLI (103, 48.4%)	Y	UK	UK
Tsai et al. [108]	MC retrospective cohort, 2005–2012, Taiwan	47/47	UTI (24, 51%) Pneumonia (9, 19.1%) SSTI (7, 14.9%) CVC (5, 10.6%) IIA (3, 6.4%) Primary bacteraemia (2, 4.3%)	*P. mirabilis* (47, 100%)	UK	DTC (40, 85.1%)	Carbapenem (21, 52.5%) BL/BLI (13, 32.5%) Other antibiotic therapy (6, 15%)	Y	UK	UK
Tumbarello et al. [109]	SC retrospective cohort, 1999–2004, Italy	186/186	Primary bacteraemia (86, 46.2%) UTI (53, 28.4%) IIA (24, 12.9%) SSTI (20, 10.7%) Pneumonia (6, 3.2%) CVC (5, 2.7%)	*E. coli* (104, 55.9%) *K. pneumoniae* (58, 31.2%) *P. mirabilis* (24, 12.9%)	UK	ETC (186 100%) DTC (171, 91.9%)	BL/BLI (45, 24.2%) Fluoroquinolones (45, 24.2%) Cephalosporins (38, 20.9%) Carbapenems (29, 15.4%) Aminoglycosides (29, 15.4%) Carbapenems (61, 35.7%) BL/BLI (55, 32.2%) Aminoglycosides (30, 17.5%) Fluoroquinolones (25, 14.6%)	Y	UK	UK
Tuon et al. [110]	SC retrospective cohort, 2006–2009, Brazil	28/58	UK	*E. cloacae* (28, 100%)	UK	DTC (25, 89.2%)	Carbapenems (15, 60%) BL/BLI (4, 16%) Non-BL/BLI (6, 24%)	N	UK	UK

Table 1 continued

Author/year of publication	Study design, region	No. of patients, ESBL/total	Type of infection (*n*, %)	Bacteria (*n*, %)	ICU (*n*, %)	ETC/DTC	Treatment (*n*, %)	MIC	Administration (CI, PI or II)	Posology
Tuon et al. [90]	SC retrospective cohort, 2006–2009, Brazil	63/104	UK	*K. pneumoniae* (63, 100%)	UK	DTC (62, 98.4%)	Carbapenems (43, 69.3%) Non-BL/BLI (17, 27.4%) BL/BLI (2, 3.1%)	N	UK	UK
Wang et al. [95]	MC, prospective cohort, 2006–2015, USA	68/68	CVC (30, 44.1%) UTI (21, 30.9%) IIA (15, 22.1%) Pneumonia (10, 14.7%) SSTI (2, 2.9%)	*Klebsiella sp.* (42, 62%) *E. coli* (24, 34%) *P. mirabilis* (2, 3%)	Y (20, 29%)	ETC (68, 100%)	Carbapenem (51, 75%) Cephalosporins (17, 25%)	N	UK	UK

BL/BLI beta-lactam/beta-lactamase inhibitor, *CVC* central venous catheter, *DTC* definitive therapy cohort, *ETC* empirical therapy cohort, *ICU* intensive care unit, *IIA* intra-abdominal infection, *MC* multicentric, *SC* single center, *SSTI* skin and soft tissue infection, *UK* unknown, *UTI* urinary tract infection

ill patients with ESBL-PE infection from non-urinary sources.

Finally 7/11 (63%) studies compared BL/BLIs to carbapenems as definitive therapy, of which 4 (36.3%) compared BL/BLIs as the only alternative to carbapenems [12, 19, 20, 22, 51]. It should be noted that only one of these studies took into account MICs [20], whereas none took into account dosages and modalities of administration for assessing the effectiveness of therapy [19].

Ecological studies

While initial research suggested the relative safety of imipenem–cilastatin on the intestinal microbiota [56], the recent analysis of rectal colonization of large number of ICU patients found that even a brief exposure to imipenem is a risk factor for carriage of resistant GNB in the intestinal flora [6].

The effect of non-carbapenem antibiotics on the emergence of multidrug-resistant bacteria and specifically carbapenem resistance is a major issue. In animal models, imipenem–cilastatin had no effect on the indigenous microflora [56]. In a mouse model, clindamycin and piperacillin–tazobactam promoted colonization, while ertapenem did not promote the establishment of intestinal colonization with KPC-Kp [57]. Also several authors highlighted the risk associated with the emergence/selection of resistant strains when using Pip–Taz. Firstly, in vitro/in vivo studies [27] suggested that Pip–Taz seems to be less resistant to the inoculum effect comparing to carbapenems. Secondly, several clinical studies [58] underlined the risk of promoting vancomycin-resistant enterococci (VRE) colonization. Finally the emergence of carbapenem-resistant PE has been documented for a variety of antibiotics in the clinical setting [59] (Table 2): Fluoroquinolones [60, 61], extended-spectrum cephalosporin [62], antipseudomonal penicillins [63] and β-lactams/β-lactamase inhibitors [64] have all been identified as risk factors for carbapenem resistance in *Klebsiella pneumoniae.*

Whether carbapenem is the only antibiotic class associated with the selection of carbapenem-resistant gram-negative isolates is an important issue, especially regarding the worldwide spread of carbapenemase-producing Enterobacteriaceae (CPE). These data suggest that antibiotics that disturb the intestinal anaerobic microflora and lack significant activity against KPC-Kp may promote colonization by this organism [65] (Table 3).

Discussion and conclusion

In our review of BL/BLI for the treatment of ESBL-PE, we found that they may be an alternative to carbapenems in a selected number of cases, based on antibiogram and CMI data, and always with pk/pd optimization.

The use of alternatives for empirical therapy in suspected ESBL-related infections is usually limited by the level of resistance [66], the risk of selecting resistant mutants [6] and clinical effectiveness [19]. We focused on BL/BLIs, chiefly piperacillin–tazobactam. Indeed, based on epidemiological data, the use of third- or fourth-generation cephalosporins such as cefepime is limited because of a high proportion of resistant isolates [66] that varies between 10 and 50% and concerns on their clinical efficacy with the associated risks of adverse patient outcomes [54]. The use of other alternatives such as temocillin is limited by unfavorable PK/PD parameters in critically ill patients [49].

The efficacy of Pip/Taz antibiotics on ESBL-PE depends on the variety and amount of enzyme produced by the isolates (Table 4). Overall, the rate of susceptibility of ESBL-PE to Pip/Taz is around 80% [28]. It may be reduced when the organisms produce multiple ESBLs, particularly if they also harbor an AmpC beta-lactamase [67]. Also it will vary within and between beta-lactamases classes [68]. The presence of additional resistance mechanisms may further decrease the activity of Pip/Taz against ESBL-producing organisms.

In the absence of a well-designed prospective randomized study comparing carbapenems to non-carbapenems in ICU patients infected with ESBL-PE, we must rely on the evidence provided by observational data. Observational studies considering the empirical treatment of ESBL-related infections with BL/BLIs have infrequently included ICU patients [12] and more often involved urinary or biliary tract infection caused by *E. coli* species [51]. Although several studies suggested no difference in mortality [12, 51, 69], 2 publications raise the warning of a potential negative impact of BL/BLI when used in patients with ESBL-PE [19, 20].

Furthermore, when analyzing those publications with a focus on the use of alternatives to carbapenems for definitive therapy, a number of limitations hamper the interpretation of studies comparing BL/BLI to carbapenems.

Firstly most of these studies were not designed to compare different antibiotic strategies. Secondly, the authors did not take into account the severity of underlying diseases, delays to antimicrobial treatment and effectiveness source control, which are all major predictors of outcome [70]. Thirdly, patients included differed largely across studies, with regard to sources of bacteremia, species involved and type of beta-lactamases; moreover, various antibiotics and different daily doses administered were included in the "alternative" group.

Fourthly, most of the studies included infections related to ESBL-producing *Escherichia coli* and did not account for the impact of MICs and pharmacodynamics data. The impact of MIC seems to be crucial for therapeutic

Table 2 Studies addressing the risk related to previous antibiotic therapy and emergence of carbapenem-resistant Enterobacteriaceae

	Year	Study design	Type of infection	Antibiotic concerned	OR, 95 % CI
Wang [62]	2016	Retrospective case–case–control	Nosocomial infection	Third–fourth-generation cephalosporins Carbapenems	4.557 (1.971–10.539) 4.058 (1.753–9.397)
Mittal G [80]	2016	Prospective	Colonization	Aminoglycosides	4.14 (1.14–14.99)
Ling [81]	2015	Retrospective case–control	Infection or colonization	Penicillins Glycopeptides	4.640 (1.529–14.079) 5.162 (1.377–19.346)
Jiao Y [82]	2015	Retrospective case–control	Infection or colonization	Glycopeptides Cefoperazone plus sulbactam	43.84 (1.73–1111.9) 49.56, (1.42–1726.72)
Candevir [83]	2015	Retrospective cohort	Infection	Meropenem Third-generation cephalosporins	3.244 (1.193–8.819) 3.590 (1.056–12.209)
Gómez Rueda [84]	2014	Retrospective case–case–control	Infection	Carbapenems	3.3 (1.2–9.3)
Ahn [85]	2014	Retrospective case–control	Colonization/infection	Fluoroquinolones Carbapenems	2.82 (1.14–6.99) 4.56 (1.44–14.46)
Mantzarlis [86]	2013	Prospective cohort	Pneumonia	Colistin*	1.156 per day (1.010–1.312)
Dizbay [87]	2013	Prospective cohort	Nosocomial infection	Imipenem	3.35 (1.675–6.726)
Orsi [88]	2013	Retrospective case control	BSI	Carbapenem	7.74 (1.70–35.2)
Chang [89]	2011	Retrospective case–control	BSI	Carbapenem	29.17 (1.76–484.70)
Falagas [63]	2007	Retrospective case control	KPC infection	Fluoroquinolones Antipseudomonal antibiotics	4.54 (1.18–11.54) 2.6 (1.00–6.71)
Schwaber [61]	2008	Retrospective case–case–control	CRKp colonization	Antibiotics Fluoroquinolones	4.4 (1–19.2) 7.2 (1.1–49.4)
Gasink [60]	2009	Retrospective case–control	KPC infection/colonization	Fluoroquinolones Third-generation cephalosporin	3.39 (1.5–7.66) 2.55 (1.18–5.22)
Papadimitriou [64]	2012	Prospective cohort	CRKp colonization	BL/BLI Carbapenems	6.7 (1–26.2) 5.2 (1–32.9)
Tuon [90]	2012	Retrospective case–control	KPC bacteremia	Fluoroquinolones	28.9 (1.85–454.6)
Papadimitriou [91]	2014	Prospective cohort	KPC bacteremia	Aminoglycosides	2.3 (1.1–4.7)
Gagliotti [79]	2014	Case–control	KPC colonization	Carbapenems Any antibiotic (other than carbapenems)	3.67 (1.37–9.83) 2.83 (1.10–7.31)
Maseda [92]	2016	Retrospective	CPE isolate colonization	Third–fourth-generation cephalosporins BL/BLI	27.96 (6.88–113.58) 11.71 (4.51–30.43)

KPC Klebsiella pneumoniae-producing carbapenemase, *CRKp* carbapenem-resistant *Klebsiella pneumoniae*, *BL/BLI* beta-lactams associated with beta-lactamase inhibitors, *BSI* bloodstream infection

efficacy when using alternatives to carbapenems as the cornerstone of treatment. Several studies [12] emphasize the risk of treatment failure when using a BL/BLI or third-generation cephalosporin for therapy of infection with isolates having MICs higher than the breakpoints. Indeed, as suggested by a recent pharmacological study, the efficacy of BL/BLI in the treatment of ESBL-related infections is related to the concentration reached in the plasma and at the site of infection [71]. However, as demonstrated by several authors [72] the probability of attaining therapeutic drug levels in ICU patients is low and variable depending on the antibiotic considered and dosing strategies [35]. Also it seems important to have MIC for piperacillin–tazobactam before using this class of antibiotic. Considering several problems related to piperacillin–tazobactam gradient tests and differences noted between gradient tests and broth microdilution, it is recommended now to use broth microdilution.

There are now enough published data on the pk/pd of piperacillin/tazobactam to recommend the use of high daily doses and prolonged infusion ICU patients and in all cases of difficult to treat pathogens such as ESBL-PE.

The ecological consequences of a given antibiotic class depend on the amount of drug reaching the different microbiota. The net result depends on both the antibiotic concentrations achieved and the susceptibility of bacterial species in the microbiota. All antibiotics alter the composition, diversity and density of the microbiota

Table 3 (Adapted from [14, 15]) usual breakpoints and susceptibility of ESBL-producing Enterobacteriaceae

	Susceptibility (%)	Breakpoints (mg/L)	Ecological impact	Comments
Third-generation cephalosporins	*Escherichia coli*: < 10% *Klebsiella* species: 3%	EUCAST: S ≤ 1 CLSI: S ≤ 1	+++	Only for targeted therapy or de-escalation MIC required
Cefepime	*E. coli*: 5–30% *K. pneumoniae*: 5–60%	EUCAST: S < 1 CLSI: S ≤ 2	+++	Frequent failure if MICs > 1 mg/L MIC required
Cefoxitin	*E. coli*: 80%	EUCAST: NA	++	PK optimization
Ceftolozane–tazobactam	*E. coli*: 85–95% *K. pneumoniae*: 40–65%	EUCAST: S ≤ 1 CLSI: S ≤ 8	?	
Ceftazidime–avibactam	*E. coli*: 98–100% *K. pneumoniae*: 90–100%	EUCAST: S ≤ 8 CLSI: S ≤ 8	?	Probably as effective as carbapenems
Temocillin	*E. coli* 61% (CMI ≤ 8) *E. coli* 99% (CMI ≤ 32)	EUCAST: S ≤ 8 EUCAST: S ≤ 32 (urinary) CLSI: S ≤ 8 CLSI: S ≤ 32 (urinary)	±	PK optimization (high dosage and prolonged infusion)

CLSI Clinical and Laboratory Standard Institute, *EUCAST* European Committee on Antimicrobial Susceptibility Testing, *MIC* minimum inhibitory concentration, *NA* not applicable, *PK* pharmacokinetic, *VAP* ventilator-associated pneumonia

Table 4 (Adapted from Bonomo and Van Duin) Activity in clinical practice of different beta-lactamase inhibitors, according to type of enzymes [68, 111]

Enzymes	Class	Substrates	Clavulanic acid	Sulbactam	Tazobactam	Avibactam
TEM-1, TEM-2, SHV-1	A	Penicillins, early cephalosporins	+	–	+	+
TEM-3, SHV-2 CTX-M-14	A	Extended-spectrum cephalosporins, monobactams	–	–	+	+
KPC-2, KPC-3	A	Broad spectrum including carbapenems	–	–	–	+
IMP-1, NDM-1, VIM-1	B	Broad spectrum including carbapenems, but not monobactams	–	–	–	–
Escherichia coli AmpC	C	Cephalosporins	–	–	±	+
OXA-48	D	Carbapenem	–	–	–	+

and select for antibiotic resistance [73]. The "ecological consequences," however, may differ according to the antibiotic used. Increasing consumption of carbapenems raises concerns on the spread of carbapenem-resistant Enterobacteriaceae and specifically carbapenemase-producing Enterobacteriaceae (CPE) [74]. Also, there are some discrepancies between the first published studies [75, 76] and the more recent ones [6] regarding the ecological effect of carbapenems. There is a significant correlation between carbapenem consumption and rates of *Pseudomonas aeruginosa* resistance to imipenem and meropenem [6, 53]. However, this mechanism of resistance is not due to the effect of antibiotics on the microbiota, but the consequence of chromosomal mutation. Earlier human studies [77] and animal models [78] suggested a limited impact on the microbiota of this class of antibiotics. However, whatever the antibiotic used, selective antibiotic pressure is an important determinant of emergence and dissemination of antibiotic resistance [61, 62], and the increasing use of carbapenems will necessarily be associated with the increase in multidrug-resistant organisms [65]. Our review underlines the fact that the administration of several other antibiotics can also be associated with the emergence of carbapenem-resistant organisms [60–64, 79–92]. Nevertheless, the heterogeneity of studies makes their comparison difficult. Indeed, all these studies are subject to several limitations, including inadequate adjustment for important confounding variables, control group selection, extent of prior antibiotic exposure and measurements of resistance outcomes.

One of the limitations of our study lies in the fact that we did not mentioned the two recent BL/BLIs approved by FDA and EMA, ceftolozane–tazobactam and ceftazidime–avibactam which are active in vitro against ESBL-producing Enterobacteriaceae. Several recent studies highlighted the in vitro efficacy of these two antibiotics on ESBL-producing Enterobacteriaceae [67, 93]. Also clinical data are scarce. Indeed for nosocomial pneumonia, a phase III study (MK-7625A-008) is currently leaded using ceftolozane–tazobactam.

A definitive answer to the question addressed in this review would need a randomized study conducted in ICU, including severe infections related to ESBL-PE. Cases should be selected according to the results of antibiotic susceptibility tests, and the trial should compare carbapenems to BL/BLI as definitive therapy. Pending such a trial, piperacillin–tazobactam should be used with caution for treatment of ESBL-PE-related infections. In ICU patients, empirical use should be avoided, and definitive therapy should be reserved to patients in clinical stable condition, after microbial documentation and results of susceptibility tests, together with adapting the administered dose and modalities of infusion to the MIC of the infecting microorganism in order to reach pharmacological targets.

Abbreviations

ADE: antimicrobial de-escalation; BL/BLI: beta-lactam/beta-lactamase inhibitor; CLSI: Clinical and Laboratory Standards Institute; CRB: carbapenem-resistant bacteria; CRE: carbapenem-resistant Enterobacteriaceae; EMA: European Medicine Agency; ESAC: European Surveillance of Antimicrobial Consumption; EUCAST: European Committee on Antimicrobial Susceptibility Testing; FDA: Food and Drug Administration; ICU: intensive care unit; KPC: *Klebsiella*-producing carbapenemase; MIC: minimal inhibitory concentration; OR: odds ratio; PD: pharmacodynamic; PK: pharmacokinetic; TDM: therapeutic drug monitoring; TID: three times in a day.

Authors' contributions

BP contributed to conception and design of the study, responsible for the "clinical studies" portion and gave final approval of the version to be published. VJ contributed to conception and design of the study, responsible for the "pharmacokinetics and pharmacodynamic studies" portion and gave final approval of the version to be published. AT revised the manuscript critically for important intellectual content and gave final approval of the version to be published. JRZ contributed to conception and design of the study, responsible for the "ecological studies" portion and gave final approval of the version to be published. CBB involved in design of the study, revised it critically for important intellectual content and gave final approval of the version to be published.

Author details

[1] Service de maladies infectieuses et tropicales, Hôpital Necker Enfants malades, Service de maladies infectieuses et tropicales, Université Paris Descartes, Paris, France. [2] Equipe mobile de microbiologie clinique, Groupe Hospitalier Paris Saint-Joseph, Paris, France. [3] Service de Pharmacologie, Hôpital Européen Georges Pompidou, Université Paris Descartes, Paris, France. [4] INSERM U1129, Paris, France. [5] Intensive Care Unit, The Redcliffe Hospital, Brisbane, Australia. [6] Burns, Trauma and Critical Care Research Centre, The University of Queensland, Brisbane, Australia. [7] Département de Microbiologie Clinique, Unité de Contrôle et de Prévention du risque Infectieux, Groupe Hospitalier Paris Seine Saint-Denis, AP-HP, CHU Avicenne, 125 rue de Stalingrad, 9300 Bobigny, France. [8] Infection Control Unit, IAME, UMR 1137, Université Paris 13, Sorbonne Paris Cité, Paris, France. [9] Réanimation médicale, Hôpital Henri Mondor, Université Paris Est Créteil (UPEC), Créteil, France.

Acknowledgements

Not applicable.

Competing interests

BP, AT and CBB declare that they have no competing interests. VJ has received research grants from Astellas, Sanofi-Aventis, Biocodex and travel Grants from MSD. JRZ has participated in an advisory board for MSD.

References

1. Arpin C, Quentin C, Grobost F, Cambau E, Robert J, Dubois V, et al. Nationwide survey of extended-spectrum {beta}-lactamase-producing enterobacteriaceae in the French community setting. J Antimicrob Chemother. 2009;63:1205–14.
2. Meier S, Weber R, Zbinden R, Ruef C, Hasse B. Extended-spectrum β-lactamase-producing Gram-negative pathogens in community-acquired urinary tract infections: an increasing challenge for antimicrobial therapy. Infection. 2011;39:333–40.
3. Prinapori R, Guinaud J, Khalil A, Lecuyer H, Gendrel D, Lortholary O, et al. Risk associated with a systematic search of extended-spectrum β-lactamase-producing Enterobacteriaceae. Am J Infect Control. 2013;41:259–60.
4. Barbier F, Pommier C, Essaied W, Garrouste-Orgeas M, Schwebel C, Ruckly S, et al. Colonization and infection with extended-spectrum β-lactamase-producing enterobacteriaceae in ICU patients: what impact on outcomes and carbapenem exposure? J Antimicrob Chemother. 2016;71:1088–97.
5. http://ecdc.europa.eu/en/eaad/antibiotics-news/Documents/antimicrobial-consumption-ESAC-Net-summary-2015.pdf.
6. Armand-Lefèvre L, Angebault C, Barbier F, Hamelet E, Defrance G, Ruppé E, et al. Emergence of imipenem-resistant gram-negative bacilli in intestinal flora of intensive care patients. Antimicrob Agents Chemother. 2013;57:1488–95.
7. Tabah A, Cotta MO, Garnacho-Montero J, Schouten J, Roberts JA, Lipman J, et al. A systematic review of the definitions, determinants, and clinical outcomes of antimicrobial de-escalation in the intensive care unit. Clin Infect Dis Off Publ Infect Dis Soc Am. 2016;62:1009–17.
8. Kalil AC, Metersky ML, Klompas M, Muscedere J, Sweeney DA, Palmer LB, et al. Management of adults with Hospital-acquired and ventilator-associated pneumonia: 2016 clinical practice guidelines by the infectious diseases society of America and the American thoracic society. Clin Infect Dis. 2016;63:e61–111.
9. Rhodes A, Evans LE, Alhazzani W, Levy MM, Antonelli M, Ferrer R, et al. Surviving sepsis campaign: international guidelines for management of sepsis and septic shock: 2016. Intensive Care Med. 2017;43:304–77.
10. Paterson DL. Recommendation for treatment of severe infections caused by Enterobacteriaceae producing extended-spectrum beta-lactamases (ESBLs). Clin Microbiol Infect Off Publ Eur Soc Clin Microbiol Infect Dis. 2000;6:460–3.
11. Piroth L, Aubé H, Doise JM, Vincent-Martin M. Spread of extended-spectrum beta-lactamase-producing *Klebsiella pneumoniae*: are beta-lactamase inhibitors of therapeutic value? Clin. Infect. Dis. Off. Publ. Infect. Dis. Soc. Am. 1998;27:76–80.
12. Rodríguez-Baño J, Navarro MD, Retamar P, Picón E, Pascual Á. Extended-Spectrum Beta-Lactamases—Red Española de Investigación en Patología Infecciosa/Grupo de Estudio de Infección Hospitalaria Group. β-Lactam/β-lactam inhibitor combinations for the treatment of bacteremia due to extended-spectrum β-lactamase-producing *Escherichia coli*: a post hoc analysis of prospective cohorts. Clin Infect Dis Off Publ Infect Dis Soc Am. 2012;54:167–74.
13. Ng TM, Khong WX, Harris PNA, De PP, Chow A, Tambyah PA, et al. Empiric piperacillin–tazobactam versus carbapenems in the treatment of bacteraemia due to extended-spectrum beta-lactamase-producing enterobacteriaceae. PLOS ONE. 2016;11:e0153696.
14. EUCAST: Clinical breakpoints [cited 2015 Aug 18]. http://www.eucast.org/clinical_breakpoints/.
15. CLSI Publishes New Antimicrobial Susceptibility Testing Standards—CLSI [cited 2016 Aug 5]. http://clsi.org/blog/2015/01/08/clsi-publishes-new-antimicrobial-susceptibility-testing-standards/.
16. Du B, Long Y, Liu H, Chen D, Liu D, Xu Y, et al. Extended-spectrum beta-lactamase-producing *Escherichia coli* and *Klebsiella pneumoniae* bloodstream infection: risk factors and clinical outcome. Intensive Care Med. 2002;28:1718–23.
17. Kang C-I, Kim S-H, Park WB, Lee K-D, Kim H-B, Kim E-C, et al. Bloodstream infections due to extended-spectrum beta-lactamase-producing *Escherichia coli* and *Klebsiella pneumoniae*: risk factors for mortality and treatment outcome, with special emphasis on antimicrobial therapy. Antimicrob Agents Chemother. 2004;48:4574–81.

18. Wang R, Cosgrove SE, Tschudin-Sutter S, Han JH, Turnbull AE, Hsu AJ, et al. Cefepime therapy for cefepime-susceptible extended-spectrum β-lactamase-producing enterobacteriaceae bacteremia. Open Forum Infect Dis. 2016;3:ofw132.
19. Tamma PD, Han JH, Rock C, Harris AD, Lautenbach E, Hsu AJ, et al. Carbapenem therapy is associated with improved survival compared with piperacillin–tazobactam for patients with extended-spectrum β-lactamase bacteremia. Clin Infect Dis Off Publ Infect Dis Soc Am. 2015;60:1319–25.
20. Ofer-Friedman H, Shefler C, Sharma S, Tirosh A, Tal-Jasper R, Kandipalli D, et al. Carbapenems versus piperacillin–tazobactam for bloodstream infections of nonurinary source caused by extended-spectrum beta-lactamase-producing enterobacteriaceae. Infect Control Hosp Epidemiol. 2015;36:981–5.
21. Lee C-C, Lee N-Y, Yan J-J, Lee H-C, Chen P-L, Chang C-M, et al. Bacteremia due to extended-spectrum-beta-lactamase-producing *Enterobacter cloacae*: role of carbapenem therapy. Antimicrob Agents Chemother. 2010;54:3551–6.
22. Harris PN, Tambyah PA, Paterson DL. β-lactam and β-lactamase inhibitor combinations in the treatment of extended-spectrum β-lactamase producing *Enterobacteriaceae*: time for a reappraisal in the era of few antibiotic options? Lancet Infect Dis. 2015;15:475–85.
23. Roberts JA, Roberts MS, Robertson TA, Dalley AJ, Lipman J. Piperacillin penetration into tissue of critically ill patients with sepsis—bolus versus continuous administration? Crit Care Med. 2009;37:926–33.
24. Dulhunty JM, Roberts JA, Davis JS, Webb SAR, Bellomo R, Gomersall C, et al. Continuous infusion of beta-lactam antibiotics in severe sepsis: a multicenter double-blind, randomized controlled trial. Clin Infect Dis Off Publ Infect Dis Soc Am. 2013;56:236–44.
25. Roberts JA, Kirkpatrick CMJ, Roberts MS, Robertson TA, Dalley AJ, Lipman J. Meropenem dosing in critically ill patients with sepsis and without renal dysfunction: intermittent bolus versus continuous administration? Monte Carlo dosing simulations and subcutaneous tissue distribution. J Antimicrob Chemother. 2009;64:142–50.
26. Carlier M, Noë M, De Waele JJ, Stove V, Verstraete AG, Lipman J, et al. Population pharmacokinetics and dosing simulations of amoxicillin/clavulanic acid in critically ill patients. J Antimicrob Chemother. 2013;68:2600–8.
27. Wu N, Chen BY, Tian SF, Chu YZ. The inoculum effect of antibiotics against CTX-M-extended-spectrum β-lactamase-producing *Escherichia coli*. Ann Clin Microbiol Antimicrob. 2014;13:45.
28. Lob SH, Nicolle LE, Hoban DJ, Kazmierczak KM, Badal RE, Sahm DF. Susceptibility patterns and ESBL rates of *Escherichia coli* from urinary tract infections in Canada and the United States, SMART 2010–2014. Diagn Microbiol Infect Dis. 2016;85:459–65.
29. Jean S-S, Coombs G, Ling T, Balaji V, Rodrigues C, Mikamo H, et al. Epidemiology and antimicrobial susceptibility profiles of pathogens causing urinary tract infections in the Asia-Pacific region: results from the Study for Monitoring Antimicrobial Resistance Trends (SMART), 2010–2013. Int J Antimicrob Agents. 2016;47:328–34.
30. Sader HS, Farrell DJ, Flamm RK, Jones RN. Antimicrobial susceptibility of gram-negative organisms isolated from patients hospitalised with pneumonia in US and European hospitals: results from the SENTRY Antimicrobial Surveillance Program, 2009–2012. Int J Antimicrob Agents. 2014;43:328–34.
31. Lodise TP, Lomaestro B, Drusano GL. Piperacillin–tazobactam for *Pseudomonas aeruginosa* infection: clinical implications of an extended-infusion dosing strategy. Clin Infect Dis Off Publ Infect Dis Soc Am. 2007;44:357–63.
32. Roberts JA, Ulldemolins M, Roberts MS, McWhinney B, Ungerer J, Paterson DL, et al. Therapeutic drug monitoring of β-lactams in critically ill patients: proof of concept. Int J Antimicrob Agents. 2010;36:332–9.
33. Sturm AW, Allen N, Rafferty KD, Fish DN, Toschlog E, Newell M, et al. Pharmacokinetic analysis of piperacillin administered with tazobactam in critically ill, morbidly obese surgical patients. Pharmacotherapy. 2014;34:28–35.
34. De Waele JJ, De Neve N. Aminoglycosides for life-threatening infections: a plea for an individualized approach using intensive therapeutic drug monitoring. Minerva Anestesiol. 2014;80:1135–42.
35. De Waele JJ, Carrette S, Carlier M, Stove V, Boelens J, Claeys G, et al. Therapeutic drug monitoring-based dose optimisation of piperacillin and meropenem: a randomised controlled trial. Intensive Care Med. 2014;40:380–7.
36. Felton TW, McCalman K, Malagon I, Isalska B, Whalley S, Goodwin J, et al. Pulmonary penetration of piperacillin and tazobactam in critically ill patients. Clin Pharmacol Ther. 2014;96:438–48.
37. McKinnon PS, Paladino JA, Schentag JJ. Evaluation of area under the inhibitory curve (AUIC) and time above the minimum inhibitory concentration (T > MIC) as predictors of outcome for cefepime and ceftazidime in serious bacterial infections. Int J Antimicrob Agents. 2008;31:345–51.
38. Sádaba B, Azanza JR, Campanero MA, García-Quetglas E. Relationship between pharmacokinetics and pharmacodynamics of beta-lactams and outcome. Clin Microbiol Infect Off Publ Eur Soc Clin Microbiol Infect Dis. 2004;10:990–8.
39. Felton TW, Roberts JA, Lodise TP, Van Guilder M, Boselli E, Neely MN, et al. Individualization of piperacillin dosing for critically ill patients: dosing software to optimize antimicrobial therapy. Antimicrob Agents Chemother. 2014;58:4094–102.
40. Abdul-Aziz MH, Lipman J, Akova M, Bassetti M, De Waele JJ, Dimopoulos G, et al. Is prolonged infusion of piperacillin/tazobactam and meropenem in critically ill patients associated with improved pharmacokinetic/pharmacodynamic and patient outcomes? An observation from the Defining antibiotic levels in intensive care unit patients (DALI) cohort. J Antimicrob Chemother. 2016;71:196–207.
41. Ulldemolins M, Martín-Loeches I, Llauradó-Serra M, Fernández J, Vaquer S, Rodríguez A, et al. Piperacillin population pharmacokinetics in critically ill patients with multiple organ dysfunction syndrome receiving continuous venovenous haemodiafiltration: effect of type of dialysis membrane on dosing requirements. J Antimicrob Chemother. 2016;71:1651–9.
42. Shotwell MS, Nesbitt R, Madonia PN, Gould ER, Connor MJ, Salem C, et al. Pharmacokinetics and pharmacodynamics of extended infusion versus short infusion piperacillin–tazobactam in critically ill patients undergoing CRRT. CJASN. 2016;11:1377–83.
43. Connor MJ, Salem C, Bauer SR, Hofmann CL, Groszek J, Butler R, et al. Therapeutic drug monitoring of piperacillin–tazobactam using spent dialysate effluent in patients receiving continuous venovenous hemodialysis. Antimicrob Agents Chemother. 2011;55:557–60.
44. Thompson MI, Russo ME, Matsen JM, Atkin-Thor E. Piperacillin pharmacokinetics in subjects with chronic renal failure. Antimicrob Agents Chemother. 1981;19:450–3.
45. Giron JA, Meyers BR, Hirschman SZ, Srulevitch E. Pharmacokinetics of piperacillin in patients with moderate renal failure and in patients undergoing hemodialysis. Antimicrob Agents Chemother. 1981;19:279–83.
46. Francke EL, Appel GB, Neu HC. Pharmacokinetics of intravenous piperacillin in patients undergoing chronic hemodialysis. Antimicrob Agents Chemother. 1979;16:788–91.
47. Guet-Revillet H, Emirian A, Groh M, Nebbad-Lechani B, Weiss E, Join-Lambert O, et al. Pharmacological study of cefoxitin as an alternative antibiotic therapy to carbapenems in treatment of urinary tract infections due to extended-spectrum-β-lactamase-producing *Escherichia coli*. Antimicrob Agents Chemother. 2014;58:4899–901.
48. Vincent J-L, Bassetti M, François B, Karam G, Chastre J, Torres A, et al. Advances in antibiotic therapy in the critically ill. Crit Care Lond Engl. 2016;20:133.
49. Laterre P-F, Wittebole X, Van de Velde S, Muller AE, Mouton JW, Carryn S, et al. Temocillin (6 g daily) in critically ill patients: continuous infusion versus three times daily administration. J Antimicrob Chemother. 2015;70:891–8.
50. Chopra T, Marchaim D, Veltman J, Johnson P, Zhao JJ, Tansek R, et al. Impact of cefepime therapy on mortality among patients with bloodstream infections caused by extended-spectrum-β-lactamase-producing *Klebsiella pneumoniae* and *Escherichia coli*. Antimicrob Agents Chemother. 2012;56:3936–42.

51. Gutiérrez-Gutiérrez B, Pérez-Galera S, Salamanca E, de Cueto M, Calbo E, Almirante B, et al. β-lactam/β-lactamase inhibitor combinations for the treatment of bloodstream infections due to extended-spectrum β-lactamase-producing enterobacteriaceae: a multinational, pre-registered cohort study. Antimicrob Agents Chemother. 2016;11:AAC-00365.
52. Apisarnthanarak A, Kiratisin P, Mundy LM. Predictors of mortality from community-onset bloodstream infections due to extended-spectrum beta-lactamase-producing *Escherichia coli* and *Klebsiella pneumoniae*. Infect Control Hosp Epidemiol. 2008;29:671–4.
53. Lee C-H, Su L-H, Tang Y-F, Liu J-W. Treatment of ESBL-producing *Klebsiella pneumoniae* bacteraemia with carbapenems or flomoxef: a retrospective study and laboratory analysis of the isolates. J Antimicrob Chemother. 2006;58:1074–7.
54. Lee N-Y, Lee C-C, Huang W-H, Tsui K-C, Hsueh P-R, Ko W-C. Cefepime therapy for monomicrobial bacteremia caused by cefepime-susceptible extended-spectrum beta-lactamase-producing enterobacteriaceae: MIC matters. Clin Infect Dis Off Publ Infect Dis Soc Am. 2013;56:488–95.
55. Paterson DL, Ko W-C, Von Gottberg A, Mohapatra S, Casellas JM, Goossens H, et al. Antibiotic therapy for *Klebsiella pneumoniae* bacteremia: implications of production of extended-spectrum beta-lactamases. Clin Infect Dis Off Publ Infect Dis Soc Am. 2004;39:31–7.
56. Nord CE, Heimdahl A, Kager L, Malmborg AS. The impact of different antimicrobial agents on the normal gastrointestinal microflora of humans. Rev Infect Dis. 1984;6(Suppl 1):S270–5.
57. Perez F, Pultz MJ, Endimiani A, Bonomo RA, Donskey CJ. Effect of antibiotic treatment on establishment and elimination of intestinal colonization by KPC-producing *Klebsiella pneumoniae* in mice. Antimicrob Agents Chemother. 2011;55:2585–9.
58. Efe Iris N, Sayıner H, Yildirmak T, Simsek F, Arat ME. Vancomycin-resistant Enterococcus carrier status in the reanimation units and related risk factors. Am J Infect Control. 2013;41:261–2.
59. Donskey CJ. Antibiotic regimens and intestinal colonization with antibiotic-resistant gram-negative bacilli. Clin Infect Dis Off Publ Infect Dis Soc Am. 2006;43(Suppl 2):S62–9.
60. Gasink LB, Edelstein PH, Lautenbach E, Synnestvedt M, Fishman NO. Risk factors and clinical impact of *Klebsiella pneumoniae* carbapenemase-producing K. pneumoniae. Infect Control Hosp Epidemiol. 2009;30:1180–5.
61. Schwaber MJ, Klarfeld-Lidji S, Navon-Venezia S, Schwartz D, Leavitt A, Carmeli Y. Predictors of carbapenem-resistant *Klebsiella pneumoniae* acquisition among hospitalized adults and effect of acquisition on mortality. Antimicrob Agents Chemother. 2008;52:1028–33.
62. Wang Q, Zhang Y, Yao X, Xian H, Liu Y, Li H, et al. Risk factors and clinical outcomes for carbapenem-resistant Enterobacteriaceae nosocomial infections. Eur J Clin Microbiol Infect Dis Off Publ Eur Soc Clin Microbiol. 2016;35:1679–89.
63. Falagas ME, Rafailidis PI, Kofteridis D, Virtzili S, Chelvatzoglou FC, Papaioannou V, et al. Risk factors of carbapenem-resistant *Klebsiella pneumoniae* infections: a matched case control study. J Antimicrob Chemother. 2007;60:1124–30.
64. Papadimitriou-Olivgeris M, Marangos M, Fligou F, Christofidou M, Bartzavali C, Anastassiou ED, et al. Risk factors for KPC-producing *Klebsiella pneumoniae* enteric colonization upon ICU admission. J Antimicrob Chemother. 2012;67:2976–81.
65. Stiefel U, Pultz NJ, Donskey CJ. Effect of carbapenem administration on establishment of intestinal colonization by vancomycin-resistant enterococci and *Klebsiella pneumoniae* in mice. Antimicrob Agents Chemother. 2007;51:372–5.
66. Antimicrobial resistance interactive database (EARS-Net) [cited 2016 Sep 20]. http://ecdc.europa.eu/en/healthtopics/antimicrobial-resistance-and-consumption/antimicrobial_resistance/database/Pages/table_reports.aspx.
67. Li H, Estabrook M, Jacoby GA, Nichols WW, Testa RT, Bush K. In vitro susceptibility of characterized β-lactamase-Producing strains tested with avibactam combinations. Antimicrob Agents Chemother. 2015;59:1789–93.
68. Drawz SM, Bonomo RA. Three decades of beta-lactamase inhibitors. Clin Microbiol Rev. 2010;23:160–201.
69. Kang C-I, Park SY, Chung DR, Peck KR, Song J-H. Piperacillin–tazobactam as an initial empirical therapy of bacteremia caused by extended-spectrum β-lactamase-producing *Escherichia coli* and *Klebsiella pneumoniae*. J Infect. 2012;64:533–4.
70. Bloos F, Rüddel H, Thomas-Rüddel D, Schwarzkopf D, Pausch C, Harbarth S, et al. Effect of a multifaceted educational intervention for anti-infectious measures on sepsis mortality: a cluster randomized trial. Intensive Care Med. 2017. http://doi.org/10.1007/s00134-017-4782-4
71. Guet-Revillet H, Tomini E, Emirian A, Join-Lambert O, Lécuyer H, Zahar J-R, et al. Piperacillin/tazobactam as an alternative antibiotic therapy to carbapenems in the treatment of urinary tract infections due to extended-spectrum β-lactamase-producing enterobacteriaceae: an in silico pharmacokinetic study. Int. J. Antimicrob Agents. 2016;49:62–6.
72. Roberts JA, Abdul-Aziz MH, Lipman J, Mouton JW, Vinks AA, Felton TW, et al. Individualised antibiotic dosing for patients who are critically ill: challenges and potential solutions. Lancet Infect Dis. 2014;14:498–509.
73. Pettigrew MM, Johnson JK, Harris AD. The human microbiota: novel targets for hospital-acquired infections and antibiotic resistance. Ann Epidemiol. 2016;26:342–7.
74. Gharbi M, Moore LSP, Gilchrist M, Thomas CP, Bamford K, Brannigan ET, et al. Forecasting carbapenem resistance from antimicrobial consumption surveillance: lessons learnt from an OXA-48-producing *Klebsiella pneumoniae* outbreak in a West London renal unit. Int J Antimicrob Agents. 2015;46:150–6.
75. Plüss-Suard C, Pannatier A, Kronenberg A, Mühlemann K, Zanetti G. Impact of antibiotic use on carbapenem resistance in *Pseudomonas aeruginosa*: is there a role for antibiotic diversity? Antimicrob Agents Chemother. 2013;57:1709–13.
76. Wexler HM, Finegold SM. Impact of imipenem/cilastatin therapy on normal fecal flora. Am J Med. 1985;78:41–6.
77. DiNubile MJ, Chow JW, Satishchandran V, Polis A, Motyl MR, Abramson MA, et al. Acquisition of resistant bowel flora during a double-blind randomized clinical trial of ertapenem versus piperacillin–tazobactam therapy for intraabdominal infections. Antimicrob Agents Chemother. 2005;49:3217–21.
78. Pultz MJ, Donskey CJ. Effects of imipenem-cilastatin, ertapenem, piperacillin–tazobactam, and ceftriaxone treatments on persistence of intestinal colonization by extended-spectrum-beta-lactamase-producing *Klebsiella pneumoniae* strains in mice. Antimicrob Agents Chemother. 2007;51:3044–5.
79. Gagliotti C, Giordani S, Ciccarese V, Barozzi A, Giovinazzi A, Pietrantonio AM, et al. Risk factors for colonization with carbapenemase-producing *Klebsiella pneumoniae* in hospital: a matched case-control study. Am J Infect Control. 2014;42:1006–8.
80. Mittal G, Gaind R, Kumar D, Kaushik G, Gupta KB, Verma PK, et al. Risk factors for fecal carriage of carbapenemase producing enterobacteriaceae among intensive care unit patients from a tertiary care center in India. BMC Microbiol. 2016;16:138.
81. Ling ML, Tee YM, Tan SG, Amin IM, How KB, Tan KY, et al. Risk factors for acquisition of carbapenem resistant enterobacteriaceae in an acute tertiary care hospital in Singapore. Antimicrob Resist Infect Control. 2015;4:26.
82. Jiao Y, Qin Y, Liu J, Li Q, Dong Y, Shang Y, et al. Risk factors for carbapenem-resistant *Klebsiella pneumoniae* infection/colonization and predictors of mortality: a retrospective study. Pathog Glob Health. 2015;109:68–74.
83. Candevir Ulu A, Kurtaran B, Inal AS, Kömür S, Kibar F, Yapıcı Çiçekdemir H, et al. Risk factors of carbapenem-resistant *Klebsiella pneumoniae* infection: a serious threat in ICUs. Med Sci Monit Int Med J Exp Clin Res. 2015;21:219–24.
84. Gómez Rueda V, Zuleta Tobón JJ. Risk factors for infection with carbapenem-resistant *Klebsiella pneumoniae*: a case-case-control study. Colomb Méd Cali Colomb. 2014;45:54–60.
85. Ahn JY, Song JE, Kim MH, Choi H, Kim JK, Ann HW, et al. Risk factors for the acquisition of carbapenem-resistant *Escherichia coli* at a tertiary care center in South Korea: a matched case-control study. Am J Infect Control. 2014;42:621–5.
86. Mantzarlis K, Makris D, Manoulakas E, Karvouniaris M, Zakynthinos E. Risk factors for the first episode of *Klebsiella pneumoniae* resistant to carbapenems infection in critically ill patients: a prospective study. Biomed Res Int. 2013;2013:850547.

87. Dizbay M, Guzel Tunccan O, Karasahin O, Aktas F. Emergence of carbapenem-resistant *Klebsiella* spp infections in a Turkish university hospital: epidemiology and risk factors. J Infect Dev Ctries. 2014;8:44–9.
88. Orsi GB, Bencardino A, Vena A, Carattoli A, Venditti C, Falcone M, et al. Patient risk factors for outer membrane permeability and KPC-producing carbapenem-resistant *Klebsiella pneumoniae* isolation: results of a double case-control study. Infection. 2013;41:61–7.
89. Chang H-J, Hsu P-C, Yang C-C, Kuo A-J, Chia J-H, Wu T-L, et al. Risk factors and outcomes of carbapenem-nonsusceptible *Escherichia coli* bacteremia: a matched case-control study. J Microbiol Immunol Infect Wei Mian Yu Gan Ran Za Zhi. 2011;44:125–30.
90. Tuon FF, Rocha JL, Toledo P, Arend LN, Dias CH, Leite TM, et al. Risk factors for KPC-producing *Klebsiella pneumoniae* bacteremia. Braz J Infect Dis Off Publ Braz SocInfect Dis. 2012;16:416–9.
91. Papadimitriou-Olivgeris M, Marangos M, Christofidou M, Fligou F, Bartzavali C, Panteli ES, et al. Risk factors for infection and predictors of mortality among patients with KPC-producing *Klebsiella pneumoniae* bloodstream infections in the intensive care unit. Scand J Infect Dis. 2014;46:642–8.
92. Maseda E, Salgado P, Anillo V, Ruiz-Carrascoso G, Gómez-Gil R, Martín-Funke C, et al. Risk factors for colonization by carbapenemase-producing enterobacteria at admission to a Surgical ICU: a retrospective study. Clin: Enferm Infecc Microbiol; 2016.
93. Popejoy MW, Paterson DL, Cloutier D, Huntington JA, Miller B, Bliss CA, et al. Efficacy of ceftolozane/tazobactam against urinary tract and intra-abdominal infections caused by ESBL-producing *Escherichia coli* and *Klebsiella pneumoniae*: a pooled analysis of Phase 3 clinical trials. J Antimicrob Chemother. 2017;72:268–72.
94. Balakrishnan I, Awad-El-Kariem FM, Aali A, Kumari P, Mulla R, Tan B, et al. Temocillin use in England: clinical and microbiological efficacies in infections caused by extended-spectrum and/or derepressed AmpC β-lactamase-producing Enterobacteriaceae. J Antimicrob Chemother. 2011;66:2628–31.
95. Bin C, Hui W, Renyuan Z, Yongzhong N, Xiuli X, Yingchun X, et al. Outcome of cephalosporin treatment of bacteremia due to CTX-M-type extended-spectrum beta-lactamase-producing *Escherichia coli*. Diagn Microbiol Infect Dis. 2006;56:351–7.
96. Chaubey VP, Pitout JD, Dalton B, Ross T, Church DL, Gregson DB, et al. Clinical outcome of empiric antimicrobial therapy of bacteremia due to extended-spectrum beta-lactamase producing *Escherichia coli* and *Klebsiella pneumoniae*. BMC Res Notes. 2010;3:116.
97. Chung H-C, Lai C-H, Lin J-N, Huang C-K, Liang S-H, Chen W-F, et al. Bacteremia caused by extended-spectrum-β-lactamase-producing *Escherichia coli* sequence type ST131 and non-ST131 clones: comparison of demographic data, clinical features, and mortality. Antimicrob Agents Chemother. 2012;56:618–22.
98. De Rosa FG, Pagani N, Fossati L, Raviolo S, Cometto C, Cavallerio P, et al. The effect of inappropriate therapy on bacteremia by ESBL-producing bacteria. Infection. 2011;39:555–61.
99. Endimiani A, Luzzaro F, Brigante G, Perilli M, Lombardi G, Amicosante G, et al. Proteus mirabilis bloodstream infections: risk factors and treatment outcome related to the expression of extended-spectrum beta-lactamases. Antimicrob Agents Chemother. 2005;49:2598–605.
100. Ferrández O, Grau S, Saballs P, Luque S, Terradas R, Salas E. Mortality risk factors for bloodstream infections caused by extended-spectrum beta-lactamase-producing microorganisms. Rev Clín Esp. 2011;211:119–26.
101. Gudiol C, Calatayud L, Garcia-Vidal C, Lora-Tamayo J, Cisnal M, Duarte R, et al. Bacteraemia due to extended-spectrum beta-lactamase-producing *Escherichia coli* (ESBL-EC) in cancer patients: clinical features, risk factors, molecular epidemiology and outcome. J Antimicrob Chemother. 2010;65:333–41.
102. Harris PNA, Yin M, Jureen R, Chew J, Ali J, Paynter S, et al. Comparable outcomes for β-lactam/β-lactamase inhibitor combinations and carbapenems in definitive treatment of bloodstream infections caused by cefotaxime-resistant *Escherichia coli* or *Klebsiella pneumoniae*. Antimicrob Resist Infect Control. 2015;4:14.
103. Lee C-H, Lee Y-T, Kung C-H, Ku W-W, Kuo S-C, Chen T-L, et al. Risk factors of community-onset urinary tract infections caused by plasmid-mediated AmpC β-lactamase-producing Enterobacteriaceae. J Microbiol Immunol Infect. 2015;48:269–75.
104. Matsumura Y, Yamamoto M, Nagao M, Komori T, Fujita N, Hayashi A, et al. Multicenter retrospective study of cefmetazole and flomoxef for treatment of extended-spectrum-β-lactamase-producing *Escherichia coli* bacteremia. Antimicrob Agents Chemother. 2015;59:5107–13.
105. Qureshi ZA, Paterson DL, Pakstis DL, Adams-Haduch JM, Sandkovsky G, Sordillo E, et al. Risk factors and outcome of extended-spectrum β-lactamase-producing *Enterobacter cloacae* bloodstream infections. Int J Antimicrob Agents. 2011;37:26–32.
106. Pilmis B, Parize P, Zahar JR, Lortholary O. Alternatives to carbapenems for infections caused by ESBL-producing enterobacteriaceae. Microbiol: Eur J Clin Microbiol Infect Dis Off Publ Eur Soc Clin; 2014.
107. Retamar P, López-Cerero L, Muniain MA, Pascual Á, Rodríguez-Baño J, ESBL-REIPI/GEIH Group. Impact of the MIC of piperacillin–tazobactam on the outcome of patients with bacteremia due to extended-spectrum-β-lactamase-producing *Escherichia coli*. Antimicrob Agents Chemother. 2013;57:3402–4.
108. Tsai H-Y, Chen Y-H, Tang H-J, Huang C-C, Liao C-H, Chu F-Y, et al. Carbapenems and piperacillin/tazobactam for the treatment of bacteremia caused by extended-spectrum β-lactamase-producing Proteus mirabilis. Diagn Microbiol Infect Dis. 2014;80:222–6.
109. Tumbarello M, Sanguinetti M, Montuori E, Trecarichi EM, Posteraro B, Fiori B, et al. Predictors of mortality in patients with bloodstream infections caused by extended-spectrum-beta-lactamase-producing Enterobacteriaceae: importance of inadequate initial antimicrobial treatment. Antimicrob Agents Chemother. 2007;51:1987–94.
110. Tuon FF, Bianchet LC, Penteado-Filho SR. Epidemiology of extended spectrum beta-lactamase producing enterobacter bacteremia in a brazilian hospital. Rev Soc Bras Med Trop. 2010;43:452–4.
111. van Duin D, Bonomo RA. Ceftazidime/avibactam and ceftolozane/tazobactam: second-generation β-lactam/β-lactamase inhibitor combinations. Clin Infect Dis Off Publ Infect Dis Soc Am. 2016;63:234–41.

11

Procalcitonin-guided antibiotic therapy in intensive care unit patients

Hui-Bin Huang[1,2], Jin-Min Peng[1], Li Weng[1], Chun-Yao Wang[1], Wei Jiang[1] and Bin Du[1*]

Abstract

Background: Serum procalcitonin (PCT) concentration is used to guide antibiotic decisions in choice, timing, and duration of anti-infection therapy to avoid antibiotic overuse. Thus, we performed a systematic review and meta-analysis to seek evidence of different PCT-guided antimicrobial strategies for critically ill patients in terms of predefined clinical outcomes.

Methods: We searched for relevant studies in PubMed, Embase, Web of Knowledge, and the Cochrane Library up to 25 February 2017. Randomized controlled trials (RCTs) were included if they reported data on any of the predefined outcomes in adult ICU patients managed with a PCT-guided algorithm or according to standard care. Results were expressed as risk ratio (RR) or mean difference (MD) with accompanying 95% confidence interval (CI).

Data synthesis: We included 13 trials enrolling 5136 patients. These studies used PCT in three clinical strategies: initiation, discontinuation, or combination of antibiotic initiation and discontinuation strategies. Pooled analysis showed a PCT-guided antibiotic discontinuation strategy had fewer total days with antibiotics (MD − 1.66 days; 95% CI − 2.36 to − 0.96 days), longer antibiotic-free days (MD 2.26 days; 95% CI 1.40–3.12 days), and lower short-term mortality (RR 0.87; 95% CI 0.76–0.98), without adversely affecting other outcomes. Only few studies reported data on other PCT-guided strategies for antibiotic therapies, and the pooled results showed no benefit in the predefined outcomes.

Conclusions: Our meta-analysis produced evidence that among all the PCT-based strategies, only using PCT for antibiotic discontinuation can reduce both antibiotic exposure and short-term mortality in a critical care setting.

Keywords: Procalcitonin, Antibiotic strategies, Meta-analysis, Systematic review, Intensive care unit

Background

Timely diagnosis and appropriate antimicrobial treatment of infection remain a major challenge in critical care settings. Delay in diagnosis due to lack of specific clinical signs in the early stage of infection may withhold or delay antibiotic therapy. On the other hand, concern of not treating potentially life-threatening infection and the risk of recurrence frequently leads clinicians to antimicrobial overuse in intensive care unit (ICU) [1, 2]. Studies have demonstrated that up to 50% of antibiotics prescribed in hospital settings are either unnecessary or inappropriate [3]. Nowadays, long-term antimicrobial regimens applied to critically ill patients are common and often based on empiric rules [4, 5]. This may result in increased medical costs, emergence of resistant pathogens, prolonged length of stay (LOS), and risk of mortality [6, 7].

Recently, procalcitonin (PCT) has shown to be a promising biomarker for identification of bacterial infections and is correlated with the severity of infection [8–11]. The 2016 Surviving Sepsis Campaign (SSC) guidelines offered a weak recommendation (low quality of evidence), favouring that measurement of procalcitonin levels can be used to support shortening the duration of antimicrobial therapy in sepsis patients [12]. However,

*Correspondence: dubin98@gmail.com

[1] Medical ICU, Peking Union Medical College Hospital, Peking Union Medical College and Chinese Academy of Medical Sciences, 1 Shuai Fu Yuan, Beijing 100730, People's Republic of China

Full list of author information is available at the end of the article

one recent large study failed to show any benefit of daily PCT measurement with regard to time to appropriate therapy or survival, but resulted in a longer antibiotic course and ICU stay [13]. To date, several meta-analyses have assessed the value of PCT to guide antibiotic stewardship in ICU patients [14–22]. Findings of these reports showed that utilizing PCT to guide antibiotic decisions could significantly reduce antibiotics use, but did not improve patient outcomes, such as mortality, hospital, or ICU LOS. However, one major limitation of these meta-analyses was unexplainable significant heterogeneity among included trials, possibly due to the fact that the different PCT guidance strategies (including antibiotic initiation, discontinuation, or combination of antibiotic initiation and discontinuation strategies) had been evaluated in these trials. Since the considerable differences in methodologies and research purposes associated with the different PCT-guided strategies, the previous meta-analyses might not accurately evaluate the effects of PCT-based algorithms (Additional file 1: Table S1). Recently, two large-scale randomized controlled trials (RCTs) of PCT-guided antibiotic strategy in ICU patients have been published, with inconsistent results [23, 24]. Of note, the study by de Jong et al., the largest PCT trial to date, demonstrated an unexpected and significant survival benefit, in addition to less antibiotic exposure.

Therefore, with the aid of increased power of meta-analytic techniques, we sought to expand the previous analyses by including studies published recently, stratifying different strategies to have a more accurate analysis of the influence of different PCT algorithms to guide antimicrobial decisions.

Methods

Search strategy and selection criteria

This systematic review and meta-analysis were conducted in accordance with the PRISMA guidance [25]. We searched RCTs in PubMed, Embase, Web of Science, and Cochrane Central Register of Controlled Trials from inception through 25 February 2017 to identify potentially relevant studies. Search included the following key words: ("Procalcitonin" OR "PCT") AND ("intensive care" OR "critically ill" OR "critical care"). No language restriction was imposed. Reference lists of relative articles were also reviewed.

Studies were included if they are enrolling adult ICU patients, with confirmed or suspected infection, assigned to either a PCT-guided therapeutic strategy group or a standard care group. Standard care referred to antimicrobial regimens based on clinical signs, laboratory results, and empiric rules or guidelines, without consideration of PCT level. We excluded studies enrolling children or patients without any evidence of infection and studies without mentioning of PCT assay methods. Articles available only in abstract form or meeting reports were also excluded.

Data extraction and outcomes

Two reviewers independently extracted data from included studies on the first author, year of publication, country, sample size, study design, ICU type, compared protocols, methods of PCT assay, methodological quality, as well as all outcomes of interest.

We stratified different PCT-guided strategies according to medical decision with regards to antimicrobial therapy. In brief, strategy of antibiotic initiation referred to the decision to or not to start antibiotics, and decision of the intensified monitoring, diagnostic efforts, and interventions to explore uncontrolled sources of infection based on a predefined threshold of baseline PCT concentration, while strategy of antibiotic discontinuation meant making the decision to stop antibiotics according to a predefined threshold of PCT concentration, or the PCT level dropped by a certain proportion predefined compared with the previous value. The primary outcomes were the duration of antibiotic use and the short-term mortality, while the latter was defined as ICU or hospital or 28-day mortality [26, 27]. Secondary outcomes included ICU and hospital LOS.

Quality assessment

Two independent reviewers evaluated the quality of studies using the risk of bias tool recommended by the Cochrane Collaboration [28]. We assigned a value of high, unclear, or low to the following items: sequence generation; allocation concealment; blinding; incomplete outcome data; selective outcome reporting; and other sources of bias. Discrepancies were identified and resolved through discussion.

Statistical analysis

The results from all relevant studies were combined to estimate the pooled risk ratio (RR) and associated 95% confidence intervals (CIs) for dichotomous outcomes. As to the continuous outcomes, mean differences (MD) and 95% CI were estimated as the effect results. Heterogeneity was tested by using the I^2 statistic. An $I^2 < 50\%$ was considered to indicate insignificant heterogeneity, and a fixed-effect model was used, whereas a random-effect model was used in cases of significant heterogeneity ($I^2 > 50\%$). Before data analysis, we estimated mean from median and standard deviations (SD) from IQR using the methods described in previous studies [29]. Sensitivity analyses were performed by excluding trials that potentially biased the results of primary outcomes. Publication bias was evaluated by visually inspecting funnel plots. All analyses were performed using Review Manager version 5.3.

Results

Study selection

The literature search yielded 881 records through database searching, and 13 RCTs fulfilled inclusion criteria were eligible for the final analysis [13, 23, 24, 30–39]. The overview of the study selection process is presented in Fig. 1. In the study by Jensen et al., some patients without infection were also included [13]; therefore, we only included patients with severe sepsis or septic shock that fulfilled our inclusion criteria from this study. The Cochrane risk of bias score for each citation varied across the studies (Additional file 2: Table S2).

Study characteristics

The main characteristics and predefined outcomes of the 13 included studies are shown in Table 1 and Additional file 3: Table S3. The degree of non-compliance with PCT algorithm recommendations for antibiotics varied among the included RCTs (Additional file 4: Table S4). Of these included studies, seven were multicenter studies. A total of 5136 patients comprised 2588 in the PCT-guided group and 2548 in the standard care group. These studies evaluated the effects of PCT-guided strategies in antibiotic discontinuation (n = 8) [23, 24, 31–34, 37, 39], antibiotic initiation (n = 3) [13, 30, 36], or the combination of the antibiotic initiation and discontinuation (n = 2) [35, 38]. Study population included surgical patients (n = 3) [30, 31, 33] and mixed medical–surgical patients (n = 10) [13, 23, 24, 32, 34–39]. PCT assays adopted varied across the included studies.

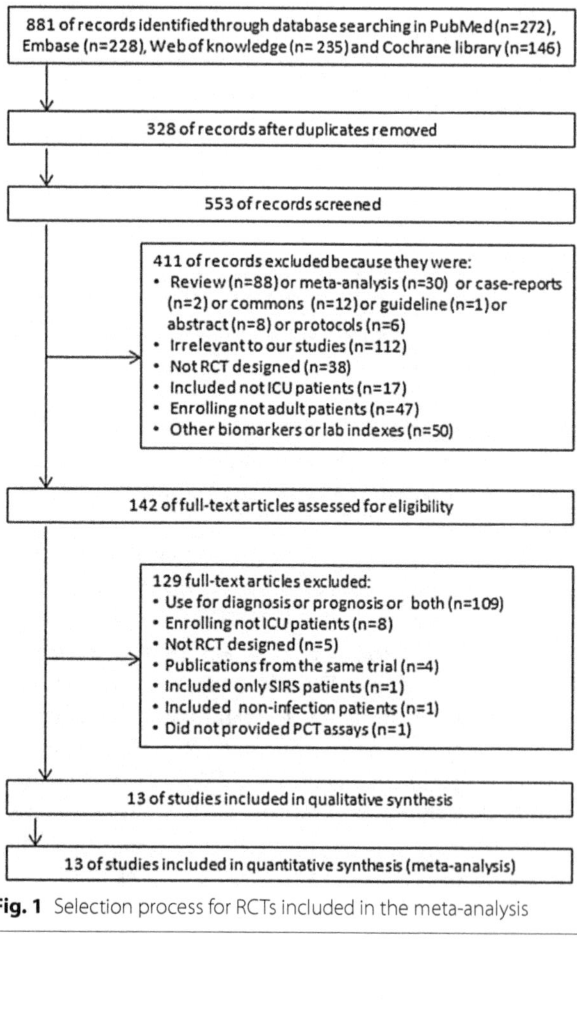

Fig. 1 Selection process for RCTs included in the meta-analysis

Data synthesis

Procalcitonin-guided discontinuation of antibiotics

The use of a PCT algorithm compared with standard care to guide antibiotic discontinuation in critically ill patients was evaluated in eight RCTs [23, 24, 31–34, 37, 39]. All eight studies reported outcomes including total days with antibiotics or antibiotic-free days. The aggregated data suggested that the duration of antibiotic treatment was 1.67 days shorter in PCT-guided group (n = 3404; MD − 1.66 days; 95% CI − 2.36 to − 0.96; I^2 = 71%; P < 0.00001) [23, 24, 31–34, 37, 39] (Fig. 2), while antibiotic-free days were 2.26 days longer (n = 2120; MD 2.26 days; 95% CI 1.40–3.12; I^2 = 0%; P < 0.00001) [23, 24, 32, 34] when compared with that of standard care group. Results showed patients in PCT-guided group had lower short-term mortality than standard care group (n = 3414; RR 0.86; 95% CI 0.76–0.98; I^2 = 0%; P = 0.02) [23, 24, 31–34, 37, 39] (Fig. 3), while no differences were found in ICU LOS (n = 3326; MD − 0.00 days; 95% CI − 0.58 to 0.58; I^2 = 0%; P = 0.99) [23, 24, 31–33, 37, 39] and hospital LOS (n = 3290; MD 0.43 days; 95% CI − 0.83 to 1.70; I^2 = 30.4%; P = 0.50) [23, 24, 32, 34, 37, 39]. There was significant heterogeneity in the outcome of duration of antibiotic treatment between the pooled studies. Therefore, we conducted sensitivity analyses to explore potential sources of heterogeneity. Exclusion of the trial by Bloos and colleagues resolved the heterogeneity without alerting the result (n = 2338; MD − 1.97 days; 95% CI − 2.27 to − 1.68; I^2 = 0%; P < 0.00001) [24, 31–34, 37, 39].

Procalcitonin-guided initiation of antibiotics

Three studies examined the efficacy of PCT-guided initiation of antibiotics [13, 30, 36]. Only one study examined the efficacy of PCT-guided initiation of antibiotics. In this case, antibiotic consumption was comparable between groups with the treatment days represented 62.6% and 57.7% of ICU stays in the PCT and standard care groups, respectively (P = 0.11) [36]. There was no statistically significant difference between groups in the

Table 1 Characteristics of included studies

Study/year	Trial design	Population	Type of ICU	*N* PCT/Ctrl	PCT-guided group protocol	Control group protocol	PCT assay
Svoboda et al. [30]	SC, P, R, OL	Postoperative severe sepsis	Surgical	38/34	AI: prompted change of ABT and catheter (≥ 2 ng/ml), prompted to repeated radiographic and/or surgical evaluation (< 2 ng/ml)	Standard evaluation by consultant surgeon	PCT-Q
Schroeder et al. [31]	SC, P, R, OL	Postoperative severe sepsis	Surgical	14/13	AD: if clinic signs and symptoms improved and PCT < 1 ng/ml or 25–35% of baseline	According to clinical signs and empiric rules	LIA
Nobre et al. [32]	SC, P, R, OL	Sepsis	Mixed	39/40	AD: if baseline PCT > 1 μg/L, re-evaluation at day 5. ABT discontinuation if PCT < 0.25 μg/L or PCT dropped by > 90% from the baseline peak level. If baseline PCT < 1 μg/L, re-evaluation at day 3. ABT discontinuation if PCT < 0.1 μg/L and careful clinical evaluation	Regimens according to guidelines	Kryptor
Hochreiter et al. [33]	SC, P, R, OL	Infection	Surgical	53/57	AD: if clinic signs and symptoms improved and PCT < 1 ng/ml or 25–35% of initial value over 3 days	Standard regimen over 8 days	LIA
Stolz et al. [34]	MC, P, R, OL	Ventilator-associated pneumonia	Mixed	51/50	AD: strongly encouraged (< 0.25 μg/L), encouraged (0.25–0.5 μg/L or a decrease ≥ 80%), discouraged (0.5–1.0 μg/L or a decrease < 80%) or strongly discouraged (> 1.0 μg/L)	According to clinical signs and empiric rules	Kryptor
Bouadma et al. [35]	MC, P, R, OL	Bacterial infection or sepsis	Mixed	311/319	AI: ABT was strongly discouraged (< 0.25 μg/L), discouraged (0.25–0.49 μg/L), encouraged (0.5–0.99 μg/L) or strongly encouraged (≥ 1 μg/L) AD: strongly encouraged (< 0.25 μg/L), encouraged (0.25–0.49 μg/L). continuing of ABT was encouraged (0.25–0.5 μg/L or > 80% peak) and change of ABT (> peak concentration and > 0.5 μg/L)	Regimens according to international and local guidelines	Kryptor
Jensen et al. [13]	MC, P, R, OL	Severe sepsis/septic shock	Mixed	212/247	AI: if PCT ≥ 1 μg/L that was not decreasing by at least 10% from previous day: increasing the antimicrobial spectrum and intensifying diagnostic efforts to find uncontrolled sources of infection	According to current guidelines	Kryptor
Layios et al. [36]	SC, P, R, OL	Infection	Mixed	258/251	AI: ABT was strongly discouraged (< 0.25 μg/L), discouraged (0.25–0.5 μg/L), encouraged (0.5–1.0 μg/L) or strongly encouraged (> 1.0 μg/L)	No reports	Kryptor
Annane et al. [38]	MC, P, R, OL	Septic shock	Mixed	31/31	AI/AD: ABT was not to be started or was to be discontinuation (< 0.25 μg/L); strongly discouraged (≥ 0.25 to < 0.5 μg/L); was recommended (≥ 0.5 to < 5 μg/L) and was strongly recommended (≥ 5 μg/L). For patients enrolled ≤ 48 h after surgery, the respective PCT cut-offs were < 4 μg/L, 4–9 μg/L and ≥ 9 μg/L	ABT at the discretion of the patient's physician	Kryptor

Table 1 continued

Study/year	Trial design	Population	Type of ICU	*N* PCT/Ctrl	PCT-guided group protocol	Control group protocol	PCT assay
Deliberato et al. [39]	SC, P, R, OL	Sepsis	Mixed	42/39	AD: if PCT dropped > 90% from the peak level or the absolute value < 0.5 ng/ml	The possible source of infection and local susceptibility profile	Vidas
Shehabi et al. [23]	MC, P, R, SB	Bacterial infection or sepsis	Mixed	200/200	AD: cease ABT when PCT < 0.1 ng/ml or PCT was 0.1–0.25 ng/ml and infection is highly unlikely or PCT level decreased > 90% from baseline	According to the ABT guidelines	Automated immunoassay analysers
De Jong et al. [24]	MC, P, R, OL	Infection	Mixed	776/799	AD: if PCT value decreased over 80% or PCT value lower than 0.5 µg/L	Guidelines and the discretion of attending physicians	Vidas, Roche or Kryptor machine
Bloos et al. [37]	MC, P, R, OL	Severe sepsis/septic shock	Mixed	587/593	AD: stopping ABT if PCT level on day 7 or later < 1 ng/ml r or dropped > 50% from the previous value	According to the local sepsis guidelines	Kryptor

ABT **antibiotics,** ***AD*** **antibiotic discontinuation,** ***AI*** **antibiotic initiation,** ***Ctrl*** **control,** ***ICU*** **intensive care unit,** ***LIA*** **immunoluminometric assay,** ***MC*** **multi-centre,** ***Mixed*** **surgical and medical intensive care unit,** ***OL*** **open label,** ***P*** **prospective,** ***PCT*** **procalcitonin,** ***PCT-Q*** **procalcitonin immunochromatographic technology,** ***R*** **RCT,** ***SC*** **single centre**

Study or Subgroup	PCT Mean	PCT SD	PCT Total	Control Mean	Control SD	Control Total	Weight	Mean Difference IV, Random, 95% CI
1.8.1 discontinuation algorithm								
Bloos 2016	7	6.7	529	7	6.7	537	14.3%	0.00 [-0.80, 0.80]
De Jong 2016	5	4.4	761	7	5.2	785	15.9%	-2.00 [-2.48, -1.52]
Deliberato 2013	10	26.7	42	11	31.9	39	0.4%	-1.00 [-13.86, 11.86]
Hochreiter 2009	5.9	1.7	57	7.9	0.5	53	15.9%	-2.00 [-2.46, -1.54]
Nobre 2008	6	23	39	9.5	23	40	0.6%	-3.50 [-13.64, 6.64]
Schroeder 2008	6.6	1.1	14	8.3	0.7	13	14.9%	-1.70 [-2.39, -1.01]
Shehabi 2014	9	10.4	196	11	11.9	198	7.3%	-2.00 [-4.21, 0.21]
Stolz 2009	10	7.4	51	15	9.6	50	4.2%	-5.00 [-8.35, -1.65]
Subtotal (95% CI)			**1689**			**1715**	**73.5%**	**-1.66 [-2.36, -0.96]**
Heterogeneity: Tau² = 0.48; Chi² = 24.16, df = 7 (P = 0.001); I² = 71%								
Test for overall effect: Z = 4.65 (P < 0.00001)								
1.8.2 discontinuation and initiation algorithm								
Annane 2013	5	2.2	30	5	1.5	28	13.5%	0.00 [-0.96, 0.96]
Bouadma 2010	6.1	6	307	9.9	7.1	314	13.1%	-3.80 [-4.83, -2.77]
Subtotal (95% CI)			**337**			**342**	**26.5%**	**-1.90 [-5.62, 1.83]**
Heterogeneity: Tau² = 6.96; Chi² = 27.80, df = 1 (P < 0.00001); I² = 96%								
Test for overall effect: Z = 1.00 (P = 0.32)								
Total (95% CI)			**2026**			**2057**	**100.0%**	**-1.76 [-2.55, -0.98]**
Heterogeneity: Tau² = 0.96; Chi² = 51.96, df = 9 (P < 0.00001); I² = 83%								
Test for overall effect: Z = 4.39 (P < 0.0001)								
Test for subgroup differences: Chi² = 0.01, df = 1 (P = 0.90), I² = 0%								

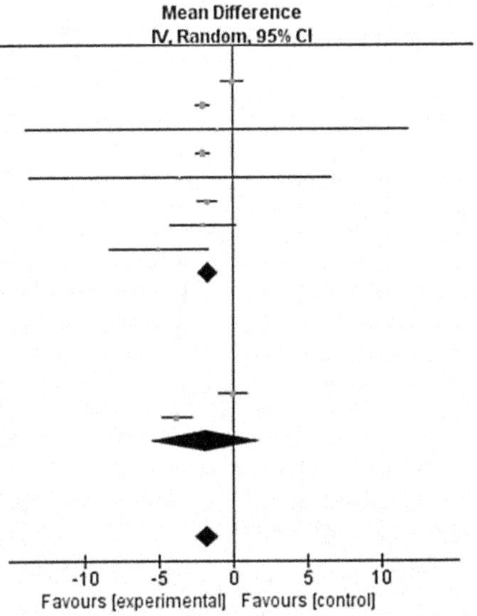

Fig. 2 Effects of PCT-guided antimicrobial strategies on total days of antibiotics

Study or Subgroup	PCT Events	PCT Total	Control Events	Control Total	Weight	Risk Ratio M-H, Fixed, 95% CI
1.17.1 Initiation algorithm						
Jensen 2011	90	247	76	212	12.4%	1.02 [0.80, 1.30]
Layios 2012	56	258	53	251	8.2%	1.03 [0.74, 1.43]
Svoboda 2007	10	38	10	34	1.6%	0.89 [0.42, 1.88]
Subtotal (95% CI)		**543**		**497**	**22.2%**	**1.01 [0.84, 1.23]**
Total events	156		139			
Heterogeneity: Chi² = 0.11, df = 2 (P = 0.94); I² = 0%						
Test for overall effect: Z = 0.12 (P = 0.90)						
1.17.2 Discontinuation algorithm						
Bloos 2016	140	547	149	529	23.0%	0.91 [0.75, 1.11]
De Jong 2016	149	761	196	785	29.4%	0.78 [0.65, 0.95]
Deliberato 2013	2	42	4	39	0.6%	0.46 [0.09, 2.39]
Hochreiter 2009	15	57	14	53	2.2%	1.00 [0.53, 1.86]
Nobre 2008	9	39	9	40	1.4%	1.03 [0.46, 2.31]
Schroeder 2008	3	14	3	13	0.5%	0.93 [0.23, 3.81]
Shehabi 2014	35	196	31	198	4.7%	1.14 [0.73, 1.77]
Stolz 2009	10	51	14	50	2.2%	0.70 [0.34, 1.43]
Subtotal (95% CI)		**1707**		**1707**	**63.9%**	**0.86 [0.76, 0.98]**
Total events	363		420			
Heterogeneity: Chi² = 4.06, df = 7 (P = 0.77); I² = 0%						
Test for overall effect: Z = 2.35 (P = 0.02)						
1.17.3 Initiation and discontinuation algorithm						
Annane 2013	7	31	10	30	1.5%	0.68 [0.30, 1.55]
Bouadma 2010	92	307	82	314	12.3%	1.15 [0.89, 1.48]
Subtotal (95% CI)		**338**		**344**	**13.9%**	**1.10 [0.86, 1.39]**
Total events	99		92			
Heterogeneity: Chi² = 1.43, df = 1 (P = 0.23); I² = 30%						
Test for overall effect: Z = 0.74 (P = 0.46)						
Total (95% CI)		**2588**		**2548**	**100.0%**	**0.93 [0.84, 1.02]**
Total events	618		651			
Heterogeneity: Chi² = 9.53, df = 12 (P = 0.66); I² = 0%						
Test for overall effect: Z = 1.54 (P = 0.12)						
Test for subgroup differences: Chi² = 3.95, df = 2 (P = 0.14), I² = 49.3%						

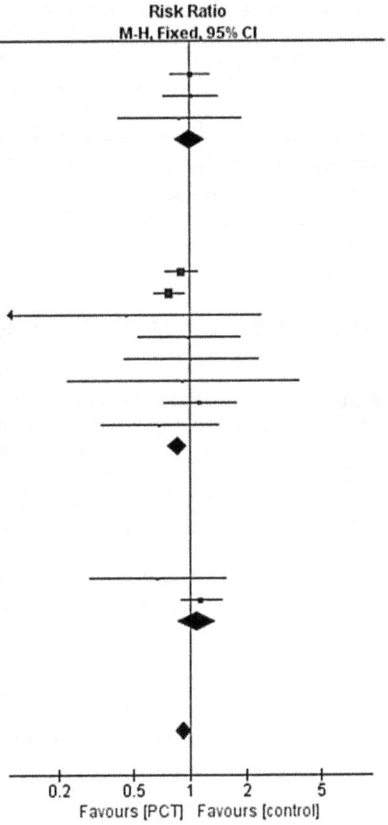

Fig. 3 Effects PCT-guided antimicrobial strategies on short-term mortality

risk of short-term mortality ($n = 1040$; RR 1.01; 95% CI 0.84–1.23; $I^2 = 0\%$; $P = 0.90$) [13, 30, 36] (Fig. 3) or ICU LOS ($n = 581$; MD − 1.22 days; 95% CI − 4.34 to 1.90; $I^2 = 60\%$; $P = 0.44$) [30, 36].

Procalcitonin-guided antibiotic initiation and discontinuation

Two studies employed a PCT-guided strategy of antibiotic initiation and discontinuation [35, 38]. No differences were observed between the PCT and standard care group in total days with antibiotics ($n = 679$; MD − 1.90 days, 95% CI − 5.62 to 1.83; $I^2 = 96\%$; $P = 0.32$) (Fig. 2), antibiotic-free days ($n = 679$; MD 1.31 days; 95% CI − 1.34 to 3.95; $I^2 = 90\%$; $P = 0.33$), short-term mortality ($n = 682$; RR 1.10; 95% CI 0.86–1.39; $I^2 = 30\%$; $P = 0.46$) (Fig. 3), the ICU LOS ($n = 682$; MD − 1.45 days; 95% CI − 0.91 to 3.80; $I^2 = 0\%$; $P = 0.23$), and hospital LOS ($n = 679$; MD − 0.43 days; 95% CI − 3.36 to 2.49; $I^2 = 0\%$; $P = 0.77$) [35, 38].

Summary of findings for the effect of PCT-guided strategy antibiotic on predefined outcomes in ICU patients is described in Table 2. We did not assess the publication bias because of the limited number of studies included in each analysis.

Discussion

PCT-guided strategies had been examined in multiple studies to optimize antibiotic treatment, with conflicting results. The current meta-analysis justified a low PCT level to discontinue antibiotic treatment, which would result in a shorter duration of antibiotic treatment of about 1.67 days, as well as lower short-term mortality compared with standard care. Due to the insufficient evidence, a baseline PCT value should not be used as a marker to guide antibiotic initiation.

Our study had several strengths. The current meta-analysis provided robust evidence to support and expand the weak suggestion in the 2016 SSC guidelines, i.e. use of low PCT level to assist the clinician in the discontinuation of empiric antibiotic [12]. In addition to those RCTs in previous meta-analyses, we had included three additional RCTs recently published, and this added to the statistical power by having 3414 cases to evaluate the primary outcome. Moreover, we had stratified enrolled RCTs according to different PCT-guided strategies, in order to eliminate the potential confounding factors caused by different strategies. Though significant heterogeneity was observed among these studies, our sensitivity analyses demonstrated that the heterogeneity was resulted from the trial by Bloss et al. [23]. This study was different from the other trials in some aspects. On the one hand, it was designed as a 2 × 2 factorial trial and the interaction between the two treatment factors was unclear; on the other hand, in the trial [23], the clinicians used a 50% decrease from previous value as a stopping rule, which was lower than that of other studies. As a result, we also demonstrated a significant improvement in short-term mortality associated with PCT-guided antibiotic discontinuation. This had added robustness to findings of reduction in antibiotics usage, since studies have demonstrated

Table 2 Summary of findings for the effect of procalcitonin-guided strategy on predefined outcomes in intensive care unit patients

PCT-guided strategy	Predefined outcome	Number of trials	N	Estimated benefit with antibiotic	I^2 (%)	P value
ABT discontinuation	Duration of antibiotic use	8	3404	− 1.66 days (− 2.36, − 0.96)	71	$P < 0.0001$
	Antibiotic-free days	4	2120	2.26 days (1.40, 3.12)	0	$P < 0.0001$
	Short-term mortality	8	3414	0.86 (0.76, 0.98)	0	0.02
	Length of stay in ICU	7	3326	− 0.00 days (− 0.58, 0.58)	0	0.99
	Length of stay in hospital	6	3290	0.43 days (− 0.83, 1.70)	30	0.50
ABT initiation	Duration of antibiotic use	–	–	–	–	–
	Antibiotic-free days	–	–	–	–	–
	Short-term mortality	3	1040	1.01 (0.84, 1.23)	0	0.90
	Length of stay in ICU	2	581	− 1.22 days (− 4.34, 1.90)	60	0.44
	Length of stay in hospital	–	–	–	–	–
ABT initiation and discontinuation	Duration of antibiotic use	2	679	− 1.90 days (− 5.62, 1.83)	96	0.32
	Antibiotic-free days	2	679	1.31 days (− 1.34, 3.95)	90	0.33
	Short-term mortality	2	682	1.10 (0.86, 1.39)	30	0.46
	Length of stay in ICU	2	682	− 1.45 days (− 0.91, 3.80)	0	0.23
	Length of stay in hospital	2	750	− 0.43 days (− 3.36, 2.49)	0	0.77

ABT antibiotics, *PCT* procalcitonin, *ICU* intensive care unit

that strategies aiming at restricting antibiotic overuse could help improve survival [40, 41]. Our findings that short-term mortality was significantly reduced in the PCT-guided discontinuation group contrasted those of previous meta-analyses. Despite the fact that no heterogeneity was detected, the beneficial effect was clearly driven by the study results of de Jong et al. [24]. However, as the authors acknowledged, this study was a non-inferiority study; therefore, the beneficial effect of mortality in PCT-guided group was unexpected, which merited cautious interpretation and further validation.

As for a PCT strategy that combined initiation and discontinuation of antibiotics, we found no beneficial effect with regard to any predefined outcomes. The reason for this failure may be that only two trials (one positive [35] and one negative [38]) investigated the combined strategies varying in objective and the methodology. On the other hand, reported non-compliance rate was high. For example, in a prospective, multicenter, open-label randomized trial (PRORATA trial) involving 630 non-surgical patients with suspected bacterial infections [35], patients in the PCT group had significantly more antibiotic-free days. However, the algorithm-guided treatment recommendation was not strictly followed in 53% of patients in the PCT group. Moreover, this trial [35] reported a higher standard deviation with regard to duration of antibiotic treatment as well as antibiotic-free days (possibly due to reported higher non-compliance rate), compared to that in the negative trial [38], which weaken its statistic weight in the meta-analysis. Interestingly, it was noteworthy that initial antibiotic prescription rate was similar in PCT and standard care groups, suggesting that the improvement in antibiotic-free days was more likely the result of antibiotic discontinuation, while it was less likely due to exclusion of potential infection.

In our study, we could not verify the efficacy of PCT-based antibiotic initiation strategy because we found only three RCT through the literature search [13, 30, 36]. Of these trials, only the trial by Layios and coworkers reported the antibiotics exposure and concluded that PCT measuring for the initiation of antibiotics failed to decrease the antibiotic consummation [36]. The reasons for this failure may be that almost half of PCT serum samples were > 1 μg/L, thus encouraging the antibiotic treatment, and the relative low proportion of patient-days with antibiotic treatment in the control group (57%). Another reason could be related to the high non-compliance rate with the PCT-guided antibiotic initiation strategy described in the study. The authors reported that nearly 64% of patients in the PCT group received antibiotics regardless of a normal PCT level (< 0.5 μg/L).

The incidence of non-compliance with the recommendations based on PCT algorithm, as reported in some, but not all RCTs, showed significant variability, ranging from 0 to 59%. In most case of non-compliance, physicians were reluctant to stop antibiotics, even with a very low PCT level (Additional file 4: Table S4), possibly due to the concerns about the accuracy of single PCT value as a biomarker of infection [42, 43]. This might lead to unnecessarily prolonged exposure of antibiotics, which supported the robustness of our findings that implementation of PCT algorithm was associated with shorter duration of antibiotic treatment and longer antibiotic-free days.

Our meta-analysis has some limitations. First, studies examining the PCT-guided strategies other than discontinuation of antibiotic treatment were scarce, with limited number of studies available as well as small number of enrolled patients. As such, data on these strategies were insufficient to draw solid conclusions. Second, the high exclusion rate of screened patients in the included studies (such as immunosuppressed patients and those requiring long-term antibiotic therapy) precluded generalization of the study results. Third, antibiotic strategy in the control group (indications to initiate and discontinue antibiotics) was not specified in most studies. Whether the variation in antibiotic strategy, if any, in the control group might have affected the results of our meta-analysis is unclear. Thus, a more uniform approach to evaluating and reporting standard care related to antibiotic use would be needed in future studies. Fourth, the uneven distribution of different underlying diseases among included studies might also exert a prognostic value. Of note, in the two recently published systematic reviews and individual patient data meta-analysis [44, 45], Schuetz et al. demonstrated with sufficient evidence that PCT-guided antibiotic treatment in patients with acute respiratory infections reduced antibiotic exposure and side effects and improved survival. Finally, different cut-off values of PCT and different PCT measurements were reported across included studies, which might also lead to bias in our results. We had originally tried to perform subgroup analyses exploring studies according to all the diversities. However, there were insufficient data.

Conclusions

In summary, based on the results of our meta-analysis, we recommend use of PCT to guide antibiotic discontinuation, which was associated with a reduction in antibiotic exposure and lower short-term mortality. Further studies are needed to define the optimal cut-off value of PCT for antibiotic discontinuation and to generalize our findings in other patient population including immunocompromised patients and those received long-term antibiotic therapy in ICU.

Abbreviations

CI: confidence interval; ICU: intensive care unit; IQR: interquartile range; LOS: length of stay; MD: mean difference; PCT: procalcitonin; RR: risk ratio; RCTs: randomized controlled trials; SD: standard deviations; VAP: ventilator-associated pneumonia.

Authors' contributions

H-BH contributed to the conception of the study, data collection, analysis, and drafting of the article. WJ and C-YW contributed to data collection and analysis. LW and J-MP contributed to design and revisions of this manuscript. BD was responsible for the integrity of the work as a whole, from inception to publication of the article. All authors read and approved the final manuscript.

Author details

[1] Medical ICU, Peking Union Medical College Hospital, Peking Union Medical College and Chinese Academy of Medical Sciences, 1 Shuai Fu Yuan, Beijing 100730, People's Republic of China. [2] Department of Critical Care Medicine, The First Affiliated Hospital of Fujian Medical University, Fuzhou, China.

Acknowledgements

We thank Jing-Chao Luo, MD, for his assistance in searching the literature.

Competing interests

The authors declare that they have no competing interests.

Funding

Cams Innovation Fund for Medical Sciences (2016-12M-1-014).

References

1. Braykov NP, Morgan DJ, Schweizer ML, et al. Assessment of empirical antibiotic therapy optimisation in six hospitals: an observational cohort study. Lancet Infect Dis. 2014;14(14):1220–7.
2. Llor C, Bjerrum L. Antimicrobial resistance: risk associated with antibiotic overuse and initiatives to reduce the problem. Ther Adv Drug Saf. 2014;5(6):229–41.
3. Dellit TH, Owens RC, McGowan JE Jr, et al. Infectious Diseases Society of America and the Society for Healthcare Epidemiology of America guidelines for developing an institutional program to enhance antimicrobial stewardship. Clin Infect Dis. 2007;44(4):263–4.
4. Dimopoulos G, Poulakou G, Pneumatikos IA, Armaganidis A, Kollef MH, Matthaiou DK. Short- vs long-duration antibiotic regimens for ventilator-associated pneumonia: a systematic review and meta-analysis. Chest. 2013;144(6):1759–67.
5. Najafi A, Khodadadian A, Sanatkar M, et al. The comparison of procalcitonin guidance administer antibiotics with empiric antibiotic therapy in critically ill patients admitted in intensive care unit. Acta Medica Iranica. 2015;53(9):562–7.
6. Evans HL, Lefrak SN, Lyman J, et al. Cost of gram-negative resistance. Crit Care Med. 2007;35(1):89–95.
7. Vincent JL, Rello J, Marshall J, et al. International study of the prevalence and outcomes of infection in intensive care units. J Am Med Assoc. 2009;302(21):2323–9.
8. Luyt CE, Combes A, Reynaud C, et al. Usefulness of procalcitonin for the diagnosis of ventilator-associated pneumonia. Intensive Care Med. 2008;34(8):1434–40.
9. Simon L, Lacroix J. Serum procalcitonin and C-reactive protein levels as markers of bacterial infection: a systematic review and meta-analysis. Clin Infect Dis. 2004;39:206–17.
10. Wacker C, Prkno A, Brunkhorst FM, Schlattmann P. Procalcitonin as a diagnostic marker for sepsis: a systematic review and meta-analysis. Lancet Infect Dis. 2013;13(5):426–35.
11. Schuetz P, Muller B, Christ-Crain M, et al. Procalcitonin to initiate or discontinue antibiotics in acute respiratory tract infections. Evid Based Child Health. 2013;8:1297–371.
12. Rhodes A, Evans LE, Alhazzani W, et al. Surviving sepsis campaign: international guidelines for management of sepsis and septic shock. Crit Care Med. 2017;45(3):486–552.
13. Jensen JU, Hein L, Lundgren B, et al. Procalcitonin-guided interventions against infections to increase early appropriate antibiotics and improve survival in the intensive care unit: a randomized trial. Crit Care Med. 2011;39(9):2048–58.
14. Kopterides P, Siempos II, Tsangaris I, Tsantes A, Armaganidis A. Procalcitonin-guided algorithms of antibiotic therapy in the intensive care unit: a systematic review and meta-analysis of randomized controlled trials. Crit Care Med. 2010;38(11):2229–41.
15. Heyland DK, Johnson AP, Reynolds SC, Muscedere J. Procalcitonin for reduced antibiotic exposure in the critical care setting: a systematic review and an economic evaluation. Crit Care Med. 2011;39(7):1792–9.
16. Agarwal R, Schwartz DN. Procalcitonin to guide duration of antimicrobial therapy in intensive care units: a systematic review. Clin Infect Dis. 2011;53(4):379–87.
17. Schuetz P, Chiappa V, Briel M, Greenwald JL. Procalcitonin algorithms for antibiotic therapy decisions: a systematic review of randomized controlled trials and recommendations for clinical algorithms. Arch Intern Med. 2011;171(15):1322–31.
18. Soni NJ, Pitrak DL, Aronson N, Samson DJ, Galaydick JL, Vats V. Procalcitonin-guided antibiotic therapy. Agency for Healthcare Research and Quality. 2012.
19. Matthaiou DK, Ntani G, Kontogiorgi M, Poulakou G, Armaganidis A, Dimopoulos G. An ESICM systematic review and meta-analysis of procalcitonin-guided antibiotic therapy algorithms in adult critically ill patients. Intensive Care Med. 2012;38(6):940–9.
20. Tang H, Huang T, Jing J, Shen H, Cui W. Effect of procalcitonin-guided treatment in patients with infections: a systematic review and meta-analysis. Infection. 2009;37(6):497–507.
21. Prkno A, Wacker C, Brunkhorst FM, Schlattmann P. Procalcitonin-guided therapy in intensive care unit patients with severe sepsis and septic shock—a systematic review and meta-analysis. Crit Care. 2013;17(6):R291.
22. Westwood M, Ramaekers B, Whiting P, et al. Procalcitonin testing to guide antibiotic therapy for the treatment of sepsis in intensive care settings and for suspected bacterial infection in emergency department settings: a systematic review and cost-effectiveness analysis. Health Technol Assess. 2015;19(96):1–236.
23. Bloos F, Trips E, Nierhaus A, et al. Effect of sodium selenite administration and procalcitonin-guided therapy on mortality in patients with severe sepsis or septic shock: a randomized clinical trial. JAMA Intern Med. 2016;176(9):1266–76.
24. de Jong E, van Oers JA, Beishuizen A, et al. Efficacy and safety of procalcitonin guidance in reducing the duration of antibiotic treatment in critically ill patients: a randomised, controlled, open-label trial. Lancet Infect Dis. 2016;16(7):819–27.
25. Moher D, Liberati A, Tetzlaff J, Altman DG, Group TP. Preferred reporting items for systematic reviews and meta-analyses: the PRISMA statement. J Chin Integr Med. 2010;8(5):336–41.
26. Huang H, Li Y, Ariani F, Chen X, Lin J. Timing of tracheostomy in critically ill patients: a meta-analysis. PLoS ONE. 2014;9(3):e92981.
27. Wang F, Wu Y, Bo L, et al. The timing of tracheotomy in critically ill patients undergoing mechanical ventilation: a systematic review and meta-analysis of randomized controlled trials. Chest. 2011;140(140):1456–65.
28. Higgins JP, Altman DG, Gotzsche PC, et al. The Cochrane Collaboration's tool for assessing risk of bias in randomised trials. BMJ. 2011;343(oct18 2):d5928.
29. Wan X, Wang W, Liu J, Tong T. Estimating the sample mean and standard deviation from the sample size, median, range and/or interquartile range. BMC Med Res Methodol. 2014;14(8):735–46.
30. Svoboda P, Kantorová I, Scheer P, Radvanova J, Radvan M. Can procalcitonin help us in timing of re-intervention in septic patients after multiple trauma or major surgery? Hepatogastroenterology. 2007;54(74):359–63.
31. Schroeder S, Hochreiter M, Koehler T, et al. Procalcitonin (PCT)-guided algorithm reduces length of antibiotic treatment in surgical intensive care patients with severe sepsis: results of a prospective randomized study. Langenbecks Arch Surg. 2009;394(2):221–6.
32. Nobre V, Harbarth S, Graf JD, Rohner P, Pugin J. Use of procalcitonin to shorten antibiotic treatment duration in septic patients: a randomized trial. Am J Respir Crit Care Med. 2008;177(5):498–505.

33. Hochreiter M, Kohler T, Schweiger AM, et al. Procalcitonin to guide duration of antibiotic therapy in intensive care patients: a randomized prospective controlled trial. Crit Care. 2009;13(3):R83.
34. Stolz D, Smyrnios N, Eggimann P, et al. Procalcitonin for reduced antibiotic exposure in ventilator-associated pneumonia: a randomised study. Eur Respir J. 2009;34(6):1364–75.
35. Bouadma L, Luyt CE, et al. Use of procalcitonin to reduce patients' exposure to antibiotics in intensive care units (PRORATA trial): a multicentre randomised controlled trial. Lancet. 2010;375(9713):463–74.
36. Layios N, Lambermont B, Canivet JL, et al. Procalcitonin usefulness for the initiation of antibiotic treatment in intensive care unit patients. Crit Care Med. 2012;40(8):2304–9.
37. Shehabi Y, Sterba M, Garrett PM, et al. Procalcitonin algorithm in critically ill adults with undifferentiated infection or suspected sepsis. A randomized controlled trial. Am J Respir Crit Care Med. 2014;190(10):1102–10.
38. Annane D, Maxime V, Faller JP, et al. Procalcitonin levels to guide antibiotic therapy in adults with non-microbiologically proven apparent severe sepsis: a randomised controlled trial. BMJ Open. 2013;3(2):e002186.
39. Deliberato RO, Marra AR, Sanches PR, et al. Clinical and economic impact of procalcitonin to shorten antimicrobial therapy in septic patients with proven bacterial infection in an intensive care setting. Diagn Microbiol Infect Dis. 2013;76(3):266–71.
40. Levy SB, Marshall B. Antibacterial resistance worldwide: causes, challenges and responses. Nat Med. 2004;10(12 suppl):S122–9.
41. Cohen ML. Epidemiology of drug resistance: implications for a post-antimicrobial era. Science. 1992;257(257):1050–5.
42. Schuetz P, Affolter B, Hunziker S, et al. Serum procalcitonin, C-reactive protein and white blood cell levels following hypothermia after cardiac arrest: a retrospective cohort study. Eur J Clin Invest. 2010;40(4):376–81.
43. Jung B, Molinari N, Nasri M, et al. Procalcitonin biomarker kinetics fails to predict treatment response in perioperative abdominal infection with septic shock. Crit Care. 2013;17(5):R25.
44. Schuetz P, Wirz Y, Sager R, et al. Procalcitonin to initiate or discontinue antibiotics in acute respiratory tract infections. Cochrane Database Syst Rev. 2017;10:CD007498.
45. Schuetz P, Wirz Y, Sager R et al. Effect of procalcitonin-guided antibiotic treatment on mortality in acute respiratory infections: a patient level meta-analysis. Lancet Infect Dis. 2017. https://doi.org/10.1016/S1473-3099(17)30592-3.

12

The 2014 updated version of the Confusion Assessment Method for the Intensive Care Unit compared to the 5th version of the Diagnostic and Statistical Manual of Mental Disorders and other current methods used by intensivists

Gérald Chanques[1,2*†], E. Wesley Ely[3,4†], Océane Garnier[1], Fanny Perrigault[5], Anaïs Eloi[5], Julie Carr[1], Christine M. Rowan[3], Albert Prades[1], Audrey de Jong[1,2], Sylvie Moritz-Gasser[5,6], Nicolas Molinari[7] and Samir Jaber[1,2]

Abstract

Background: One third of patients admitted to an intensive care unit (ICU) will develop delirium. However, delirium is under-recognized by bedside clinicians without the use of delirium screening tools, such as the Intensive Care Delirium Screening Checklist (ICDSC) or the Confusion Assessment Method for the ICU (CAM-ICU). The CAM-ICU was updated in 2014 to improve its use by clinicians throughout the world. It has never been validated compared to the new reference standard, the Diagnostic and Statistical Manual of Mental Disorders 5th version (DSM-5).

Methods: We made a prospective psychometric study in a 16-bed medical–surgical ICU of a French academic hospital, to measure the diagnostic performance of the 2014 updated CAM-ICU compared to the DSM-5 as the reference standard. We included consecutive adult patients with a Richmond Agitation Sedation Scale (RASS) ≥ -3, without preexisting cognitive disorders, psychosis or cerebral injury. Delirium was independently assessed by neuropsychological experts using an operationalized approach to DSM-5, by investigators using the CAM-ICU and the ICDSC, by bedside clinicians and by ICU patients. The sensitivity, specificity, positive and negative predictive values were calculated considering neuropsychologist DSM-5 assessments as the reference standard (primary endpoint). CAM-ICU inter-observer agreement, as well as that between delirium diagnosis methods and the reference standard, was summarized using κ coefficients, which were subsequently compared using the *Z*-test.

Results: Delirium was diagnosed by experts in 38% of the 108 patients included for analysis. The CAM-ICU had a sensitivity of 83%, a specificity of 100%, a positive predictive value of 100% and a negative predictive value of 91%. Compared to the reference standard, the CAM-ICU had a significantly ($p < 0.05$) higher agreement ($\kappa = 0.86 \pm 0.05$) than the physicians,' residents' and nurses' diagnoses ($\kappa = 0.65 \pm 0.09$; 0.63 ± 0.09; 0.61 ± 0.09, respectively), as well as the patient's own impression of feeling delirious ($\kappa = 0.02 \pm 0.11$). Differences between the ICDSC ($\kappa = 0.69 \pm 0.07$)

*Correspondence: g-chanques@chu-montpellier.fr
†Gérald Chanques and E. Wesley Ely contributed equally to this study
[1] Department of Anaesthesia and Critical Care Medicine, University of Montpellier Saint Eloi Hospital, 80, avenue Augustin Fliche, 34295 Montpellier Cedex 5, France
Full list of author information is available at the end of the article

and CAM-ICU were not significant ($p = 0.054$). The CAM-ICU demonstrated a high reliability for inter-observer agreement ($\kappa = 0.87 \pm 0.06$).

Conclusions: The 2014 updated version of the CAM-ICU is valid according to DSM-5 criteria and reliable regarding inter-observer agreement in a research setting. Delirium remains under-recognized by bedside clinicians.

Keywords: Delirium, Intensive care unit, Critical care

Background

Nearly one third of patients admitted to an intensive care unit (ICU) will develop delirium [1], which is subsequently associated with sedation–analgesia management issues [2–4], an increased duration of mechanical ventilation, length of stay in the ICU and hospital, risk of death, as well as of having long-term neurocognitive dysfunction [1, 5]. Guidelines recommend the routine use of validated clinical tools for the early recognition and treatment of delirium by medical and nursing ICU teams, even if they are not expert neuropsychologists [6].

Among the delirium diagnosis tools that can be used by ICU clinicians in routine practice, the Confusion Assessment Method for the ICU (CAM-ICU) [7, 8] and the Intensive Care Delirium Screening Checklist (ICDSC) [9] have been extensively studied for more than 15 years, demonstrating good psychometric properties in a research setting [6]. In 2014, the CAM-ICU and its training manual were updated to avoid any misinterpretation by users (Table 1). Also, the original version of the CAM-ICU [7, 8] was validated against the American Psychiatric Association's fourth edition of the Diagnostic and Statistical Manual of Mental Disorders (DSM-IV). Differences between the 4th and the new 5th versions (DSM-5) regarding delirium assessment are still under debate [10, 11].

The primary objective of this study was to measure the ability of the 2014 updated version of the CAM-ICU to diagnose delirium according to the most updated neuropsychological reference standard, i.e., the DSM-5 method. Secondary objectives were (1) to measure inter-observer agreement for the CAM-ICU, and (2) within the context of a comprehensive investigation of delirium assessment in a real-life intensive care setting, to compare the diagnostic accuracy of the CAM-ICU to the ICDSC and to physician, resident and nurse recognition of delirium, as well as to common orientation questions and to the patient's own impression of feeling delirious.

Methods

Ethics and consent

The protocol was approved by an independent ethics committee [*Comité de Protection des Personnes (CPP) Sud Méditerranée.IV* (N°ID-RCB: 2015-A01084-45; Protocol version 1: 06/23/2015)] and was conducted in accordance with the Declaration of Helsinki (clinicaltrials.gov: NCT02760446). Written consent was required from the patient or the legally authorized representative or a proxy/surrogate decision maker (patient's next of kin) who gave consent on the patient's behalf, followed by the patient's consent as soon they could communicate.

Table 1 Principal changes made in the 2014 updated version of the CAM-ICU training manual

Features	Changes in the 2014 updated version
Feature 1 = *Acute onset or fluctuating course of mental status*	The term "sedation level" was intertwined with the "level of consciousness" throughout the method because some clinicians used these two terms interchangeably, but others were confused by the fact that patients could not receive sedatives. Note that RASS can be used in patients sedated or non-sedated
Feature 2 = *Inattention*	Another new 10-letter set (C–A–S–A–B–L–A–N–C–A) is now provided to allow for international understanding
Feature 3 = *Altered level of consciousness*	Following many institutions, the former feature #3 (disorganized thinking) was switched with former feature #4 (altered level of consciousness). The new feature #3 (level of consciousness) is often sufficient to rate a CAM-ICU as positive, while the new feature #4 (disorganized thinking) is less often necessary to perform in the end
Feature 4 = *Disorganized thinking*	This feature was rewritten to avoid any confusion in the total number of errors required among the 4 questions and 1 command: > 1 error = feature #4 present
Supporting materials	The updated method was associated with a 32-page complete training manual (available at www.icudelirium.org), including an extensive Frequently Asked Questions section, new case studies and links to the ICUDelirium.org Web site that was completely remodeled

CAM-ICU Confusion Assessment Method for the Intensive Care Unit, *RASS* Richmond Agitation Sedation Scale

Population

The study took place in the 16-bed medical–surgical ICU of the University of Montpellier Saint Eloi Hospital, an academic tertiary-care hospital, from November 2015 to April 2016. All consecutive French-speaking patients ≥ 18-year old were eligible for enrollment if they had a Richmond Agitation Sedation Scale (RASS) ≥ −3 [12–14]. Exclusion criteria were preexisting cognitive disorder/psychosis (baseline cognitive status is often unknown early in the ICU stay, precluding accurate evaluation of change in mental status, a key feature of delirium), visual/hearing loss without helpers, pregnancy (according to French law), patients under tutelage, withdrawal of consent or change in clinical status that would preclude a complete cognitive testing.

Study conduct

All consecutive patients admitted to our ICU were screened by the ICU research team every morning including weekends, until they reached the inclusion criteria during a period of 5 months (November 2015–March 2016). After having obtained consent and enrolling the patient, the ICU research team contacted one of two neuropsychological experts participating in the study to independently perform a neuropsychological assessment of delirium. Figure 1 summarizes the timing of delirium assessments by the neuropsychological experts and the ICU research team.

Data collection

Delirium

Delirium was assessed once, the same day, in five ways that occurred as close together as possible in time, but strictly independent of each other. Separate clinical research forms were used to assure independence between observers.

1. ICU delirium tools: CAM-ICU and ICDSC The ICU research team used the French versions of the 2014 updated CAM-ICU training manual and the ICDSC [9, 15]. The CAM-ICU was assessed by two independent investigators to estimate inter-observer agreement.

2. Expert neuropsychological assessment of delirium (the reference standard) The neuropsychological experts were members of the speech and language therapy team, usually in charge of neuropsychological testing in the neurology/neurosurgery/neuro-ICU departments of the Neurosciences University Hospital of Montpellier. A standardized method for diagnosing delirium was used based on the DSM-5 [16] using the Montreal Cognitive Assessment (MOCA) [17], Dubois' 5-word test [18], Language Screening Test (LAST) [19], with helpers for intubated ICU patients (see Additional file 1: Supplemental Digital Content).

3. Bedside–clinician assessment of delirium When immediately available, the patient's bedside ICU team

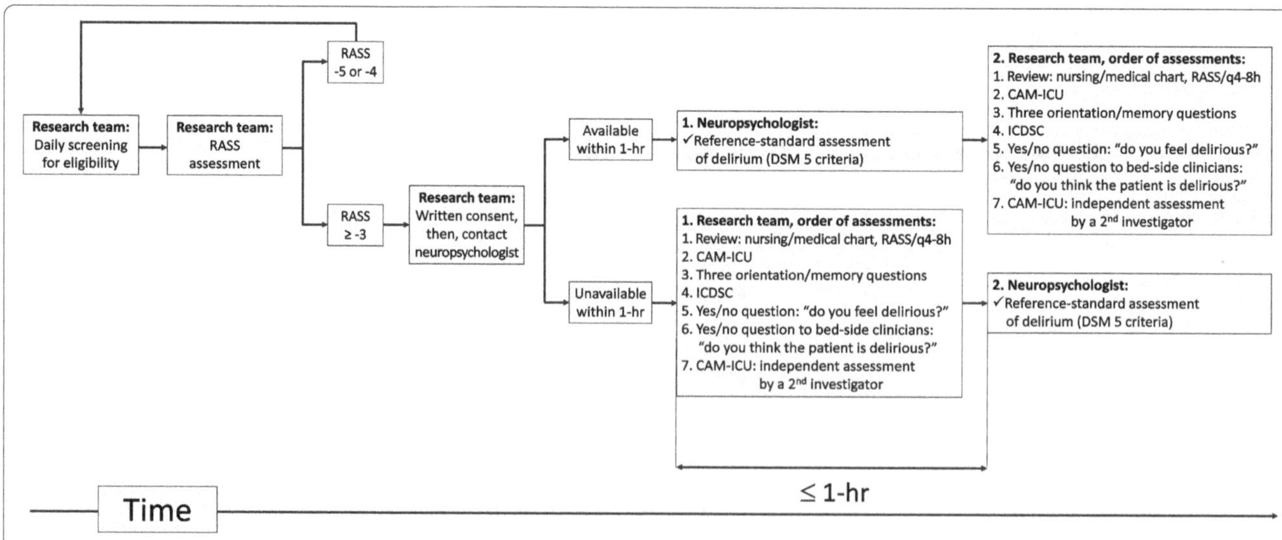

Fig. 1 Study design. The order of assessments by the research team was determined to check both the patient's eligibility and the presence of some CAM-ICU and ICDSC features (i.e., fluctuating course of mental status assessed by RASS ratings). ICDSC was assessed after CAM-ICU because ICDSC included some CAM-ICU features (i.e., inattention). *RASS* Richmond Agitation Sedation Scale, *CAM-ICU* Confusion Assessment Method for the Intensive Care Unit, *ICDSC* Intensive Care Delirium Screening Checklist, *DSM-5* 5th version of the Diagnostic and Statistical Manual of Mental Disorders

(i.e., the patient's nurse, resident and attending physician) were contacted by the ICU research team to get their personal feeling about the presence or absence of delirium.

4. The 3 simple orientation/memory questions for the assessment of delirium The ICU research team also assessed delirium by asking three simple questions commonly used to assess delirium at our institution: Where are you? What day is it today? Who is the president? (because long-term memory is frequently altered in delirium) [20]. The number of incorrect and absent response(s) was recorded.

5. The patient's own feeling At the end of testing, the patients were asked by the ICU research team if they had the impression they were confused.

Demographic and medical data

Age, gender, comorbidities and the reason for ICU admission were recorded. The Simplified Acute Physiological Score II (SAPS-II) score [21] and the Sequential Organ Failure Assessment (SOFA) score [22] were calculated within 24 h after ICU admission and upon enrollment. In case enrollment occurred before 24 h, the SAPS-II score took into account the worst value available during the 24 h preceding enrollment. Therapeutics such as sedation, mechanical ventilation and the use of vasopressors were collected upon enrollment.

Data presentation and statistical analysis

Psychometric properties of the CAM-ICU

Validity (primary endpoint) The performance of the CAM-ICU for diagnosing delirium was assessed by measuring the sensitivity, specificity, positive predictive value (PPV) and negative predictive value (NPV) according to standardized definitions [23, 24]. Expert assessments were used as the reference standard.

Reliability The kappa coefficient was calculated between the two ICU research investigators. Kappa coefficients above 0.80, 0.60 and 0.40 are considered as measuring 'near perfect,' 'strong' and 'moderate' levels of agreement [25], respectively.

The diagnostic performance of other methods commonly used to assess delirium (ICSDC, bedside clinician assessments, 3-question test), as well as patients' impressions)

The sensitivity, specificity, PPV and NPV were also calculated using the expert assessments as the reference standard. To compare all five methods for diagnosing delirium, kappa coefficients were calculated between the expert assessments and the other methods. Kappa coefficient comparisons between methods were made using the *Z*-test [26]. A p value of < 0.05 was considered statistically significant.

Power analysis The study sample size was determined in relation to the primary endpoint. For expected values [8] of sensitivity and specificity at 85 and 75%, respectively, a desired level of precision set at 10% and the prevalence of delirium set at 50%, the number of patient inclusions required for achieving appropriate power would be 95. Taking into account possible post-enrollment exclusions, 115 patients needed to be enrolled in the study. The prevalence of delirium ranged from 30 to 90% in the literature [1]. Thus, we set the prevalence of delirium at 50% which is conservative regarding the number of patients needed to be analyzed, in order to maximize the power.

Data presentation Quantitative data are shown as medians and 25th–75th percentiles. Data were analyzed using SAS version 9.2 (SAS Institute, Cary, NC).

Results

A total of 108 patients were included for analysis among the 115 patients enrolled in the study. A Standards for Reporting of Diagnostic Accuracy (STARD) diagram for patient enrollment is shown in Additional file 1: Supplemental Digital Content. Table 2 summarizes patient demographic and medical characteristics. Delirium was diagnosed by the neuropsychological experts for 41 of the 108 patients (38%).

Validation of the 2014 updated CAM-ICU

A positive CAM-ICU was found for 34 (31%) patients. Compared to expert assessments, there were 7 misclassified CAM-ICU ratings among the 108 ratings, of which there were 7 false negatives and no false positives. Compared to expert assessments, the CAM-ICU had a sensitivity of 83% [95% confidence interval 71–94], a specificity of 100% [100–100], a PPV of 100% [100–100] and a NPV of 91% [84–97].

To measure the inter-observer reliability of the CAM-ICU, 98 patients were assessed by a second investigator. For the ten remaining patients, a second assessment was impossible because of changes in vigilance status or clinical condition. The kappa coefficient for inter-observer reliability was 0.87 (SD $\pm$ 0.06) demonstrating strong agreement. There were no significant differences between the 5 ICU investigators and the 2 neuropsychological experts (kappa coefficients ranging from 0.82 $\pm$ 0.1 to 0.88 $\pm$ 0.2). First and second CAM-ICU investigators obtained similar agreement with experts' assessments (kappa coefficients = 0.86 $\pm$ 0.1 and 0.85 $\pm$ 0.1, respectively).

Table 2 Demographic and medical characteristics of the 108 patients included for analysis

Characteristics	Median [IQR] or *n* (%)
Upon ICU admission	
Age (years)	62 [54–68]
Sex [*n* (%)]	
Male	64 (59%)
Female	44 (41%)
Body mass index (kg/m^{-2})	25 [23–29]
Type of admission	
Unplanned surgical (from operating room) [*n* (%)]	26 (24%)
Planned surgical (from operating room) [*n* (%)]	15 (14%)
Surgical (from ward) [*n* (%)]	5 (05%)
Medical [*n* (%)]	62 (57%)
SAPS II score	39 [31–49]
SOFA score	7 [4–9]
Sepsis at admission [*n* (%)]	47 (44%)
Intubation at admission [*n* (%)]	70 (65%)
Upon study enrollment	
Time between ICU admission and enrollment (days)	3 [2–5]
SAPS II score	29 [23–38]
SOFA score	4 [2–7]
Vigilance status	
Median RASS level	0 [0–0]
RASS level = +2 [*n* (%)]	2 (2%)
RASS level = +1 [*n* (%)]	8 (7%)
RASS level = 0 [*n* (%)]	76 (70%)
RASS level = −1 [*n* (%)]	13 (12%)
RASS level = −2 [*n* (%)]	4 (4%)
RASS level = −3 [*n* (%)]	5 (5%)
Therapeutics	
Invasive mechanical ventilation [*n* (%)]	23 (21%)
Noninvasive mechanical ventilation [*n* (%)]	8 (07%)
Vasopressors [*n* (%)]	18 (17%)
Sedation (propofol) [*n* (%)]	12 (11%)
At ICU discharge	
Total duration of mechanical ventilation (days)	1.6 [0.3–5.5]
ICU length of stay (days)	6.5 [3.0–12.4]

BMI body mass index, *ICU* Intensive Care Unit, *IQR* inter-quartile range, *RASS* Richmond Agitation Sedation Scale, *SAPS II* Simplified Acute Physiological Score II, *SOFA* Sequential Organ Failure Assessment score

Diagnostic performance of commonly used methods for assessing delirium

Table 3 presents the statistical measurement of performance regarding delirium recognition via the CAM-ICU, and the ICDSC, by nurses, residents and physicians, as well as via three simple questions. The CAM-ICU demonstrated good performance, while the 3 simple questions demonstrated poor performance. The 3 simple questions demonstrated the highest sensitivity for a false or absent response, but with the lowest specificity and PPV. The ICDSC and clinicians' diagnosis demonstrated similar performances.

Figure 2 shows the graphic representation of kappa coefficients for each of the methods used to assess delirium. The kappa coefficient measured the agreement between each of the methods and the assessment by the neuropsychological experts using DSM-5 criteria (reference standard). There was a significant difference between the level of agreement found for the CAM-ICU (kappa 0.86 ± 0.05) and that found for other methods ($p < 0.047$), except the ICDSC (0.69 ± 0.07, $p = 0.054$, Z-test). Detailed data regarding CAM-ICU/ICDSC procedures are provided in Additional file 1: Supplemental Digital Content.

The 3 simple questions and the patient's own impression had the lowest agreements with experts and demonstrated significant differences with other methods.

Patient's own impression of feeling delirious

Among the 108 patients, 77 (71%) were able to answer the question as to whether they felt delirious or not (all had a RASS level ≥ -1). Among these patients, 27 (35%) answered that they were. The patient's sensitivity for recognizing delirium compared to expert assessments was 38%, with a specificity of 66%, a PPV of 22% and a NPV of 80%.

Discussion

The main finding of this study is that the 2014 updated version of the CAM-ICU was valid compared to the DSM-5 reference standard, with strong inter-observer agreement. CAM-ICU and ICDSC agreed with experts' opinion without significant difference. The CAM-ICU had superior performance for diagnosing delirium compared to the bedside–clinicians' opinion, as well as compared to simple questions that are commonly used to assess delirium. Patient impressions of feeling delirious are not accurate, with a false-positive rate at 78%.

Delirium is multifactorial and frequent in critically ill ICU patients [6, 27–35]. It is diagnosed in 10–90% of ICU patients, depending on the diagnosis tool, the timing of assessment (during or after interrupting sedation), as well as the frequency of assessment (one-point assessment for validation studies or throughout the ICU stay) [6, 36]. A recent review of 42 studies estimated the prevalence of delirium at 5280 (31.8%) out of 16,595 critically ill patients [1]. The prevalence of delirium in the present study is close to this result: 38% according to neuropsychological assessment and 31% according to the CAM-ICU. Although frequent, delirium is under-recognized

Table 3 Patients' clinical diagnosis and simple orientation questions

Measurement	ICU delirium tools		Patients' clinician diagnosis[a]			3 Simple orientation questions			
	CAM-ICU	ICDSC	Physician	Resident	Nurse	1 false or absent response	2 false or absent responses	1 false response[b]	2 false responses[b]
Sensitivity	83% [71–94]	83% [71–94]	79% [65–94]	68% [52–83]	70% [54–86]	90% [81–99]	68% [54–83]	78% [59–97]	28% [7–48]
Specificity	100% [100–100]	87% [78–95]	85% [75–96]	93% [86–100]	89% [82–97]	66% [54–77]	82% [73–91]	73% [62–85]	92% [85–99]
PPV	100% [100–100]	79% [67–91]	79% [65–94]	85% [72–99]	78% [62–93]	62% [49–74]	70% [56–84]	47% [29–65]	50% [19–81]
NPV	91% [84–97]	89% [82–97]	85% [75–96]	82% [72–92]	85% [76–94]	92% [84–99]	81% [72–90]	92% [84–99]	81% [72–90]
Delirium diagnosis by non experts	31%	40%	41%	31%	31%	56%	37%	38%	13%
by experts	38%	38%	41%	39%	34%	38%	38%	21%	21%
Agreement with experts ($\kappa \pm$ SD)[c]	0.86 ± 0.05	0.69 ± 0.07	0.65 ± 0.09	0.63 ± 0.09	0.61 ± 0.09	0.51 ± 0.08	0.51 ± 0.09	0.41 ± 0.10	0.23 ± 0.13

The statistical measurement of performance is expressed as the percentage and its 95% confidence interval. *CAM-ICU* Confusion Assessment Method for the Intensive Care Unit, *ICDSC* Intensive Care Delirium Screening Checklist, *PPV* positive predictive value, *NPV* negative predictive value

[a] Among the 108 patients included for analysis, patients' clinicians were available upon study completion for 91 patient nurses (84%), 89 patient residents (82%) and 71 patient physicians (66%). Among the clinicians participating in the study, the 4 nurses, 1 resident and 1 physician who could not answer the question whether the patient was or was not delirious were not taken into account for the analysis

[b] Analysis was performed among the 78 patients (72%) who were able to answer all three simple questions

[c] The agreement between each method of delirium diagnosis and the assessment by the neuropsychological experts using DSM-5 criteria (reference standard) was measured using kappa coefficients

by both physicians and nurses [37]. Compared to the CAM-ICU, clinician sensitivity for diagnosing delirium is about 30% [38, 39]. The recognition of delirium by physicians and nurses in the present study was better, with a sensitivity of nearly 70%, suggesting that there might have been an increase in clinician awareness regarding delirium in the ICU over the past decade [40]. However, with PPVs under 80% and NPVs under 90% in the present study, clinicians should still use an ICU delirium tool to improve their diagnostic performance, according to current guidelines [6]. In the present study, agreement with expert diagnosis was not significantly different between the CAM-ICU and the ICDSC. In previous studies, the pooled sensitivity and specificity were 76 and 96%, respectively, for the CAM-ICU, and 80 and 75% for the ICDSC [41]. Sensitivity and specificity were slightly higher for both tools in the present study. This could be due to the study setting where a research team with experience in conducting research in the area of sedation–analgesia was available to conduct this psychometric study. Indeed, performance measurements for ICU delirium tools are higher in research settings than in real life [41]. However, the original study validating the CAM-ICU reported higher sensitivity and specificity than in the present study, with a sensitivity ranging from 93 to 100% and a specificity ranging from 98 to 100% [8]. This could be due to differences in the studied populations. In the original study [8], patients had a median Glasgow score of 7 at enrollment, while in the present study, 80% of patients had a RASS level ≥ 0, suggesting they were more alert. It has been reported that the CAM-ICU could have a lower sensitivity in alert patients, possibly because of better cognitive function [42, 43]. Because delirium prevalence and recognition may depend on the level of consciousness, some authors recommend stratifying delirium assessments for sedation score using a cutoff of RASS $-$ 2 [44]. In the present study also, when taking into account only the 99 patients who had a RASS level of > -2 for a sensitivity analysis, the delirium prevalence was lower than in the overall population (32% instead of 38% according to the experts, 25% instead of 31%, according to the CAM-ICU). The CAM-ICU had a slightly lower sensitivity (78%, instead of 83%), while conserving the same specificity, positive and negative predictive values. Similar findings were obtained when excluding from the analysis the 12 patients who were sedated (8 of them having a RASS level of > -2).

Our study has several limitations. For example, all the methods for diagnosing delirium were assessed within a short time. This may have tired patients and decreased their cognitive functions. The research team planned the assessments within the space of an hour to increase

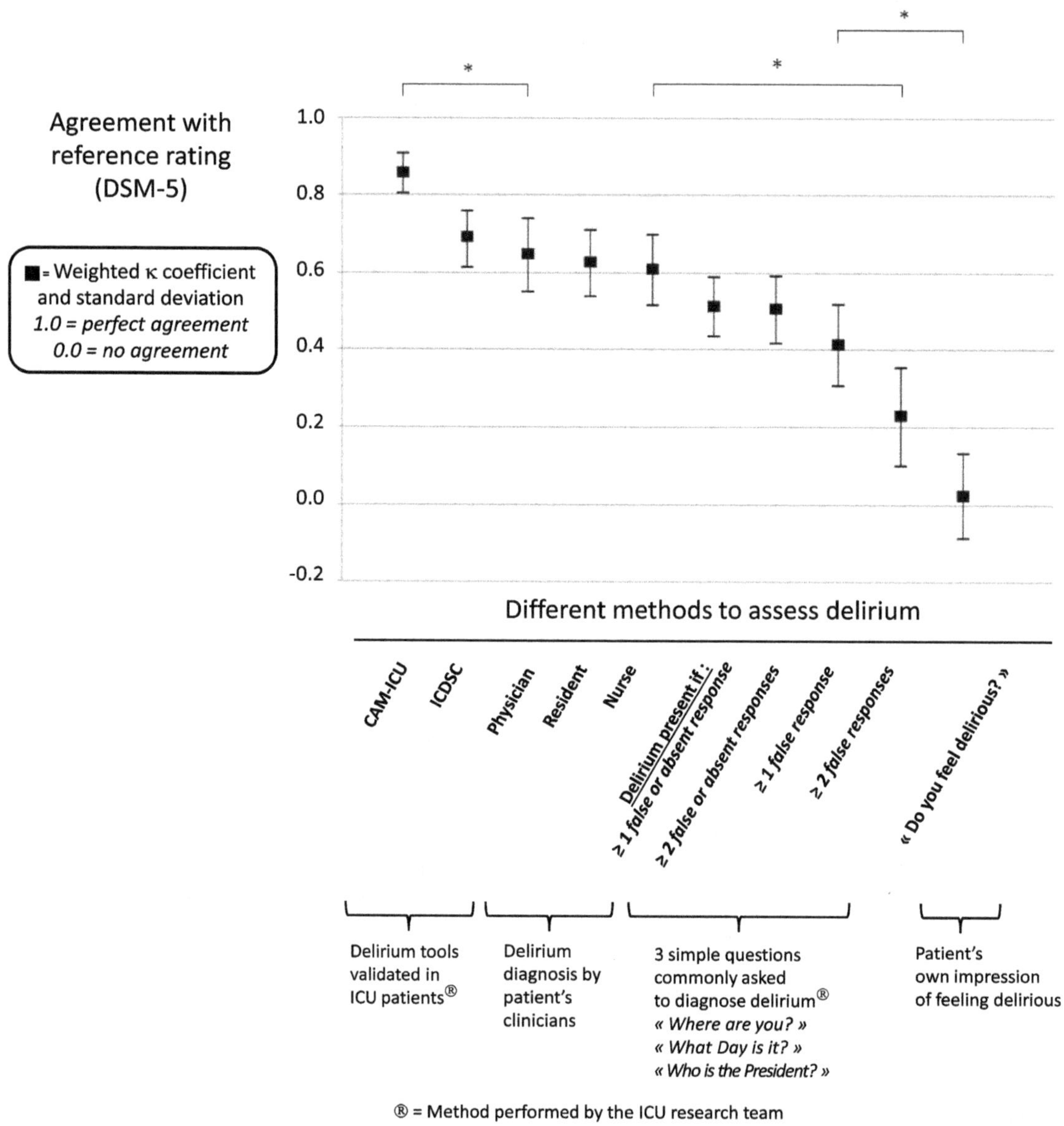

Fig. 2 Agreement between different delirium assessment methods and the neurological experts' reference rating using the DSM-5 criteria. This figure shows the graphic representation of kappa coefficients and their standard deviations for each of the methods used to assess delirium. The kappa coefficient measured the agreement between each of the methods and the assessment by the neuropsychologist experts using DSM-5 criteria (reference standard). For simple questions, we did not decide a priori how to analyze the answers. Because some patients answered some questions but did not answer other ones, we decided a posteriori to analyze these data following two approaches: including all patients and including only the patients able to answer all the questions. Several thresholds were tested, i.e., delirium was defined in all patients if they gave at least 1 or 2 false or no response(s), or, among the patients who were able to answer all simple questions, if the patients gave at least 1 or 2 false response(s). There was a significant difference ($p < 0.047$) between the CAM-ICU and each of the other methods, except the ICDSC ($p = 0.054$). There were significant differences between "all methods from CAM-ICU to ≥ 1 false response to simple questions" and "patient's own impression of feeling delirious," as well as between "all methods from CAM-ICU to nurse diagnosis" and "≥ 2 false responses to simple questions" or "patient's own impression of feeling delirious." *: Significant difference ($p < 0.05$); *CAM-ICU* Confusion Assessment Method for the Intensive Care Unit, *ICDSC* Intensive Care Delirium Screening Checklist

the chance of measuring delirium at the same time for a given patient (Fig. 1). The agreement between the neuropsychological expert and the CAM-ICU was not significantly different whether the expert performed the assessment before or after the research team (kappa coefficient 0.86 ± 0.1 vs 0.85 ± 0.1, respectively). Secondly, except ICDSC, many other validated delirium tools [42] were not performed in order to make the duration of assessment feasible. In the same way, the ICDSC could have demonstrated higher sensitivity and specificity if it had been performed in more alert patients, and by the patient's clinicians rather than by the research team. To perform the ICDSC, the research team took into account all nursing/medical charts (Fig. 1) but performed only "punctual" cognitive evaluations instead of evaluations over a nursing shift. The ICDSC was not performed by the patient's clinicians to avoid any bias regarding their raw opinion about the presence or the absence of delirium. In other words, clinicians did not use a validated delirium tool which is to take into account for the interpretation of the data. The primary goal of the present study was to validate the 2014 updated version of the CAM-ICU. Measuring the psychometric properties of the ICDSC was only informative because it is a second recommended tool for assessing delirium and therefore frequently used throughout the world [6]. Moreover, the present study demonstrated no significant difference between the ICDSC and CAM-ICU regarding the agreement between the ICU research team and the neuropsychological experts (Fig. 2). However, this study was not calibrated to measure this difference. A longer period of evaluation could have resulted in a higher sensitivity for ICDS. Similarly, repeated measurements of delirium on a longer period of time could have lead to a higher sensitivity. Regarding the expert's assessment, DSM-5 interpretations and use as a reference standard for delirium are a source of debate and thus may vary according to assessor [10, 11]. Finally, all the causes of delirium were not investigated because this was out of the scope of this psychometric study. Sepsis was present in 44% of patients at admission, and 11% of patients received sedatives at enrollment. Thus, a few intubated patients were included, due to a strategy of "early-sedation-interruption." This study should be further performed in different settings/ICU populations.

Study strengths include the reference standard method used by experts to diagnose delirium, which was provided for the first time in detail to facilitate study reproducibility (see Additional file 1: Supplemental Digital Content). Aside from the expert assessment, a pragmatic approach for diagnosing delirium was also evaluated in order to reflect real-life situations in intensive care. This included nurse, resident and physician diagnoses, as well as commonly used simple orientation/memory questions. These questions are not appropriate for diagnosing delirium. This might be due to patient disorientation, which can be related to environment (absence of windows). The recommendation to use a validated delirium tool is reinforced by the fact that the ICU team is used to conducting clinical research and quality improvement projects in the area of agitation, sedation and analgesia [45–47]. Even in such an "a priori" favorable setting for the early recognition of delirium, bedside–clinicians still need to use a validated tool during their routine practice, repeatedly during the day and throughout the ICU stay. This is paramount for treating the factors associated with delirium [6, 27–35] as soon as possible, especially when taking into account the negative outcomes associated with delirium [5, 6]. A comprehensive approach [48] integrating delirium management with analgesia, sedation, mechanical ventilation, mobility/exercise and family engagement/empowerment has shown a positive impact on increasing ventilatory-free days [49, 50], decreasing delirium incidence [49–51] and improving hospital mortality [51].

Finally, the study investigated the patient's ability to recognize delirium. Though delusional memories are frequent in ICU survivors, they have not been investigated during hospitalization in the ICU setting [52–54]. Recent studies found no significant association between delirium in the ICU and mental disorders in survivors [55–57]. However, memories of being delirious in the ICU are associated with anxiety [56]. The link between delirium recollection, feelings of being delirious while in the ICU (which is possibly theoretically wrong or too abstract for some patients) and long-term psychological outcomes thus requires further exploration.

Conclusions

The 2014 updated version of the CAM-ICU is a valid tool for delirium diagnosis in a research setting in critically ill patients according to the DSM-5 criteria used by neuropsychological experts. It demonstrated important inter-observer reliability, and better performance for diagnosing delirium in ICU patients than physicians, residents and nurses, despite increased awareness regarding delirium in the ICU for many years. Future studies should investigate the discrepancies between validated methods to diagnose delirium (DSM-5, CAM-ICU, ICDSC) and the ICU team. Moreover, the patient's own ability to report delirium might be inaccurate. Ethics committees should pay attention to delirium assessment when checking for patient's ability to consent to participate in ICU studies [58]. This suggests also that delusional memories reported by survivors should be investigated in regard to a valid assessment of delirium during the ICU stay. In the ICU, patients should be asked about feeling delirious, comforted if they are not, but be taken care of regarding what could make them feel so.

Abbreviations

CAM-ICU: Confusion Assessment Method for the Intensive Care Unit; DSM-5: 5th version of the Diagnostic and Statistical Manual of Mental Disorders; ICDSC: Intensive Care Delirium Screening Checklist; ICU: Intensive care unit; NPV: negative predictive value; PPV: positive predictive value; RASS: Richmond Agitation Sedation Scale; SAPS II: Simplified Acute Physiological Score II score; SOFA: Sequential Organ Failure Assessment.

Authors' contributions

GC, EWE, CMR, SMG and SJ contributed to study concept and design; OG, FP, AE and AP contributed to data acquisition; GC, EWE, SMG and SJ contributed to data analysis and interpretation; GC, ADJ and NM contributed to statistical methods and statistical data analysis; GC, EWE and JC contributed to manuscript preparation and drafting; CMR, ADJ, SMG and SJ contributed to manuscript critique and review. All authors read and approved the final manuscript.

Author details

[1] Department of Anaesthesia and Critical Care Medicine, University of Montpellier Saint Eloi Hospital, 80, avenue Augustin Fliche, 34295 Montpellier Cedex 5, France. [2] PhyMedExp, INSERM U1046, CNRS, UMR 9214, University of Montpellier, Montpellier, France. [3] Department of Medicine, Division of Allergy, Pulmonary, and Critical Care Medicine and the Center for Health Services Research, Vanderbilt University School of Medicine, Nashville, TN, USA. [4] Geriatric Research Education Clinical Center (GRECC), Department of Veterans Affairs, Tennessee Valley Healthcare System, Nashville, TN, USA. [5] Department of Speech and Language Therapy, School of Medicine, University of Montpellier, Montpellier, France. [6] Institute of Neurosciences of Montpellier, INSERM U105, University of Montpellier, Montpellier, France. [7] Department of Statistics, University of Montpellier Hospitals, Montpellier, France.

Acknowledgements

We would like to thank all patients who participated in the study and the families who gave their consent for participation, as well as the clinical and research staff. We also thank Dr. Carey M. Suehs for her help with English corrections.

Competing interests

In contexts unrelated to the present work, Pr Jaber has consulted for and received honorarium from the following companies: Dräger, Hamilton, Maquet and Fisher Paykel. No other conflicts of interest related to this article exist for the other authors.

Funding

Support for this study was provided solely via institutional and/or departmental sources (Montpellier University Hospitals; 34000, France).

References

1. Salluh JI, Wang H, Schneider EB, Nagaraja N, Yenokyan G, Damluji A, et al. Outcome of delirium in critically ill patients: systematic review and meta-analysis. BMJ. 2015;350:h2538.
2. Chanques G, Tarri T, Ride A, Prades A, De Jong A, Carr J, et al. Analgesia nociception index for the assessment of pain in critically ill patients: a diagnostic accuracy study. Br J Anaesth. 2017;119:812–20.
3. Chanques G, Payen JF, Mercier G, de Lattre S, Viel E, Jung B, et al. Assessing pain in non-intubated critically ill patients unable to self report: an adaptation of the Behavioral Pain Scale. Intensive Care Med. 2009;35:2060–7.
4. Wang PP, Huang E, Feng X, Bray CA, Perreault MM, Rico P, et al. Opioid-associated iatrogenic withdrawal in critically ill adult patients: a multi-center prospective observational study. Ann Intensive Care. 2017;7:88.
5. Pandharipande PP, Girard TD, Jackson JC, Morandi A, Thompson JL, Pun BT, et al. Long-term cognitive impairment after critical illness. N Engl J Med. 2013;369:1306–16.
6. Barr J, Fraser GL, Puntillo K, Ely EW, Gelinas C, Dasta JF, et al. Clinical practice guidelines for the management of pain, agitation, and delirium in adult patients in the intensive care unit. Crit Care Med. 2013;41:278–80.
7. Ely EW, Margolin R, Francis J, May L, Truman B, Dittus R, et al. Evaluation of delirium in critically ill patients: validation of the Confusion Assessment Method for the Intensive Care Unit (CAM-ICU). Crit Care Med. 2001;29:1370–9.
8. Ely EW, Inouye SK, Bernard GR, Gordon S, Francis J, May L, et al. Delirium in mechanically ventilated patients: validity and reliability of the confusion assessment method for the intensive care unit (CAM-ICU). JAMA. 2001;286:2703–10.
9. Bergeron N, Dubois MJ, Dumont M, Dial S, Skrobik Y. Intensive Care Delirium Screening Checklist: evaluation of a new screening tool. Intensive Care Med. 2001;27:859–64.
10. Adamis D, Rooney S, Meagher D, Mulligan O, McCarthy G. A comparison of delirium diagnosis in elderly medical inpatients using the CAM, DRS-R98, DSM-IV and DSM-5 criteria. Int Psychogeriatr. 2015;27:883–9.
11. Meagher DJ, Morandi A, Inouye SK, Ely W, Adamis D, Maclullich AJ, et al. Concordance between DSM-IV and DSM-5 criteria for delirium diagnosis in a pooled database of 768 prospectively evaluated patients using the delirium rating scale-revised-98. BMC Med. 2014;12:164.
12. Sessler CN, Gosnell MS, Grap MJ, Brophy GM, O'Neal PV, Keane KA, et al. The Richmond Agitation–Sedation Scale: validity and reliability in adult intensive care unit patients. Am J Respir Crit Care Med. 2002;166:1338–44.
13. Ely EW, Truman B, Shintani A, Thomason JW, Wheeler AP, Gordon S, et al. Monitoring sedation status over time in ICU patients: reliability and validity of the Richmond Agitation–Sedation Scale (RASS). JAMA. 2003;289:2983–91.
14. Chanques G, Jaber S, Barbotte E, Verdier R, Henriette K, Lefrant J, et al. Validation of the French translated Richmond vigilance-agitation scale. Ann Fr Anesth Reanim. 2006;25:696–701.
15. Chanques G, Garnier O, Carr J, Conseil M, de Jong A, Rowan CM, et al. The CAM-ICU has now a French "official" version. The translation process of the 2014 updated Complete Training Manual of the Confusion Assessment Method for the Intensive Care Unit in French (CAM-ICU.fr). Anaesth Crit Care. Pain Med. 2017;36:297–300.
16. American Psychiatric Association: Diagnostic and Statistical Manual of Mental Disorders. 5th edition. Arlington, VA; 2013.
17. Nasreddine ZS, Phillips NA, Bedirian V, Charbonneau S, Whitehead V, Collin I, et al. The Montreal Cognitive Assessment, MoCA: a brief screening tool for mild cognitive impairment. J Am Geriatr Soc. 2005;53:695–9.
18. Dubois B, Touchon J, Portet F, Ousset PJ, Vellas B, Michel B. "The 5 words": a simple and sensitive test for the diagnosis of Alzheimer's disease. Presse Med. 2002;31:1696–9.
19. Flamand-Roze C, Falissard B, Roze E, Maintigneux L, Beziz J, Chacon A, et al. Validation of a new language screening tool for patients with acute stroke: the Language Screening Test (LAST). Stroke. 2011;42:1224–9.
20. Meagher D, Adamis D, Trzepacz P, Leonard M. Features of subsyndromal and persistent delirium. Br J Psychiatry. 2012;200:37–44.
21. Legall J-R, Lemeshow S, Saulnier F. New Simplified Acute Physiology Score (SAPS II) based on a European/North American Multicenter Study. JAMA. 1993;270:2957–63.
22. Vincent J, de Mendonça A, Cantraine F, Moreno R, Takala J, Suter P, et al. Use of the SOFA score to assess the incidence of organ dysfunction/failure in intensive care units: results of a multicenter, prospective study. Working group on "sepsis-related problems" of the European Society of Intensive Care Medicine. Crit Care Med. 1998;26:1793–800.
23. Altman DG, Bland JM. Diagnostic tests 2: predictive values. BMJ. 1994;309:102.
24. Altman DG, Bland JM. Diagnostic tests. 1: sensitivity and specificity. BMJ. 1994;308:1552.
25. Landis J, Koch G. The measurement of observer agreement for categorical data. Biometrics. 1977;33:159–74.
26. Altman DG, editor. Practical statistics for medical research. London: Chapman and Hall; 1991.
27. Page VJ, Davis D, Zhao XB, Norton S, Casarin A, Brown T, et al. Statin use and risk of delirium in the critically ill. Am J Respir Crit Care Med. 2014;189:666–73.
28. Van Rompaey B, Elseviers MM, Van Drom W, Fromont V, Jorens PG. The effect of earplugs during the night on the onset of delirium and sleep perception: a randomized controlled trial in intensive care patients. Crit Care. 2012;16:R73.
29. Kamdar BB, Niessen T, Colantuoni E, King LM, Neufeld KJ, Bienvenu OJ, et al. Delirium transitions in the medical ICU: exploring the role of sleep quality and other factors. Crit Care Med. 2015;43:135–41.

30. Serafim RB, Dutra MF, Saddy F, Tura B, de Castro JE, Villarinho LC, et al. Delirium in postoperative nonventilated intensive care patients: risk factors and outcomes. Ann Intensive Care. 2012;2:51.
31. Rafat C, Flamant M, Gaudry S, Vidal-Petiot E, Ricard JD, Dreyfuss D. Hyponatremia in the intensive care unit: How to avoid a Zugzwang situation? Ann Intensive Care. 2015;5:39.
32. Delaney LJ, Van Haren F, Lopez V. Sleeping on a problem: the impact of sleep disturbance on intensive care patients—a clinical review. Ann Intensive Care. 2015;5:3.
33. Dittrich T, Tschudin-Sutter S, Widmer AF, Ruegg S, Marsch S, Sutter R. Risk factors for new-onset delirium in patients with bloodstream infections: independent and quantitative effect of catheters and drainages—a four-year cohort study. Ann Intensive Care. 2016;6:104.
34. van Ewijk CE, Jacobs GE, Girbes ARJ. Unsuspected serotonin toxicity in the ICU. Ann Intensive Care. 2016;6:85.
35. Neuville M, El-Helali N, Magalhaes E, Radjou A, Smonig R, Soubirou JF, et al. Systematic overdosing of oxa- and cloxacillin in severe infections treated in ICU: risk factors and side effects. Ann Intensive Care. 2017;7:34.
36. Patel SB, Poston JT, Pohlman A, Hall JB, Kress JP. Rapidly reversible, sedation-related delirium versus persistent delirium in the intensive care unit. Am J Respir Crit Care Med. 2014;189:658–65.
37. SRLF Trial Group. Sedation in French intensive care units: a survey of clinical practice. Ann Intensive Care. 2013;3:24.
38. Spronk PE, Riekerk B, Hofhuis J, Rommes JH. Occurrence of delirium is severely underestimated in the ICU during daily care. Intensive Care Med. 2009;35:1276–80.
39. van Eijk MM, van Marum RJ, Klijn IA, de Wit N, Kesecioglu J, Slooter AJ. Comparison of delirium assessment tools in a mixed intensive care unit. Crit Care Med. 2009;37:1881–5.
40. Patel RP, Gambrell M, Speroff T, Scott TA, Pun BT, Okahashi J, et al. Delirium and sedation in the intensive care unit: survey of behaviors and attitudes of 1384 healthcare professionals. Crit Care Med. 2009;37:825–32.
41. Neto AS, Nassar AP Jr, Cardoso SO, Manetta JA, Pereira VG, Esposito DC, et al. Delirium screening in critically ill patients: a systematic review and meta-analysis. Crit Care Med. 2012;40:1946–51.
42. Luetz A, Heymann A, Radtke FM, Chenitir C, Neuhaus U, Nachtigall I, et al. Different assessment tools for intensive care unit delirium: which score to use? Crit Care Med. 2010;38:409–18.
43. Mitasova A, Kostalova M, Bednarik J, Michalcakova R, Kasparek T, Balabanova P, et al. Poststroke delirium incidence and outcomes: validation of the Confusion Assessment Method for the Intensive Care Unit (CAM-ICU). Crit Care Med. 2012;40:484–90.
44. Haenggi M, Blum S, Brechbuehl R, Brunello A, Jakob SM, Takala J. Effect of sedation level on the prevalence of delirium when assessed with CAM-ICU and ICDSC. Intensive Care Med. 2013;39:2171–9.
45. Chanques G, Jaber S, Barbotte E, Violet S, Sebbane M, Perrigault P, et al. Impact of systematic evaluation of pain and agitation in an intensive care unit. Crit Care Med. 2006;34:1691–9.
46. de Jong A, Molinari N, de Lattre S, Gniadek C, Carr J, Conseil M, et al. Decreasing severe pain and serious adverse events while moving intensive care unit patients: a prospective interventional study (the NURSE-DO project). Crit Care. 2013;17:R74.
47. Dodek P, Chanques G, Brown G, Norena M, Grubisic M, Wong H, et al. Role of organisational structure in implementation of sedation protocols: a comparison of Canadian and French ICUs. BMJ Qual Saf. 2012;21:715–21.
48. Ely EW. The ABCDEF bundle: science and philosophy of how ICU liberation serves patients and families. Crit Care Med. 2017;45:321–30.
49. Balas MC, Vasilevskis EE, Olsen KM, Schmid KK, Shostrom V, Cohen MZ, et al. Effectiveness and safety of the awakening and breathing coordination, delirium monitoring/management, and early exercise/mobility bundle. Crit Care Med. 2014;42:1024–36.
50. Chanques G, Conseil M, Roger C, Constantin JM, Prades A, Carr J, et al. Immediate interruption of sedation compared with usual sedation care in critically ill postoperative patients (SOS-Ventilation): a randomised, parallel-group clinical trial. Lancet Respir Med. 2017;5:795–805.
51. Barnes-Daly MA, Phillips G, Ely EW. Improving hospital survival and reducing brain dysfunction at seven California community hospitals: implementing PAD guidelines via the ABCDEF bundle in 6,064 patients. Crit Care Med. 2017;45:171–8.
52. Jones C, Bäckman C, Capuzzo M, Flaatten H, Rylander C, Griffiths RD. Precipitants of post-traumatic stress disorder following intensive care: a hypothesis generating study of diversity in care. Intensive Care Med. 2007;33:978–85.
53. Jones C, Griffiths RD, Humphris G, Skirrow PM. Memory, delusions, and the development of acute posttraumatic stress disorder-related symptoms after intensive care. Crit Care Med. 2001;29:573–80.
54. Parker AM, Sricharoenchai T, Raparla S, Schneck KW, Bienvenu OJ, Needham DM. Posttraumatic stress disorder in critical illness survivors: a metaanalysis. Crit Care Med. 2015;43:1121–9.
55. Wolters AE, Peelen LM, Welling MC, Kok L, de Lange DW, Cremer OL, et al. Long-term mental health problems after delirium in the ICU. Crit Care Med. 2016;44:1808–13.
56. Svenningsen H, Egerod I, Christensen D, Tonnesen EK, Frydenberg M, Videbech P. Symptoms of posttraumatic stress after intensive care delirium. Biomed Res Int. 2015;2015:876947.
57. Jackson JC, Pandharipande PP, Girard TD, Brummel NE, Thompson JL, Hughes CG, et al. Depression, post-traumatic stress disorder, and functional disability in survivors of critical illness in the BRAIN-ICU study: a longitudinal cohort study. Lancet Respir Med. 2014;2:369–79.
58. Fan E, Shahid S, Kondreddi VP, Bienvenu OJ, Mendez-Tellez PA, Pronovost PJ, et al. Informed consent in the critically ill: a two-step approach incorporating delirium screening. Crit Care Med. 2008;36:94–9.

13

Removal of totally implanted venous access ports for suspected infection in the intensive care unit

Marie Lecronier[1*], Sandrine Valade[2], Naike Bigé[3], Nicolas de Prost[4], Damien Roux[5], David Lebeaux[6,7], Eric Maury[3], Elie Azoulay[2], Alexandre Demoule[1,8], Martin Dres[1,8]
and on behalf of the GrrrOH (Group for Research in Respiratory Intensive Care Onco-Hematology)

Abstract

Background: While no data support this practice, international guidelines recommend the removal of totally implanted venous access ports (TIVAPs) in patients with suspicion of TIVAP-related bloodstream infection admitted in the intensive care unit (ICU) for a life-threatening sepsis.

Methods: During this multicenter, retrospective and observational study, we included all patients admitted in five ICU for a life-threatening sepsis in whom a TIVAP was removed between January 2012 and December 2014. We aimed (1) at determining the proportion of confirmed TIVAP-related infections and (2) at assessing short- and long-term survival of patients with and without TIVAP-related infections.

Results: One hundred and fifty-one patients (58 ± 14 years, 62% males) were included between 2012 and 2014. TIVAP-related infections were confirmed in 68 patients (45%). Demographic characteristics were similar between patients with and without TIVAP-related infections. SOFA score on admission per point increase [odd ratio (OR), 0.86 interval confidence (IC) 95% (0.8–0.9), $p < 0.01$] and local signs of infection [OR 4.0, IC 95% (1.1–15.6), $p = 0.04$] were significantly associated with TIVAP-related infection. Patients with TIVAP-related infection had lower ICU and 6-month mortality as compared to their counterparts (9 vs. 40%, respectively, $p < 0.01$; and 50 vs. 66%, respectively, $p = 0.04$). TIVAP-related infection was significantly associated with ICU survival [OR 0.2, IC 95% (0.05–0.5), $p < 0.01$].

Conclusions: TIVAP-related infection was confirmed in nearly one out of two cases of life-threatening sepsis in patients in whom it has been removed. TIVAP-related infection was associated with a good prognosis, as compared to patients with other causes of infection.

Keywords: Sepsis, Intensive care unit, Totally implantable venous access ports

Background

Totally implanted venous access ports (TIVAPs) are commonly used for patients requiring long-term or iterative treatments such as antineoplastic chemotherapy, parenteral nutrition and transfusion [1–3]. Even if TIVAPs are associated with a low risk of infection, they still remain a source of infections potentially leading to life-threatening sepsis and subsequent admission in the intensive care unit (ICU) [4, 5].

In case of tunnel or port-pocket infection, TIVAP-related bloodstream infection is obviously strongly suspected and the device should be promptly removed [6]. However, local signs of infection are frequently lacking [7–10]. International guidelines support the removal

*Correspondence: marie.lecronier@aphp.fr
[1] Service de Pneumologie et Réanimation Médicale (Département "R3S"), Groupe Hospitalier Pitié-Salpêtrière Charles Foix, Assistance Publique-Hôpitaux de Paris, 75013 Paris, France
Full list of author information is available at the end of the article

of TIVAP in case of TIVAP-related bloodstream infection, with complication like severe sepsis or/and septic shock (use of vasopressors) [6, 11], although no data support this practice. Removal of TIVAP may have deleterious consequences in critically ill patients. First, patients with TIVAP are frequently frail and exposed to uncontrolled bleeding (low platelets and coagulation disorders). Second, removal of TIVAP is a surgical procedure that may interfere with the management of the ongoing sepsis [12–15]. Eventually, removing TIVAP may defer administration of chemotherapy or specific treatments once patients are discharged from the ICU. Therefore, removal of TIVAP is an important decision that should be supported by clinical evidences, but predictive factors of TIVAP-related infections are lacking in ICU patients. Likewise, no study regarding the prognosis of TIVAP-related infections has been conducted outside the ICU [16–20]. In light with this, the present study was designed to address three main objectives: (1) to determine the proportion of confirmed TIVAP-related infections in a population of patients admitted in the ICU in whom a TIVAP was removed for life-threatening sepsis, (2) to identify predictive factors of confirmed TIVAP infection in patients admitted to the ICU and (3) to assess short- and long-term outcome of patients with TIVAP-related infection and compare them with their counterparts in whom TIVAP was removed without confirmation of infection.

Patients and methods

This retrospective, multicenter, observational study was conducted in five ICU located in academic hospitals. The study period extended from January 2012 through December 2014. The Institutional Review Board of the French Intensive Care Society approved the study (CE SRLF15-52).

Selection of patients

Using clinical microbiology laboratory databases, we identified retrospectively all the patients admitted in participating ICU in whom a TIVAP was removed during the ICU stay and sent to the microbiology laboratory. Each patient's record was analyzed by two investigators (ML and MD) and those patients who fulfilled the following criteria were entered into the study: (1) age > 18 years, (2) sepsis, severe sepsis or septic shock, defined according to criteria of the Surviving Sepsis Campaign's definition [21], as the main reason for TIVAP removal. Of notice, peripherally inserted central catheters and surgically inserted long-term central venous catheters others than TIVAP were not considered for the study. In addition, patients with TIVAP removed before ICU admission or for another reason than sepsis (thrombosis, uselessness) were also not included in the study.

Data collection

The following data were extracted from each patient's medical record: age, gender, clinical and biological variables on admission. Simplified Acute Physiology Score (SAPS) 2 [22] and Sequential Organ Failure Assessment (SOFA) [23] were calculated upon ICU admission. Predisposing risk factors for TIVAP-related infections were also collected: immunosuppression status (i.e., hematological malignancies, solid organ transplant, recent antineoplastic chemotherapy for cancer or HIV infection), time since TIVAP insertion, main indication of the TIVAP (antineoplastic chemotherapy, parenteral nutrition), date of last antineoplastic chemotherapy and delay between ICU admission and removal of the device. We also looked through each patient's record for local signs of infection (induration or erythema, warmth and pain or tenderness along the tract of a catheterized vein) whenever it was described and general sign of infection (fever defined as temperature ≥38°3, hypothermia defined as temperature <36°, hypotension defined as systolic blood pressure <90 mmHg or mean blood pressure <65 mmHg). Advanced life support measures taken during the ICU stay (mechanical ventilation and vasopressors) and antibiotics regimens were recorded for each patient. Microbiological data were collected as follows: positive culture of TIVAP catheter tip or port reservoir, positive blood culture from the TIVAP and from a peripheral vein with the differential time to positivity. We also collected information regarding use of appropriate antibiotic in initial regimen (antibiotics with in vitro activity against the infecting agent). Finally, we recorded length of ICU stay, time spent under invasive mechanical ventilation and vasopressors. Mortality was determined in the ICU, at 28 days and 6 months after ICU admission.

Definitions

Culture of TIVAP was considered as positive if the tip or port reservoir (indoor or outdoor) was positive. Positivity of TIVAP tip culture was defined according to the same modality across all the microbiological laboratories of participating centers. It was defined on blood agar plate by quantitative method after vortexing or sonication (taking into account pathogens present in their inner or outer surfaces) with a cutoff of ≥1000 colony-forming units (CFU)/mL [24–26]. Growth of <1000 CFU/mL from a catheter by quantitative method was considered as catheter contamination. TIVAP box culture was performed according to each clinical microbiology laboratory-own protocol, such as immersion of the case in broth and then sowing on blood agar plate or chocolate plate, needle puncture and aspiration of the case contents then sowing, or swab from outside the case then sowing. In all these techniques, a qualitative culture was performed.

Definition of TIVAP-related infection was adapted from the Infectious Diseases Society of America (IDSA) guidelines [6] as one of the following conditions:

1. TIVAP-related bloodstream infection, defined as (1) a positive culture of the TIVAP (catheter tip or reservoir's port) associated with a positive peripheral blood culture with the same microorganism (same species and same antibiotic susceptibility testing) or (2) a differential time to positivity of a blood culture drawn from the catheter versus from a peripheral vein (positivity of the catheter blood sample at least 2 h before the peripheral blood sample) [27, 28];
2. Local or general (fever ≥38°3 or <36° and chills) signs of infection, positive culture of TIVAP (catheter tip or the reservoir's port) and regression of clinical signs of infection after TIVAP removal despite a negative peripheral blood culture.

We also included patients who did not meet the two above conditions but who had positive blood culture without other suspected infection and regression of clinical signs of infection after TIVAP removal despite negative culture of TIVAP (catheter tip or the reservoir's port).

Exclusive TIVAP-related infection was defined by TIVAP-related infection that was not associated with any other documented source of infection among lower respiratory, digestive or urinary tract infection.

Statistical analysis

Continuous variables are expressed as mean ± standard deviation or median (interquartile range). Categorical variables are expressed as number and relative frequencies. Patients were categorized a posteriori into two groups according to microbiologic findings: patients with or without TIVAP-related infection. Continuous variables were tested for normality using the Shapiro–Wilk test. Gaussian variables were compared using a *t* test and non-normally distributed variables using a Mann–Whitney test. Categorical variables were compared with Chi-square test. The primary endpoint was the prevalence of TIVAP-related infection. A stepwise logistic regression analysis was performed to identify variables associated with TIVAP-related infection and with ICU and 28-day mortality. Variables found to have univariate association ($p < 0.05$) with the outcome of interest were considered in the final model. Kaplan–Meier survival curves for patients with and without TIVAP-related infections were computed for 6-month mortality. For all final comparisons, a two-tailed p value less than or equal to 0.05 was considered statistically significant. The statistical analysis was performed with SAS statistical V9.3 software (SAS Institute Inc., Cary, NC, USA).

Results

Characteristics upon ICU admission

Over the study period, 151 patients met the inclusion criteria and were retained in the analysis (see flowchart, Additional file 1: Figure S1). Main characteristics of the patients are presented in Table 1. One hundred and forty-eight (98%) patients were immunosuppressed, and 50 patients (33%) had neutropenia. Antineoplastic chemotherapy was administrated in 131 patients (87%) in the last 6 months, and 18 (12%) of the patients were receiving parenteral nutrition. Severe sepsis was present in 48 patients (32%) and septic shock in 93 (62%).

Proportion and features of TIVAP-related infection

TIVAP-related infection was found in 68 patients (45%). Among these 68 patients, the diagnosis of TIVAP-related infection was retained because of (1) TIVAP-related bloodstream infection with the association of a positive peripheral blood culture with a positive culture of the TIVAP (tip or reservoir) in 33 patients (48%) or a differential time to positivity of a blood culture drawn from the catheter versus from a peripheral vein in 11 patients (16%); (2) a positive culture of the TIVAP and the regression of clinical signs of infection after TIVAP removal in 12 (18%) patients (negative peripheral blood culture) or (3) a positive blood culture associated with favorable outcome after TIVAP removal in 12 (18%) patients (negative tip or reservoir culture of the TIVAP). A growth of 100 CFU/mL of *Staphylococcus epidermidis* was found in two patients who were classified as catheter contamination (without TIVAP-related infection).

Regarding microbiological findings, TIVAP-related infections were associated with 53% (36/68) of Gram-negative rods, 44% (30/68) of Gram-positive cocci and 7% (5/68) of *Candida* sp. (see Table 2). Sixty-nine percent of patients with TIVAP-related infection had no other focus of infection and were subsequently classified as exclusive TIVAP-related infection (see Additional file 1: Table S1). Among patients with infectious other than TIVAP-related infections, 65% had positive microbiological samples (see Table 3; Additional file 1: Table S2).

Characteristics of the patients according to the presence or absence of TIVAP-related infections

Demographic characteristics of patients with and without TIVAP-related infections were not different (Table 1). Parenteral nutrition was more frequent in patients with TIVAP-related infections. In addition, SAPS2 and SOFA

Table 1 Clinical characteristics and laboratory features upon intensive care unit admission

Characteristic	All $n=151$	TIVAP-related infection $n=68$	No TIVAP-related infection $n=83$	p value
Age, year	58±14	57±14	58±14	0.58
Female gender, n (%)	58 (38)	30 (44)	28 (34)	0.19
Transfer from the emergency room, n (%)	47 (31)	21 (31)	26 (31)	1.00
Transfer from the ward, n (%)	104 (69)	47 (69)	57 (69)	1.00
SAPS2	52±17	47±15	56±17	<0.01
SOFA	9±4	7±4	10±4	<0.01
TIVAP-related infection risk factors, n (%)				
Immunosuppression	148 (98)	66 (97)	82 (99)	0.44
Hematological malignancies	72 (48)	28 (41)	44 (53)	0.14
Solid organ cancer	71 (47)	35 (51)	36 (43)	0.32
Metastatic cancer	44 (29)	24 (35)	20 (24)	0.13
Recent chemotherapy (<6 months)	131 (87)	58 (85)	73 (88)	0.63
Parenteral nutrition	18 (12)	14 (21)	4 (5)	<0.01
Clinical signs				
Temperature <36 or ≥38.3 °C, n (%)	111 (74)	55 (81)	56 (67)	0.08
Systolic blood pressure, mmHg	98±27	97±29	99±25	0.54
Mean blood pressure, mmHg	69±20	69±23	70±18	0.77
Glasgow Score Scale	13±3	14±3	13±4	0.04
Local sign of infection, n (%)	15 (10)	12 (18)	3 (4)	<0.01
Biological signs				
White blood cells <1 Giga/l, n (%)	50 (33)	19 (28)	31 (37)	0.22
Platelet counts, Giga/l	116±113	124±99	110±123	0.45
Prothrombin time, %	64±17	69±17	60±17	<0.01
Serum creatinine, µmol/l	142±119	126±113	155±123	0.13
Bicarbonate, mmol/l	20±5	21±5	20±6	0.05
Arterial lactate, mmol/l	3.4±3.2	3.3±3.0	3.6±3.3	0.61

Categorical variables are expressed as no. (%) and continuous variables as mean±SD

SAPS2 Simplified Acute Physiology Score, *SOFA* Sepsis-Related Organ Failure Assessment, *TIVAP* totally implanted venous access port

score were higher in patients with infectious other than TIVAP-related infections as compared to their counterparts. Local signs of infection were present in 18% of the patients with a TIVAP-related infection versus 4% for their counterparts ($p<0.01$). There was no difference regarding the presence of neutropenia upon admission between patients with TIVAP-related infection and patients without.

By multivariate logistic regression analysis, two factors were independently associated with TIVAP-related infection: SOFA score upon admission per point increase [odd ratio (OR) 0.86 interval confidence (IC) 95% (0.80–0.90), $p<0.01$] and local signs of infection [OR 4.0 IC 95% (1.1–15.6), $p=0.04$].

Therapeutic management and outcome

Patients with infections other than TIVAP-related infections received more vasopressors and were more likely to require mechanical ventilation than their counterparts (Table 4). There was no significant difference in terms of antibiotics management between both groups. The duration of ICU stay was similar between patients with and without TIVAP-related infections. Overall ICU mortality was 26%. Patients with TIVAP-related infection had lower ICU, 28-day and 6-month mortality as compared to their counterparts (Table 4; Fig. 1). In addition, patients with exclusive TIVAP-related infection had a lower ICU mortality as compared to patients who had TIVAP-related infection and another focus of infection: 2% (1/47) versus 24% (5/21), respectively ($p<0.01$).

Table 5 displays the variables associated with 28-day mortality, and Tables 2 and 3 show microbiological findings associated with 28-day mortality among patients with and without TIVAP-related infections, respectively. By multivariate logistic regression analysis, three factors were independently associated with higher 28-day mortality: SOFA at admission per point increase [OR 1.3 IC 95% (1.1–1.6), $p<0.01$], the use of mechanical ventilation [OR 11 IC 95% (2.8–41.2), $p<0.01$] and hematological malignancies [OR 3.2 IC 95% (1.1–9.1), $p=0.03$].

Table 2 Microbiological findings in patients with totally implanted venous access ports-related infections and association with 28-day mortality (univariate analysis)

	All $n=68$	Alive $n=54$	Dead $n=14$	*p* value
Gram-negative bacilli, *n* (%)	36 (53)	32 (59)	4 (29)	0.07
Enterobacteriaceae	27 (40)	25 (46)	2 (14)	0.03
Escherichia coli	8 (12)	8 (15)	0 (0)	0.19
Klebsiella pneumoniae	7 (10)	6 (11)	1 (7)	0.99
Enterobacter cloacae	7 (10)	7 (13)	0 (0)	0.33
Other *Enterobacteriaceae*	6 (9)	5 (9)	1 (7)	0.99
Pseudomonas aeruginosa	8 (12)	6 (11)	2 (14)	0.99
Stenotrophomonas maltophilia	1 (2)	1 (2)	0 (0)	0.99
Acinetobacter sp.	1 (2)	1 (2)	0 (0)	0.99
Gram-positive cocci, *n* (%)	30 (44)	21 (39)	9 (64)	0.13
Staphylococcus aureus	9 (13)	5 (9)	4 (29)	0.09
Coagulase-negative staphylococci	19 (28)	15 (28)	4 (29)	0.99
Enterococcus sp.	2 (3)	1 (2)	1 (7)	0.37
Other Gram-positive cocci	1(2)	1 (2)	0 (0)	0.99
Candida sp., *n* (%)	5 (7)	2 (4)	3 (21)	0.06
Polymicrobial, *n* (%)	6 (9)	4 (7)	2 (14)	0.59

Data are expressed as *n* (%)

Table 3 Microbiological findings in patients without TIVAP (totally implanted venous access port)-related infections and association with 28-day mortality (univariate analysis)

	All $n=83$	Alive $n=43$	Dead $n=40$	*p* value
Gram-negative bacilli, *n* (%)	34 (41)	17 (40)	17 (43)	0.83
Enterobacteriaceae	26 (31)	15 (35)	11 (28)	0.49
Escherichia coli	14 (17)	7 (16)	7 (18)	0.99
Klebsiella pneumoniae	7 (9)	4 (9)	3 (8)	0.99
Enterobacter cloacae	3 (4)	2 (5)	1 (3)	0.99
Other *Enterobacteriaceae*	9 (11)	7 (16)	2 (5)	0.16
Pseudomonas aeruginosa	6 (7)	1 (2)	5 (13)	0.10
Acinetobacter sp.	2 (3)	1 (2)	1 (3)	0.99
Gram-positive cocci, *n* (%)	22 (27)	8 (19)	14 (35)	0.13
Staphylococcus aureus	4 (5)	2 (5)	2 (5)	0.99
Coagulase-negative staphylococci	4 (5)	0 (0)	4 (10)	0.05
Enterococcus sp.	10 (12)	3 (7)	7 (18)	0.18
Other Gram-positive cocci	5 (6)	3 (7)	2 (5)	0.99
Other bacteria, *n* (%)	4 (5)	4 (9)	0 (0)	0.12
Candida sp., *n* (%)	8 (10)	4 (9)	4 (10)	0.99
Polymicrobial, *n* (%)	16 (19)	7 (16)	9 (23)	0.58

Data are expressed as *n* (%)

One factor, TIVAP-related infection, was independently associated with lower 28-day mortality [OR 0.2 IC 95% (0.1–0.7), $p=0.02$].

Additional file 1: Table S3 displays the variables associated with ICU mortality. By multivariate logistic regression analysis, two factors were independently associated with higher ICU mortality: SOFA at admission per point increase [OR 1.4 IC 95% (1.2–1.7), $p<0.01$] and the use of mechanical ventilation [OR 14.0 IC 95% (3.6–56.0), $p<0.01$]. One factor, TIVAP-related infection, was independently associated with lower ICU mortality [OR 0.16 IC 95% (0.05–0.5), $p<0.01$].

Discussion

This study is seemingly the first reporting characteristics and outcome of patients admitted for a life-threatening sepsis in the ICU whose TIVAP has been removed. Our findings can be summarized as follows: (1) TIVAP-related infection was confirmed in almost half of the patients; (2) except for a low value of SOFA score and local signs of infection, no other variable was found to be independently associated with TIVAP-related infection upon admission; and (3) patients with TIVAP-related infection had a better prognosis than patients with other source of infection.

Proportion of TIVAP-related infection

The proportion of patients in whom a TIVAP-related infection was confirmed was 45%. Being the first study addressing this issue in the ICU, our results are hardly comparable. Indeed, most of previous studies were conducted outside the ICU [4, 5, 10, 17, 19, 20, 29]. For instance, in two studies [8, 9], among patient whose TIVAP was removed because of a suspected infection, TIVAP-related infection was confirmed in two thirds of the patients (19/29 and 15/23, respectively). Based on our findings, the remaining key question is whether this 45% rate is high enough to justify TIVAP removal as supported by international guidelines [6] or whether these recommendations should be questioned. A higher rate (>80%) would have made clearly acceptable the TIVAP removal (and all its consequences), whereas a lower rate (<20%) would have discouraged current practices in term of potential harmful effects. While this 45% rate of TIVAP-related infection could be considered disappointing, it might represent the lower bounder of the proportion of patients with TIVAP-related infection. Indeed, all our patients received antibiotics prior ICU admission, a condition that could easily lead to false-negative microbiological findings [30]. As a matter of fact, this could have artificially underestimated the rate of patients with confirmed TIVAP-related infections. A randomized controlled trial might be necessary to definitively support the removal of TIVAP in case of severe sepsis or septic shock.

Another important finding is that a concomitant infection focus was evidenced in approximately one-third of

Table 4 Therapeutic management and outcome of patients with and without TIVAP (totally implanted venous access port)-related infection

Characteristic	All patients $n=151$	TIVAP-related infections $n=68$	No TIVAP-related infections $n=83$	p value
Time between ICU admission and TIVAP withdrawal, days	1 (0–2)	1 (0–1)	1 (0–2)	0.09
Antibiotics				
Beta lactam antibiotic, n (%)	143 (95)	63 (93)	80 (96)	0.49
Glycopeptide/linezolid, n (%)	78 (52)	38 (57)	40 (48)	0.29
Use of MV, n (%)	74 (49)	24 (35)	50 (60)	<0.01
MV duration, days	0 (0–5)	0 (0–3)	2 (0–7)	0.26
Vasopressors, n (%)	103 (68)	37 (55)	66 (80)	<0.01
Vasopressors, days	2 (0–3)	1 (0–2)	2 (1–4)	0.04
ICU length of stay, days	5 (3–10)	4 (3–6)	6 (3–12)	0.40
ICU mortality, n (%)	39 (26)	6 (9)	33 (40)	<0.01
28-day mortality, n (%)	54 (36)	14 (20.5)	40 (48)	<0.01
6-Month mortality, n (%)	89 (59)	34 (50)	55 (66)	0.04

Categorical variables are expressed as no. (%) and continuous variables as median (interquartile range)

TIVAP totally implanted venous access port, *ICU* intensive care unit, *MV* mechanical ventilation

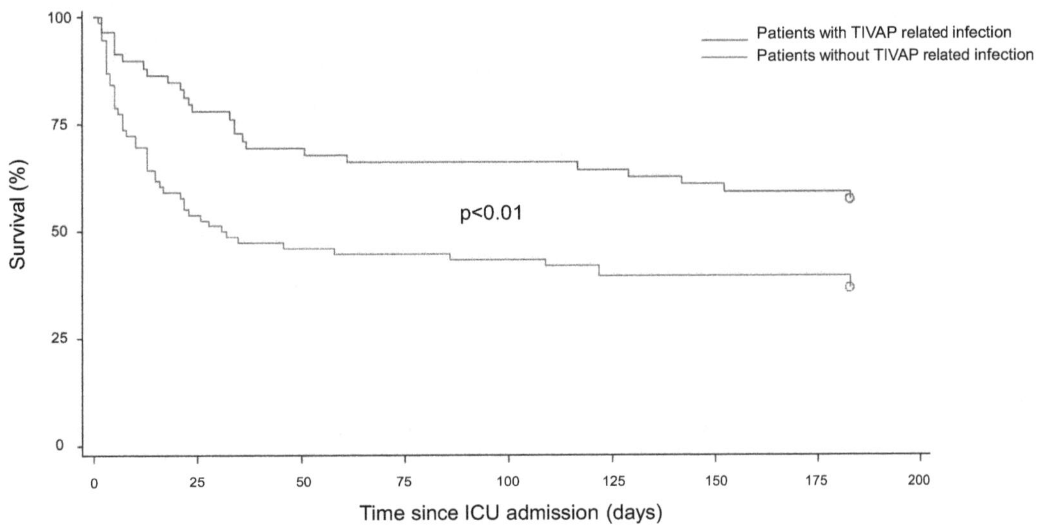

Fig. 1 Kaplan–Meier survival curve with 6-month mortality in patients with and without totally implanted venous access port (TIVAP)-related infections

patients with TIVAP-related infection. In half of these cases, the same pathogen was responsible (Additional file 1: Table S1). Whether this focus was the primary source or an hematogenous seeding from the TIVAP-related infection is unknown. This finding points out the importance of an extensive investigation even though a TIVAP infection is identified.

Factors associated with TIVAP-related infection

While a 45% rate of confirmed TIVAP-related infection may be acceptable, identifying associated factors of TIVAP-related infection upon admission would be helpful to prevent patients from undue procedures. Unfortunately, our study failed at providing new insightful clues in this purpose. Immunosuppression, a known risk factor for infection [4, 31–33], was equally present in both groups. By contrast, the use of parenteral nutrition, another recognized risk factor for TIVAP-related infection [34–36], was used more frequently in patients with TIVAP-related infection, but this finding remained infrequent and was not confirmed in multivariate analysis. While local signs of infection have been reported to be

Table 5 Variables associated with 28-day mortality

	All $n=151$	Alive $n=97$	Dead $n=54$	p value
Age, year	58±14	57±15	59±13	0.40
Female gender, *n* (%)	58 (38)	41 (43)	17 (32)	0.71
SAPS2	52±17	47±13	62±19	<0.01
SOFA	9±4	7±3.5	11±4.5	<0.01
TIVAP-related infection	68 (45)	55 (57)	13 (24)	<0.05
TIVAP-related infection risk factors, *n* (%)				
Immunosuppression	148 (98)	97 (100)	51 (95)	0.99
Hematological malignancies	72 (48)	43 (44)	29 (54)	<0.05
Solid organ cancer	71 (47)	52 (54)	19 (35)	0.12
Metastatic cancer	44 (29)	31 (32)	13 (24)	0.55
Recent chemotherapy (<6 months)	131 (87)	88 (91)	43 (80)	0.85
Parenteral nutrition	18 (12)	13 (14)	5 (9)	0.34
Initial presentation				
Systolic blood pressure, mmHg	98±27	98±27	101±28	0.55
Mean blood pressure, mmHg	69±20	69±19	72±24	0.44
Glasgow Score Scale	13±3	14±3	13±3	0.20
White blood cells, Giga/l	7.6±13.2	7.6±15.6	7.6±10.2	0.98
Platelet counts, Giga/l	116±113	128±110	91±114	<0.05
Prothrombin time, %	64±17	68±15	55±19	<0.01
Serum creatinine, µmol/l	142±119	125±106	176±137	0.01
Bicarbonate, mmol/l	20±5	21±6	19±5	<0.01
Arterial blood lactate, mmol/l	3.4±3.2	2.7±2.2	5±4	<0.01
Treatments				
Time between ICU admission and device withdrawal, days	1.8±3.5	1.6±2.8	2.2±4.5	0.35
Use of MV, *n* (%)	74 (49)	37 (38)	37 (69)	<0.01
MV duration, days	4±7	4±7	5±5	0.32
Use of vasopressors, *n* (%)	103 (68)	62 (64)	41 (76)	<0.01
Vasopressors duration, days	3±4	2±3	4±5	<0.01
ICU stay, days	8±9	9±10	8±7	0.53

Categorical variables are expressed as no. (%) and continuous variables as mean ± SD

ICU intensive care unit, *SOFA* Sepsis-Related Organ Failure Assessment, *SAPS2* Simplified Acute Physiology Score, *TIVAP* totally implanted venous access port, *MV* mechanical ventilation

present from 7 to 33% of the cases [8–10, 17, 20], in our patient series, only few had local sign of infection (18%). But it's important to specify that information about local signs of infection is difficult to collect in a retrospective study. They are not systematically looked for and their identification may vary between healthcare providers when clear definitions are not used. Interestingly, it was independently associated with TIVAP-related infection in our study.

TIVAP-related infections: impact on prognosis

While ICU mortality of sepsis is still high, up to 20% in latest publications [37–39], it reaches even higher rates in immunocompromised patients, between 40 and 60% [40]. In the present study, we report a lower mortality: 26% for ICU mortality and 36% at 28 days. While expected mortality (predicted by SAPS2 score) was around 40%, patients with TIVAP-related infections had a much lower mortality (9%). Moreover, ICU mortality was 2% in patients with exclusive TIVAP-related infection (no other infection focus). TIVAP-related infection was significantly associated with highest ICU and 28-day survival, whereas high SOFA score upon admission and the need for mechanical ventilation were significantly associated with ICU mortality and at 28 days. The low mortality observed in patients with exclusive TIVAP-related infections may be explained by the strong experience in the management of immunocompromised patients of participating ICUs. As a matter of fact, the precociousness of source control was probably a major driver of such a favorable outcome. In agreement with other studies, neutropenia was not significantly related to mortality [41–44]. Interestingly, patients who had both TIVAP-related infections and another focus had a worst prognosis than patients who had only TIVAP-related infection. In light with this, our study provides an important message for physicians managing immunosuppressed patients with severe presentation (septic shock, need for mechanical ventilation). While admission in the ICU of such patients is sometimes questioned, our findings suggest that in case of TIVAP-related infection, those patients have a short ICU stay and good prognosis. Likewise, our findings suggest that in patients admitted for a suspected TIVAP-related infection who do not recover shortly, this diagnosis should be questioned.

Limits

While reporting the first cohort of TIVAP-related infections in the ICU, this retrospective study has some limitations. As we obtained data from patient's medical charts, we cannot pretend to be exhaustive in data collection. Important information such as presence of thrombosis or endocarditis associated with TIVAP-related infection would have been interesting, but not all patients had a Doppler ultrasonography at time of admission. Then, it is likely that all patients with TIVAP admitted in participating ICU were not enrolled in the study since the main inclusion criteria was TIVAP removal. As a matter of fact, our inclusion criteria could have biased the true incidence of TIVAP-related infection toward overestimation. Due to the retrospective nature of the study, it was not possible to systematically identify patients who may have been admitted in our ICUs with a TIVAP in place that was not removed. The fact that positive blood cultures were available prior TIVAP removal may have also influenced clinicians' decision. However, ICUs participating in the study had homogeneous practices regarding admission policy of immunocompromised patients and the decision to remove TIVAP in case of life-threatening sepsis. Last, the definition of TIVAP-related infection was extended to patients with positive blood culture without other suspected infection ($n = 12$) and regression of clinical signs of infection after TIVAP removal despite negative culture of TIVAP (catheter tip or the reservoir's port). Since all our patients received antibiotics prior TIVAP removal, a condition that could fairly lead to misclassification, we estimated legitimate to consider these twelve patients as having TIVAP-related infection.

Conclusion

In almost one out of two cases, TIVAP-related infection was evidenced in immunosuppressed patients admitted in the ICU for sepsis and in whom the device has been removed. With the exception of local signs of infection, no other associated factor could have been identified. TIVAP-related infection was associated with a good prognosis, as compared to patients with other causes of infection.

Abbreviations

TIVAP: totally implanted venous access port; ICU: intensive care unit; SAPS II: Simplified Acute Physiology Score II; SOFA: Sequential Organ Failure Assessment; HIV: human immunodeficiency virus; IDSA: Infectious Diseases Society of America; CFU: colony-forming unit; OR: odd ratio; CI: confidence interval.

Authors' contributions

ML participated in the conception and design of the study, performed the literature search, performed the data analysis and drafted the manuscript. SV helped to collect data. NB helped to collect data. NdeP helped to collect data and helped to revise the manuscript. DR helped to collect data and helped to revise the manuscript. DL, EM, EA and AD helped to revise the manuscript. MD designed the study, helped to draft the manuscript and helped to revise the manuscript. All authors read and approved the final manuscript.

Author details

[1] Service de Pneumologie et Réanimation Médicale (Département "R3S"), Groupe Hospitalier Pitié-Salpêtrière Charles Foix, Assistance Publique-Hôpitaux de Paris, 75013 Paris, France. [2] Service de Réanimation médicale, Groupe Hospitalier Saint-Louis – Lariboisière – Fernand-Widal, Assistance Publique-Hôpitaux de Paris, Paris, France. [3] Service de Réanimation médicale, Groupe Hospitalier Est Parisien, Hôpital Saint-Antoine Paris, Assistance Publique-Hôpitaux de Paris, Paris, France. [4] Service de Réanimation médicale, Groupe Hospitalier Henri Mondor, Assistance Publique-Hôpitaux de Paris, Créteil, France. [5] Service de Réanimation médico-chirurgicale, Groupe Hospitalier Paris Nord, Hôpital Louis-Mourier, Assistance Publique-Hôpitaux de Paris, Colombes, France. [6] Service de Microbiologie, Unité Mobile de Microbiologie Clinique, Hôpital Européen Georges Pompidou, Assistance Publique-Hôpitaux de Paris, Paris, France. [7] Université Paris Descartes, Sorbonne Paris Cité, Paris, France. [8] INSERM, UMRS1158 Neurophysiologie respiratoire expérimentale et clinique, Sorbonne Universités, UPMC Univ Paris 06, Paris, France.

Acknowledgements

The authors would like to thank all the microbiologist from each center, for providing the clinical microbiology laboratory data to identify and include the patients.

Competing interests

Alexandre Demoule has signed research contracts with Medtronic (Dublin, Ireland), Maquet (Solna, Sweden) and Philips (Carlsbad, CA); he has also received personal fees from Medtronic (Dublin, Ireland), Maquet (Solna, Sweden), Fisher&Paykel (Kingston, Milton Keynes, UK), Resmed, Hamilton and MSD (Courbevoie, France). Martin Dres received personal fees from Pulsion Medical System (Feldkirchen, Germany) and Astra Zeneca (Cambridge, UK). Jean-Damien Ricard received travel expenses from Fisher&Paykel (Kingston, Milton Keynes, UK) to attend scientific meetings. Damien Roux received personal fees from Astellas (Levallois-Perret, France). The other authors declare that they have no competing interests.

Funding

MD was supported by the French Intensive Care Society, Paris, France (bourse de mobilité 2015); The 2015 Short Term Fellowship Program of the European Respiratory Society, Lausanne, Switzerland; The 2015 Bernhard Dräger Award for advanced treatment of acute respiratory failure of the European Society of Intensive Care Medicine, Brussels, Belgium; the Assistance Publique-Hôpitaux de Paris, Paris, France; and the Fondation pour la Recherche Médicale, Paris, France (FDM 20150734498).

References

1. Niederhuber JE, Ensminger W, Gyves JW, Liepman M, Doan K, Cozzi E. Totally implanted venous and arterial access system to replace external catheters in cancer treatment. Surgery. 1982;92:706–12.
2. Biffi R, Toro A, Pozzi S, Di Carlo I. Totally implantable vascular access devices 30 years after the first procedure. What has changed and what is still unsolved? Support Care Cancer. 2014;22:1705–14.
3. Barbetakis N, Asteriou C, Kleontas A, Tsilikas C. Totally implantable central venous access ports. Analysis of 700 cases. J Surg Oncol. 2011;104:654–6.
4. Groeger JS, Lucas AB, Thaler HT, Friedlander-Klar H, Brown AE, Kiehn TE, et al. Infectious morbidity associated with long-term use of venous access devices in patients with cancer. Ann Intern Med. 1993;119:1168–74.
5. Chang L, Tsai J-S, Huang S-J, Shih C-C. Evaluation of infectious complications of the implantable venous access system in a general oncologic population. Am J Infect Control. 2003;31:34–9.
6. Mermel LA, Allon M, Bouza E, Craven DE, Flynn P, O'Grady NP, et al. Clinical practice guidelines for the diagnosis and management of intravascular catheter-related infection: 2009 Update by the Infectious Diseases Society of America. Clin Infect Dis. 2009;49:1–45.
7. Safdar N, Maki DG. Inflammation at the insertion site is not predictive of catheter-related bloodstream infection with short-term, noncuffed central venous catheters. Crit Care Med. 2002;30:2632–5.
8. Whitman ED, Boatman AM. Comparison of diagnostic specimens and methods to evaluate infected venous access ports. Am J Surg. 1995;170:665–9.
9. Douard MC, Arlet G, Longuet P, Troje C, Rouveau M, Ponscarme D, et al. Diagnosis of venous access port-related infections. Clin Infect Dis. 1999;29:1197–202.
10. Hsu J-F, Chang H-L, Tsai M-J, Tsai Y-M, Lee Y-L, Chen P-H, et al. Port type is a possible risk factor for implantable venous access port-related bloodstream infections and no sign of local infection predicts the growth of gram-negative bacilli. World J Surg Oncol. 2015;13:288.
11. Timsit J-F. Updating of the 12th consensus conference of the Société de Réanimation de langue française (SRLF): catheter related infections in the intensive care unit. Ann Fr Anesth Réanim. 2005;24:315–22.
12. Seymour CW, Kahn JM, Martin-Gill C, Callaway CW, Yealy DM, Scales D, et al. Delays from first medical contact to antibiotic administration for sepsis. Crit Care Med. 2017;45:759–65.
13. Bagshaw SM, Lapinsky S, Dial S, Arabi Y, Dodek P, Wood G, et al. Acute kidney injury in septic shock: clinical outcomes and impact of duration of hypotension prior to initiation of antimicrobial therapy. Intensive Care Med. 2009;35:871–81.
14. Kumar A, Roberts D, Wood KE, Light B, Parrillo JE, Sharma S, et al. Duration of hypotension before initiation of effective antimicrobial therapy is the critical determinant of survival in human septic shock. Crit Care Med. 2006;34:1589–96.
15. Lundberg JS, Perl TM, Wiblin T, Costigan MD, Dawson J, Nettleman MD, et al. Septic shock: an analysis of outcomes for patients with onset on hospital wards versus intensive care units. Crit Care Med. 1998;26:1020–4.
16. Lebeaux D, Fernández-Hidalgo N, Chauhan A, Lee S, Ghigo J-M, Almirante B, et al. Management of infections related to totally implantable venous-access ports: challenges and perspectives. Lancet Infect Dis. 2014;14:146–59.
17. Lebeaux D, Larroque B, Gellen-Dautremer J, Leflon-Guibout V, Dreyer C, Bialek S, et al. Clinical outcome after a totally implantable venous access port-related infection in cancer patients: a prospective study and review of the literature. Medicine (Baltimore). 2012;91:309–18.
18. Raad I, Hanna H, Maki D. Intravascular catheter-related infections: advances in diagnosis, prevention, and management. Lancet Infect Dis. 2007;7:645–57.
19. Sotir MJ, Lewis C, Bisher EW, Ray SM, Soucie JM, Blumberg HM. Epidemiology of device-associated infections related to a long-term implantable vascular access device. Infect Control Hosp Epidemiol. 1999;20:187–91.
20. Vidal M, Genillon JP, Forestier E, Trouiller S, Pereira B, Mrozek N, et al. Outcome of totally implantable venous-access port-related infections. Méd Mal Infect. 2016;46:32–8.
21. Dellinger RP, Levy MM, Rhodes A, Annane D, Gerlach H, Opal SM, et al. Surviving sepsis campaign: international guidelines for management of severe sepsis and septic shock: 2012. Crit Care Med. 2013;41:580–637.
22. Le Gall JR, Lemeshow S, Saulnier F. A new Simplified Acute Physiology Score (SAPS II) based on a European/North American multicenter study. JAMA. 1993;270:2957–63.
23. Vincent JL, Moreno R, Takala J, Willatts S, De Mendonça A, Bruining H, et al. The SOFA (Sepsis-related Organ Failure Assessment) score to describe organ dysfunction/failure. On behalf of the Working Group on Sepsis-Related Problems of the European Society of Intensive Care Medicine. Intensive Care Med. 1996;22:707–10.
24. Brun-Buisson C, Abrouk F, Legrand P, Huet Y, Larabi S, Rapin M. Diagnosis of central venous catheter-related sepsis. Critical level of quantitative tip cultures. Arch Intern Med. 1987;147:873–7.
25. Cleri DJ, Corrado ML, Seligman SJ. Quantitative culture of intravenous catheters and other intravascular inserts. J Infect Dis. 1980;141:781–6.
26. Safdar N, Fine JP, Maki DG. Meta-analysis: methods for diagnosing intravascular device-related bloodstream infection. Ann Intern Med. 2005;142:451–66.
27. Blot F, Nitenberg G, Chachaty E, Raynard B, Germann N, Antoun S, et al. Diagnosis of catheter-related bacteraemia: a prospective comparison of the time to positivity of hub-blood versus peripheral-blood cultures. Lancet. 1999;354:1071–7.
28. Blot F, Schmidt E, Nitenberg G, Tancrède C, Leclercq B, Laplanche A, et al. Earlier positivity of central-venous-versus peripheral-blood cultures is highly predictive of catheter-related sepsis. J Clin Microbiol. 1998;36:105–9.
29. Pegues D, Axelrod P, McClarren C, Eisenberg BL, Hoffman JP, Ottery FD, et al. Comparison of infections in Hickman and implanted port catheters in adult solid tumor patients. J Surg Oncol. 1992;49:156–62.
30. Rijnders BJ, Van Wijngaerden E, Vandecasteele SJ, Stas M, Peetermans WE. Treatment of long-term intravascular catheter-related bacteraemia with antibiotic lock: randomized, placebo-controlled trial. J Antimicrob Chemother. 2005;55:90–4.
31. Howell PB, Walters PE, Donowitz GR, Farr BM. Risk factors for infection of adult patients with cancer who have tunnelled central venous catheters. Cancer. 1995;75:1367–75.
32. Adler A, Yaniv I, Steinberg R, Solter E, Samra Z, Stein J, et al. Infectious complications of implantable ports and Hickman catheters in paediatric haematology-oncology patients. J Hosp Infect. 2006;62:358–65.
33. Lebeaux D, Zarrouk V, Leflon-Guibout V, Lefort A, Fantin B. Totally implanted access port-related infections: features and management. Rev Méd Interne. 2010;31:819–27.
34. Penel N, Neu J-C, Clisant S, Hoppe H, Devos P, Yazdanpanah Y. Risk factors for early catheter-related infections in cancer patients. Cancer. 2007;110:1586–92.
35. Santarpia L, Pasanisi F, Alfonsi L, Violante G, Tiseo D, De Simone G, et al. Prevention and treatment of implanted central venous catheter (CVC)—related sepsis: a report after six years of home parenteral nutrition (HPN). Clin Nutr Edinb Scotl. 2002;21:207–11.
36. Touré A, Chambrier C, Vanhems P, Lombard-Bohas C, Souquet J-C, Ecochard R. Propensity score analysis confirms the independent effect of parenteral nutrition on the risk of central venous catheter-related bloodstream infection in oncological patients. Clin Nutr Edinb Scotl. 2013;32:1050–4.
37. Damiani E, Donati A, Serafini G, Rinaldi L, Adrario E, Pelaia P, et al. Effect of performance improvement programs on compliance with sepsis bundles and mortality: a systematic review and meta-analysis of observational studies. PLoS ONE. 2015;10:e0125827.
38. Kaukonen K-M, Bailey M, Suzuki S, Pilcher D, Bellomo R. Mortality related to severe sepsis and septic shock among critically ill patients in Australia and New Zealand, 2000–2012. JAMA. 2014;311:1308–16.
39. Stevenson EK, Rubenstein AR, Radin GT, Wiener RS, Walkey AJ. Two decades of mortality trends among patients with severe sepsis: a comparative meta-analysis. Crit Care Med. 2014;42:625–31.
40. Pène F, Percheron S, Lemiale V, Viallon V, Claessens Y-E, Marqué S, et al. Temporal changes in management and outcome of septic shock in patients with malignancies in the intensive care unit. Crit Care Med. 2008;36:690–6.
41. Azoulay E, Mokart D, Pène F, Lambert J, Kouatchet A, Mayaux J, et al. Outcomes of critically ill patients with hematologic malignancies: prospec-

tive multicenter data from France and Belgium—A Groupe de Recherche Respiratoire en Réanimation Onco-Hématologique Study. J Clin Oncol. 2013;31:2810–8.

42. Darmon M, Azoulay E, Alberti C, Fieux F, Moreau D, Le Gall J-R, et al. Impact of neutropenia duration on short-term mortality in neutropenic critically ill cancer patients. Intensive Care Med. 2002;28:1775–80.
43. Mokart D, Darmon M, Resche-Rigon M, Lemiale V, Pène F, Mayaux J, et al. Prognosis of neutropenic patients admitted to the intensive care unit. Intensive Care Med. 2015;41:296–303.
44. Vandijck DM, Benoit DD, Depuydt PO, Offner FC, Blot SI, Van Tilborgh AK, et al. Impact of recent intravenous chemotherapy on outcome in severe sepsis and septic shock patients with hematological malignancies. Intensive Care Med. 2008;34:847–55.

14

Potentially modifiable respiratory variables contributing to outcome in ICU patients without ARDS: a secondary analysis of PRoVENT

Fabienne D. Simonis[1*], Carmen S. V. Barbas[2,3], Antonio Artigas-Raventós[4], Jaume Canet[5], Rogier M. Determann[6], James Anstey[7], Goran Hedenstierna[8], Sabrine N. T. Hemmes[9], Greet Hermans[10,11], Michael Hiesmayr[12], Markus W. Hollmann[9], Samir Jaber[13], Ignacio Martin-Loeches[14,15], Gary H. Mills[16], Rupert M. Pearse[17], Christian Putensen[18], Werner Schmid[12], Paolo Severgnini[19], Roger Smith[7], Tanja A. Treschan[20], Edda M. Tschernko[12], Marcos F. Vidal Melo[21], Hermann Wrigge[22], Marcelo Gama de Abreu[23,24], Paolo Pelosi[25], Marcus J. Schultz[1,26], Ary Serpa Neto[1,2], For the PRoVENT investigators, The PROVE Network investigators

Abstract

Background: The majority of critically ill patients do not suffer from acute respiratory distress syndrome (ARDS). To improve the treatment of these patients, we aimed to identify potentially modifiable factors associated with outcome of these patients.

Methods: The PRoVENT was an international, multicenter, prospective cohort study of consecutive patients under invasive mechanical ventilatory support. A predefined secondary analysis was to examine factors associated with mortality. The primary endpoint was all-cause in-hospital mortality.

Results: 935 Patients were included. In-hospital mortality was 21%. Compared to patients who died, patients who survived had a lower risk of ARDS according to the 'Lung Injury Prediction Score' and received lower maximum airway pressure (P_{max}), driving pressure (ΔP), positive end-expiratory pressure, and FiO_2 levels. Tidal volume size was similar between the groups. Higher P_{max} was a potentially modifiable ventilatory variable associated with in-hospital mortality in multivariable analyses. ΔP was not independently associated with in-hospital mortality, but reliable values for ΔP were available for 343 patients only. Non-modifiable factors associated with in-hospital mortality were older age, presence of immunosuppression, higher non-pulmonary sequential organ failure assessment scores, lower pulse oximetry readings, higher heart rates, and functional dependence.

Conclusions: Higher P_{max} was independently associated with higher in-hospital mortality in mechanically ventilated critically ill patients under mechanical ventilatory support for reasons other than ARDS.

Trial Registration ClinicalTrials.gov (NCT01868321).

Keywords: Mechanical ventilation, Outcome, Mortality, Ventilator settings

*Correspondence: f.d.simonis@amc.uva.nl; f.d.simonis@gmail.com

[1] Department of Intensive Care and Lab. of Experimental Intensive Care and Anesthesiology (L E I C A), Academic Medical Center, Meibergdreef 9, 1105 AZ Amsterdam, The Netherlands

Full list of author information is available at the end of the article

Introduction

Mechanical ventilation is a potentially life-saving intervention, though there is an increasing body of evidence for potential harm from this intervention in critically ill patients [1, 2]. Too high tidal volumes (V_T) and airway pressures have been shown to be associated with worse outcomes in patients with acute respiratory distress syndrome (ARDS) [3, 4], and there is increasing evidence for the injurious effects of too high V_T in ventilated patients without ARDS [5, 6]. While inadequately too low positive end-expiratory pressures (PEEP) have been demonstrated to worsen outcome of patients with ARDS, especially in moderate or severe cases [7], patients without ARDS likely do not benefit from higher PEEP [8]. More recently, a positive association between driving pressures (ΔP) and mortality was demonstrated in patients with ARDS [9], but it is unclear whether ΔP is associated with a worse outcome also in patients without ARDS.

Results from the 'Large observational study to UNderstand the Global impact of Severe Acute respiratory FailurE' (LUNG SAFE) [10], a prospective cohort study undertaken in 459 intensive care units (ICUs) in 50 countries, as well as the more recent 'PRactice of VENTilation in patients without ARDS study' (PRoVENT) [11], a prospective cohort study undertaken in 119 ICUs in 16 countries, convincingly showed that the practice of invasive mechanical ventilatory support in ICUs has changed remarkably over the recent years [10–12]. First, V_T size decreased over time, not only in patients with ARDS [10, 12–14], but also in patients at risk of ARDS [11]. Presently, V_T above 10 to 12 ml/kg predicted body weight (PBW) is seldom used. The median PEEP level that is set has increased over time in patients without ARDS [11, 13, 14]. In patients with ARDS, higher levels of PEEP usually are restricted to patients with more severe hypoxemia [7, 10, 15]. Both investigations, though, suggested there is still potential for improvement in ventilatory management in critically ill patients [10, 11], and one recently published secondary analysis of LUNG SAFE showed that lower PEEP, higher peak inspiratory (P_{peak}), plateau (P_{plat}), ΔP, and increased respiratory rate represent potentially modifiable factors contributing to worse outcome in patients with ARDS [16].

The aim of the present study was to identify modifiable respiratory variables that could potentially change outcome in critically ill patients under invasive mechanical ventilatory support without ARDS. Specifically, we hypothesized that there are several modifiable respiratory variables associated with all-cause in-hospital mortality.

Methods

Study design

PRoVENT was an investigator-initiated international multicenter study; details of its methods have been published elsewhere [11, 17]. Details on study population and data collection are described in the supplement. PRoVENT was registered at Clinicaltrials.gov (NCT01868321).

Patients

Consecutive patients under invasive mechanical ventilatory support were eligible for participation if admitted in a predefined period lasting one week. Inclusion criteria were: (1) age $\geq$ 18 years and (2) under invasive mechanical ventilatory support, which could have been initiated outside the hospital, in the emergency room, in the normal ward or in the operating room, or start of invasive mechanical ventilatory support in the ICU, after admission. Patients in whom mechanical ventilatory support was started before the study recruitment week of PRoVENT, patients receiving only noninvasive mechanical ventilatory support or transferred from another hospital under invasive mechanical ventilatory support were excluded. Although data were also collected from patients who fulfilled the Berlin definition for ARDS [18] at start of ventilation, data of those patients were not used in the present analysis.

Definitions and calculations

The risk of death was derived from acute physiology and chronic health evaluation (APACHE) II scores [19] or simplified acute physiology score (SAPS) III [20].

Under the assumption that the maximum airway pressure (P_{max}) during pressure-controlled assist modes of invasive mechanical ventilatory support is similar to P_{plat} during volume-controlled assist modes [21, 22], P_{max} was defined as P_{max} in pressure-controlled assist modes and plateau pressure in volume-controlled assist modes, when available. Also, ΔP was calculated by subtracting PEEP from P_{max} during pressure-controlled and volume-controlled ventilation, respectively. This, however, was only done when set and measured respiratory rates were equal, indicating the absence of spontaneous breathing.

V_T size was expressed as a volume normalized for predicted body weight (ml/kg PBW). The PBW of male patients was calculated as equal to $50 + 0.91$(centimeters of height—152.4); that of female patients was calculated as equal to $45.5 + 0.91$(centimeters of height—152.4) [23]. Dead space fraction was calculated as (partial pressure of carbon dioxide in arterial blood ($PaCO_2$)–end-tidal carbon dioxide ($etCO_2$))/$PaCO_2$, and static compliance of the respiratory system as $V_T/\Delta P$. 'Non-pulmonary' sequential organ failure assessment (SOFA) was calculated by leaving out the pulmonary component and amending the denominator accordingly. The presence of acidosis was split into respiratory and metabolic acidosis to include separately in the univariate analysis, under the assumption that a respiratory acidosis could be modifiable by adjusting respiratory minute volume as opposed to metabolic acidosis. Immunosuppression was defined as the presence of human immunodeficiency virus or the use of chemotherapy, systemic steroids (> 1 mg/kg of prednisone or equivalent), or other immunosuppressive agents.

Outcomes

The primary outcome was all-cause in-hospital mortality, defined as mortality at hospital discharge, or at 90 days after start of invasive mechanical ventilatory support while still in hospital, whichever occurred first. The secondary outcome was ICU mortality, defined as mortality at ICU discharge or at 90 days after start of mechanical ventilatory support while still in ICU, whichever occurred first.

Statistical analysis

Daily-collected variables, including P_{max} or P_{plat}, ΔP, PEEP, V_T, oxygen fraction of inspired air (FiO_2), respiratory rate, dead space fraction, and compliance, and blood gas analysis parameters such as partial pressure of oxygen in arterial blood (PaO_2), $PaCO_2$, pH, and bicarbonate level, were presented as medians with their interquartile ranges. Proportions were compared using Chi-square or Fisher's exact tests, and continuous variables were compared using the *t* test or Wilcoxon rank sum test, as appropriate. Since the amount of missing data were low, no assumptions were made for missing data.

In all descriptive analyses, survivors were separated from non-survivors according to all-cause in-hospital mortality. In univariate analyses assessing the impact of ventilatory variables on outcome, relative risk (RR) of in-hospital mortality was estimated for patients dividing the study sample according to the median of P_{max} (≤ 18 vs. > 18 cm H_2O), ΔP (≤ 12 vs. > 12 cm H_2O), PEEP (≤ 5 vs. > 5 cm H_2O), and V_T (≤ 7.9 vs. > 7.9 ml/kg PBW), as measured at the first day of ventilation. For this specific analysis, two separate groups were included: patients not at risk and patients at risk of ARDS according to the Lung Injury Prediction Score (LIPS), where a LIPS ≥ 4 was considered 'at risk of ARDS' and a LIPS < 4 'not at risk of ARDS.'

To identify potentially modifiable and non-modifiable factors contributing to hospital mortality, a multivariable model was built using demographic factors, comorbidities, illness severities, and respiratory and laboratorial variables at the first day of ventilation. Since P_{max} and ΔP have a high collinearity, we chose to include only P_{max} in the main model. We conducted multilevel analyses to adjust for clustering of the data. Therefore, a multilevel logistic regression was used to identify factors contributing to mortality by modeling it as the dependent variable. Variables were selected when the univariate analysis *p* value was < 0.2. Then, a multilevel multivariable logistic model was built with centers treated as random effect. The cluster effects induced by the structure of the data were taken into account through random effects. In the multivariable model, statistical significance was set at a $p < 0.05$. Results are shown as odds ratios (ORs) with 95% confidence intervals (CI).

The odds ratio for hospital mortality of P_{max} was plotted in curves showing the odds ratios according to increases of one standard deviation of the P_{max}. These curves were divided according to the risk of ARDS and adjusted for the variables included the final model and reported in Table 3. A similar curve was made using ICU mortality as outcome.

We performed a secondary analysis in which we replaced P_{max} with ΔP in the multivariate model for in-hospital and ICU mortality. Since we lacked reliable values for ΔP for a large group of patients, this analysis had a much smaller sample size, increasing the risk of losing power to show an association between ΔP and in-hospital mortality. To test this, we performed one post hoc analysis in which we used P_{max} instead of ΔP, but only for patients for whom we had a reliable ΔP.

Statistical significance was considered to be at two-sided $p < 0.05$. All analyses were performed with SPSS v.20 (IBM SPSS Statistics for Windows, Version 20·0. Armonk, NY: IBM Corp.), and R v.2·12·0 (http://www.r-project.org).

Results

Participating centers and patients

One hundred and nineteen ICUs from 16 countries in four continents enrolled 1021 patients under invasive mechanical ventilatory support. Excluding 86 patients who were admitted to ICU with ARDS, we analyzed the data from a total of 935 patients (Fig. 1). All-cause in-hospital mortality was 21% in all patients. Patients who survived had lower derived risk scores for mortality, were younger, and had lower SOFA scores; patients who died were more often functionally dependent and more often admitted for a medical condition or for emergency surgery (Table 1).

Ventilation characteristics

Patients who survived had a lower P_{max} or P_{plat}, lower ΔP, lower PEEP, and lower FiO_2 levels than patients who died, but a similar V_T (Table 2). PaO_2/FiO_2, pulse oximetry, and arterial pH were higher and $PaCO_2$ levels were lower in patients who survived (Table 2). The unadjusted impact of ventilatory parameters in the overall cohort and in each group of risk of ARDS is shown in Fig. 2. Mortality

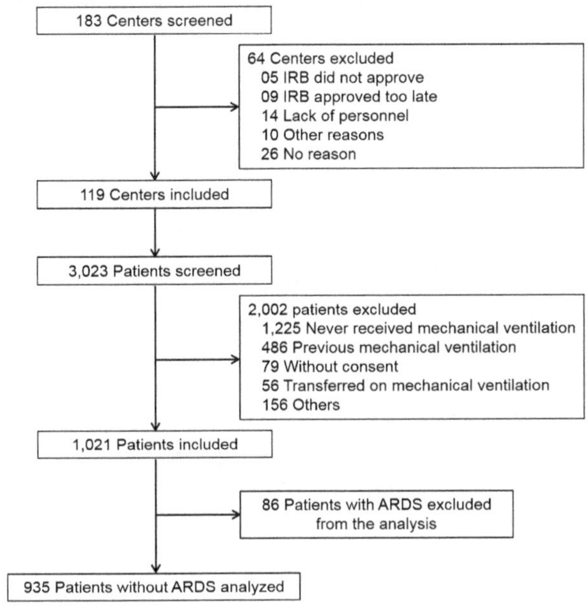

Fig. 1 Flowchart of inclusion

risk was similar in patients stratified according tidal volume and ΔP. In the overall cohort, patients receiving higher PEEP had higher risk of hospital mortality (Fig. 2). Patients ventilated with higher P_{max} had a higher risk of hospital mortality in the overall cohort and in patients at risk of ARDS (Fig. 2).

Factors associated with in-hospital mortality

The results of the univariable analysis of factors associated with in-hospital mortality are provided in Additional file 1: Table S1. In multivariable analysis, P_{max} was the only ventilatory variable associated with higher in-hospital mortality; in this analysis, the ΔP was excluded due to the collinearity with P_{max} (Table 3). Non-modifiable factors associated with worse outcome were older age, presence of immunosuppression, higher non-pulmonary SOFA, lower pulse oximetry readings, higher heart rates, and functional dependency (Table 3).

Figure 3 shows the odds ratio for hospital mortality per increase in one standard deviation in P_{max} for patients not at risk of ARDS and patients at risk of ARDS and adjusted for the variables indicated in Table 3.

Factors associated with ICU mortality

Results of the univariable analysis of factors associated with ICU mortality are provided in Additional file 1: Table S2. After multivariable adjustments, P_{max} was the only ventilatory variable associated with worse outcome (Additional file 1: Table S2); non-modifiable factors associated with worse outcome were history of COPD, presence of immunosuppression, higher non-pulmonary SOFA scores, and functional dependency.

Additional file 1: Figure S1 shows the odds ratio for ICU mortality per increase in one standard deviation in P_{max} for patients not at risk of ARDS and patients at risk of ARDS and adjusted for the variables indicated in Additional file 1: Table S2.

Driving pressure

The analysis including ΔP was only possible in 343 patients for whom ΔP could be calculated in a reliable way. When considering ΔP instead of P_{max} in the model, there was an association between ΔP and ICU (Additional file 1: Table S3), but not between ΔP and in-hospital mortality (Additional file 1: Table S4). The lack of an association between ΔP and in-hospital mortality could very well have been caused by the smaller sample size, since the post hoc analysis in which we used P_{max} in the model, now using the same number of patients as done for the analysis including ΔP, also showed no association between P_{max} and in-hospital mortality (Additional file 1: Table S5), while the association between P_{max} and ICU mortality remained present (Additional file 1: Table S6).

Discussion

In the present study, older age, presence of immunosuppression, a more dependent premorbid condition, and severity of illness markers such as the pulse oximetry, the non-pulmonary SOFA score, and a higher heart rate were all independently associated with increased in-hospital mortality. In the present analysis, P_{max} was the single ventilator factor associated with in-hospital mortality, suggesting this is the only potentially modifiable factor in these patients. Parts of our findings are in line with prior studies in this field. Older age is independently associated with worse outcome in patients with ARDS [16, 24, 25] and patients without ARDS [13], and also immunosuppression is a risk factor for mortality in our study and in trials that included patients with ARDS [16, 25]. Severity of illness factors associated with outcome was a higher heart rate and higher non-pulmonary SOFA score, consistent with previous studies in patients with [16, 25], as well as in patients without ARDS [13]. In addition to the results of the LUNG SAFE [16], we here show that, irrespective of the presence of ARDS, older patients, patients with immunosuppression, patients with high non-pulmonary SOFA score, and higher heart rate are at increased risk of worse outcomes. Ventilatory support with a higher P_{max} was independently associated with both increased hospital mortality and ICU mortality. This finding is in accordance with previous studies where higher P_{max} was associated with worse outcomes, for example increased risk of ventilator-induced lung injury (VILI) [26, 27], and

Table 1 Demographic characteristics of patients without ARDS receiving mechanical ventilation, comparison of survivors and non-survivors

	All ($n = 935$)	Survivors ($n = 738$)	Non-survivors ($n = 197$)	p value[a]
Age (years)	65.0 (52.0–75.0)	63.0 (50.0–73.0)	72.0 (60.0–79.0)	< 0.001
Gender (male)	570/910 (62.6)	453/713 (36.5)	117/197 (40.6)	0.287
Ethnic				0.366
African	11/903 (1.2)	7/708 (1.0)	4/195 (2.1)	
Afro-Caribbean	11/903 (1.2)	8/708 (1.1)	3/195 (1.5)	
Asian	57/903 (6.3)	40/708 (5.6)	17/195 (8.7)	
Caucasian	760/903 (84.2)	603/708 (85.2)	157/195 (80.5)	
Latin American	64/903 (7.1)	50/708 (7.1)	14/195 (7.2)	
BMI (kg/m^2)	25.5 (22.9–29.2)	25.7 (23.0–29.3)	24.7 (22.5–27.9)	0.019
PBW (kg)	64.2 (54.2–71.5)	64.6 (54.2–72.4)	64.2 (52.8–70.6)	0.143
Smoker				
Never	298/902 (33.0)	238/706 (33.7)	60/196 (30.6)	0.044
Previous	153/902 (17.0)	122/706 (17.3)	31/196 (15.8)	
Former	31/902 (3.4)	26/706 (3.7)	5/196 (2.6)	
Current	174/902 (19.3)	144/706 (20.4)	30/196 (15.3)	
Unknown	246/902 (27.3)	176/706 (24.9)	70/196 (35.7)	
Functional status				
Independent	675/900 (75.0)	569/705 (80.7)	106/195 (54.4)	< 0.001
Partially dependent	158/900 (17.6)	96/705 (13.6)	62/195 (31.8)	
Totally dependent	40/900 (4.4)	26/705 (3.7)	14/195 (7.2)	
Unknown	27/900 (3.0)	14/705 (2.0)	13/195 (6.7)	
Reason for ICU admission				
Planned surgery	313/902 (34.7)	292/706 (41.4)	21/196 (10.7)	< 0.001
Emergency surgery	187/902 (20.7)	138/706 (19.5)	49/196 (25.0)	
Clinical condition	402/902 (44.6)	276/706 (39.1)	126/196 (64.3)	
NIV before intubation	69/900 (7.7)	46/705 (6.5)	23/195 (11.8)	0.022
Duration (min)	240.0 (75.0–720.0)	285.0 (74.2–626.2)	180.0 (60.0–690.0)	0.013
Risk of death* (%)	12.7 (7.0–35.1)	12.0 (4.1–30.0)	34.5 (12.9–56.8)	< 0.001
LIPS	3.5 (2.0–6.0)	2.5 (1.0–5.0)	4.5 (2.5–7.0)	< 0.001
Limitation of treatment	30/892 (3.4)	17/696 (2.4)	13/196 (6.6)	0.004
Unplanned admission	483/900 (53.7)	341/704 (48.4)	142/196 (72.4)	< 0.001
Reason for intubation**				
Cardiac arrest	79/900 (8.8)	46/704 (6.5)	33/196 (16.8)	< 0.001
Anesthesia for surgery (planned)	467/900 (51.9)	412/703 (58.6)	55/196 (28.1)	< 0.001
Depressed level of consciousness	239/900 (26.6)	179/703 (25.5)	60/196 (30.6)	0.148
Respiratory failure	255/900 (28.4)	159/702 (22.6)	96/196 (49.0)	< 0.001
Chronic comorbidity**				
Hypertension	381/894 (42.6)	287/700 (41.0)	94/194 (48.5)	0.063
Diabetes mellitus	166/896 (18.5)	125/702 (17.8)	41/194 (21.1)	0.290
Heart failure	158/894 (17.7)	109/700 (15.6)	49/194 (25.3)	0.001
Chronic kidney failure	94/897 (10.5)	60/703 (8.5)	34/194 (17.5)	< 0.001
Cirrhosis	33/896 (3.7)	22/702 (3.1)	11/194 (5.7)	0.096
COPD	107/888 (12.0)	66/695 (9.5)	41/194 (21.2)	< 0.001
Oxygen at home	16/935 (1.7)	6/738 (0.8)	10/197 (5.1)	< 0.001
Cancer	219/896 (24.4)	170/702 (24.2)	49/194 (25.3)	0.765
Former	65/888 (7.3)	49/695 (7.1)	16/193 (8.3)	0.835
Current	146/888 (16.4)	114/695 (16.4)	32/193 (16.6)	
Neuromuscular disease	19/895 (2.1)	20/701 (2.8)	4/194 (2.1)	0.726

Table 1 continued

	All ($n = 935$)	Survivors ($n = 738$)	Non-survivors ($n = 197$)	p value[a]
Immunosuppression	70/895 (7.8)	41/702 (5.8)	29/193 (15.0)	< 0.001
Use of NIV at home	11/892 (1.2)	7/698 (1.0)	4/194 (2.1)	0.237
Severity of illness, SOFA score[b]				
Total	6.0 (4.0–9.0)	5.0 (3.0–8.0)	8.0 (6.0–11.0)	< 0.001
Non-pulmonary SOFA	4.0 (2.0–7.0)	4.0 (2.0–6.0)	6.0 (4.0–9.0)	< 0.001
Pulmonary	2.0 (0.0–3.0)	1.0 (0.0–3.0)	2.0 (1.0–3.0)	< 0.001
Hematologic	0.0 (0.0–1.0)	0.0 (0.0–1.0)	0.0 (0.0–1.0)	0.032
Liver	0.0 (0.0–0.0)	0.0 (0.0–0.0)	0.0 (0.0–1.0)	0.005
Circulation	1.0 (0.0–3.0)	1.0 (0.0–3.0)	2.0 (0.0–4.0)	< 0.001
Neurology	2.0 (0.0–4.0)	2.0 (0.0–4.0)	3.0 (1.0–4.0)	< 0.001
Renal	0.0 (0.0–1.0)	0.0 (0.0–1.0)	0.0 (0.0–2.0)	< 0.001

BMI body mass index, *PBW* predicted body weight, *ICU* intensive care unit, *NIV* noninvasive ventilation, *LIPS* Lung Injury Prediction Score, *COPD* chronic obstructive pulmonary disease, *SOFA* sequential organ failure assessment, *ARDS* acute respiratory distress syndrome

*Risk of death was derived from scores on APACHE II or SAPS III

**Patient can have more than one diagnosis

[a] p value is related to comparison between survivors and non-survivors

[b] For all SOFA scores for which data points were missing, this value was omitted and the denominator adjusted accordingly

increased mortality in patients without ARDS [13] and those with ARDS [16, 21, 28, 29].

ΔP was only associated with ICU mortality and not with in-hospital mortality. It should be recognized, though, that that analysis was only possible for 343 patients, and this smaller sample size may have reduced the power so that there was no association between ΔP and in-hospital mortality. This could also be concluded from the results of the post hoc analysis of P_{max}, using the same smaller cohort of patients. Nevertheless, the finding that ΔP was not associated with in-hospital mortality is in line with a recently published investigation in a cohort of patients without ARDS [30]. In addition, the small range of tidal volumes used in this cohort also led to a small range of ΔP, which could blunt the effect of ΔP on mortality, which may be much subtler than is found in patients with ARDS [9]. Similar findings came from a recently published study that failed to find an association between ΔP and mortality, even though their results show a trend for higher mortality rates with each cm H_2O increase of ΔP [30]. Yet the influence of ΔP on outcome is consistent with previous reports exposing the importance of ΔP on development of pulmonary complications also in patients without ARDS undergoing general anesthesia for surgery [31], and on ventilator-induced diaphragmatic injury in critically patients receiving mechanical ventilation [32]. Similarly, experimental studies suggested an association between higher ΔP and development of VILI. In studies considering patients with ARDS, ΔP was the ventilation variable that best stratified mortality risk, even in those undergoing ECMO for refractory hypoxemia [9, 16, 28, 33, 34].

While higher V_T was related to worse outcomes in critically ill patients without ARDS [5, 6, 35], and with pulmonary complications in patients undergoing general anesthesia for surgery [36–38], in this analysis as well as the earlier reported primary analysis of PRoVENT [11], such an association was not found. The lack of a relationship between V_T and outcome in the present study likely reflects the widespread adoption of lower V_T ventilation, as V_T in our cohort concentrated in a narrow range around a median of 7.9 ml/kg PBW. With less patients receiving ventilation with high V_T, the association between V_T and outcome was no longer present. This finding is in line with the abovementioned recently published investigation in a cohort of patients without ARDS [30]. We are awaiting the results from two randomized controlled trials (RCT) testing different V_T in patients without ARDS [39, 40].

A higher PEEP level was not associated with outcome in our study, and this is similar to previous findings [8, 11, 41]. However, one small randomized controlled trial found that application of 'prophylactic' PEEP in non-hypoxemic ICU patients not only reduced the number of hypoxemic episodes, but also the incidence of ventilator-associated pneumonia [42]. Nevertheless, most trials performed so far that addressed the effects of PEEP on outcomes in ICU patients without ARDS were relatively small and mainly assessed other outcomes than mortality, for example development of pulmonary complications [8]. Well-designed RCT are needed to address the true impact of PEEP in ICU patients without ARDS.

We suggest that the risk of ARDS can act as an additive to 'injurious' ventilation, which can be explained by a smaller inspiratory capacity in these patients. When

Table 2 Characteristics of critically ill patients without ARDS receiving mechanical ventilation, comparison of survivors and non-survivors

	All ($n=935$)	Survivors ($n=738$)	Non-survivors ($n=197$)	p value[a]
Ventilator settings				
Mode of ventilation				
Volume-controlled	116/849 (13.7)	85/657 (12.9)	31/192 (16.1)	0.075
Pressure-controlled	193/849 (22.7)	151/657 (23.0)	42/192 (21.9)	
Pressure support	80/849 (9.4)	68/657 (10.4)	12/192 (6.3)	
SIMV	223/849 (26.3)	178/657 (27.1)	45/192 (23.4)	
BiPAP/APRV	185/849 (21.8)	138/657 (21.0)	47/192 (24.5)	
ASV	17/849 (2.0)	16/657 (2.4)	1/192 (0.5)	
PAV	0/849 (0.0)	0/657 (0.0)	0/192 (0.0)	
NAVA	1/849 (0.1)	1/657 (0.2)	0/192 (0.0)	
VAPS	8/849 (0.9)	4/657 (0.6)	4/192 (2.1)	
PRVC	23/849 (2.7)	14/657 (2.1)	9/192 (4.7)	
Other	3/849 (0.4)	2/657 (0.3)	1/192 (0.5)	
Ventilatory variables				
Maximum airway pressure (cm H_2O)	18.0 (15.0–22.0)	18.0 (15.0–22.0)	20.0 (16.0–24.0)	0.001
Plateau pressure (cm H_2O)[b]	16.0 (13.0–20.0)	15.0 (12.0–19.0)	17.0 (14.0–21.0)	0.005
No of patients	343/935 (36.7)	259/738 (35.1)	113/197 (57.4)	< 0.001
Tidal volume (ml)	500 (440–575)	500 (450–580)	500 (414–568)	0.229
Tidal volume (ml/kg PBW)	7.9 (6.8–9.1)	7.9 (6.8–9.1)	8.1 (6.7–9.2)	0.622
Controlled vent mode	7.7 (6.7–8.9)	7.7 (6.8–8.9)	7.8 (6.4–9.2)	0.958
Spontaneous vent mode	8.0 (6.8–9.2)	7.9 (6.8–9.2)	8.1 (6.9–9.3)	0.616
p value (controlled vs. spontaneous)	0.089	0.161	0.340	
≤ 7	242/811 (29.8)	188/627 (30.0)	54/184 (29.3)	0.181
7–8	347/811 (42.8)	271/627 (43.2)	76/184 (41.3)	
9–10	161/811 (19.9)	116/627 (18.5)	45/184 (24.5)	
> 10	61/811 (7.5)	52/627 (8.3)	9/184 (4.9)	
PEEP (cm H_2O)	5.0 (5.0–8.0)	5.0 (5.0–8.0)	6.0 (5.0–8.0)	0.004
≤ 5	450/830 (54.2)	365/642 (56.9)	85/188 (45.2)	0.003
6–8	253/830 (30.5)	185/642 (28.8)	68/188 (36.2)	
9–10	86/830 (10.4)	57/642 (8.9)	29/188 (15.4)	
> 10	41/830 (4.9)	35/642 (5.5)	6/188 (3.2)	
Driving pressure (cm H_2O)	12.0 (9.0–15.0)	12.0 (9.0–15.0)	13.0 (10.0–16.0)	0.020
Respiratory rate (bpm)	15.0 (12.0–18.0)	15.0 (12.0–18.0)	15.0 (12.0–18.0)	0.753
FiO_2	0.5 (0.4–0.6)	0.4 (0.4–0.5)	0.5 (0.4–0.7)	< 0.001
Static compliance (ml/cm H_2O)	54.2 (36.9–77.1)	55.4 (40.0–84.0)	54.3 (32.4–76.3)	0.121
Indexed static compliance (ml/cm H_2O PBW)	0.83 (0.65–1.27)	0.85 (0.66–1.33)	0.80 (0.49–1.09)	0.069
Minute ventilation (l/min)	7.4 (6.2–8.9)	7.5 (6.2–8.9)	7.2 (6.1–8.9)	0.409
Vital signs				
SpO_2 (%)	99 (97–100)	99 (98–100)	98 (95–100)	< 0.001
Heart rate (bpm)	87 (75–100)	85 (73–98)	95 (80–110)	< 0.001
Mean arterial pressure (mmHg)	78 (69–90)	79 (70–92)	73 (64–86)	< 0.001
$etCO_2$ (mmHg)	36 (30–42)	36 (30–41)	36 (30–45)	0.976
V_D/V_T^*	20.0 (10.5–28.5)	19.2 (9.3–25.9)	21.5 (12.4–33.6)	0.077
Laboratory data				
PaO_2/FiO_2 (mmHg)	261 (165–367)	285 (187–393)	232 (139–342)	< 0.001
$PaCO_2$ (mmHg)	38.0 (34.0–45.0)	37.5 (34.0–45.0)	40.0 (35.0–52.0)	0.003
pH	7.36 (7.30–7.42)	7.37 (7.31–7.43)	7.34 (7.25–7.41)	< 0.001
HCO_3 (mEq/l)	22.0 (20.0–25.0)	22.0 (20.0–25.0)	22.0 (18.0–25.0)	0.090

Table 2 continued

	All ($n=935$)	Survivors ($n=738$)	Non-survivors ($n=197$)	p value[a]
Clinical outcome				
Duration of ventilation (days)	2 (1–4)	2 (1–4)	2 (1–4)	0.974
ICU length of stay (days)	4 (2–10)	3 (2–8)	8 (3–16)	< 0.001
Hospital length of stay (days)	16 (9–35)	16 (9–34)	17 (7–37)	0.583

ARDS acute respiratory distress syndrome, *SIMV* synchronized intermittent mandatory ventilation, *BiPAP* biphasic positive airway pressure, *APRV* airway pressure release ventilation, *ASV* adaptive support ventilation, *PAV* proportional assist ventilation, *NAVA* neurally adjusted ventilatory assist, *VAPS* volume-assured pressure support, *PRVC* pressure-regulated volume control, *PEEP* positive end-expiratory pressure, *$etCO_2$* end-tidal carbon dioxide, *FiO_2* inspired fraction of oxygen, *PaO_2* partial pressure of oxygen, *$PaCO_2$* partial pressure of carbon dioxide, *HCO_3* bicarbonate, *PBW* predicted body weight, *BPM* beats per minute, V_D/V_T dead space fraction, *SpO_2* pulse oximetry, *ICU* intensive care unit

*V_D/V_T calculated as $(PaCO_2-etCO_2)/PaCO_2$

[a] p value is related to comparison between survivors and non-survivors

[b] Plateau pressure values are limited to patients in whom this value was reported and in whom either an assist control mode was used or in whom a mode permitting spontaneous ventilation was used

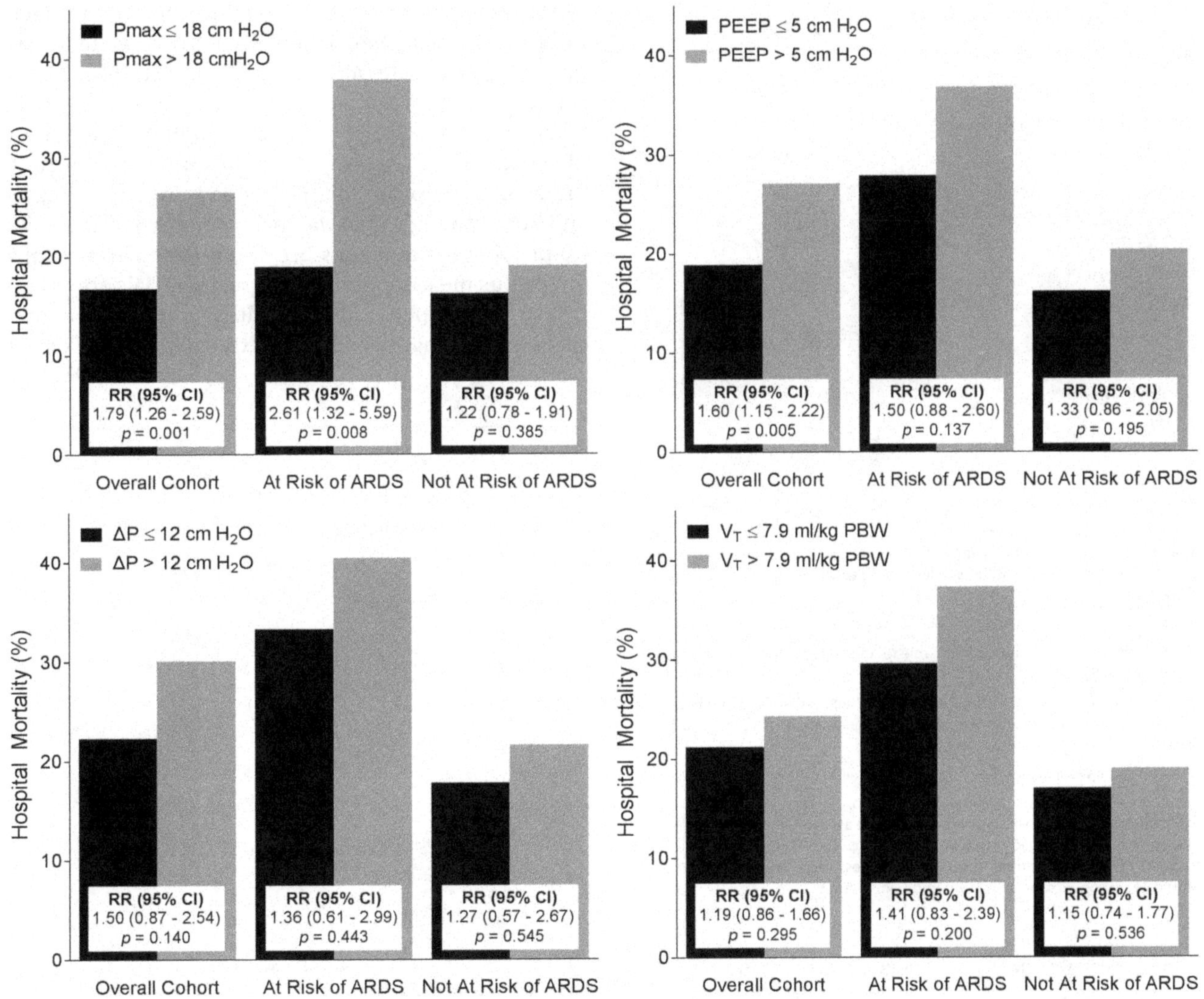

Fig. 2 Unadjusted relative risks of hospital mortality in the overall cohort and in patients at risk and not at risk of ARDS and according to the median of the: **a** P_{max}; **b** PEEP; **c** ΔP; and **d** tidal volume. Abbreviations: P_{max}: maximum airway pressure; PEEP: positive end-expiratory pressure; V_T: tidal volume; ΔP: driving pressure; RR: relative risk; CI: confidence interval

Table 3 Factors associated with in-hospital mortality in patients without ARDS receiving mechanical ventilation

	Odds ratio (95% CI)	p value
Clinical characteristics and comorbidities		
Age	1.03 (1.01–1.04)	0.001
Functional status		
Independent	1 (Reference)	
Partially dependent	2.18 (1.31–3.63)	0.003
Totally dependent	2.04 (0.83–5.03)	0.120
Hypertension	1.00 (0.63–1.59)	0.984
Heart failure	0.96 (0.57–1.63)	0.888
Chronic kidney disease	1.04 (0.56–1.91)	0.904
COPD	1.67 (0.93–3.00)	0.086
Immunosuppression	4.21 (2.12–8.36)	< 0.001
Severity of illness		
Non-pulmonary SOFA	1.14 (1.07–1.22)	< 0.001
LIPS	1.10 (1.02–1.20)	0.019
Management		
Use of NIV before intubation	1.09 (0.52–2.29)	0.824
Maximum airway pressure (cm H_2O)	1.05 (1.01–1.10)	0.020
PEEP (cm H_2O)	0.93 (0.83–1.04)	0.200
FiO_2	1.00 (0.99–1.01)	0.817
Laboratory parameters		
PaO_2/FiO_2 (mmHg)	1.00 (0.99–1.01)	0.247
$PaCO_2$ (mmHg)	0.99 (0.98–1.01)	0.886
Acidosis		
No	1 (Reference)	
Respiratory	1.35 (0.66–2.79)	0.412
Metabolic/Mixed	1.26 (0.76–2.10)	0.369
Vital signs		
SpO_2 (%)	0.95 (0.91–0.99)	0.027
Heart rate (bpm)	1.01 (1.00–1.02)	0.020
Mean arterial pressure (mmHg)	0.99 (0.98–1.00)	0.153

Mortality is defined as mortality at hospital discharge or at 90 days after start of invasive mechanical ventilatory support while still in hospital, whichever occurred first

All parameters were measured in the first day of ventilation

V_D/V_T was not included in the multivariable model because there were many missing values (68.8%)

Static compliance corrected by the PBW was not included in the model due to many missing values (64.8%) and to multicollinearity with P_{max} ($r = -0.351$; $p < 0.001$)

Driving pressure was excluded due to the multicollinearity with P_{max}

CI confidence interval, *NIV* noninvasive ventilation, *COPD* chronic obstructive pulmonary disease, *SOFA* sequential organ failure assessment, *PEEP* positive end-expiratory pressure, *FiO_2* inspired fraction of oxygen, *SpO_2* oxygen saturation, *BPM* beats per minute, *PaO_2* partial pressure of oxygen, *$PaCO_2$* partial pressure of carbon dioxide, *LIPS* Lung Injury Prediction Score

the inspiratory capacity is exceeded, stress failure occurs [43, 44]; thus, the level of a certain ventilation parameter could be well within the inspiratory capacity of a patient not at risk, while exceeding the smaller capacity of a patient at risk. These findings are particularly important since PRoVENT found differences between the ventilatory management of patients at risk and not at risk of ARDS [11]. While within the inspiratory capacity, the only independent variable for VILI is dynamic strain, i.e., V_T, above the inspiratory capacity, the combination of all ventilation parameters can lead to VILI and worse outcome [43, 44].

The present analysis has several limitations. It is important to note that we classified pulse oximetry as non-modifiable; however, one could argue that this is modifiable through adjustment of FiO_2. Also, although respiratory variables are potentially modifiable, adjustment of the ventilator can be influenced by certain non-modifiable factors that are present at the time of adjustment. For example, PEEP is affected by hypoxemia; some protocols allow higher plateau pressures in the presence of severe acidemia, and ΔP is directly influenced by changes in the respiratory system compliance. These interactions are complex, and ventilator settings may not always turn out to be modifiable when treating a patient. Another limitation is the use of maximal airway pressure in pressure-controlled mode as a surrogate for the plateau pressure to calculate ΔP, although this was only done when there was no proof of spontaneous breathing efforts to minimize erroneous measurements. Prospective trials are needed investigating specifically the directly measured pressures in the lung, including the transpulmonary driving

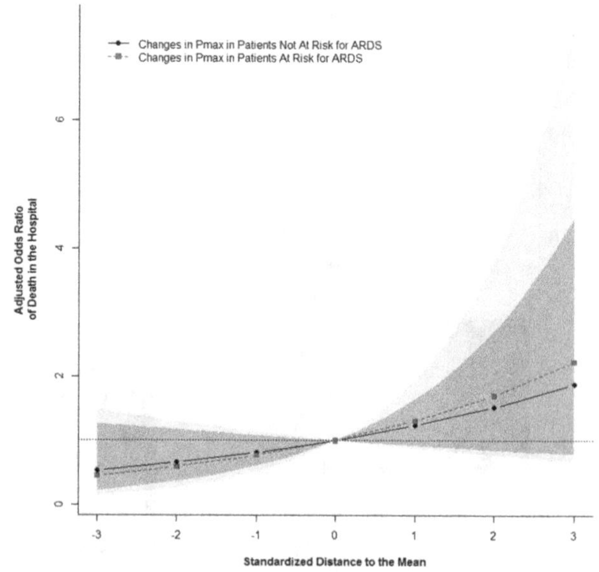

Fig. 3 Odds ratio of hospital mortality according to increases in one standard deviation of P_{max} and in the patients at risk and not at risk of ARDS. All curves are adjusted by the same set of variables described in Table 3

pressure, to explore their effect on outcome in patients without ARDS.

By identifying potentially modifiable factors in care of ICU patients, we indicate what future implementation studies should focus on to actually prove benefit of the suggested strategies on outcome. The identification of non- or less-modifiable factors points out which patients are more vulnerable and potentially may benefit most from an early start of protective treatment strategies.

Conclusion

The present analysis of a large prospective observational study suggests that higher P_{max} was a potentially modifiable factor associated with increased in-hospital mortality in critically ill patients without ARDS. Whether ΔP is also a potentially modifiable factor associated with increased in-hospital mortality needs further testing in larger patient cohorts.

Additional file

Additional file 1. List of PRoVENT network collaborators. **Table S1** Univariable analysis of factors associated with in-hospital mortality in patients without ARDS receiving mechanical ventilation. **Table S2** Analysis of factors associated with ICU mortality in patients without ARDS receiving mechanical ventilation. **Table S3** Analysis of factors associated with ICU mortality in patients without ARDS receiving mechanical ventilation considering driving pressure in the model instead of maximum airway pressure. **Table S4** Analysis of factors associated with in-hospital mortality in patients without ARDS receiving mechanical ventilation considering driving pressure in the model instead of maximum airway pressure. **Table S5** Analysis of factors associated with in-hospital mortality in patients without ARDS receiving mechanical ventilation considering maximum airway pressure in the subset of 343 patients in whom driving pressure could be reliably measured. **Table S6** Analysis of factors associated with ICU mortality in patients without ARDS receiving mechanical ventilation considering maximum airway pressure in the subset of 343 patients in whom driving pressure could be reliably measured. **Figure S1** Odds ratio of ICU mortality according to increases in one standard deviation of Pmax and in the patients at risk and not at risk of ARDS.

Abbreviations

APACHE: acute physiology and chronic health evaluation; ARDS: acute respiratory distress syndrome; ECMO: extracorporeal membrane oxygenation; $etCO_2$: end-tidal carbon dioxide; FiO_2: fraction of inspired oxygen; ICU: intensive care unit; LIPS: Lung Injury Prediction Score; PBW: predicted body weight; $PaCO_2$: partial pressure of carbon dioxide (in arterial blood); PaO_2: partial pressure of oxygen (in arterial blood); PEEP: positive end-expiratory pressure; P_{max}: maximum airway pressure; P_{peak}: peak pressure; P_{plat}: plateau pressure; RCT: randomized controlled trial; SAPS: simplified acute physiology score; SOFA: sequential organ failure assessment; VILI: ventilator-induced lung injury; V_T: tidal volume; ΔP: driving pressure.

Authors' contributions

The members of the Steering Committee of the 'PRactice of VENTilation in patients without ARDS study' (PRoVENT) designed and overviewed conduct of the study and this secondary analysis. PRoVENT collaborators, consisting of National and Local Investigators, collected the data. The study report was written by the PRoVENT Writing Committee and revised by the PRoVENT Steering Committee. ASN and MJS had complete access to all study data and performed the analyses, with support from FDS, MGdA, and PP. FDS, ASN, MGdA, PP, and MJS made the final decision to submit the report for publication. ASN was the study coordinator. FDS, ASN, MGdA, PP, and MJS contributed equally to this secondary analysis of PRoVENT. All authors read and approved the final manuscript.

Author details

[1] Department of Intensive Care and Lab. of Experimental Intensive Care and Anesthesiology (L E I C A), Academic Medical Center, Meibergdreef 9, 1105 AZ Amsterdam, The Netherlands. [2] Department of Intensive Care Medicine, Hospital Israelita Albert Einstein, São Paulo, Brazil. [3] Department of Pulmonology, Faculdade de Medicina da Universidade de São Paulo, São Paulo, Brazil. [4] Department of Intensive Care Medicine and CIBER de Enfermedades Respiratorias, Hospital de Sabadell, Corporació Sanitaria I Universitària Parc Taulí, Sabadell, Spain. [5] Department of Anesthesiology, Hospital Universitari Germans Trias I Pujol, Barcelona, Spain. [6] Department of Critical Care, Westfriesgasthuis, Hoorn, The Netherlands. [7] Department of Intensive Care, St Vincent's Hospital, Melbourne, Australia. [8] Department of Medical Sciences, Uppsala University, Uppsala, Sweden. [9] Department of Anesthesiology, Academic Medical Center, Amsterdam, The Netherlands. [10] Medical Intensive Care Unit, Division of General Internal Medicine, University Hospital Leuven, Louvain, Belgium. [11] Laboratory of Intensive Care Medicine, Department of Cellular and Molecular Medicine, KU Leuven, Louvain, Belgium. [12] Division of Cardiac, Thoracic, and Vascular Anesthesia and Intensive Care, Medical University Vienna, Vienna, Austria. [13] Department of Critical Care Medicine and Anesthesiology (SAR B), Saint Eloi University Hospital, Montpellier, France. [14] Department of Clinical Medicine, Trinity Centre for Health Sciences, Multidisciplinary Intensive Care Research Organization (MICRO), Welcome Trust, HRB Clinical Research, St James's University Hospital Dublin, Dublin, Ireland. [15] Irish Centre for Vascular Biology, Irish Centre for Vascular Biology (ICVB), Dublin, Ireland. [16] Department of Anaesthesia and Critical Care Medicine, Sheffield Teaching Hospital, Sheffield, UK. [17] Barts and the London School of Medicine and Dentistry, Queen Mary University of London, London, UK. [18] Department of Anesthesiology and Intensive Care Medicine, University Hospital Bonn, Bonn, Germany. [19] Department of Biotechnologies and Sciences of Life, Insubria University, Varese, Italy. [20] Department of Anaesthesiology, Düsseldorf University Hospital, Düsseldorf, Germany. [21] Department of Anesthesia, Critical Care and Pain Medicine, Massachusetts General Hospital, Harvard Medical School, Boston, USA. [22] Department of Anesthesiology and Intensive Care Medicine, University of Leipzig, Leipzig, Germany. [23] Pulmonary Engineering Group, Department of Anesthesiology and Intensive Care Medicine, University Hospital Carl Gustav Carus, Dresden, Germany. [24] Pulmonary Engineering Group, Department of Anesthesiology and Intensive Care Medicine, Technische Universität Dresden, Dresden, Germany. [25] Department of Surgical Sciences and Integrated Diagnostics, Ospedale Policlinico per la Oncologia, IRCCS per l'Oncologia, University of Genoa, Genoa, Italy. [26] Mahidol Oxford Research Unit (MORU), Mahidol University, Bangkok, Thailand.

Acknowledgements

We are indebted to all participating research nurses, nurses, physicians, and our patients. Without this support, PRoVENT and its secondary analysis would have never have been successful.

PRoVENT: 'PRactice of VENTilation in critically ill patients without ARDS at onset of ventilation study' (https://sites.google.com/site/proventtrial/home).

PROVE Network: 'PROtective VEntilation Network' (http://www.provenet.eu). The PRoVENT Steering Committee members & Writing Committee members are listed below; Collaborators are listed in the Additional supplement.

Members of the PRoVENT Steering Committee

Ary Serpa Neto (Academic Medical Center, University of Amsterdam, Amsterdam, Netherlands; Hospital Israelita Albert Einstein, São Paulo, Brazil); Carmen SV Barbas (Hospital Israelita Albert Einstein, São Paulo, Brazil); Antonio Artigas-Raventós (Corporació Sanitaria i Universitaria Parc Taulí, Sabadell, Spain); Jaume Canet (Hospital Universitari Germans Trias I Pujol, Barcelona, Spain); Rogier M Determann (Academic Medical Center, University of Amsterdam, Amsterdam, Netherlands); Barry Dixon (St. Vincent's Hospital, Melbourne, Australia); Goran Hedenstierna (Uppsala University, Uppsala, Sweden); Sabrine NT Hemmes (Academic Medical Center, University of Amsterdam, Amsterdam, Netherlands); Greet Hermans (University Hospital Leuven, Leuven, Belgium; KU Leuven, Leuven, Belgium); Michael Hiesmayr (Medical University Vienna, Vienna, Austria); Markus W Hollmann (Academic Medical Center, University of Amsterdam, Amsterdam, Netherlands); Samir Jaber (Saint Eloi University Hospital, Montpellier, France); Ignacio Martin-Loeches (Corporació Sanitaria i

Universitaria Parc Taulí, Sabadell, Spain); Gary H Mills (Sheffield Teaching Hospital and University of Sheffield, Sheffield, UK); Rupert M Pearse (Queen Mary University of London, London, UK); Christian Putensen (University Hospital Bonn, Bonn, Germany); Werner Schmid (Medical University Vienna, Vienna, Austria); Paolo Severgnini (Insubria University, Varese, Italy); Roger Smith (St. Vincent's Hospital, Melbourne, Australia); Tanja A Treschan (Düsseldorf University Hospital, Düsseldorf, Germany); Edda M Tschernko (Medical University Vienna, Vienna, Austria); Marcos F Vidal Melo (Massachusetts General Hospital, Harvard Medical School, Boston, USA); Hermann Wrigge (University of Leipzig, Leipzig, Germany); Marcelo Gama de Abreu (University Hospital Dresden, Technische Universität Dresden, Dresden, Germany); Paolo Pelosi (Ospedale Policlinico per la Oncologia, IRCCS per l'Oncologia, University of Genoa, Genoa, Italy); and Marcus J. Schultz (Academic Medical Center, University of Amsterdam, Amsterdam, Netherlands & Mahidol University, Bangkok, Thailand).

Members of the PRoVENT Writing Committee of this manuscript
Fabienne D. Simonis (Academic Medical Center, University of Amsterdam, Amsterdam, Netherlands); Ary Serpa Neto (Hospital Israelita Albert Einstein, São Paulo, Brazil); Marcelo Gama de Abreu (University Hospital Dresden, Technische Universität Dresden, Dresden, Germany); Paolo Pelosi (IRCCS AOU San Martino IST Hospital, University of Genoa, Genoa, Italy); Marcus J. Schultz (Academic Medical Center, University of Amsterdam, Amsterdam, Netherlands & Mahidol University, Bangkok, Thailand).

Competing interests
Rupert Pearse holds research grants and has given lectures and/or performed consultancy work for Nestle Health Sciences, Braun, Medtronic, Glaxo Smithkline, and Edwards Lifesciences and is a member of the associate editorial board of the British Journal of Anaesthesia. All other authors declared no conflicts of interest with respect to this analysis.

Funding
None.

References

1. Slutsky AS, Ranieri VM. Ventilator-induced lung injury. N Engl J Med. 2013;369:2126–36.
2. Sutherasan Y, Vargas M, Pelosi P. Protective mechanical ventilation in the non-injured lung: review and meta-analysis. Crit Care. 2014;18:211.
3. Putensen C, Theuerkauf N, Zinserling J, et al. Meta-analysis: ventilation strategies and outcomes of the acute respiratory distress syndrome and acute lung injury. Ann Intern Med. 2009;151:566–76.
4. Burns KEA, Adhikari NKJ, Slutsky AS, et al. Pressure and volume limited ventilation for the ventilatory management of patients with acute lung injury: a systematic review and meta-analysis. PLoS ONE. 2011;6:e14623. https://doi.org/10.1371/journal.pone.0014623.
5. Serpa Neto A, Simonis FD, Barbas CSV, et al. Association between tidal volume size, duration of ventilation, and sedation needs in patients without acute respiratory distress syndrome: an individual patient data meta-analysis. Intensive Care Med. 2014;40:950–7.
6. Serpa Neto A, Simonis FD, Barbas CSV, et al. Lung-protective ventilation with low tidal volumes and the occurrence of pulmonary complications in patients without acute respiratory distress syndrome. Crit Care Med. 2015;43:2155–63.
7. Briel M, Meade M, Mercat A, et al. Higher vs lower positive end-expiratory pressure in patients with acute lung injury and acute respiratory distress syndrome: systematic review and meta-analysis. JAMA. 2010;303:865–73.
8. Serpa Neto A, Filho RR, Cherpanath T, et al. Associations between positive end-expiratory pressure and outcome of patients without ARDS at onset of ventilation: a systematic review and meta-analysis of randomized controlled trials. Ann Intensive Care. 2016;6:109.
9. Amato MBP, Meade MO, Slutsky AS, et al. Driving pressure and survival in the acute respiratory distress syndrome. N Engl J Med. 2015;372:747–55. https://doi.org/10.1056/NEJMsa1410639.
10. Bellani G, Laffey JG, Pham T, et al. Epidemiology, patterns of care, and mortality for patients with acute respiratory distress syndrome in intensive care units in 50 countries. JAMA. 2016;315:788–800.
11. Serpa Neto A, Barbas CSV, Simonis FD, et al. Epidemiological characteristics, practice of ventilation, and clinical outcome in patients at risk of acute respiratory distress syndrome in intensive care units from 16 countries (PRoVENT): an international, multicentre, prospective study. Lancet Respir Med. 2016;4:882–93.
12. Thompson BT, Hayden D, Matthay MA, et al. Clinicians' approaches to mechanical ventilation in acute lung injury and ARDS. Chest. 2001;120:1622–7. https://doi.org/10.1378/chest.120.5.1622.
13. Esteban A, Anzueto A, Frutos F, et al. Characteristics and outcomes in adult patients receiving mechanical ventilation. JAMA. 2002;287:345–55.
14. Esteban A, Frutos-Vivar F, Muriel A, et al. Evolution of mortality over time in patients receiving mechanical ventilation. Am J Respir Crit Care Med. 2013;188:220–30.
15. Britos M, Smoot E, Liu KD, et al. The value of positive end-expiratory pressure and Fio_2 criteria in the definition of the acute respiratory distress syndrome. Crit Care Med. 2011;39:2025–30.
16. Laffey JG, Bellani G, Pham T, et al. Potentially modifiable factors contributing to outcome from acute respiratory distress syndrome: the LUNG SAFE study. Intensive Care Med. 2016. https://doi.org/10.1007/s00134-016-4571-5.
17. Serpa Neto A, Barbas CS, Artigas-Raventós A, et al. Rationale and study design of Provent-An international multicenter observational study on practice of ventilation in critically Ill patients without ARDS. J Clin Trials. 2013;3:2–7.
18. The ARDS Definition Task Force. Acute respiratory distress syndrome: the Berlin definition. JAMA. 2012;307:2526–33.
19. Zimmerman JE, Kramer AA, McNair DS, et al. Acute Physiology and Chronic Health Evaluation (APACHE) IV: hospital mortality assessment for today's critically ill patients. Crit Care Med. 2006;34:1297–310.
20. Le Gall JR, Lemeshow S, Saulnier F. A new Simplified Acute Physiology Score (SAPS II) based on a European/North American multicenter study. JAMA. 1993;270:2957–63.
21. Bos LD, Schouten LR, Cremer OL, et al. External validation of the APPS, a new and simple outcome prediction score in patients with the acute respiratory distress syndrome. Ann Intensive Care. 2016;6:89.
22. Chatburn RL, Volsko TA. Documentation issues for mechanical ventilation in pressure-control modes. Respir Care. 2010;55:1705–16.
23. Acute Respiratory Distress Syndrome Network. Ventilation with lower tidal volumes as compared with traditional tidal volumes for acute lung injury and the acute respiratory distress syndrome. The Acute Respiratory Distress Syndrome Network. N Engl J Med. 2000;342:1301–8.
24. Rubenfeld GD, Caldwell E, Peabody E, et al. Incidence and outcomes of acute lung injury. N Engl J Med. 2005;353:1685–93. https://doi.org/10.1056/NEJMoa050333.
25. Brun-Buisson C, Minelli C, Bertolini G, et al. Epidemiology and outcome of acute lung injury in European intensive care units Results from the ALIVE study. Intensive Care Med. 2004;30:51–61.
26. Dreyfuss D, Basset GUY, Soler P, et al. Intermittent Positive-Pressure Hyperventilation with High Inflation Pressures Produces Pulmonary Microvascular Injury in Rats. Am Rev Respir Dis. 1985;132:880–4.
27. Webb HH, Tierney DF. Experimental pulmonary edema due to intermittent positive pressure ventilation with high inflation pressures. Protection by positive end-expiratory pressure. Am Rev Respir Dis. 1974;110:556–65.
28. Amato MB, Barbas CS, Medeiros DM, et al. Effect of a protective-ventilation strategy on mortality in the acute respiratory distress syndrome. N Engl J Med. 1998;338:347–54.
29. Kregenow DA, Rubenfeld GD, Hudson LD, et al. Hypercapnic acidosis and mortality in acute lung injury. Crit Care Med. 2006;34:1–7.
30. Schmidt MFS, Amaral ACKB, Fan E, et al.: Driving pressure and hospital mortality in patients without ARDS: a cohort study. Chest 2017; 1–9.
31. Serpa Neto A, Hemmes SNT, Barbas CSV, et al. Association between driving pressure and development of postoperative pulmonary complications in patients undergoing mechanical ventilation for general anaesthesia: a meta-analysis of individual patient data. Lancet Respir Med. 2016;4:272–80.
32. Goligher EC, Fan E, Herridge MS, et al. Evolution of diaphragm thickness during mechanical ventilation. Impact of inspiratory effort. Am J Respir Crit Care Med. 2015;192:1080–8. https://doi.org/10.1164/rccm.201503-0620OC.
33. Estenssoro E, Dubin A, Laffaire E, et al. Incidence, clinical course, and outcome in 217 patients with acute respiratory distress syndrome. Crit Care Med. 2002;30:2450–6.
34. Serpa Neto A, Schmidt M, Azevedo LCP, et al. Associations between ventilator settings during extracorporeal membrane oxygenation for

refractory hypoxemia and outcome in patients with acute respiratory distress syndrome: a pooled individual patient data analysis. Intensive Care Med. 2016;42:1672–84. https://doi.org/10.1007/s00134-016-4507-0.

35. Serpa Neto A, Cardoso SO, Manetta JA, et al. Association between use of lung-protective ventilation with lower tidal volumes and clinical outcomes among patients without acute respiratory distress syndrome: a meta-analysis. JAMA. 2012;308:1651–9.
36. Serpa Neto A, Hemmes SNT, Barbas CSV, et al. Incidence of mortality and morbidity related to postoperative lung injury in patients who have undergone abdominal or thoracic surgery: a systematic review and meta-analysis. Lancet Respir Med. 2014;2:1007–15.
37. Serpa Neto A, Hemmes SNT, Barbas CSV, et al. Protective versus conventional ventilation for surgery. Anesthesiology. 2015;123:66–78.
38. Futier E, Constantin J-M, Paugam-Burtz C, et al. A trial of intraoperative low-tidal-volume ventilation in abdominal surgery. N Engl J Med. 2013;369:428–37.
39. Simonis FD, Binnekade JM, Braber A, et al. PReVENT–protective ventilation in patients without ARDS at start of ventilation: study protocol for a randomized controlled trial. Trials. 2015;16:226.
40. Corporacion Parc Tauli: Corporacion Parc Tauli. Preventive Strategies in Acute Respiratory Distress Syndrome (ARDS) (EPALI). In: ClinicalTrials.gov NLM Identifier: NCT02070666.
41. PROVE Network Investigators for the Clinical Trial Network of the European Society of Anaesthesiology, Hemmes SNT, Gama de Abreu M, et al. High versus low positive end-expiratory pressure during general anaesthesia for open abdominal surgery (PROVHILO trial): a multicentre randomised controlled trial. Lancet (London, England). 2014;384:495–503.
42. Manzano F, Fernández-Mondéjar E, Colmenero M, et al. Positive-end expiratory pressure reduces incidence of ventilator-associated pneumonia in nonhypoxemic patients. Crit Care Med. 2008;36:2225–31.
43. Protti A, Andreis DT, Milesi M, et al. Lung anatomy, energy load, and ventilator-induced lung injury. Intensive Care Med Exp. 2015;3:34.
44. Nieman GF, Satalin J, Andrews P, et al. Lung stress, strain, and energy load: engineering concepts to understand the mechanism of ventilator-induced lung injury (VILI). Intensive Care Med Exp. 2016;4:16.

15

Point-of-care ultrasonography in Brazilian intensive care units: a national survey

José Augusto Santos Pellegrini[1], Ricardo Luiz Cordioli[2,3,7*], Ana Cristina Burigo Grumann[4], Patrícia Klarmann Ziegelmann[5] and Leandro Utino Taniguchi[6]

Abstract

Background: Point-of-care ultrasonography (POCUS) has recently become a useful tool that intensivists are incorporating into clinical practice. However, the incorporation of ultrasonography in critical care in developing countries is not straightforward.

Methods: Our objective was to investigate current practice and education regarding POCUS among Brazilian intensivists. A national survey was administered to Brazilian intensivists using an electronic questionnaire. Questions were selected by the Delphi method and assessed topics included organizational issues, POCUS technique and training patterns, machine availability, and main applications of POCUS in daily practice.

Results: Of 1533 intensivists who received the questionnaire, 322 responded from all of Brazil's regions. Two hundred and five (63.8%) reported having access to an ultrasound machine dedicated to the intensive care unit (ICU); however, this was more likely in university hospitals than in non-university hospitals (80.6 vs. 59.6%; risk ratio [RR] = 1.35 [1.16–1.58], $p = 0.002$). The main applications of POCUS were ultrasound-guided central vein catheterization (49.4%) and bedside echocardiographic assessment (33.9%). Two hundred and fifty-eight (80.0%) reported having at least one POCUS-trained intensivist in their staff (trained units). Trained units were more likely to perform routine ultrasound-guided jugular vein catheterization than non-trained units (38.6 vs. 16.4%; RR = 2.35 [1.31–4.23], $p = 0.001$). The proportion of POCUS-trained intensivists and availability of a dedicated ultrasound machine were both independently associated with performing ultrasound-guided jugular vein catheterization (RR = 1.91 [1.32–2.77], $p = 0.001$) and (RR = 2.20 [1.26–3.29], $p = 0.005$), respectively.

Conclusions: A significant proportion of Brazilian ICUs had at least one intensivist with POCUS capability in their staff. Although ultrasound-guided central vein catheterization constitutes the main application of POCUS, adherence to guideline recommendations is still suboptimal.

Keywords: Ultrasonography, Critical care, Survey

Background

Point-of-care ultrasonography (POCUS) has recently become a useful and widely disseminated tool that intensivists are incorporating into clinical practice. Assimilation timeframe varies according to the geographic, economic, and structural characteristics in which the practitioner is working. POCUS assists physicians to diagnose different causes of clinical deterioration and respiratory and/or hemodynamic failure, to tailor medical interventions (e.g., fluid therapy and mechanical ventilation adjustments), and to guide invasive procedures [1–3].

Despite guidelines that recommend the use of POCUS in different scenarios of critical care [3, 4], the incorporation of ultrasonography into clinical practice is not

*Correspondence: rlcordioli@gmail.com
[7] Department of Intensive Care Unit, Hospital Israelita Albert Einstein, 627, Albert Einstein St., São Paulo 05652-900, Brazil
Full list of author information is available at the end of the article

straightforward. For central venous catheterization (CVC), recent data showed that 18% of French intensivists reported that they routinely use ultrasonography [5], while 44% and 37% of emergency medicine specialists [6] and anesthesiologists [7], respectively, reported never using ultrasonography for CVC guidance.

Previous studies assessed the implementation of POCUS in critical care [5, 8–10]. Methodologies for collecting data were varied: while some authors applied electronic mailing and waited for spontaneous return, or based their findings on self-reported previous experience, others adopted cross-sectional epidemiological sampling consisting of punctual observations [9]. Similar studies revealing ultrasonographic patterns of use in intensive care units (ICUs) in developing regions are still lacking.

Brazil's large territory and policies of public health system organization lead to challenges in access of health care personnel to the population, access to medical education, and the incorporation of new technologies into clinical practice. Therefore, precise information about regionalization, training methods, and preferential applications could help guide national entities in achieving more efficient dissemination of ultrasonography across Brazilian ICUs, potentially improving the quality of delivered care.

Surveys are standard tools that are increasingly used for assessing various aspects of health care, including educational, technological, and organizational aspects [11], as well as for investigating translation from scientific research to clinical practice [12]. Consisting of descriptive or explanatory questions, surveys can support the incorporation of medical evidence in current patient care.

Therefore, the purpose of our study was to utilize a survey to assess current practice and education of POCUS by Brazilian intensivists, as well as to assess the dissemination of ultrasonography and main applications in ICUs across Brazil. By evaluating the frequency of use and barriers of implementing ultrasonography, we can identify gaps in medical education and incorporate recommended clinical practices to critical care.

Methods

This study was conducted with the logistic support of AMIBNet (the Brazilian network of research in intensive care) and *Ecografia em Terapia Intensiva* (ECOTIN), the national training program of POCUS for intensivists. No financial support was received from any source.

The ECOTIN program is an initiative of the Brazilian Intensivists Medical Association (AMIB), which was conceived in 2010. It consists of a board of POCUS experts who developed a teaching method and conduct short duration courses throughout Brazil. The ECOTIN course encompasses physical principles of ultrasound, knobology, echocardiographic and lung ultrasound basic techniques, as well as incorporating supervised, practical activities to allow participants to demonstrate expertise acquisition.

Questions were selected using the Delphi method. Four of the authors developed a set of questions of interest, which were then subjected to three rounds of appreciation. One author served as a facilitator, assessing agreement among the other three authors and providing feedback between rounds. Rounds were stopped when consensus was reached for all questions in the set. No physical meetings occurred. All of the panel members are formally certified intensivists and well-known experts in POCUS techniques and teaching. Three of the panel members are from the board of the ECOTIN group.

The survey consisted of 32 questions (Additional file 1) assessing the geographic location, type of hospital and type of ICU, availability of an ultrasound (US) machine, training in POCUS techniques, use and daily practice of US-guided CVC and other applications of POCUS (e.g., echocardiography, measuring the optic nerve sheath diameter, lung and abdominal studies), medical residents' education in POCUS, and perceived barriers to the implementation of ultrasonography. All questions focused on POCUS performed by intensivists, not on complementary exams done by other physicians (e.g., radiologist or cardiologist). Skip logic was used when appropriate to ease the burden on respondents.

A web-based platform (SurveyMonkey®, www.surveymonkey.com) was used for the survey according to recent recommendations [12]. Initially, a group of 12 ICU physicians tested the questionnaire. After an interval of 3 weeks, a retest was performed by the same 12 physicians to verify reliability. The survey was physician-centered and was directly sent to intensivists subscribed to the AMIBnet mailing list. The questionnaire was available for 6 months (from September 2016 to March 2017). Reminders were sent via e-mail to potential participants on three occasions, every 2 months.

Survey respondents were stratified according to the training status of POCUS: trained versus non-trained. Trained status was dependent on having at least one intensivist with formal POCUS training working in the ICU staff. Additionally, questions gathered data on the proportion of staff that were trained in POCUS.

Statistical analysis

Categorical variables were presented as absolute numbers and percentages and compared using the Chi-square test with standardized adjusted residuals analysis (for tables larger than 2×2) and the Fisher exact test (for 2×2 comparisons). A two-sided p value < 0.05 was considered statistically significant. Risk ratios (RRs) and 95% confidence intervals were calculated for associated measurements.

Multivariate analysis through Poisson linear models with robust estimation were constructed to identify variables that are independently associated with an important quality-of-care marker: US-guided internal jugular vein (IJV) puncture, in compliance with international guidelines [13–15]. A priori interest factors were those plausibly associated: the type of institution (university vs. non-university), presence of an intensivist on a daily basis, availability of a dedicated US machine, intensivists' formal certification in critical care, proportion of POCUS-trained intensivists (low vs. high level), and payoff. For the construction of the multivariate model, we used forced simultaneous entry—all candidate variables remained in the model regardless of statistical significance. Outputs from this analysis are summarized as RRs.

All analyses were performed using Statistical Package for Social Science (SPSS), version 21.0 (IBM Corp., Armonk, NY, USA).

Results

Characteristics of the study population

From September 2016 to March 2017, 1533 intensivists were contacted by electronic mail. Of these, 322 responded (20.7% response rate) from all Brazilian regions. Of the units where respondents were working, private hospitals represented 46% while clinical-surgical units represented 72%. Three hundred and three units (94%) had a certified ICU physician attending daily rounds (Table 1).

Two hundred and five (63.8%) of the respondents stated that they had access to a US machine dedicated to the ICU (Table 2). There were disparities throughout Brazil's territory in this subject ($p=0.017$). Availability of a dedicated US machine was more likely in university than in non-university hospitals (80.6 vs. 59.6%, respectively; RR = 1.35 [1.16–1.58], $p=0.002$).

US-guided CVC was the main indication of POCUS, representing 49.4% of indications, followed by bedside echocardiography (33.9%). Pleuropulmonary and abdominal ultrasonographic examinations were infrequently reported (8.5 and 8.2%, respectively). According to 59% of the respondents, chest x-rays are performed on a daily basis in more than 50% of the patients. This was negatively associated with the frequency of lung ultrasound examination ($p=0.028$).

Sixteen respondents (5.1%) stated that they use a prespecified form for summarizing data concerning examinations. The exam results images and clips) were electronically recorded 14.6% of the time.

Table 1 Baseline characteristics of the study population

Characteristic	*n* (322)
Region within Brazil	
Southwest	191 (59.7)
South	58 (18.1)
Northeast	43 (13.4)
Central-West	19 (5.9)
North	9 (2.8)
Hospital's type	
Private	148 (46)
Public	107 (33.2)
University	67 (20.8)
ICU type	
Mixed, clinico-surgical	231 (72)
Clinical	43 (13.4)
Pediatrics	22 (6.8)
Surgical	13 (4.0)
Trauma	12 (3.7)
Number of beds	
< 10	130 (40.5)
11–20	107 (33.2)
21–40	47 (14.6)
>41	37 (11.5)
Attendance of a certified intensivist during daily rounds	
Full-time (morning and afternoon)	151 (46.9)
Part time (morning or afternoon)	152 (47.2)
None	19 (5.9)

ICU intensive care unit

Competence and training of POCUS

Two hundred fifty-eight (80.0%) respondents reported to have at least one intensivist with formal POCUS training working in their staff (Table 3). We designated these as trained units for the following comparisons. We did not identify significant differences across Brazil's territory according to training. The most frequently reported training structure was one- to two-day courses (65%).

ECOTIN trained 53% of the participants. The implementation of the ECOTIN training method was associated with the type of hospital: 67 and 49% of university and non-university hospital workers reported ECOTIN training, respectively (RR = 1.35 [1.1–1.67], $p=0.013$). ECOTIN training prevalence was heterogeneous among Brazil's regions ($p=0.001$).

Medical residents were present in 69% of the units, including critical care medicine residents in 44%. There were no structured training modules for US-guided CVC in 54% of cases. Twenty-six respondents (8.1%) said that their residents use simulation techniques to learn how to perform US-guided CVC.

Table 2 POCUS characteristics

Characteristic	n (322)
Dedicated ultrasound machine availability	
No	116 (36.1)
Yes, without Doppler imaging	35 (10.9)
Yes, with Continuous and Pulsatile Doppler	63 (19.6)
Yes, with Continuous, Pulsatile and Tissue Doppler	107 (33.3)
Proportion of patients assessed by POCUS on a regular basis	
< 10%	124 (39)
11–25%	100 (31.4)
26–50%	55 (17.3)
51–75%	22 (6.9)
> 75%	17 (5.3)
POCUS type	
US-guided CVC insertion	156 (49.4)
Cardiac assessment	107 (33.9)
Lung	27 (8.5)
Abdominal	26 (8.2)
POCUS recording	
No recording	170 (54.5)
Registered on patient's records	102 (32.7)
Electronically stored and registered on patient's records	47 (14.6)
Medical report formally provided	16 (5.1)
Payoffs	
None	278 (90.3)
Only for the institution	13 (4.2)
Only for the physician	4 (1.3)
For both the institution and the physician	13 (4.2)

POCUS point-of-care ultrasound, *US* ultrasound, *CVC* central vein catheterization

Table 3 Medical trainment in POCUS

Characteristic	n (322)
Trainment status	
Yes—ECOTIN	60 (18.7)
Yes—ECOTIN and other courses	111 (34.6)
Yes—only other courses	87 (27.1)
None	63 (19.6)
Trainment modality	
1–2 days courses	163 (65.2)
2 days–1 week	46 (18.4)
1 week–1 month	8 (3.2)
> 1 month	33 (13.2)
Proportion of medical staff trained in POCUS	
< 10%	125 (50)
11–25%	68 (27.2)
26–50%	38 (15.2)
51–75%	11 (4.4)
> 76%	8 (3.2)
Medical residents	
Yes—Critical care medicine	138 (44.1)
Yes—Other specialties	76 (24.3)
None	99 (31.6)
Medical residents POCUS training modality	
Practice-based only	118 (54.1)
Lecture-based trainment available	44 (20.2)
Simulation-based	26 (11.9)
No trainment	30 (13.8)

POCUS point-of-care ultrasound, *ECOTIN* ecografia em terapia intensiva

As aforementioned, we stratified respondents and their respective units into trained versus non-trained units based on self-reporting of training. We observed that the training status in POCUS affected the pattern of some answers (Table 4), such as availability of a dedicated US machine, proportion of patients assessed by POCUS and the density of certified intensivists.

The most frequent POCUS applications were distinct according to individual capability ($p < 0.001$; Fig. 1a): US-guided CVC and pulmonary ultrasonography was positively associated with trained individuals.

The status of POCUS training was negatively associated with exam payoff: fourteen (5.6%) of the trained units reported payoffs, compared to 27.6% of the non-trained units (RR = 0.20 [0.11–0.39], $p < 0.001$).

US-guided CVC

According to the study participants, 58.5% of the units dealt with a monthly incidence density of less than 200 catheter-days and, in 54.5% of the cases, a catheter-related bloodstream infection of less than 2 events per 1000 catheter-days. The two most common approaches for CVC were the US-guided IJV (36.2%) and landmark-guided subclavian vein approaches (35.6%).

Respondents were questioned about the frequency with which CVC is US-guided in their units. In 22.8% of cases, IJV catheterization was "always" guided (in line with international guidelines). The most frequent answer was "only in specific situations" (45%). One hundred thirty-one (40.7%) of the participants classified the recommendations for routine use of ultrasonography when catheterizing the IJV as "weak". For subclavian access, 78% of the respondents reported "rarely" using US, while 5% reported routinely using it; two hundred twenty-seven (70.5%) physicians classified the recommendation supporting US for subclavian puncture as "weak".

Patterns of preferences for CVC according to training status are represented in Fig. 1b. US-guided IJV was the first choice for trained individuals (41%), in contrast to the landmark-guided subclavian approach (48.4%) for those not trained. Overall, eighty-five percent of non-trained individuals preferred landmark-guided CVC.

Table 4 Competence and POCUS

Characteristic	Trained (258)	Not trained (63)	Risk Ratio (95% CI)	*p* value
Dedicated ultrasound machine	184 (71.3)	22 (34.9)	2.04 (1.44–2.89)	< 0.001
High intensity of certified intensivists	160 (62)	21 (33.3)	1.86 (1.29–2.67)	< 0.001
> 10% of patients assessed by POCUS on daily basis	165 (64.7)	29 (46.8)	1.38 (1.04–1.83)	0.013
Routine US-guided IJV catheterization	96 (38.6)	10 (16.4)	2.35 (1.31–4.23)	0.001
Payoff	14 (5.6)	16 (27.6)	0.20 (0.11–0.39)	< 0.001

POCUS point-of-care ultrasound, *CI* confidence interval, *US* ultrasound, *IJV* internal jugular vein

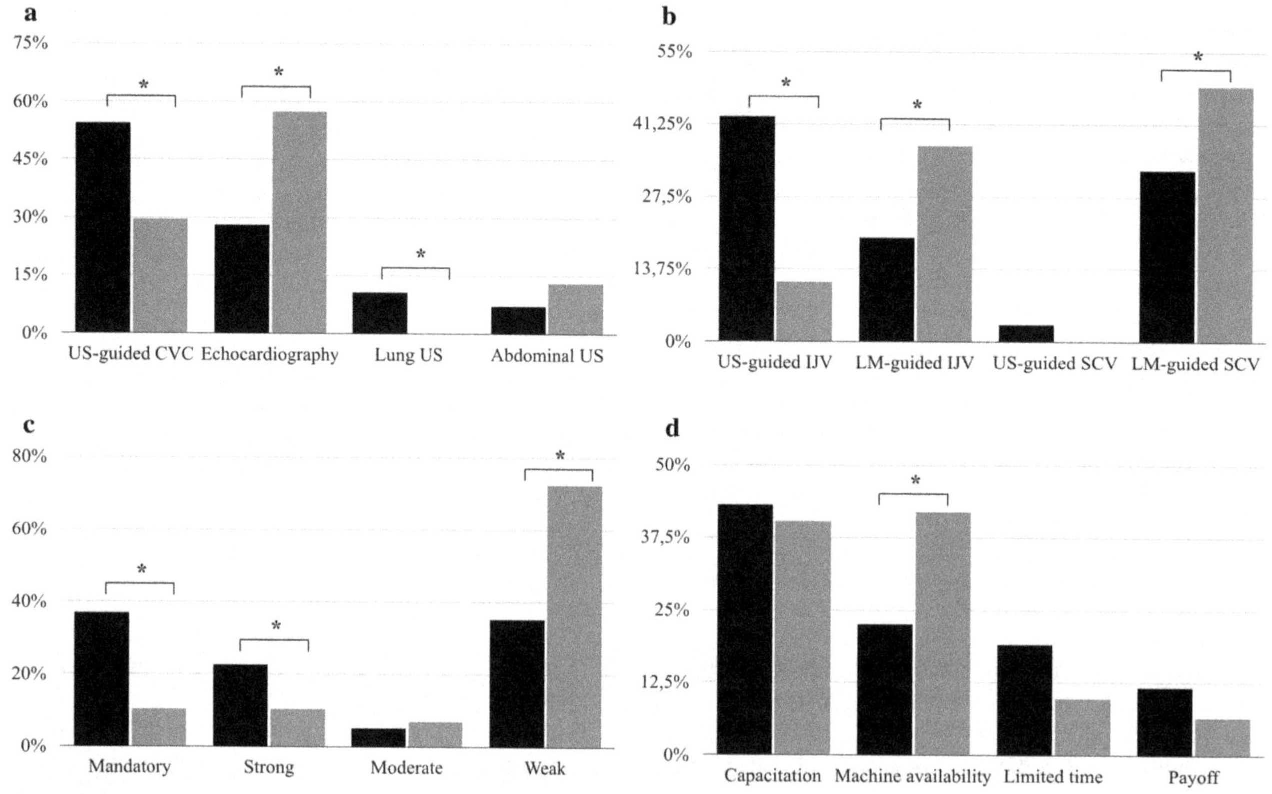

Fig. 1 Black bars represent trained units; gray bars represent non-trained units. **a** main types of POCUS application; **b** preferential venous access site; **c** perceived strength of recommendation for US-guided jugular vein catheterization; and **d** main barriers for ultrasound dissemination. See text for full explanation. *differences in prevalences with $p < 0.05$. *US* ultrasound, *CVC* central vein catheterization, *IJV* internal jugular vein, *SCV* subclavian vein, *LM* landmark

Physicians' perception about strength of recommendation for US-guided IJV catheterization appears to be affected by their training status. While answers of "routine use" or "strong recommendation" were associated with trained units, "weak recommendation" was associated with non-trained units ($p < 0.001$; Fig. 1c). For the subclavian route, the same pattern was identified ($p < 0.001$).

Other invasive procedures that were reported to be "usually" US-guided included thoracentesis (49%), paracentesis (31.5%), and arterial line insertion (27%).

Routine US-guided IJV puncture

Routine US (defined as more than two-thirds of the time) was used by 38.6% of the trained individuals compared to 16.4% of the non-trained ones (RR = 2.35 [1.31–4.23], $p = 0.001$).

Most of the factors plausibly associated with routine US-guided IJV puncture (as defined above) were statistically associated in univariate analysis (all factors except payoff). Considering multivariate analysis, two factors maintained independent association: dedicated ultrasound machine availability (RR = 2.20 [1.26–3.29],

$p=0.005$) and proportion of POCUS-trained intensivists (RR = 1.91 [1.32 - 2.77], $p=0.001$) (Additional file 2: Table S1).

Barriers for nationwide dissemination of POCUS

One hundred thirty-three (41.3%) of the respondents answered that physicians' training was the greatest barrier in the dissemination of ultrasonography across the Brazilian territory. When comparing the types of institutions, private hospitals responded differently ($p=0.012$); in these institutions, limited intensivist time when considering other tasks was more relevant than medical capability or other limitations.

Main barriers to the dissemination of ultrasonography according to the training status are represented in Fig. 1d. Non-trained respondents were more likely to classify the availability of a dedicated US machine as the most relevant barrier (not training itself) ($p=0.021$).

Discussion

The main findings of this survey can be summarized as follows: (1) availability of a dedicated US machine in Brazilian ICUs is still suboptimal; (2) US-guided CVC insertion is the main application of POCUS, followed by echocardiography, and lung ultrasonography is rarely performed; (3) a large proportion of assessed intensivists are trained in POCUS, but as there is a predominance of courses with a short duration and workshop structure, medical residents are being trained in POCUS in an unstructured fashion); and 4) training is associated with several aspects of POCUS application, including US-guided IJV catheterization, an important marker of quality of care regarding ultrasonography in critical care medicine.

Availability of a dedicated US machine is obviously a fundamental aspect for the dissemination of POCUS. While two-thirds of the respondents in this study reported having this machine in their units, authors in other countries [8, 16] have reported higher rates. Some specific regions in Brazil and non-university hospitals were less likely to have a dedicated US machine. Our results indicated that a dedicated US machine is independently associated with adherence to US-guided IJV catheterization.

Similar rates of training in POCUS were reported from 70 to 81% in Europe and the United States [6, 8, 9], although precise information concerning the training structure and specific curriculum is scarce. Other authors [5] have reported even higher rates. Our results on this subject, however, are unique: although previous studies [5, 6, 8] have focused on specific areas within POCUS education (e.g., US-guided venous catheterization or echocardiography), we assessed general aspects of ultrasonography of the critically ill. Additionally, we aimed to directly assess the intensivists and their self-perception of training, in contrast to previous studies [9] that designed questionnaires for ICU coordinators regarding their medical staff's capability. Medical residents in Brazil are beginning to learn ultrasonography in their education, although this is done in an unstructured and potentially heterogeneous way.

POCUS training issues are one of the major challenges of ultrasound dissemination in Brazil and other low- and middle-income countries. When heterogeneous training modalities coexist, it is difficult to ensure that all kinds of training provide comparable efficacy and competence acquisition. Standardization of training structures, both for medical residents and for those already working as intensivists, is needed, as those training structures influence intensivists' perceptions and use of evidence-based practices.

Reaching a balance between uniform accessibility to US machines and achieving minimum requirements of quality in care delivery remains an important future objective for Brazil. Realistic simulation should be provided in a method that is scalable and replicable. Medical associations of developing countries should contextualize international recommendations on POCUS training [17, 18] for specific guidelines in Brazilian (and other developing country) contexts.

Zielezkiewicz et al. [9] demonstrated in a 1-day prevalence study in Europe that 13% of the POCUS examinations performed were for central venous puncture, and that nearly half of the CVCs were US-guided. In the present survey, we assessed physicians' self-reporting practice, not real procedures; nevertheless, US-guided CVC insertion was identified as the major indication for POCUS by Brazilian intensivists. This behavior was also more pronounced in environments with a high level of training: the proportion of trained staff was identified as independently associated with adherence to US-guided IJV puncture. Overall adherence to routine US-guided IJV catheterization recommendations was relatively low (22.8%), compared to other critical care scenarios [19–21].

Lung ultrasonography, although infrequently reported, also showed a positive association with educational status. Lung ultrasound prevalence was negatively associated with routine chest x-ray, indicating a potential role of POCUS in reducing radiation exposure. This finding, however, is exploratory due to low adherence to lung ultrasound examination in this study. Other authors have previously reported similar data [22, 23].

Our results contrast with other studies, as US-guided CVC insertion represents the major indication for POCUS in Brazil. This could be explained by several reasons: the evidence concerning CVC guidance is solid, reducing adverse event rates and improving procedural success; the learning curve for US-guided IJV catheterization appears to be smoother than, for example, cardiac assessment and hemodynamic monitoring; some of the US machines available in Brazilian ICUs are relatively basic technology, and do not offer Doppler techniques or cardiac assessment software.

Our study has several limitations. First, inherent self-selection bias can influence our results. Physicians who already use ultrasonography were more likely to complete the survey; however, we obtained answers from a wide range of respondents from all Brazilian regions, representing private and public institutions, as well as clinical, surgical, and mixed units. Second, self-reporting, while providing direct answers from the practitioner, risks data precision. Instead of obtaining objective real-time measures, our study was based on physicians' impressions, which could be a distorted representation of actual practices. This limitation has been previously recognized [24]. Third, as we obtained direct responses from the intensivists, large ICUs could be redundantly represented, which could also bias our results. Nevertheless, our sample consisted of intensivists working in small units (40.5% had less than 10 beds) with part time intensivist presence (47.2%), indicating that although some degree of redundancy may have occurred, it was likely of minor influence to our results. Finally, we aimed to construct direct, objective questions that could reduce misunderstanding as much as possible. Our intention was to minimize the survey burden effect [25] that could potentially minimize our return rate. Nevertheless, our questionnaire was validated in a standard way, as previously described [12].

Conclusions

The rate of dissemination of POCUS in Brazilian ICUs is nearing rates reported in other countries. Although US-guided CVC insertion constitutes the main application of POCUS, adherence to international recommendations remains suboptimal. POCUS training, although including various relevant aspects of care, is heterogeneous, as is medical resident education regarding POCUS. Future research could address these gaps and help to better achieve POCUS dissemination in developing countries.

Abbreviations

CVC: central venous catheterization; ECOTIN: Ecografia em Terapia Intensiva (ultrasonography in intensive care); ICU: intensive care unit; IJV: internal jugular vein; POCUS: point-of-care ultrasonography; RR: risk ratio; US: ultrasound.

Authors' contributions

Drs. JASP and LUT had full access to all data and take responsibility for the writing of the manuscript, the integrity of the data and the accuracy of the final analysis. Dr. Ziegelmann was responsible for biostatistical consultation and data interpretation. Dr. Cordioli and Grumann contributed substantially to the study design, data acquisition, and analysis and interpretation of the results. All authors read and approved the final manuscript.

Author details

[1] Department of Critical Care Medicine, Hospital de Clínicas de Porto Alegre, Universidade Federal do Rio Grande do Sul, Porto Alegre, Brazil. [2] Department of Critical Care Medicine, Hospital Israelita Albert Einstein, São Paulo, Brazil. [3] Department of Critical Care Medicine, Alemão Oswaldo Cruz Hospital, São Paulo, Brazil. [4] Department of Critical Care Medicine, Nereu Ramos Hospital, Florianópolis, Brazil. [5] Statistics Department and Post-Graduation Program in Epidemiology, Universidade Federal do Rio Grande do Sul, Porto Alegre, Brazil. [6] Department of Critical Care Medicine, Hospital das Clínicas de São Paulo, FMUSP, São Paulo, Brazil. [7] Department of Intensive Care Unit, Hospital Israelita Albert Einstein, 627, Albert Einstein St., São Paulo 05652-900, Brazil.

Acknowledgements

The authors would like to thank the FIPE-HCPA (Fundo de Incentivo à Pesquisa of Hospital de Clínicas de Porto Alegre) for their support in manuscript publication.

Competing interests

The authors declare that they have no competing interests.

References

1. Lichtenstein D, van Hooland S, Elbers P, Malbrain ML. Ten good reasons to practice ultrasound in critical care. Anaesthesiol Intensive Ther. 2014;46(5):323–35.
2. Cardenas-Garcia J, Mayo PH. Bedside ultrasonography for the intensivist. Crit Care Clin. 2015;31(1):43–66.
3. Frankel HL, Kirkpatrick AW, Elbarbary M, Blaivas M, Desai H, Evans D, et al. Guidelines for the appropriate use of bedside general and cardiac ultrasonography in the evaluation of critically ill patients—part I: general ultrasonography. Crit Care Med. 2015;43(11):2479–502.
4. Levitov A, Frankel HL, Blaivas M, Kirkpatrick AW, Su E, Evans D, et al. Guidelines for the appropriate use of bedside general and cardiac ultrasonography in the evaluation of critically ill patients—part II: cardiac ultrasonography. Crit Care Med. 2016;44(6):1206–27.
5. Maizel J, Bastide MA, Richecoeur J, Frenoy E, Lemaire C, Sauneuf B, et al. Practice of ultrasound-guided central venous catheter technique by the French intensivists: a survey from the BoReal study group. Ann Intensive Care. 2016;6(1):76.
6. Soni NJ, Reyes LF, Keyt H, Arango A, Gelfond JA, Peters JI, et al. Use of ultrasound guidance for central venous catheterization: a national survey of intensivists and hospitalists. J Crit Care. 2016;36:277–83.
7. Bailey PL, Glance LG, Eaton MP, Parshall B, McIntosh S. A survey of the use of ultrasound during central venous catheterization. Anesth Analg. 2007;104(3):491–7.
8. Quintard H, Philip I, Ichai C. French survey on current use of ultrasound in the critical care unit: ECHOREA. Ann Fr Anesth Reanim. 2011;30(11):e69–73.
9. Zieleskiewicz L, Muller L, Lakhal K, Meresse Z, Arbelot C, Bertrand PM, et al. Point-of-care ultrasound in intensive care units: assessment of 1073 procedures in a multicentric, prospective, observational study. Intensive Care Med. 2015;41(9):1638–47.
10. Berlet T, Fehr T, Merz TM. Current practice of lung ultrasonography (LUS) in the diagnosis of pneumothorax: a survey of physician sonographers in Germany. Crit Ultrasound J. 2014;6(1):16.
11. Estenssoro E, Alegria L, Murias G, Friedman G, Castro R, Nin Vaeza N, et al. Organizational issues, structure, and processes of care in 257 ICUs in Latin America: a study from the Latin America intensive care network. Crit Care Med. 2017;45(8):1325–36.
12. Burns KE, Duffett M, Kho ME, Meade MO, Adhikari NK, Sinuff T, et al. A guide for the design and conduct of self-administered surveys of clinicians. CMAJ. 2008;179(3):245–52.

13. Lamperti M, Bodenham AR, Pittiruti M, Blaivas M, Augoustides JG, Elbarbary M, et al. International evidence-based recommendations on ultrasound-guided vascular access. Intensive Care Med. 2012;38(7):1105–17.
14. American Society of Anesthesiologists Task Force on Central Venous A, Rupp SM, Apfelbaum JL, Blitt C, Caplan RA, Connis RT, et al. Practice guidelines for central venous access: a report by the American Society of Anesthesiologists Task Force on Central Venous Access. Anesthesiology. 2012;116(3):539–73.
15. Troianos CA, Hartman GS, Glas KE, Skubas NJ, Eberhardt RT, Walker JD, et al. Special articles: guidelines for performing ultrasound guided vascular cannulation: recommendations of the American Society of Echocardiography and the Society of Cardiovascular Anesthesiologists. Anesth Analg. 2012;114(1):46–72.
16. Eisen LA, Leung S, Gallagher AE, Kvetan V. Barriers to ultrasound training in critical care medicine fellowships: a survey of program directors. Crit Care Med. 2010;38(10):1978–83.
17. Mayo PH, Beaulieu Y, Doelken P, Feller-Kopman D, Harrod C, Kaplan A, et al. American College of Chest Physicians/La Societe de Reanimation de Langue Francaise statement on competence in critical care ultrasonography. Chest. 2009;135(4):1050–60.
18. Expert Round Table on Echocardiography in ICU. International consensus statement on training standards for advanced critical care echocardiography. Intensive Care Med. 2014;40(5):654–66.
19. Jain MK, Heyland D, Dhaliwal R, Day AG, Drover J, Keefe L, et al. Dissemination of the Canadian clinical practice guidelines for nutrition support: results of a cluster randomized controlled trial. Crit Care Med. 2006;34(9):2362–9.
20. Reschreiter H, Maiden M, Kapila A. Sedation practice in the intensive care unit: a UK national survey. Crit Care. 2008;12(6):R152.
21. Safdar N, Musuuza JS, Xie A, Hundt AS, Hall M, Wood K, et al. Management of ventilator-associated pneumonia in intensive care units: a mixed methods study assessing barriers and facilitators to guideline adherence. BMC Infect Dis. 2016;16:349.
22. Peris A, Tutino L, Zagli G, Batacchi S, Cianchi G, Spina R, et al. The use of point-of-care bedside lung ultrasound significantly reduces the number of radiographs and computed tomography scans in critically ill patients. Anesth Analg. 2010;111(3):687–92.
23. Oks M, Cleven KL, Cardenas-Garcia J, Schaub JA, Koenig S, Cohen RI, et al. The effect of point-of-care ultrasonography on imaging studies in the medical ICU: a comparative study. Chest. 2014;146(6):1574–7.
24. Brunkhorst FM, Engel C, Ragaller M, Welte T, Rossaint R, Gerlach H, et al. Practice and perception—a nationwide survey of therapy habits in sepsis. Crit Care Med. 2008;36(10):2719–22.
25. Crawford SDCM, Lamias MJ. Web surveys: perceptions of burden. Soc Sci Comput Rev. 2001;19:146–62.

16

The safety and efficacy of nicotine replacement therapy in the intensive care unit

Ben de Jong[1*], Anne Sophie Schuppers[2], Arriette Kruisdijk-Gerritsen[2], Maurits Erwin Leo Arbouw[3], Hubertus Laurentius Antonius van den Oever[2] and Arthur R. H. van Zanten[1]

Abstract

Background: Studies evaluating nicotine replacement therapy (NRT) to prevent nicotine withdrawal symptoms in ICU patients have yielded conflicting results. We performed a randomised controlled double-blind pilot study to assess the safety and efficacy of NRT in critically ill patients. Mechanically ventilated patients admitted to two medical–surgical intensive care units and smoking more than 10 cigarettes per day before ICU admission were enrolled in this study. Participants were randomised to transdermal NRT (14 or 21 mg per day) or placebo until ICU discharge or day 30. Smoking status was confirmed by the biomarkers serum cotinine and urinary NNAL. The primary endpoint was 30-day mortality. Among secondary endpoints and post hoc endpoints, 90-day mortality, safety, time spent without delirium, sedation and coma, and patient destination at day 30 were addressed.

Results: We enrolled 47 patients. No differences were found between NRT and control group patients concerning 30-day mortality (9.5 vs. 7.7%, $p=0.84$) and 90-day mortality (14.3 vs. 19.2%, $p=0.67$). The number of serious adverse events was comparable between groups (NRT: 4, control: 11, $p=0.13$). At day 20, average time alive without delirium, sedation and coma was 16.6 days among NRT patients versus 12.6 days among control patients ($p=0.03$). At day 30, more NRT group patients were discharged from the ICU or hospital compared with controls ($p=0.03$).

Conclusions: NRT did not affect mortality or the number of (serious) adverse events compared with placebo. Time alive without delirium, sedation and coma at day 20 in NRT patients was longer than in control patients. An adequately powered randomised controlled trial to further study safety and efficacy of NRT in ICU patients seems feasible and is warranted.

Trial registration ClinicalTrials.gov, number NCT01362959, registered 1 June 2011

Keywords: Smoking, NNAL, Cotinine, Delirium, Agitation, Withdrawal

Background

Tobacco use is the leading cause of preventable deaths worldwide, killing 6 million people annually and reducing life expectancy by an average of 10 years [1, 2]. In 2015, 19% of the Dutch and 11% of the US population were daily smokers [3, 4]. For patients admitted to the intensive care unit (ICU), this is even higher and 25–47% are active smokers [5–7].

Active smokers admitted to an ICU, present more agitation, self-removal of devices, need for physical restraint and receive higher doses of sedatives, neuroleptics and analgesics [5]. Agitated behaviour might be a consequence of nicotine withdrawal, but may also be due to delirium or abstinence of concomitant alcohol and/or drug use. Until now it is unclear whether tobacco use confers higher risk of delirium during ICU stay [8].

Neuroadaptation leads to withdrawal symptoms in the abstinence of nicotine. Furthermore, smoking itself may

*Correspondence: benjongde@gmail.com
[1] Department of Intensive Care Medicine, Gelderse Vallei Hospital, Willy Brandtlaan 10, 6716 RP Ede, The Netherlands
Full list of author information is available at the end of the article

also lead to a variety of pathological changes in organ systems (e.g. cardiovascular diseases) and affect multiple biological pathways, potentially increasing the risk for agitated behaviour [9, 10].

Nicotine replacement therapy (NRT) has been shown to reduce withdrawal symptoms in nicotine-dependent subjects who quit smoking [11, 12]. Research addressing the efficacy of NRT during critical illness shows conflicting results [13–22]. However, irrespective of its potential side effects and in the presence of inconsistent data on safety and efficacy, NRT is prescribed to prevent withdrawal symptoms or to treat agitated behaviour in smoking patients admitted to the ICU [23].

We designed a randomised controlled double-blind pilot study to assess the safety and efficacy of NRT in mechanically ventilated and actively smoking ICU patients.

Methods

Trial design

We performed a randomised, controlled, double-blind, pilot study between July 2012 and June 2016 that was approved by the Medical Research Ethics Committee (MREC) of the University Medical Centre of Utrecht and registered at ClinicalTrials.gov, number NCT01362959.

Participants

Mechanically ventilated and actively smoking patients admitted to the medical–surgical ICU of two University-affiliated teaching hospitals, Gelderse Vallei Hospital (17 beds, GVH) and Deventer Hospital (12 beds, DH) were eligible for inclusion.

Exclusion criteria were: age <18 years, last smoking >72 h before inclusion, smoking ≤10 cigarettes/day, >48 h after hospital admission admitted to the ICU, expected duration of mechanical ventilation ≤48 h, pregnant or breastfeeding, history of dementia or psychosis, neurologic disease on admission such as traumatic brain injury, intracranial haemorrhage, seizures, meningitis, encephalitis, intracranial tumour, cerebrovascular accident, NRT<2 weeks before ICU admission, acute myocardial infarction, severe cardiac arrhythmia, unstable angina pectoris, generalised skin diseases, severe hearing deficiency, hypersensibility to nicotine or patches, insufficient Dutch language skills, imminent death or participation in another intervention study. Apart from regular exclusion criteria, we excluded factors interfering with the trial assessments and/or outcome or being a contraindication as mentioned in the Summary of Product Characteristics of the nicotine patches.

Written informed consent was obtained from all patients or their legal representatives. Retrospective written informed consent was obtained from the patient once mental capacity had regained.

Procedures and interventions

After inclusion and before the start of study drugs, blood and urine samples were taken to determine serum cotinine levels (Immulite 2000 nicotine metabolite assay, Siemens Healthcare Diagnostics Limited) and urine 4-(methylnitrosamino)-1-(3-pyridyl)-1-butanol (NNAL) concentrations (analysis according to Xia et al. [24]) to confirm inclusion of actively smoking patients [25, 26]. For women of fertile age, a pregnancy test was performed. Patient characteristics were recorded including age, sex, weight, length, medical history including medication and allergies, Charlson Comorbidity Index (CCI), patient type (surgical/medical), Sequential Organ Failure Assessment (SOFA) score, Acute Physiology and Chronic Health Evaluation (APACHE) II and IV scores.

Treatment allocation was performed using restricted randomisation with blocks of four, with a 1:1 ratio to NRT or placebo. Patients were stratified to patient type (medical or surgical), nicotine exposure (<21 cigarettes or ≥21 cigarettes/day) and study site (GVH or DH). After enrolment, healthcare workers not involved in ICU patient care performed randomisation. Randomisation codes were unknown to the investigators, ICU staff, patients and relatives.

Patients were treated with nicotine patches (Nicotinell® TTS 20 and 30, Novartis Consumer Health) or similar size and shape, placebo patches (DuoDerm® Extra Thin, ConvaTec), both subsequently covered by an opaque plaster (Fixomull® stretch, BSN medical). Patches and covers were applied and replaced every 24 h until ICU discharge or day 30 by nurses not involved in ICU patient care, while ICU staff was not present. Patients smoking <21 cigarettes/day received patches delivering 14 mg nicotine/24 h those smoking ≥21 cigarettes/day received patches delivering 21 mg nicotine/24 h.

Both hospitals involved in this study used sedation and agitation management protocols.

Trial assessments

After inclusion, patients or legal representatives completed the Alcohol Use Disorders Identification Test (AUDIT) and the Fagerström Test of Nicotine Dependence (FTND) to assess alcohol consumption and nicotine dependency.

Part of routine ICU care was the daily assessment of the Richmond Agitation and Sedation Scale (RASS) score, Confusion Assessment Method for the ICU (CAM-ICU) score, Delirium Observation Scale (DOS) score, Behaviour Pain Scale (BPS) and the Numeric Rating Scale (NRS) at 08:00, 14:00 and 21:00. During the intervention period (day 1 until discharge from the ICU or day 30), hours of physical restraint was recorded as well as self-removal of catheters, self-extubations, nosocomial infections according to CDC-criteria [27], medication prescribed and hours of mechanical ventilation.

At day 30 and day 90, patient destination and survival status was confirmed by reviewing the electronic medical record (EMR) or by telephone interviews with the patient or their representatives.

Serious adverse events (SAEs) were reported by attending physicians to the principal investigator (PI). Potential relationships to the treatment were determined according to the definitions from the Guideline for Good Clinical Practice (version November 2016). All EMRs were screened for adverse events by the investigators.

Outcomes

The primary endpoint was 30-day mortality. Secondary endpoints were 90-day mortality, ICU and in-hospital mortality, ICU and hospital length of stay (LOS), patient destination at day 30 and 90 (home, ICU, general hospital ward, nursing home, rehabilitation centre, deceased), hours with delirium assessed by the CAM-ICU or DOS-score, number of nosocomial infections, number of (serious) adverse events, number of self-removed catheters (i.e. arterial lines, peripheral and central venous catheters, nasogastric tubes, drains, urinary catheters), number of self-extubations, hours of physical restraint, hours without mechanical ventilation at day 30 (defined as persistent (non)invasive ventilation disconnection for at least 48 h), total dose of antipsychotics (i.e. haloperidol, olanzapine, quetiapine), RASS score and hours with RASS score outside the optimal range (score less than -3 and greater than $+1$).

A composite post hoc endpoint, reflecting return of normal brain function, was defined and assessed before unblinding the results comprising the number of hours alive without delirium, and without sedation (RASS ≥ 3) or coma. This endpoint was modified from a study addressing ICU sedation [28]. At day 10, 20 and 30, the average time spent with normal brain function between groups was compared.

Statistical analysis

In order to evaluate the feasibility of an adequately powered trial to study the safety and efficacy of NRT among mechanically ventilated patients and actively smoking before ICU admission, a pilot study was conducted, assessing time investment, safety and effect size on a smaller scale. The initial sample size was set at 70, accepting lack of statistical power for the primary outcome parameter. No interim analyses were planned.

Results and baseline characteristics were described as medians with interquartile ranges (IQR), means with standard deviations (SD) or as numbers and percentages (%) when appropriate. Continuous variables were analysed using Student's t test or the Mann–Whitney U test for normally distributed and non-normally distributed data, respectively. To analyse categorical variables Fisher's exact or Chi-Square tests were used.

Kaplan–Meier survival plots were generated for the 30-day and 90-day mortality, and the survival curves were compared with log-rank tests.

The primary outcome parameter was subjected to logistic multivariate analysis, in which the stratification variables (patient type, nicotine dosage and study site) were included.

A p value < 0.05 was considered statistically significant.

Data were collected in a database using Microsoft Office Access 2007 and were analysed using IBM SPSS Statistics 22 on an intention-to-treat basis.

Results

Between July 2012 and June 2016, eligibility was determined for 2715 admitted and mechanically ventilated ICU patients of whom 48 patients were enrolled: 27 patients at GVH and 21 at DH. As many patients met exclusion criteria, the inclusion rate was low. Therefore, after 4 years the study was stopped. The main reason for recruitment failure was elevated cardiac enzymes, often interpreted as a sign of instable angina pectoris or acute myocardial infarction, defined as exclusion criteria.

As one patient was excluded due to withdrawal of informed consent, 21 patients received NRT (of whom 62% a dose of 21 mg/day) and 26 patients received placebo. Baseline characteristics and serum cotinine and urinary NNAL concentrations were similar between groups and are shown in Table 1.

Primary endpoint

The 30-day mortality rates for patients in the NRT and control groups were 9.5 and 7.7%, respectively ($p = 0.84$, Fig. 1). Multiple logistic regression analysis using the 3 predefined stratification groups as independent variables showed no effect of NRT on 30-day mortality [OR 0.96 (0.11–8.23)].

Secondary clinical endpoints

The 90-day mortality rates for patients in the NRT and control groups were 14.3 and 19.2%, respectively ($p = 0.67$, Fig. 1). In the NRT group, fewer patients were still in the ICU or hospital at day 30 compared with the control group (1 vs. 11, $p = 0.03$), but not at day 90 (Fig. 2).

Table 1 Baseline characteristics of the patients

Characteristic	Nicotine replacement therapy ($N=21$)	Control group ($N=26$)
Age, years, mean (SD)	60.1 (10.55)	65. 2 (9.13)
Male sex, *n* (%)	12 (57)	16 (62)
BMI (m^2/kg), mean (SD)	26.4 (6.75)	27.8 (5.95)
Charlson Comorbidity Index, median (IQR)	1 (0–1)	1 (0–2.25)
APACHE-II score, mean (SD)	19.0 (5.03)	21.1 (8.60)
APACHE-IV score, mean (SD)	69.7 (19.01)	75.9 (34.20)
Admission SOFA score, mean (SD)	6.5 (2.94)	6.9 (2.94)
Patient type (medical), *n* (%)	16 (76)	15 (58)
Smoking (cigarettes/day), median (IQR)	20 (12.5–27.5)	15 (14.5–25.0)
Alcohol (units/day), median (IQR)	2 (0–4)	2 (0–4)
FTND score, median (IQR)	5.5 (4–7.75)	5.0 (4–7)
AUDIT score, median (IQR)	5.5 (0.75–12)	5.0 (1–10.75)
Receiving nicotine 21 mg/day, *n* (%)	13 (62)	NA
Serum cotinine (ng/ml), median (IQR)	70.6 (25.8–110)	80.7 (37.5–126)
Urine NNAL (pg/ml), median (IQR)	117.6 (62.5–156.4)	177.9 (116.9–325.4)
Inclusion GVH, *n* (%)	12 (57)	14 (54)

BMI body mass index, *APACHE* Acute Physiology and Chronic Health Evaluation, *SOFA* Sequential Organ Failure Assessment Score, *FTND* Fagerström Test of Nicotine Dependence [0–4 (very) low, 5 medium, 6–7 high and 8–10 very high dependence], *AUDIT* Alcohol Use Disorders Identification Test (score ≥ 8 hazardous and harmful alcohol use), *NA* not applicable, *NNAL* 4-(methylnitrosamino)-1-(3-pyridyl)-1-butanol, *GVH* Gelderse Vallei Hospital

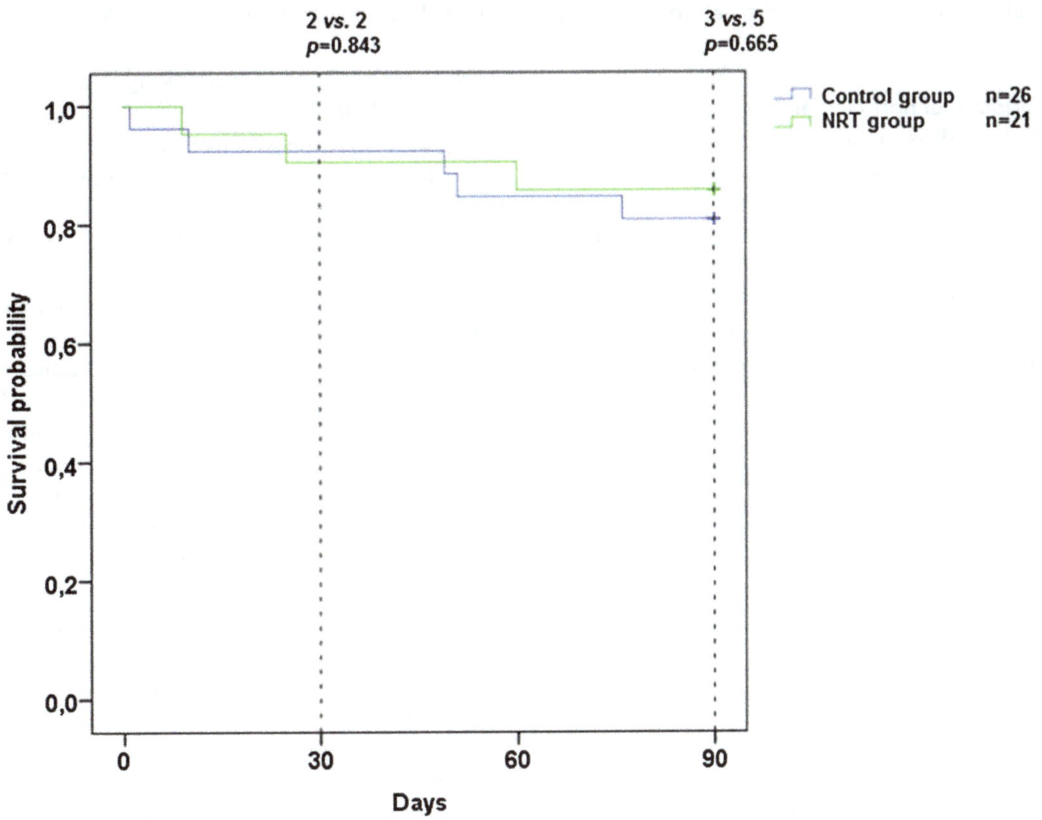

Fig. 1 30-Day and 90-day mortality comparing nicotine replacement therapy and placebo group. *NRT* nicotine replacement therapy

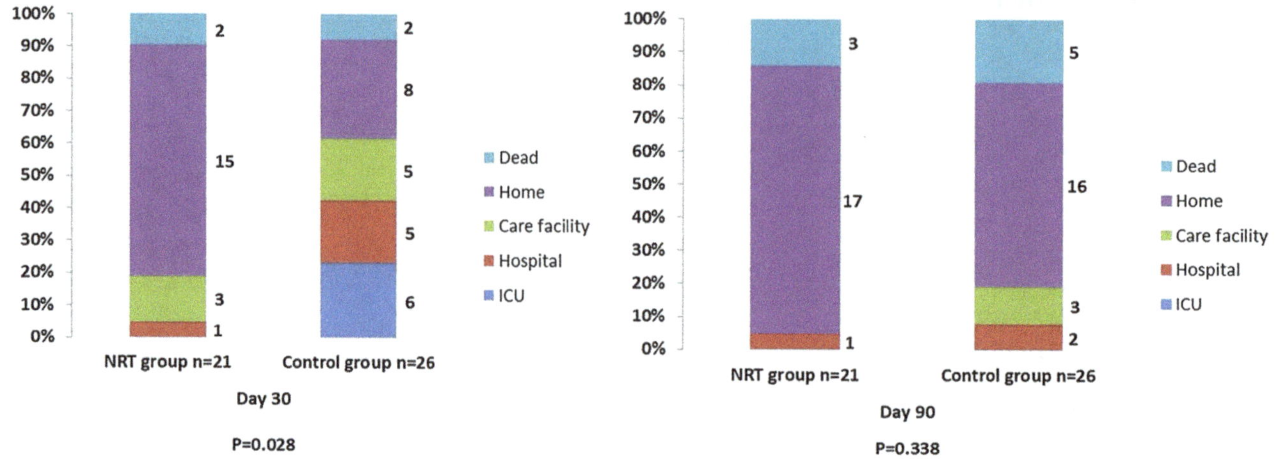

Fig. 2 Patient destinations at day 30 and day 90 comparing nicotine replacement therapy and placebo group. Data are presented as numbers. *ICU* intensive care unit, *NRT* nicotine replacement therapy

No differences were observed between NRT and control patients concerning in ICU and hospital LOS, hours without mechanical ventilation at day 30, total number of nosocomial infections, hours with delirium, time outside optimal sedation range, hours with physical restraint, number of self-removed devices and total dose of antipsychotics (Table 2).

Composite endpoint of normal brain function

During the first 10 days, patients receiving NRT on average were alive without delirium and without sedation or coma for 160 h, versus 88 h in the placebo group. The difference in time with normal brain function was 72 h, which was statistically significant ($p=0.04$). At day 20, this difference had increased to 104 h (i.e. >4 days; $p=0.03$). After 30 days, the difference was still 86 h, which was at that moment no longer significant (Fig. 3).

Adverse events

In total, 15 SAEs were reported during the study period: 4 in the NRT group and 11 in the control group. In the NRT group, two patients died due to respiratory failure after extubation, but with do-not-reintubate orders. The other SAEs were reintubation due to respiratory insufficiency after extubation and a spontaneous haemothorax in a patient admitted with a pneumonia and congestive heart failure. No SAEs were thought to be related to NRT.

The number of adverse events in the NRT group compared with the control group was similar (102 vs. 177, $p=0.10$, Table 2) as well as the number of cardiovascular adverse events (16 vs. 43).

Discussion

This pilot randomised controlled trial provides data on the efficacy and safety of nicotine replacement therapy from mechanically ventilated patients, who were actively smoking before admission. Using biomarkers to distinguish active from passive smokers (serum cotinine ≥ 3.1 ng/ml or urinary NNAL ≥ 47.3 pg/ml), all patients were classified as actively smoking [25, 26].

We could not demonstrate differences between NRT and placebo groups with respect to mortality and (serious) adverse events. However, NRT was associated with more patients being discharged from the ICU or hospital at day 30. Moreover, patients receiving NRT spent more time alive without delirium and without sedation or coma during the first 20 days. This beneficial effect lost significance at day 30.

Available cohort and case–control studies assessing the role of NRT in supposed actively smoking ICU patients have shown conflicting results. Some studies suggested that NRT was associated with clinical benefits such as less agitation or decreased mortality, while others linked NRT to adverse effects such as increased ICU and hospital LOS, more delirium and need for physical restraining, increased duration of mechanical ventilation and more use of antipsychotics and even increased hospital mortality [13–19, 21]. Due to the retrospective design of all studies except one, selection bias and confounders may have influenced the reported results. In addition, varying inclusion and exclusion criteria were used, relevant differences in baseline characteristics were observed within some studies and heterogeneous populations were studied. Furthermore, smoking history obtained from patients or their legal representatives in general underestimates tobacco use in critically ill patients and there are

Table 2 Secondary outcome parameters

Secondary outcome parameters	Nicotine replacement therapy (*N*=21)	Control group (*N*=26)	*p* value
ICU length of stay (h), median (IQR)			
Day 30	186 (127 to 278)	246 (88 to 694)	0.41
Day 90	186 (127 to 278)	246 (88 to 694)	0.392
Hospital length of stay (h), median (IQR)			
Day 30	313 (226 to 528)	408 (220 to 720)	0.356
Day 90	313 (226 to 528)	408 (220 to 885)	0.369
Mechanical ventilation-free hours at day 30, median (IQR)	559 (494 to 605)	515 (135 to 606)	0.152
Mechanical ventilation >48 h, *n* (%)	17 (81)	20 (77)	–
Only non-invasive ventilation, *n* (%)	2 (10)	1 (4)	–
Nosocomial infections, *n* (%)	7 (24)	22 (76)	0.285
Hours with delirium, median (IQR)	8 (0 to 44)	16 (0 to 86)	0.152
RASS score, median (IQR)	− 1.0 (− 2.1 to − 0.2)	− 1.3 (− 2.3 to − 0.7)	0.266
Highest score	1 (0 to 1)	1 (0 to 1)	0.615
Lowest score	− 4 (− 5 to − 2.5)	− 5 (− 5 to − 4)	0.132
Outside optimal range (h)	40 (0 to 64)	48 (14 to 122)	0.202
Physical restraint (h), median (IQR)	12.0 (0 to 85.5)	44.5 (0 to 123)	0.417
Self-removed devices, *n* (%)			
Self-extubations	1 (20)	4 (80)	0.245
Catheters	24 (40)	36 (60)	0.886
Total dose of haloperidol (mg), median (IQR)	9 (0 to 24.5)	19.5 (3.25 to 31)	0.185
Serious adverse events, *n*	4	11	0.129
Adverse events, *n*			
Electrolyte disturbances	36	49	
Gastrointestinal	27	40	
Cardiovascular	16	43	
Arrhythmia	5	19	
Hypo-/hypertension	10	18	
Cardiac ischaemia	1	5	
Elevated cardiac enzymes	0	1	
Pulmonary	5	8	
Renal	1	6	
Others[a]	17	31	
Total adverse events, *n* (%)	102 (37)	177 (63)	0.096

NRT nicotine replacement therapy, *RASS* Richmond Agitation Sedation Scale, *mg* milligram, *h* hours, catheters are urinary and vascular catheters and nasogastric tubes

[a] Others: fever, fungal infection, sinusitis, allergic reaction, skin lesion, subcutaneous emphysema, thrombocytopenia, anaemia, pancytopenia, bleeding, hypo-/hyperthermia, hypothyroidism, ICU-acquired weakness, hypoventilation (hypercapnia), hemiplegia, anxiety

no validated tools or questionnaires available to detect active smoking in ICU patients [25]. None of these studies used biomarkers such as cotinine or NNAL to confirm active smoking. Moreover, in case delirium was an outcome parameter, most studies did not use validated delirium instruments [13, 14, 19–21].

The only prospective pilot study that has addressed the effect of NRT in ICU patients ($n=40$) demonstrated no effect of NRT on the use of sedatives and analgesics or ventilator free days compared with placebo [22]. However, there was a trend towards shorter ICU stay in the NRT group compared with the control group [4.5 (±3.8) vs 7.0 (±5.8) days, $p=0.08$]. This study and our study suggested that NRT may lead to a shorter ICU and hospital LOS.

At study entry, brain dysfunction could be demonstrated in around 80% of patients in both groups. However, between admission and day 20, significantly more patients in the NRT group had regained normal brain function compared with the control group. This positive effect of NRT on brain function is in accordance with the time course of nicotine withdrawal symptoms, which peaks in the first week after abstinence and lasts for 2–4 weeks [29].

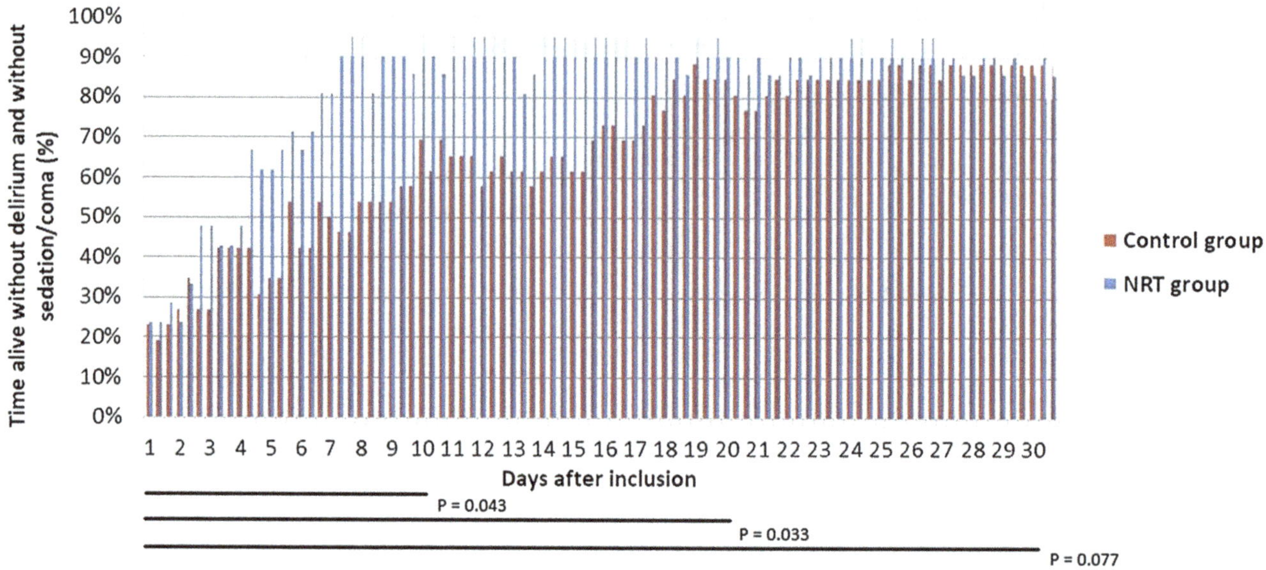

Fig. 3 Patients alive without delirium and without sedation or coma comparing nicotine replacement therapy and placebo group. Data presented as the percentage of time patients were alive without delirium and without sedation or coma (RASS ≥ -3). *NRT* nicotine replacement therapy

Our observation that the difference between groups disappeared after 3 weeks suggests that nicotine withdrawal symptoms may have vanished during the study period, and no beneficial effect of NRT on the withdrawal syndrome may be expected any longer after 3 weeks.

Strengths and limitations

Proper patient selection is essential to evaluate the safety and efficacy of NRT in critically ill patients. In our study, the smoking status had to be confirmed by a questionnaire and had to be at a minimum of 10 cigarettes per day. The FTND classified patients as smokers with medium nicotine dependency. Serum cotinine or urinary NNAL confirmed that all patients were active smokers. Thorough patient selection with subsequent biomarker confirmation assured the inclusion of actively smoking patients and increased the validity of our study.

The main limitation of the study is the sample size with increased likelihood of type-1 or type-II errors. The small number of patients in the treatment arm ($n=21$) precludes strong conclusions on safety and efficacy of NRT.

Recommendations for further research on NRT in critically ill patients

When a similar design to our study would be used, a RCT with mortality as the primary endpoint would need a sample size of at least 6000 participants to detect a 20% difference between NRT and placebo (alpha 0.05, power 80%). With respect to feasibility, we suggest to use a composite endpoint of time alive without delirium, sedation or coma as the primary endpoint in future trials. This would necessitate inclusion of around 200 patients to detect a 48-h difference (alpha 0.05, power 80%). We suggest an intervention period as long as the withdrawal syndrome lasts (3–4 weeks).

An important reason for recruitment failure was the clinical indistinctness between myocardial infarction or ischaemia and increased cardiac enzymes for other reasons. When in doubt, attending physicians chose to exclude these patients. For future research, we advise clear definitions of cardiovascular events and no exclusion in the absence of a clear diagnosis by using 12-lead ECGs, repeated measurements of troponins, echocardiography to identify regional wall movement abnormalities and eventually angiography [30].

Although in our study clear effects of the present NRT could be demonstrated, in general the dosages of NRT to be used in future research and the route of administration are still unclear. In non-ICU patients, NRT is used to maintain some of the nicotine effects, but also to reduce the addiction potential by reducing the dosage and speed of delivery. Higher doses of NRT seem to be more effective in achieving smoking abstinence compared with lower doses [31]. However, during critical illness the main reason for prescribing NRT is to prevent or treat agitated behaviour. As ICU patients might have subcutaneous oedema or are treated with vasopressors, absorption of transdermal NRT may be compromised. Thus, nicotine inhalation or an oral or nasal spray and administration at a higher dose may better mimic smoking behaviour and potentially be more effective and could be considered in future studies [9, 11]. At present, there are no scientific data on the use of non-nicotine products to treat or prevent presumed nicotine withdrawal in critically ill patients (Additional file 1).

Conclusions

Among patients, actively smoking before ICU admission and mechanically ventilated after ICU admission, transdermal nicotine replacement therapy had no effect on mortality compared with placebo, although our pilot study was underpowered to detect such difference. The numbers of (serious) adverse events between groups were comparable.

Patients in the nicotine replacement therapy group spent more time with normal brain function during the first 20 days after ICU admission compared with control patients. Moreover, at day 30, more patients in this group were discharged from the ICU or hospital compared with controls.

An adequately powered RCT to study safety and efficacy of NRT in ICU patients seems feasible and is warranted.

Abbreviations

APACHE: Acute Physiology and Chronic Health Evaluation; AUDIT: Alcohol Use Disorders Identification Test; BPS: Behaviour Pain Scale; CAM-ICU: Confusion Assessment Method for the ICU; CCI: Charlson Comorbidity Index; DH: Deventer Hospital; DOS: Delirium Observation Scale; EMR: electronic medical record; FTND: Fagerström Test of Nicotine Dependence; GVH: Gelderse Vallei Hospital; ICU: intensive care unit; IQR: interquartile ranges; LOS: length of stay; MREC: Medical Research Ethics Committee; NNAL: 4-(methylnitrosamino)-1-(3-pyridyl)-1-butanol; NRS: Numeric Rating Scale; NRT: nicotine replacement therapy; PI: principal investigator; RASS: Richmond Agitation and Sedation Scale; RCT: randomised controlled trial; SAEs: serious adverse events; SD: standard deviations; SOFA: Sequential Organ Failure Assessment.

Authors' contributions

BJ and AZ were involved in conception and design of the study. BJ, AS, HO, AK-G contributed to data collection. BJ, AS, HO, MA, AZ collected data analysis and interpretation. BJ, AS, HO, MA, AZ were involved in drafting the article. All authors were involved in critical revision of the article. All authors were involved in final approval of the version for publication. All authors agree to be accountable for all aspects of the study and manuscript. All authors read and approved the final manuscript.

Author details

[1] Department of Intensive Care Medicine, Gelderse Vallei Hospital, Willy Brandtlaan 10, 6716 RP Ede, The Netherlands. [2] Department of Intensive Care Medicine, Deventer Hospital, Nico Bolkesteinlaan 75, 7416 SE Deventer, The Netherlands. [3] Department of Clinical Pharmacy, Deventer Hospital, Nico Bolkesteinlaan 75, 7416 SE Deventer, The Netherlands.

Competing interests

All authors declare that they have no competing interests.

Funding

Not applicable.

References

1. World Health Organization. WHO report on the global tobacco epidemic, 2011: warning about the dangers of tobacco. Geneva: World Health Organization; 2011. p. 8.
2. Jha P, Ramasundarahettige C, Landsman V, et al. 21st-Century hazards of smoking and benefits of cessation in the united states. N Engl J Med. 2013;368:341–50.
3. Trend in roken volwassenen, 1990–2015. https://www.volksgezondheidenzorg.info/onderwerp/roken/cijfers-context/trends#definities. Accessed 11 Jan 2018.
4. Burden of tobacco use in de U.S.: current cigarette smoking among U.S. adults aged 18 years and older. https://www.cdc.gov/tobacco/campaign/tips/resources/data/cigarette-smoking-in-united-states.html. Accessed 11 Jan 2018.
5. Lucidarme O, Seguin A, Daubin C, et al. Nicotine withdrawal and agitation in ventilated critically ill patients. Crit Care. 2010;14(2):R58.
6. Van Rompaey B, Elseviers MM, Schuurmans MJ, et al. Risk factors for delirium in intensive care patients: a prospective cohort study. Crit Care. 2009;13(3):R77.
7. Moller AM, Pedersen T, Villebro N, et al. A study of the impact of long-term tobacco smoking on postoperative intensive care admission. Anaesthesia. 2003;58(1):55–9.
8. Zaal IJ, Devlin JW, Peelen LM, et al. A systematic review of risk factors for delirium in the ICU. Crit Care Med. 2015;43(1):40–7.
9. Benowitz NL. Nicotine addiction. N Engl J Med. 2010;362(24):2295–303.
10. National Center for Chronic Disease Prevention and Health Promotion (US) office on smoking and health. The health consequences of smoking—50 years of progress: a report of the surgeon general. Atlanta (GA): Centers for Disease Control and Prevention (US); 2014. Chapter 5 (Nicotine) and Chapter 8 (Cardiovascular Diseases).
11. Hatsukami DK, Stead LF, Gupta PC. Tobacco addiction. Lancet. 2008;371(9629):2027–38.
12. Fagerström KO, Schneider NG, Lunell E. Effectiveness of nicotine patch and nicotine gum as individual versus combined treatment for tobacco withdrawal symptoms. Psychopharmacology. 1993;111(3):271–7.
13. Mayer SA, Chong JY, Ridgway E, et al. Delirium from nicotine withdrawal in neuro-ICU patients. Neurology. 2001;57(3):551–3.
14. Honisett TD. Nicotine replacement therapy for smokers admitted to intensive care. Intensive Crit Care Nurs. 2001;17(6):18–21.
15. Lee AH, Afessa B. The association of nicotine replacement therapy with mortality in a medical intensive care unit. Crit Care Med. 2007;35(6):1517–21.
16. Paciullo CA, Short MR, Steinke DT, et al. Impact of nicotine replacement therapy on postoperative mortality following coronary artery bypass graft surgery. Ann Pharmacother. 2009;43(7):1197–202.
17. Panos NG, Tesoro EP, Kim KS, et al. Outcomes associated with transdermal nicotine replacement therapy in a neurosurgery intensive care unit. Am J Health Syst Pharm. 2010;67(16):13571361.
18. Cartin-Ceba R, Warner DO, Hays JT, et al. Nicotine replacement therapy in critically ill patients: a prospective observational cohort study. Crit Care Med. 2011;39(7):1635–40.
19. Seder DB, Schmidt JM, Badjatia N, et al. Transdermal nicotine replacement therapy in cigarette smokers with acute subarachnoid hemorrhage. Neurocrit Care. 2011;14(1):77–83.
20. Gillies MA, McKenzie CA, Whiteley C, et al. Safety of nicotine replacement therapy in critically ill smokers: a retrospective cohort study. Intensive Care Med. 2012;38(10):1683–8.
21. Kerr A, McVey JT, Wood AM, et al. Safety of nicotine replacement therapy in critically ill smokers: a retrospective cohort study. Anaesth Intensive Care. 2016;44(6):758–61.
22. Pathak V, Rendon ISH, Lupu R, et al. Outcome of nicotine replacement therapy in patients admitted to ICU: a randomized controlled double-blind prospective pilot study. Respir Care. 2013;58(10):1625–9.
23. Kowalski M, Udy AA, McRobbie HJ, et al. Nicotine replacement therapy for agitation and delirium management in the intensive care unit: a systematic review of the literature. J Intensive Care. 2016;15(4):69.
24. Xia Y, McGuffey JE, Bhattacharyya S, et al. Analysis of the tobacco-specific nitrosamine 4-(methylnitrosamino)-1-(3-pyridyl)-1-butanol in urine by extraction on a molecularly imprinted polymer column and liquid chromatography/atmospheric pressure ionization tandem mass spectrometry. Anal Chem. 2005;77(23):7639–45.

25. Hsieh SJ, Ware LB, Eisner MD, et al. Biomarkers increase detection of active smoking and secondhand smoke exposure in critically ill patients. Crit Care Med. 2011;39(1):40–5.
26. Goniewicz ML, Eisner MD, Lazcano-Ponce E, et al. Comparison of urine cotinine and the tobacco-specific nitrosamine metabolite 4-(methylnitrosamino)-1-(3-pyridyl)-1-butanol (NNAL) and their ratio to discriminate active from passive smoking. Nicotine Tob Res. 2011;13(3):202–8.
27. Horan TC, Andrus M, Duceck MA. CDC/NHSN surveillance definition of health care-associated infection and criteria for specific types of infections in the acute care setting. Am J Infect Control. 2008;36(5):309–32.
28. Pandharipande PP, Pun BT, Herr DL, et al. Effect of sedation with dexme detomidine vs lorazepam on acute brain dysfunction in mechanically ventilated patients: the MENDS randomized controlled trial. JAMA. 2007;298(22):2644–53.
29. Hughes JR. Effects of abstinence from tobacco: valid symptoms and time course. Nicotine Tob Res. 2007;9(3):315–27.
30. Carroll I, Mount T, Atkinson D. Myocardial infarction in intensive care units: a systematic review of diagnosis and treatment. J Intensive Care Soc. 2016;17(4):314–25.
31. Stead LF, Perera R, Bullen C, et al. Nicotine replacement therapy for smoking cessation. Cochrane Database Syst Rev. 2012. https://doi.org/10.1002/14651858.cd000146.pub4.

17

Hypoxemia in the ICU: prevalence, treatment, and outcome

SRLF Trial Group*

Abstract

Background: Information is limited regarding the prevalence, management, and outcome of hypoxemia among intensive care unit (ICU) patients. We assessed the prevalence and severity of hypoxemia in ICU patients and analyzed the management and outcomes of hypoxemic patients.

Methods: This is a multinational, multicenter, 1-day point prevalence study in 117 ICUs during the spring of 2016. All patients hospitalized in an ICU on the day of the study could be enrolled. Hypoxemia was defined as a PaO_2/FiO_2 ratio ≤ 300 mmHg and classified as mild (PaO_2/FiO_2 between 300 and 201), moderate (PaO_2/FiO_2 between 200 and 101), and severe ($PaO_2/FiO_2 \leq 100$ mmHg).

Results: Of 1604 patients included, 859 (54%, 95% CI 51–56%) were hypoxemic, 51% with mild ($n=440$), 40% with moderate ($n=345$), and 9% ($n=74$) with severe hypoxemia. Among hypoxemic patients, 61% ($n=525$) were treated with invasive ventilation, 10% ($n=84$) with non-invasive ventilation, 5% ($n=45$) with high-flow oxygen therapy, 22% ($n=191$) with standard oxygen, and 1.6% ($n=14$) did not receive oxygen. Protective ventilation was widely used in invasively ventilated patients. Twenty-one percent of hypoxemic patients ($n=178$) met criteria for acute respiratory distress syndrome (ARDS) including 65 patients (37%) with mild, 82 (46%) with moderate, and 31 (17%) with severe ARDS. ICU mortality was 27% in hypoxemic patients and significantly differed according to severity: 21% in mild, 26% in moderate, and 50% in patients with severe hypoxemia, $p<0.001$. Multivariate Cox regression identified moderate and severe hypoxemia as independent factors of ICU mortality compared to mild hypoxemia (adjusted hazard ratio 1.38 [1.00–1.90] and 2.65 [1.69–4.15], respectively).

Conclusions: Hypoxemia affected more than half of ICU patients in this 1-day point prevalence study, but only 21% of patients had ARDS criteria. Severity of hypoxemia was an independent risk factor of mortality among hypoxemic patients.

Keywords: Hypoxemia, Epidemiology, Critical care, ARDS-acute respiratory failure, Invasive ventilation

Background

Hypoxemia is frequent and potentially life-threatening in critically ill patients. However, the prevalence, management, and outcomes of hypoxemia in non-selected intensive care unit (ICU) patients are poorly known. Most epidemiological studies have specifically focused on patients under mechanical ventilation [1–3] or those with criteria for acute respiratory distress syndrome (ARDS) [4–9], and none covered the entire spectrum of the whole hypoxemic patients. Whereas mechanical ventilation may be needed in non-hypoxemic patients, a number of hypoxemic patients are treated with oxygen while breathing spontaneously. The proportion of hypoxemic patients treated with standard or high-flow oxygen therapy and without need for mechanical ventilation is unknown among the whole patients in the ICU. Moreover, whereas the severity of hypoxemia was directly associated with mortality in patients with ARDS [10], this relation is not demonstrated among the other hypoxemic patients, especially in non-intubated patients. Finally, the

*Correspondence: david.grimaldi@erasme.ulb.ac.be
Brussels, Belgium

relationship between respiratory support, hypoxemia severity, and outcome is not straightforward. It appears then important to provide epidemiological data regarding these gaps of knowledge that could help to design future trials on acute respiratory failure.

Therefore, we designed a large, multicenter, 1-day point prevalence study to measure the prevalence of hypoxemia (defined as a PaO_2/FiO_2 ratio ≤ 300 mmHg) among all ICU patients regardless of their oxygenation device and to stratify them according to the severity of hypoxemia (PaO_2/FiO_2 between 300 and 201 in mild, between 200 and 101 in moderate, and below or equal to 100 mmHg in severe). We also analyzed the potential impact of hypoxemia and its severity on outcome.

Patients and methods

Study design

The SPECTRUM study was a 1-day point prevalence study, endorsed by the French Intensive Care Society (Société de Réanimation de Langue Française: www.srlf.org) and conducted during the spring of 2016 in 117 ICUs in 7 French-speaking countries (62 general ICUs, 36 medical ICUs, 19 surgical ICUs). Additional file 1: Table S1 lists the participating centers and their characteristics. All patients already hospitalized in a participating ICU or newly admitted the day of the study could be enrolled. Exclusion criteria were refusal to participate and in France, being under guardianship, without social insurance, or being pregnant. Approval by the ethics committees according to the laws of each participating country was obtained (CE SRLF 15–35). In France, EC waived from written informed consent, and according to French law, the absence of opposition was obtained from patients or a next of kin before study enrollment.

Definitions

Hypoxemia was defined as a PaO_2/FiO_2 ratio of 300 mmHg or less [5]. We stratified hypoxemia severity as mild for PaO_2/FiO_2 between 300 and 201 mmHg, moderate for PaO_2/FiO_2 between 200 and 101 mmHg, and severe for PaO_2/FiO_2 below or equal to 100 mmHg. ARDS was defined according to the Berlin definition [10]. Each single criterion of the ARDS definition was collected separately in the case report form. Patients fulfilling all the criteria were classified as having ARDS. Potential causes of ARDS were collected independently of the presence of hypoxemia and ARDS. Other causes/mechanisms of hypoxemia were also collected.

Oxygenation administration was classified as: no oxygen supply (ambient air), low-flow (conventional) oxygen whatever the device used (nasal cannula, mask, tracheostomy), high-flow oxygen through nasal cannula, noninvasive ventilation (NIV) whatever the modalities of ventilation, invasive ventilation through tracheal intubation or tracheostomy, and extracorporeal oxygenation. Patients with intermittent modes were classified with the mode in use at the time of data collection.

Data collection

All data were assessed at the time of arterial blood gas measurement during the morning round. In cases where no arterial blood was drawn, data were recorded when the patient had an $SpO_2 \leq 97\%$. Follow-up was restricted to ICU stay and censored at day 90 after the study day.

PaO_2/FiO_2 determination

PaO_2 and FiO_2 were recorded simultaneously. In the case of low-flow oxygen without an FiO_2 setting device, we calculated FiO_2 as $0.21 + (\text{oxygen flow rate in liters per minute} \times 0.03)$ [11]. In the absence of PaO_2 measurement, we estimated the PaO_2/FiO_2 ratio through the SpO_2/FiO_2 ratio using the equation proposed by Rice et al. [12], using a $SpO_2 \leq 97\%$ because the Rice equation cannot infer PaO_2 at higher SaO_2 given the sigmoid relationship between SaO_2 and PaO_2.

In mechanically ventilated patients, we measured the following parameters: expired tidal volume (V_t), measured respiratory rate, set positive end expiratory pressure (PEEP) and plateau pressure and PEEP during an inspiratory and expiratory pause in patients in volume control mode without spontaneous breathing. We calculated the driving pressure by subtracting total PEEP from plateau pressure [13].

Statistical analysis

Prevalence of hypoxemia was computed using the total number of patients included as the denominator, and the 95% confidence interval was estimated (95% CI). We compared the three groups of hypoxemic patients with different degrees of severity in terms of baseline characteristics, comorbidities, and respiratory conditions. Quantitative variables were described as mean (SD) or median (25th–75th centiles), as appropriate, and compared using Student's *t* test or the Wilcoxon–Mann–Whitney test. Qualitative variables were described as counts (%) and compared using the χ^2 or the Fisher exact test, as appropriate. The completeness of the database is indicated in tables. No imputation was used for missing data.

Overall survival was estimated using the Kaplan–Meier method, and survival curves were compared according to the severity of hypoxemia using the log-rank test for categorical variables and the Wald test based on a univariate Cox model for quantitative variables. Among hypoxemic patients, Cox proportional hazards regression was performed to estimate unadjusted hazard ratios and their

95% CI. Variables associated with p values < 0.20 were selected for multivariable analyses. Confounders and interactions were tested in bivariate models. The proportional hazards assumption was assessed statistically using the Schoenfeld residuals test.

All tests were two-sided, and p values < 0.05 were considered significant. Analyses were conducted using Stata v12.1 (StataCorp LP, College Station, TX, USA).

The study was registered in Clinical trials: NCT 02722031.

Results

Characteristics of hypoxemic patients

Of the 1748 patients hospitalized in the participating ICUs the day of the study, 1604 were included. Flowchart of the study is given in Fig. 1. The general characteristics of the patients are reported in Table 1. The day of the study, 859 (54%, 95% CI 51–56%) patients were hypoxemic. Comparison between hypoxemic and non-hypoxemic patients is reported in Additional file 1: Table S2. Among the hypoxemic patients, 440 (51%) had mild, 345 (40%) moderate, and 74 (9%) severe hypoxemia. The causes and mechanisms of hypoxemia are given in Table 2. Pneumonia was the main cause of hypoxemia (53%), but there were a median of 2 [1–3] causes/mechanisms of hypoxemia per patient. A total of 178 (21%) patients fulfilled the criteria for ARDS: 65 (37%) had mild, 82 (46%) moderate, and 31 (17%) severe ARDS. ARDS exclusion criteria among the other 228 hypoxemic patients with bilateral infiltrates are shown in Additional file 1: Table S3. Even though the frequency of ARDS increased with severity of hypoxemia (p < 0.001), it represented less than 50% of severely hypoxemic patients (Table 2).

Of the 1604 patients, 1110 (69%) had an arterial blood gas analysis (ABG) the day of the study. This proportion reached 87% (n = 749) in hypoxemic patients. ABG revealed that the most severely ill patients had the highest level of $PaCO_2$ and the lowest level of PaO_2 (Table 3).

Modalities of oxygen administration are reported in Table 3. Nearly 40% of the hypoxemic patients and 25% of the most severely ill were managed with non-invasive devices. Twenty-five per cent of patients on high-flow oxygen were severely hypoxemic, compared with less than 10% on NIV. Sixteen percent of these patients required later invasive ventilation in their ICU stay whatever the mode of support received the study day (Additional file 1: Figure S1). Causes and radiological finding according to the modalities of oxygen supply are depicted in Table 4. Adjunctive therapies designed to improve oxygenation beyond ventilation were mostly used in the severely hypoxemic patients, the most frequent being neuromuscular blockers, followed by extracorporeal membrane oxygenation, inhaled nitric oxide, and prone positioning (Table 3).

Ventilator settings in patients on invasive mechanical ventilation

Among hypoxemic patients under invasive mechanical ventilation, the measured median V_t was 6.9 [6.1–7.9]

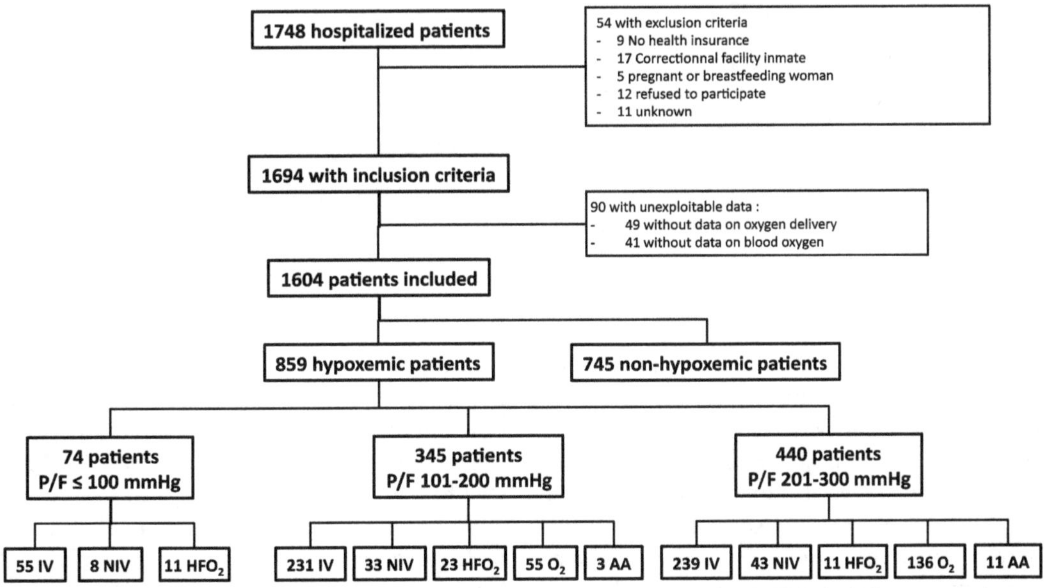

Fig. 1 Flowchart of the study. *P/F*: PaO_2/FiO_2 ratio; IV: invasive ventilation, NIV non-invasive ventilation, HFO_2: high-flow oxygen therapy, O_2: low-flow (standard) oxygen therapy, AA: ambient air

Table 1 Characteristics of hypoxemic patients according to severity of hypoxemia

	All hypoxemic patients, $n = 859$	Mild hypoxemia *P/F* 201–300 mmHg, $n = 440$	Moderate hypoxemia *P/F* 101–200 mmHg, $n = 345$	Severe hypoxemia $P/F \leq 100$ mmHg, $n = 74$	*p*
Age, years median (IQR)	64 [53–73]	65 [54–74]	65 [53–73]	58 [47–69]	0.006
Female, *N* (%)	273 (31.8)	142 (32.3)	109 (31.6)	22 (29.7)	0.91
Body mass index ($n = 844/431/341/72$)	26.1 [22.5–31.1]	26.1 [22.7–30.9]	26.0 [22.5–31.0]	27.0 [22.1–34.4]	0.83
Main diagnosis at ICU admission ($n = 858/439/345/74$)					–
Septic shock	124 (14.5)	67 (15.2)	49 (14.2)	8 (10.8)	
Other shock	47 (5.5)	24 (5.4)	17 (4.9)	6 (8.1)	
Severe trauma	20 (2.3)	14 (3.2)	6 (1.7)	0 (0)	
De novo acute respiratory failure	275 (32.0)	118 (26.9)	120 (34.8)	37 (50.0)	
Acute on chronic respiratory failure	128 (14.9)	55 (12.5)	68 (19.7)	5 (6.8)	
Coma/seizures	66 (7.7)	43 (9.8)	19 (5.5)	4 (5.4)	
Metabolic disorders	18 (2.1)	11 (2.5)	6 (1.7)	1 (1.4)	
Hepatic failure	6 (0.7)	2 (0.5)	2 (0.6)	2 (2.7)	
Cardiac arrest	30 (3.5)	15 (3.4)	12 (3.5)	3 (4.1)	
Postoperative surveillance	96 (11.2)	64 (14.6)	31 (9.0)	1 (1.3)	
Other	48 (5.6)	26 (5.9)	15 (4.4)	7 (9.5)	
Admission category ($n = 857/439/344/74$)					0.004
Medical	675 (78.8)	327 (74.5)	281 (81.7)	67 (90.5)	
Scheduled surgery	76 (8.9)	49 (11.1)	27 (7.8)	0 (0)	
Urgent surgery	92 (10.7)	53 (12.1)	32 (9.3)	7 (9.5)	
Trauma	14 (1.6)	10 (2.3)	4 (1.2)	0 (0)	
SAPS II ($n = 832/425/334/73$)	43 [31–57]	42 [30–56]	43 [31–57]	45 [34–61]	0.32
Chronic respiratory disease (obstructive) ($n = 855/440/342/73$)	288 (33.7)	141 (32.1)	127 (37.1)	20 (27.4)	0.16
Chronic respiratory disease (restrictive) ($n = 855/440/342/73$)	71 (8.3)	28 (6.4)	37 (10.8)	6 (8.2)	0.08
Obstructive sleep apnea syndrome ($n = 855/440/342/73$)	71 (8.3)	36 (8.2)	29 (8.5)	6 (8.2)	0.99
Chronic oxygen therapy ($n = 855/440/342/73$)	71 (8.3)	32 (7.3)	33 (9.7)	6 (8.2)	0.49
Long-term non-invasive ventilation ($n = 855/440/342/73$)	32 (3.7)	17 (3.9)	14 (4.1)	1 (1.4)	0.68
Chronic heart failure ($n = 855/440/342/73$)	145 (17.0)	74 (16.8)	62 (18.1)	9 (12.3)	0.48
Chronic kidney failure ($n = 855/440/342/73$)	83 (9.7)	55 (12.5)	23 (6.7)	5 (6.9)	0.02
Cirrhosis ($n = 855/440/342/73$)	45 (5.3)	25 (5.7)	15 (4.4)	5 (6.9)	0.54
Cancer ($n = 855/440/342/73$)	79 (9.2)	43 (9.8)	32 (9.4)	4 (5.5)	0.50
Immunosuppression ($n = 853/439/341/73$)	99 (11.6)	46 (10.5)	43 (12.6)	10 (13.7)	0.55
Withholding/withdrawal of treatment the day of the study	105 (12.2)	41 (9.3)	47 (13.6)	17 (23)	0.002

mL/kg of ideal body weight and 77% received a tidal volume of 8 mL/kg or less of ideal body weight. Tidal volume decreased with the severity of hypoxemia (Table 3). PEEP was set at 6 [5–10] cmH_2O in the whole cohort and increased with the severity of hypoxemia to a median of 10 [8–12] cmH_2O in the severely hypoxemic patients. Whereas plateau pressure increased with severity of hypoxemia, median driving pressure was below 15 cmH_2O and similar in the 3 groups of patients (Table 3).

Outcomes

Median ICU length of stay was 12 [5–28] days and ICU mortality was 20% in the 1604 patients of the study. In the hypoxemic population, median ICU length of stay was higher (16 [7–32] vs 8 [3–22] days in non-hypoxemic patients, $p < 0.001$) but not related to the severity of hypoxemia even when looking only at the patients leaving the ICU alive (Table 3). Patients with invasive

Table 2 Mechanisms/causes of hypoxemia[a] and radiological findings according to severity of hypoxemia on the day of the study

	All hypoxemic patients, $n=859$	Mild hypoxemia, $n=440$	Moderate hypoxemia, $n=345$	Severe hypoxemia, $n=74$	p
Pneumonia, N (%) ($n=852/440/339/73$)	453 (53.2)	189 (43.0)	204 (60.2)	60 (82.2)	<0.001
Aspiration ($n=852/440/339/73$)	74 (8.7)	30 (6.8)	33 (9.7)	11 (15.1)	0.05
Acute on chronic respiratory failure ($n=853/440/340/73$)	166 (19.5)	73 (16.6)	80 (23.5)	13 (17.8)	0.05
Cardiogenic pulmonary edema ($n=853/440/340/73$)	127 (14.9)	64 (14.6)	51 (15.0)	12 (16.4)	0.91
Pulmonary embolism ($n=853/440/340/73$)	26 (3.1)	16 (3.6)	7 (2.1)	3 (4.1)	0.37
Thoracic trauma ($n=852/440/339/73$)	21 (2.5)	9 (2.1)	11 (3.2)	1 (1.4)	0.59
Pleural effusion ($n=852/440/339/73$)	192 (22.5)	99 (22.5)	77 (22.7)	16 (21.9)	0.99
Atelectasis ($n=853/440/340/73$)	176 (20.6)	93 (21.1)	72 (21.2)	11 (15.1)	0.47
Pneumothorax ($n=853/440/340/73$)	15 (1.8)	6 (1.4)	7 (2.1)	2 (2.7)	0.49
Fluid overload ($n=853/440/340/73$)	280 (32.8)	140 (31.8)	115 (33.8)	25 (34.3)	0.81
Acute pancreatitis ($n=852/440/339/73$)	22 (2.6)	14 (3.2)	6 (1.8)	2 (2.7)	0.48
Shock, low PvO_2 ($n=853/440/340/73$)	110 (12.9)	42 (9.6)	48 (14.1)	20 (27.4)	<0.001
Smoke/toxic inhalation ($n=852/440/339/73$)	5 (0.6)	1 (0.2)	3 (0.9)	1 (1.4)	0.20
Transfusion-related acute lung injury ($n=852/440/339/73$)	44 (5.2)	32 (7.3)	9 (2.7)	3 (4.1)	0.01
Pulmonary vasculitis ($n=852/440/339/73$)	6 (0.7)	3 (0.7)	2 (0.6)	1 (1.4)	0.66
Drowning ($n=851/440/339/72$)	1 (0.1)	1 (0.2)	0 (0)	0 (0)	1
Other ($n=851/440/338/73$)	90 (10.6)	43 (9.8)	42 (12.4)	5 (6.9)	0.30
Number of causes of hypoxemia ($n=853$[b]$/440/340/73$)	2 [1–3]	2 [1–3]	2 [1–3]	2 [1–3]	<0.001
Number of causes of hypoxemia ($n=853$[b]$/440/340/73$)					<0.001
None	107 (12.5)	82 (18.6)	22 (6.5)	3 (4.1)	
1	230 (27.0)	110 (25.0)	100 (29.4)	20 (27.4)	
2	221 (25.9)	110 (25.0)	93 (27.3)	18 (24.7)	
3 or more	295 (34.6)	138 (31.4)	125 (36.8)	32 (43.8)	
Radiological infiltrates ($n=845/435/337/73$)	583 (69.0)	257 (59.1)	260 (77.2)	66 (90.4)	<0.001
Unilateral[c] ($n=581/255/260/66$)	176 (30.3)	85 (33.3)	81 (31.2)	10 (15.2)	0.02
Bilateral[c] ($n=581/255/260/66$)	406 (69.6)	171 (67.1)	179 (68.9)	56 (84.9)	0.02
ARDS	178 (20.7)	65 (14.7)	82 (23.8)	31 (41.9)	<0.001

[a] Multiple causes and mechanisms could be selected

[b] In 6 patients data on hypoxemia, causes were not recorded

[c] Among patients with radiological infiltrates

ventilation had the longest stay in the ICU and the highest mortality (Table 4).

ICU mortality was 12% in non-hypoxemic patients and 27% in hypoxemic patients ($p<0.001$). ICU mortality increased with severity of hypoxemia: 21% in mildly, 29% in moderately, and 51% in severely hypoxemic patients ($p<0.001$) (Table 3 and Fig. 2) and with invasiveness of ventilator support (Table 4). Additional file 1: Table S4 reports the ICU mortality according to ventilator support and hypoxemia class.

Multivariate analysis

Taking into account the variables associated with ICU mortality in univariate analysis (Additional file 1: Table S5), multivariate analysis using a Cox model confirmed that moderate hypoxemia and severe hypoxemia were independently associated with ICU mortality compared to mild hypoxemia (adjusted hazard ratio 1.38 [1.00–1.90] and 2.65 [1.69–4.15], respectively), as well as other classic variables (Table 5). We performed several sensitivity analyses to strengthen this result (Additional file 1: Table S6): first, including the oxygen support in the analysis, second analyzing only patients with a PaO_2/FiO_2 ratio based on actual PaO_2 and FiO_2, third excluding patients on chronic oxygen therapy or chronic NIV, and fourth excluding patients with therapeutics withholding/withdrawing. These analyses show similar results, although moderate hypoxemia was no longer significantly associated with mortality (Additional file 1: Table S6). Moreover, analyzing the PaO_2/FiO_2 ratio as a continuous variable in the same model

Table 3 Respiratory conditions and outcome according to severity of hypoxemia

	All hypoxemic patients, $n=859$	Mild hypoxemia P/F 201–300 mmHg, $n=440$	Moderate hypoxemia P/F 101–200 mmHg, $n=345$	Severe hypoxemia $P/F \leq 100$ mmHg, $n=74$	p
Respiratory rate ($n=846/432/340/74$)	23 [18–27]	22 [18–26]	24 [20–28]	25 [20–30]	0.001
Arterial blood gases	749 (87.2)	368 (83.6)	311 (90.1)	70 (94.6)	0.004
pH ($n=745/366/309/70$)	7.41 [7.36–7.46]	7.42 [7.38–7.45]	7.41 [7.36–7.46]	7.38 [7.29–7.45]	0.007
$PaCO_2$ (mmHg) ($n=749/368/311/70$)	41 [36–49]	40 [35–46]	43 [38–55]	45 [39–56]	0.001
$PaCO_2>45$ mmHg ($n=749/368/311/70$)	260 (34.7)	96 (26.1)	131 (42.1)	33 (47.1)	<0.001
PaO_2 (mmHg) ($n=749/368/311/70$)	78 [66–92]	84 [73–100]	74 [64–88]	65 [56–74]	<0.001
FiO_2 (%) ($n=749/368/311/70$)	0.40 [0.33–0.50]	0.35 [0.30–0.40]	0.50 [0.40–0.60]	1 [0.70–1]	<0.001
HCO_3-(meq/L) ($n=747/368/309/70$)	26 [23–30]	26 [22–29]	27 [23–32]	26 [23–30]	0.03
Lactates (meq/L) ($n=630/312/257/61$)	1.3 [1.0–1.9]	1.2 [0.9–1.7]	1.3 [1.0–1.9]	1.4 [1.1–2.7]	0.02
Oxygenation modalities, N (%)					<0.001
Ambient air	14 (1.6)	11 (2.5)	3 (0.9)	0 (0)	
Low-flow oxygen	191 (22.2)	136 (30.9)	55 (15.9)	0 (0)	
High-flow oxygen	45 (5.2)	11 (2.5)	23 (6.7)	11 (14.9)	
Non-invasive ventilation	84 (9.8)	43 (9.8)	33 (9.6)	8 (10.8)	
Invasive ventilation	525 (61.2)	239 (54.3)	231 (66.9)	55 (74.3)	
Ventilator settings[a]					
Tidal volume, mL/kg of ideal body weight; median IQR ($n=509/230/225/54$)	6.9 [6.1–7.9]	7.1 [6.2–8.1]	6.8 [6.0–7.6]	6.1 [4.8–6.6]	<0.001
TV ≤ 8 mL/kg of ideal body weight ($n=509/230/225/54$)	393 (77.2)	165 (71.7)	178 (79.1)	50 (92.6)	0.003
PEEP (cmH20) ($n=519/236/229/54$)	6 [5–10]	5 [5–8]	7 [5–10]	10 [8–12]	<0.001
Plateau pressure[b] (cmH20) ($n=186/66/84/36$)	22.5 [19–27]	20 [16–24]	23.5 [20–28]	25.5 [23–29.5]	<0.001
Driving pressure[b] (cmH20) ($n=186/66/84/36$)	14 [10–18]	13 [9–17]	14 [11–18]	13 [10–19]	0.31
Adjunctive therapies					
Prone positioning ($n=516/232/230/54$)	22 (4.3)	3 (1.3)	13 (5.7)	6 (11.1)	0.001
Inhaled NO ($n=513/233/226/54$)	19 (3.7)	3 (1.3)	9 (4.0)	7 (13.0)	0.001
Continuous intravenous sedation, N (%) ($n=522/237/231/54$)	321 (61.5)	121 (51.1)	159 (68.8)	41 (75.9)	<0.001
Neuromuscular blocking agents, N (%) ($n=522/237/231/54$)	83 (15.9)	11 (4.6)	44 (19.1)	28 (51.9)	<0.001
Extracorporeal oxygenation, N (%) ($n=522/237/231/54$)	26 (3.0)	5 (1.1)	7 (2.0)	14 (18.9)	<0.001
ICU length of stay (days) ($n=840/431/336/73$)	16 [7–32]	15 [7–32]	16 [8–31.5]	18 [7–37]	0.89
ICU length of stay (days) in ICU survivors ($n=625/342/246/37$)	15 [7–30]	15 [7–30]	14 [6.5–30]	20.5 [9–46.5]	0.27
ICU mortality, N (%) ($n=839/431/335/73$)	225 (26.7)	92 (21.3)	96 (28.5)	37 (50.7)	<0.001

[a] Invasively ventilated patients $n=525$

[b] Only in patients in whom plateau pressure was measurable (i.e., patients in VAC without spontaneous breathing). $n=186$

confirmed the independent association between the severity of hypoxemia and mortality (adjusted hazard ratio for each 10 mmHg decrease 1.06 [1.03–1.09], $p<0.001$).

Discussion

This large, multicenter study gives for the first time data on the prevalence of hypoxemia in non-selected ICU-hospitalized patients. Strikingly, though more

Table 4 Mechanisms/causes of hypoxemia and radiological findings according to oxygenation modalities

	Ambient air, $n=14$	Low-flow oxygen, $n=191$	High-flow oxygen, $n=45$	Non-invasive ventilation, $n=84$	Invasive ventilation, $n=525$	p
Pneumonia, *N* (%) ($n=852/14/189/45/83/521$)	3 (21.4)	62 (32.8)	34 (75.6)	37 (44.6)	317 (60.8)	<0.001
Aspiration ($n=852/14/190/45/83/520$)	0 (0)	11 (5.8)	0 (0)	3 (3.6)	60 (11.5)	0.003
Acute on chronic respiratory failure ($n=853/14/190/45/83/521$)	0 (0)	32 (16.8)	4 (8.9)	41 (49.4)	89 (17.1)	<0.001
Cardiogenic pulmonary edema ($n=853/14/190/45/83/521$)	2 (14.3)	28 (14.7)	4 (8.9)	15 (18.1)	78 (15.0)	0.75
Pulmonary embolism ($n=853/14/190/45/83/521$)	0 (0)	5 (2.6)	2 (4.4)	2 (2.4)	17 (3.3)	0.93
Thoracic trauma ($n=852/14/190/45/83/520$)	0 (0)	5 (2.6)	2 (4.4)	0 (0)	14 (2.7)	0.46
Pleural effusion ($n=852/14/189/45/83/521$)	2 (14.3)	34 (18.0)	11 (24.4)	24 (28.9)	121 (23.2)	0.3
Atelectasis ($n=853/14/190/45/83/521$)	2 (14.3)	30 (15.8)	10 (22.2)	22 (26.5)	112 (21.5)	0.27
Pneumothorax ($n=853/14/190/45/83/521$)	0 (0)	4 (2.1)	0 (0)	0 (0)	11 (2.1)	0.72
Fluid overload ($n=853/14/190/45/83/521$)	2 (14.3)	47 (24.7)	12 (26.7)	28 (33.7)	191 (36.7)	0.02
Acute pancreatitis ($n=852/14/190/45/83/520$)	0 (0)	6 (3.2)	0 (0)	1 (1.2)	15 (2.9)	0.81
Shock, low PvO_2 ($n=853/14/190/45/83/521$)	0 (0)	6 (3.2)	3 (6.7)	6 (7.2)	95 (18.2)	<0.001
Smoke/toxic inhalation ($n=852/14/190/45/83/520$)	0 (0)	0 (0)	0 (0)	0 (0)	5 (1.0)	0.63
Transfusion-related acute lung injury ($n=852/14/190/45/83/520$)	1 (7.1)	10 (5.3)	2 (4.4)	3 (3.6)	28 (5.4)	0.92
Pulmonary vasculitis ($n=852/14/190/45/83/520$)	0 (0)	1 (0.5)	0 (0)	0 (0)	5 (1.0)	1
Drowning ($n=851/14/190/45/82/520$)	0 (0)	0 (0)	0 (0)	0 (0)	1 (0.2)	1
Other ($n=851/14/190/45/83/519$)	0 (0)	21 (11.1)	11 (24.4)	9 (10.8)	49 (9.4)	0.04
Number of causes of hypoxemia ($n=853/14/190/45/83/521$)	1 [0–1]	1 [1, 2]	2 [1, 2]	2 [1–3]	2 [1–3]	<0.001
Number of causes of hypoxemia ($n=853/14/190/45/83/521$)						<0.001
None	6 (42.9)	41 (21.6)	0 (0)	6 (7.2)	54 (10.4)	
1	5 (35.7)	63 (33.1)	16 (35.6)	24 (28.9)	122 (23.4)	
2	2 (14.3)	45 (23.7)	18 (40.0)	23 (27.7)	133 (25.5)	
3 or more	1 (7.1)	41 (21.6)	11 (24.4)	30 (36.2)	212 (40.7)	
Radiological infiltrates ($n=845/14/189/45/82/515$)	4 (28.6)	101 (53.4)	37 (82.2)	57 (69.5)	384 (74.6)	<0.001
Unilateral c ($n=583/4/101/37/56/385$)	1 (25.0)	36 (35.6)	9 (24.3)	19 (33.9)	111 (28.8)	0.58
Bilateral c ($n=581/4/100/37/56/384$)	3 (75.0)	65 (65.0)	28 (75.7)	37 (66.1)	273 (71.1)	0.65
ARDS	0 (0)	0 (0)	0 (0)	9 (10.7)	169 (32.2)	<0.001
Hypoxemia class						<0.001
Mild	11 (78.6)	136 (71.2)	11 (24.4)	43 (51.2)	239 (45.5)	
Moderate	3 (21.4)	55 (28.8)	23 (51.2)	33 (39.3)	231 (44.0)	
Severe	0 (0)	0 (0)	11 (24.4)	8 (9.5)	55 (10.5)	
ICU length of stay (days) ($n=840/14/190/45/83/508$)	11 [4–21]	8 [4–17]	14 [8–23]	9 [4–18]	21 [12–40]	<0.001
ICU length of stay (days) in ICU survivors ($n=625/11/170/37/70/337$)	11 [4–16]	7.5 [4–15]	13 [8–22]	9 [4–18]	24 [12–43]	<0.001
ICU mortality, *N* (%) ($n=839/14/190/44/83/508$)	3 (21.4)	20 (10.5)	7 (15.9)	13 (15.7)	168 (33.1)	<0.001

than half of the patients hospitalized in ICUs the day of the study were hypoxemic, 79% did not fulfill the criteria of ARDS according to the Berlin definition [10]. The prevalence of ARDS, albeit greater in the most hypoxemic patients, was still less than half (42%). Our results highlight also that hypoxemia is frequent among non-ventilated patients. The other main result of our study is that among hypoxemic patients, moderate and severe hypoxemia compared to mild hypoxemia was independently associated with higher ICU mortality.

Data concerning hypoxemia in unselected ICU patients, regardless of the presence of ARDS or the use

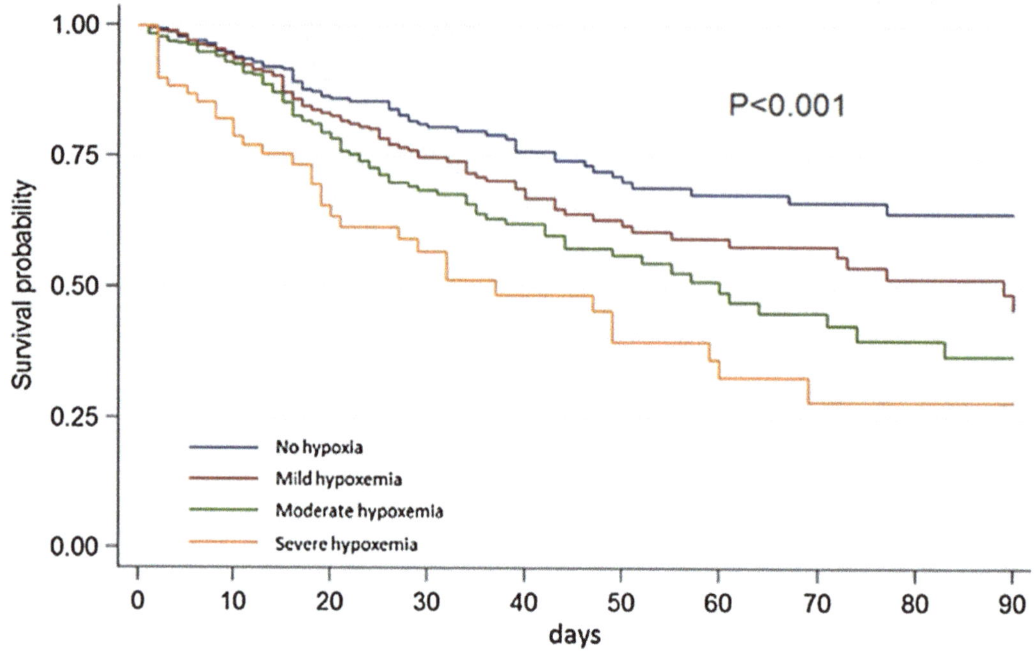

Fig. 2 Survival curve according to hypoxemia severity. Survival curves were drawn according to the severity of hypoxemia using the Kaplan–Meier method and were compared using the log-rank test. Follow-up ended at the ICU leaving or was censored at day 90

Table 5 Multivariate analysis of parameters associated with ICU survival

	Adjusted HR x [95% CI]	*p*
Age	1.01 [1.00–1.02]	0.054
Obesity	0.63 [0.45–0.89]	0.008
Main diagnosis at ICU admission		0.049
Septic shock	1.05 [0.68–1.64]	
Other shock	1.83 [1.09–3.07]	
Severe trauma	0.29 [0.04–2.13]	
De novo acute respiratory failure	1 (ref)	
Acute on chronic respiratory failure	1.56 [0.95–2.57]	
Coma/seizures	1.58 [0.89–2.78]	
Metabolic disorders	0.74 [0.25–2.19]	
Cardiac arrest	1.73 [0.88–3.40]	
Postoperative surveillance	0.67 [0.32–1.40]	
Other	0.76 [0.37–1.56]	
Chronic heart failure	1.69 [1.19–2.42]	0.004
Chronic kidney failure	1.65 [1.05–2.62]	0.032
Cirrhosis	1.71 [0.95–3.10]	0.075
SAPS II (per point)	1.01 [1.00–1.02]	0.012
Hypoxemia class		<0.001
Mild	1 (ref)	
Moderate	1.38 [1.00–1.90]	
Severe	2.65 [1.69–4.15]	

SAPS II Simplified Acute Physiology Score

Multivariate Cox analysis of variables associated with ICU survival

of mechanical ventilation, are rather scarce, and we think this is strength of the SPECTRUM study to have included patients with all types of oxygenation devices. In the LUNG-SAFE study, hypoxemia was less frequent (35%), but all the patients considered in the analysis received ventilatory support [4], unlike those analyzed in our study. In another study focusing on ARDS [5], the incidence of hypoxemia was 50% among ventilated patients, but no data on non-invasively ventilated patients were given.

The prevalence of ARDS in the SPECTRUM study was 21% in hypoxemic patients, leading to an overall prevalence of 11% of included patients. This prevalence rate is close to the incidence found in the LUNG-SAFE study, in which 10.4% of the patients admitted in the ICU (23% of the mechanically ventilated patients) met the criteria for ARDS. Other studies, using the 1994 ALI/ARDS definition, reported similar results [5] or higher incidence [7, 8].

The presence of hypoxemia was associated with higher mortality and ICU length of stay, and the association with mortality was even stronger in the group of patients with severe hypoxemia. Severe hypoxemia was still associated with mortality after adjustment on respiratory support and in several sensitivity analyses, strengthening this result. This association is not so straightforward as several interventions known to improve PaO_2/FiO_2

ratio failed to reduce mortality [14] or were even detrimental [15, 16], suggesting that improving PaO_2/FiO_2 ratio cannot be an isolated therapeutic goal. Interestingly, ICU mortality among patients with mild-to-moderate hypoxemia was lower than that reported in patients with mild-to-moderate ARDS [4]. Conversely, mortality in our severely hypoxemic patients was close to that of severe ARDS patients described in other large studies. This result may be due to the fact that ARDS accounted for almost half of the severely hypoxemic patients in our cohort but also to the fact that similar pathophysiological mechanisms may be involved in severe hypoxemic patients with or without ARDS. For instance, pneumonia and aspiration as a cause of hypoxemia were more frequent in the most severe patients compared to other frequent causes of hypoxemia (see Table 2). Further studies should try to decipher the respective roles of ARDS and hypoxemia in the prognosis.

Invasiveness of respiratory support was also associated with mortality in univariate analysis, but time-dependent multivariate analysis did not confirm this association. Indeed, roles of respiratory support and severity of hypoxemia in mortality have a complex interplay as the most severe patients received the more invasive support and as respiratory support is not fixed across disease course. Our data suggest that severity of hypoxemia assessed by the *P*/*F* ratio a given day is associated with mortality whatever the ventilator support needed in line with other study [17]. This finding may be useful in clinical practice to assess even roughly the severity of hypoxemia and the potential impact on outcomes.

We also evaluated the oxygenation devices used and the ventilator settings in hypoxemic patients. High-flow oxygen and NIV were not rare, even among severely hypoxemic patients. Almost 20% of the patients with a PaO_2/FiO_2 ratio ≤ 100 were not on invasive mechanical ventilation, despite the fact that several studies have shown that NIV for de novo hypoxemic respiratory failure is associated with a poorer outcome in patients who finally required invasive mechanical ventilation [18–20]. We included all patients in the ICU and presenting hypoxemia (both de novo acute respiratory failure and acute on chronic respiratory failure), and it may be that those patients with severe hypoxemia on NIV had severe chronic respiratory failure or severe cardiogenic pulmonary edema. High-flow oxygen therapy was recently shown to have beneficial effects in patients with a PaO_2/FiO_2 ratio ≤ 200, as compared with standard oxygen and NIV in a randomized controlled trial [11]. However, the outcome of patients with the most severe hypoxemia receiving high-flow oxygen is unknown. Interestingly, in our study, high-flow oxygen was proportionally more frequently used in the most severely ill patients.

In mechanically ventilated patients, hypoxemia was associated with the use of "protective ventilation" in most cases with low V_t and higher PEEP, permissive hypercapnia and hypoxemia resulting in median plateau and driving pressures below the commonly admitted thresholds. Whereas reduced tidal volume appeared beneficial in observational studies among non-ARDS patients [21] and is currently the object of ongoing trials, the value of other protective strategies such as reducing driving pressure, increasing PEEP, or prone positioning may deserve evaluation in this population. The use of adjunctive therapies was correlated with the degree of hypoxemia. Neuromuscular blocking agents were the most often used in line with recent ARDS guidelines [22]: half of the patients with a PaO_2/FiO_2 ratio ≤ 100 were continuously paralyzed. More surprising is the limited use of prone positioning on the day of the study in the subgroup of severely hypoxemic patients, even if not all patients fulfilled ARDS criteria. Recourse to prone positioning was, for instance, less frequent than the use of inhaled NO, whereas the level of evidence widely favors prone positioning rather than inhaled NO during ARDS [23–25].

Our study provides novel data about hypoxemia prevalence and management that could have implications for research and clinical practice. We provide an accurate prevalence of hypoxemia and stratification according to its severity even in those breathing spontaneously. This could help in the design of future interventional studies targeting these patients. In the clinical practice, physician should be alerted by the severity of hypoxemic non-intubated patients and the risk of mortality.

As we enrolled more than 90% of the screened patients, our observations were likely unbiased. However, our study has some limits. First, it was a point prevalence study and thus does not yield accurate data on incidence. By design, patients with prolonged stay had more chance to be included and are thus overrepresented in our study. Data on length of stay had then to be interpreted with caution and does not reflect accurately the mean length of stay of patients admitted in the ICU. Given the higher ICU length of stay of hypoxemic patients, one could hypothesize that the incidence of hypoxemia is lower than the prevalence. Conversely, some patients without hypoxemia on the day of study may have had hypoxemia before or after the study day during their ICU stay, and some hypoxemic patients may have been more severe. Likewise, our data on adjuvant therapies should be analyzed with caution as some, such as extracorporeal membrane oxygenation, cover a long period of time and so increase the chance of being present on the day of the study. Second, arterial blood gas was not analyzed in 31% of patients. In those cases, hypoxemia was assessed with an extrapolation of the PaO_2/FiO_2 ratio from the $SpO_2/$

FiO_2 ratio. However, most patients classified as "hypoxemic" underwent arterial blood gas analysis on the day of the SPECTRUM study. Moreover, published data show that PaO_2/FiO_2 can be accurately derived from the SpO_2/FiO_2 ratio [12, 26, 27] and sensitivity analysis including only patients with arterial blood gases was consistent with our result on mortality. Third, we conducted our study in spring to avoid the inclusion during an influenza seasonal pandemic; thus, our results could have been different in other seasons. Fourth, the inclusion of patients with limitation of treatment could impact our results as invasive devices are less likely to be used and mortality is higher in these patients. However, this allows to report in an unbiased way our epidemiological data. Lastly, the difficulty of separating ARDS from non-ARDS in hypoxemic patients is well known. In our survey, the diagnosis of ARDS was based on the Berlin criteria given in the CRF, independently of the clinical judgment of the clinician. However, chest-X ray analysis was not independently assessed. Even though we found a percentage of ARDS similar to that found in other large cohorts, it has been shown that ARDS is largely underdiagnosed, especially in its mild forms [4]. Even in the era of the Berlin definition, ARDS continues to be underrecognized, especially because of concerns about the reliable interpretation of chest radiographs [28]. Finally, although we identified an independent association between hypoxemia and mortality, our study does not provide mechanistic explanations of this finding.

Conclusion

In this 1-day point prevalence study, more than half of the patients suffered from hypoxemia, of mostly mild-to-moderate severity. ARDS criteria were present the day of data collection in only one out of five patients and were far from capturing the spectrum of hypoxemia in the ICU setting. Non-invasive methods of oxygenation were largely used even in the most hypoxemic patients. Finally, among hypoxemic patients, moderate and severe hypoxemia were independently associated with ICU survival, as compared to mild hypoxemia.

Authors' contributions

Not applicable.

Acknowledgements

The authors are deeply indebted to the patients who agreed to participate and to all physicians who took care of them. We also thank Chantal Sevens, Florence Neels, and Mathieu Lloung for their assistance. Special thanks to all involved in the collection and analysis of the data: all CERC members, all investigators, SRLF presidents and secretaries (Additional file 1: Table S1).

Writing committee: Grimaldi D (1) Hraiech S (2) Boutin E (3) Lacherade JC (4) Boissier F (5) Pham T (6) Richard JC (7) Thille AW (8) Ehrmann S (9) Lascarrou JB (10) Aissaoui N (11)

1. Intensive Care Unit, Clinique Universitaire de Bruxelles, Erasme hospital, Université Libre de Bruxelles (ULB) Route de Lennik, 808 1070, Brussels, Belgium

2. Aix-Marseille University, APHM, URMITE UMR CNRS 7278, Hôpital Nord, Réanimation des Détresses Respiratoires et Infections Sévères, Marseille, France

3. APHP, hopital Henri-Mondor, department of public health and clinical research unit (URC Mondor), 94010 Creteil Cedex, France

4. Médecine Intensive Réanimation, Centre Hospitalier Départemental de la Vendée, La Roche sur Yon, France

5. Service de Réanimation médicale, CHU de Poitiers, Poitiers, France; INSERM CIC 1402 (ALIVE group), Université de Poitiers, Poitiers, France

6. Interdepartmental Division of Critical Care Medicine, University of Toronto, Canada; Keenan Research Centre for Biomedical Science, Li Ka Shing Knowledge Institute, St. Michael's Hospital, Toronto, Canada. Sorbonne Universités, UPMC Université Paris 06, Paris, France

7. Service de Réanimation Médicale, Hôpital De La Croix Rousse, Hospices Civils de Lyon, Lyon, France. Université de Lyon, Université LYON I, Lyon, France. CREATIS INSERM 1044 CNRS 5220, Villeurbanne, FRANCE

8. CHU de Poitiers, Réanimation Médicale, Poitiers, France; INSERM CIC 1402 ALIVE, Université de Poitiers, Poitiers, France

9. Médecine Intensive Réanimation, CHRU de Tours, Tours, France; Centre d'étude des pathologies respiratoires, INSERM U1100, Aérosolthérapie et biomédicaments à visée respiratoire, Faculté de médecine, Université François Rabelais, Tours, France

10. Medical Intensive Care Unit CHU de Nantes 30 Bd. Jean Monnet 44093 Nantes cedex 1

11. Assistance Publique-Hôpitaux de Paris (AP-HP); Hôpital Européen Georges Pompidou (HEGP), Department of Critical Care Unit, Paris, France; Université Paris-Descartes, Paris, France; Paris-Cardiovascular-Research-Center, INSERM U970, Paris, France

Competing interests

The authors declare that they have no competing interests.

Funding

The study was funded by the French Intensive Care Society (Société de Réanimation de langue française: SRLF Trial Group).

References

1. Luhr OR, Antonsen K, Karlsson M, Aardal S, Thorsteinsson A, Frostell CG, et al. Incidence and mortality after acute respiratory failure and acute respiratory distress syndrome in Sweden, Denmark, and Iceland. Am J Respir Crit Care Med. 1999;159(6):1849–61.
2. Vincent J-L, Akça S, De Mendonça A, Haji-Michael P, Sprung C, Moreno R, et al. The epidemiology of acute respiratory failure in critically ill patients (*). Chest. 2002;121(5):1602–9.
3. The FINNALI-Study Group, Linko R, Okkonen M, Pettilä V, Perttilä J, Parviainen I, et al. Acute respiratory failure in intensive care units. FINNALI: a prospective cohort study. Intensive Care Med. 2009;35(8):1352–61.
4. Bellani G, Laffey JG, Pham T, Fan E, Brochard L, Esteban A, et al. Epidemiology, patterns of care, and mortality for patients with acute respiratory distress syndrome in intensive care units in 50 countries. JAMA. 2016;315(8):788.
5. Roupie E, Lepage E, Wysocki M, Fagon JY, Chastre J, Dreyfuss D, et al. Prevalence, etiologies and outcome of the acute respiratory distress syndrome among hypoxemic ventilated patients. SRLF Collaborative Group on Mechanical Ventilation. Société de Réanimation de Langue Française. Intensive Care Med. 1999;25(9):920–9.
6. Brun-Buisson C, Minelli C, Bertolini G, Brazzi L, Pimentel J, Lewandowski K, et al. Epidemiology and outcome of acute lung injury in European intensive care units. Results from the ALIVE study. Intensive Care Med. 2004;30(1):51–61.
7. Rubenfeld GD, Caldwell E, Peabody E, Weaver J, Martin DP, Neff M, et al. Incidence and outcomes of acute lung injury. N Engl J Med. 2005;353(16):1685–93.

8. Group TICCT. Acute lung injury and the acute respiratory distress syndrome in Ireland: a prospective audit of epidemiology and management. Crit Care. 2008;12(1):30.
9. on behalf of the ALIEN Network, Villar J, Blanco J, Añón JM, Santos-Bouza A, Blanch L, et al. The ALIEN study: incidence and outcome of acute respiratory distress syndrome in the era of lung protective ventilation. Intensive Care Med. 2011;37(12):1932–41.
10. ARDS Definition Task Force, Ranieri VM, Rubenfeld GD, Thompson BT, Ferguson ND, Caldwell E, Fan E, Camporota L, Slutsky AS. Acute respiratory distress syndrome: the Berlin definition. JAMA [Internet]. 2012 Jun 20 [cited 2017 Oct 6];307(23). Available from: http://jama.jamanetwork.com/article.aspx?doi=10.1001/jama.2012.5669.
11. Frat J-P, Thille AW, Mercat A, Girault C, Ragot S, Perbet S, et al. High-flow oxygen through nasal cannula in acute hypoxemic respiratory failure. N Engl J Med. 2015;372(23):2185–96.
12. Rice TW, Wheeler AP, Bernard GR, Hayden DL, Schoenfeld DA, Ware LB. Comparison of the SpO_2/FiO_2 ratio and the PaO_2/FiO_2 ratio in patients with acute lung injury or ARDS. Chest. 2007;132(2):410–7.
13. Amato MBP, Meade MO, Slutsky AS, Brochard L, Costa ELV, Schoenfeld DA, et al. Driving pressure and survival in the acute respiratory distress syndrome. N Engl J Med. 2015;372(8):747–55.
14. Taylor RW. Low-dose inhaled nitric oxide in patients with acute lung injury: a randomized controlled trial. JAMA. 2004;291(13):1603.
15. Acute Respiratory Distress Syndrome Network. Ventilation with lower tidal volumes as compared with traditional tidal volumes for acute lung injury and the acute respiratory distress syndrome. N Engl J Med. 2000;342(18):1301–8.
16. Derdak S, Mehta S, Stewart TE, Smith T, Rogers M, Buchman TG, et al. High-frequency oscillatory ventilation for acute respiratory distress syndrome in adults: a randomized, controlled trial. Am J Respir Crit Care Med. 2002;166(6):801–8.
17. Coudroy R, Frat J-P, Boissier F, Contou D, Robert R, Thille AW. Early identification of acute respiratory distress syndrome in the absence of positive pressure ventilation: implications for revision of the Berlin criteria for acute respiratory distress syndrome. Crit Care Med. 2018;46(4):540–6.
18. Demoule A, Girou E, Richard J-C, Taille S, Brochard L. Benefits and risks of success or failure of noninvasive ventilation. Intensive Care Med. 2006;32(11):1756–65.
19. Thille AW, Contou D, Fragnoli C, Córdoba-Izquierdo A, Boissier F, Brun-Buisson C. Non-invasive ventilation for acute hypoxemic respiratory failure: intubation rate and risk factors. Crit Care. 2013;17(6):R269.
20. Bellani G, Laffey JG, Pham T, Madotto F, Fan E, Brochard L, et al. Non-invasive ventilation of patients with acute respiratory distress syndrome. Insights from the LUNG SAFE Study. Am J Respir Crit Care Med. 2017;195(1):67–77.
21. Serpa Neto A, Cardoso SO, Manetta JA, Pereira VGM, Espósito DC, Pasqualucci MDOP, et al. Association between use of lung-protective ventilation with lower tidal volumes and clinical outcomes among patients without acute respiratory distress syndrome: a meta-analysis. JAMA. 2012;308(16):1651.
22. Murray MJ, DeBlock H, Erstad B, Gray A, Jacobi J, Jordan C, et al. Clinical practice guidelines for sustained neuromuscular blockade in the adult critically ill patient. Crit Care Med. 2016;44(11):2079–103.
23. Guérin C, Reignier J, Richard J-C, Beuret P, Gacouin A, Boulain T, et al. Prone positioning in severe acute respiratory distress syndrome. N Engl J Med. 2013;368(23):2159–68.
24. Adhikari NKJ, Burns KEA, Friedrich JO, Granton JT, Cook DJ, Meade MO. Effect of nitric oxide on oxygenation and mortality in acute lung injury: systematic review and meta-analysis. BMJ. 2007;334(7597):779.
25. Ruan S-Y, Wu H-Y, Lin H-H, Wu H-D, Yu C-J, Lai M-S. Inhaled nitric oxide and the risk of renal dysfunction in patients with acute respiratory distress syndrome: a propensity-matched cohort study. Crit Care [Internet]. 2016 Dec [cited 2017 Oct 6];20(1). Available from: http://ccforum.biomedcentral.com/articles/10.1186/s13054-016-1566-0.
26. Ellis RK. Determination of PO_2 from saturation. J Appl Physiol (Bethesda Md 1985). 1989;67(2):902.
27. Sanz F, Dean N, Dickerson J, Jones B, Knox D, Fernández-Fabrellas E, et al. Accuracy of PaO_2/FiO_2 calculated from SpO_2 for severity assessment in ED patients with pneumonia: PaO_2/FiO_2 from SpO_2 in pneumonia. Respirology. 2015;20(5):813–8.
28. Laffey JG, Pham T, Bellani G. Continued under-recognition of acute respiratory distress syndrome after the Berlin definition: what is the solution? Curr Opin Crit Care. 2017;23(1):10–7.

ICU physicians' and internists' survival predictions for patients evaluated for admission to the intensive care unit

Monica Escher[1,2*], Bara Ricou[3], Mathieu Nendaz[2,4], Fabienne Scherer[1], Stéphane Cullati[1], Patricia Hudelson[5] and Thomas Perneger[6]

Abstract

Background: A higher chance of survival is a key justification for admission to the intensive care unit (ICU). This implies that physicians should be able to accurately estimate a patient's prognosis, whether cared for on the ward or in the ICU. We aimed to determine whether physicians' survival predictions correlate with the admission decisions and with patients' observed survival. Consecutive ICU consultations for internal medicine patients were included. The ICU physician and the internist were asked to predict patient survival with intensive care and with care on the ward using 5 categories of probabilities (< 10%, 10–40%, 41–60%, 61–90%, > 90%). Patient mortality at 28 days was recorded.

Results: Thirty ICU physicians and 97 internists assessed 201 patients for intensive care. Among the patients, 140 (69.7%) were admitted to the ICU. Fifty-eight (28.9%) died within 28 days. Admission to intensive care was associated with predicted survival gain in the ICU, particularly for survival estimates made by ICU physicians. Observed survival was associated with predicted survival, for both groups of physicians. The discrimination of the predictions for survival with intensive care, measured by the area under the ROC curve, was 0.63 for ICU physicians and 0.76 for internists; for survival on the ward the areas under the ROC curves were 0.69 and 0.74, respectively.

Conclusions: Physicians are able to predict survival probabilities when they assess patients for intensive care, albeit imperfectly. Internists are more accurate than ICU physicians. However, ICU physicians' estimates more strongly influence the admission decision. Closer collaboration between ICU physicians and internists is needed.

Keywords: Intensive care, Survival, Prediction, Patient admission, Triage

Background

The decision to admit or not a patient to the intensive care unit (ICU) is often complex and is based on a combination of criteria [1]. They include a patient's need for life-sustaining therapies, but also patient prognosis, prehospital functional status, patient preferences, and available clinical expertise and resources. Since expected survival benefit is one of the main justifications for ICU admission, physicians must estimate and compare the patient's prognosis according to two scenarios: continued care on the ward, and care in the ICU. Most scoring systems apply to patients once admitted to the ICU and the low performance of the few existing triage scores limits their use [2]. Moreover, even validated scoring systems are not accurate enough in predicting an individual's mortality and they should not be used alone to determine level of care [1, 3, 4].

Previous research has shown that physicians predict patient survival more accurately than scoring systems [5]. However, their accuracy in prediction was generally assessed for patients already admitted to the ICU. In one French study, ICU physicians estimated patient mortality at the time of the admission decision [6]. Their predictions were higher than the observed mortality rates both for non-admitted and for admitted patients.

*Correspondence: monica.escher@hcuge.ch
[1] Pain and Palliative Care Consultation, Division of Clinical Pharmacology and Toxicology, Geneva University Hospitals, Rue Gabrielle-Perret-Gentil 4, 1211 Geneva, Switzerland
Full list of author information is available at the end of the article

Furthermore, the requesting physicians and the ICU physicians sometimes disagree about the appropriateness of an ICU admission [7, 8]. Whether this is due to differences in survival estimates or to other reasons is currently unknown.

When medical in-patients become critically ill, the need for intensive care is first assessed by the internists. They will then request an ICU consultation. The final decision about the patient's admission to the ICU belongs to the ICU physician. The ICU physician is not involved in the patient's care if he is not admitted to the ICU. The objective of this study was to compare internists' and ICU physicians' predictions of patient survival if cared on the ward or in the ICU, i.e., expected survival benefit from intensive care, and to determine whether the survival estimates correlated with the admission decisions and with observed survival. We hypothesized that agreement between the physicians would be weak to moderate, that expected survival would be greater in admitted than in non-admitted patients, and that observed survival would be associated with predicted survival. We also hypothesized that ICU physicians, who are used to care for acutely ill patients, would be more accurate in their predictions than internists.

Methods

Setting

The study took place at the Geneva University Hospitals, a tertiary care hospital of 1741 beds, including 156 internal medicine beds and 34 adult ICU beds, between August 2014 and August 2015. It was approved by the Geneva Research Ethics Committee.

Participants

All consecutive ICU consultations for patients hospitalized in the Division of General Internal Medicine were identified. The internist and the ICU physician directly involved were eligible. Upon first contact, all physicians provided written consent to participate and socio-demographic data.

Data collection

Internists and ICU physicians were contacted by phone within 12 h of the request for ICU consultation and were asked to complete a questionnaire. Questionnaires were administered orally, by phone, or by email, according to physicians' preferences. Reminders were sent 3 days later when necessary. Physicians were asked to predict patient survival (i.e., "probability that the patient survives the acute health problem") if admitted in the ICU and if staying on the ward using 5 predetermined categories of probabilities (< 10%, 10–40%, 41–60%, 61–90%, > 90%). They also rated how confident they were in their estimates on a Likert scale ranging from 1 (not at all confident) to 5 (fully confident). Internists were asked about the reason for requesting the ICU consultation and whether the patient was admitted or not. The ICU consultation was included and patient data were recorded only if both physicians completed the questionnaire. Patient data (gender, age, comorbidities) and mortality at 28 days were collected from the electronic patient file.

Sample size and statistical analysis

Sample size was driven by the main objective of the study, i.e., modeling of the decision to admit a patient to intensive care. Assuming 8 potential predictors of the decision to admit the patient, we intended to enroll 80 patients in the smaller of the 2 groups (admitted or not), and aimed for 160 patients if the admission rate was 50%. As the observed admission rate was 70%, the sample size was increased to 200.

Each patient was assigned 4 survival estimates (2 by each of the physicians: survival on the ward and in the ICU) on a 5-point ordinal scale. We compared survival predictions on the ward versus in the ICU for each physician, and survival predictions by the internist versus the intensivist for each location, using paired Wilcoxon tests. We also obtained Spearman correlation coefficients between survival predictions.

To capture the expected survival benefit of an ICU admission, we computed the difference, in survival categories, between predicted survival in the ICU and on the ward, for each physician (thus 0 indicated the same survival category in both locations, and 4 a survival > 90% in the ICU and < 10% on the ward). We cross-tabulated this expected survival benefit with the admission to the ICU, expecting that patients with the highest expected benefit would be the most likely to be admitted (Table 3).

To clarify which physician's opinion weighed more in the decision to admit the patient, we used a logistic regression model, with admission as the dependent variable, and expected survival benefit estimated by each physician as covariates (because of sparse data, expected survival benefit was grouped as −1 or 0, 1 or 2, and 3 or 4).

To assess the accuracy of physicians' predictions, we cross-tabulated predicted survival with observed survival at 28 days, stratifying on the admission decision, separately for the 2 categories of physicians. Because expected survival was on an ordinal scale, we obtained P values for linear trend (Table 4). We also obtained areas under the receiver operating characteristic (ROC) curves. The area represents the probability that predicted survival would be lower for a randomly selected patient who died than for a randomly selected patient who survived; 0.5 corresponds to a coin toss, and 1.0 to perfect discrimination. To clarify which physician's survival prediction was more accurate, we used a logistic regression model with actual survival as the dependent variable, and the 2 physicians' predictions as independent variables.

Finally, we computed mean ratings of confidence (on a 1–5 scale) in the four survival estimates and compared them across levels of survival using Kruskal–Wallis tests.

Results

During the study period, 219 patients were assessed for intensive care admission and 201 situations were included. They involved 128 men and 73 women (Table 1). Mean age was 64.9 years (SD 14.3). Among the patients, 140 (69.7%) were admitted to the ICU and 58 (28.9%) died within 28 days.

In total, 30 ICU physicians (1–14 assessments per physician) and 97 internists (1–11 assessments per physician) participated in the study (Additional file 1: Table S1). ICU physicians were mostly men (66%) and internists mostly women (61%). ICU physicians were older than internists (mean age 38 vs. 30 years, respectively). They were more experienced: mean years from graduation were 12 and 7, respectively, and mean years of experience in medical specialty were 7 and 3.5, respectively. The delay between the admission decision and physicians' prediction of survival was one day or less for 143 (71.1%) of the internists and 127 (63.2%) of the ICU physicians (McNemar test, $P=0.11$).

Predicting survival

The physicians used all five categories of survival probabilities (Table 2). Both physician groups rated expected patient survival significantly higher with care in the ICU rather than on the ward, e.g., the ICU physicians assigned 59.2% of patients to the 2 highest categories of survival (> 60%) if in the ICU, but only 24.8% to the same categories of survival on the ward. For the internists, the corresponding proportions were 67.9% and 13.9%. The internists were more optimistic about the patients' chances of survival with intensive care than the ICU physicians ($P=0.006$) and somewhat more pessimistic about survival on the ward, but the latter difference

Table 1 Patient characteristics

Characteristics	Patients, N (%)[a] ($n=201$)
Men	128 (63.7)
Age, median (IQR) (year)	67 (56–77)
Living place	
Home	191 (95)
Nursing home	10 (5)
Advanced disease	105 (52.2)
Type of disease in patients with advanced disease[b]	($n=105$)
Metastatic cancer or active hematologic malignancy	37 (35.2)
Chronic obstructive pulmonary disease (FEV ≤ 50% or non-invasive ventilation or oxygenotherapy)	38 (36.2)
Chronic heart failure (NYHA III and IV and/or LVEF ≤ 20%)	7 (6.6)
Chronic renal failure (GFR ≤ 30 ml/min)	20 (19.0)
Cirrhosis Child B or C	18 (17.1)
Number of hospitalizations in previous 12 months	
0	107 (53.2)
1	39 (19.4)
> 1	55 (27.4)
Number of days between admission to general internal medicine wards and ICU consultation, median (IQR)	3 (1–8)
Code status (2 missing): full code	104 (51.7)
Reason for calling ICU[c]	
Respiratory failure	111 (55.2)
Cardiac failure or shock (including sepsis)	55 (27.4)
Neurological symptoms	32 (15.9)
Cardiac arrest or arrhythmia	16 (8)
ICU physician's advice	48 (23.9)
Other	18 (8.9)

[a] Data are *N* (%) of patients unless otherwise indicated

[b] Total > 100% because more than one advanced disease per patient

[c] Total > 100% because more than one reason possible

Table 2 Physicians' estimated probabilities of survival for 201 patients evaluated for intensive care

Estimate	Prediction by intensive care physician		Prediction by internist	
	Survival if care in the ICU *N* (%)	Survival if care on the ward *N* (%)	Survival if care in the ICU (2 missing) *N* (%)	Survival if care on the ward *N* (%)
<10%	15 (7.5)	72 (35.8)	8 (4.0)	62 (30.8)
10–40%	34 (16.9)	47 (23.4)	19 (9.5)	62 (30.8)
41–60%	33 (16.4)	32 (15.9)	37 (18.6)	49 (24.4)
61–90%	54 (26.9)	28 (13.9)	72 (36.2)	24 (11.9)
> 90%	65 (32.3)	22 (10.9)	63 (31.7)	4 (2.0)
Within physician*	$P<0.001$		$P<0.001$	

* Wilcoxon paired test

was not statistically significant ($P = 0.079$). As expected, the survival estimates were correlated with each other, both within physician (Spearman r correlation coefficient 0.69 for the ICU physician and 0.61 for the internist) and between physicians (0.48 for survival if in the ICU, 0.44 for survival on the ward).

Estimated survival benefit

We examined the difference in expected survival categories between care in the ICU and on the ward (Table 3). For the ICU physicians, 31.4% of the patients would not increase their chances of survival if admitted to the ICU. The other patients would gain between 1 and 4 categories on the 5-level survival scale. Internists were globally more optimistic than intensive care physicians ($P < 0.001$) and classified only 11.9% of the patients as not increasing their chances of survival if admitted to the ICU.

Survival benefit and admission to the ICU

Ratings by both physicians were associated with observed proportions of admitted patients (Table 3). The probability of admission was below 40% for patients who were not expected to improve their survival if admitted, but exceeded 80% if the patient was predicted to gain 2 categories of survival or more. The linear association between survival gain and admission was highly significant for both physicians. However, ICU physicians' estimates had a greater influence on the admission decision: the adjusted odds ratios of admission were 7.6 (95% confidence interval 3.6–15.8) for a gain of 1–2 categories, and 30.8 (95% CI 3.8–247) for a gain of 3–4 categories, compared to no gain. The corresponding adjusted odds ratios for estimates made by the internist were 2.3 (95% CI 0.8–6.5) and 4.2 (95% CI 1.1–16.4).

Patient survival

Of the 140 patients admitted to the ICU, 40 (28.6%) had died at 28 days of follow-up, and of the 61 patients who were not admitted to the ICU, 18 (29.5%) had died. Observed survival was associated with predicted survival, for both groups of physicians (Table 4). Patient survival in the ICU ranged from 33.3 to 91.4% across categories of survival predicted by ICU physicians, and from 0 to 95.1% across predictions made by internists. The discrimination of the predictions, measured by the area under the ROC curve, was 0.63 and 0.76, respectively. The predictions for the patients who stayed on the ward were of similar accuracy. The gradients of observed proportions of survivors ran from 40.0 to 85.0% across estimates made by ICU physicians, and from 25.0 to 100% across estimates made by internists. The areas under the ROC curves were 0.69 and 0.74, respectively.

We compared the predictions made by the two groups of physicians in mutually adjusted logistic regression models (Table 5). For both groups of patients—those admitted to the ICU and those who stayed on the ward—the prediction of the internists was more accurate. In fact, once the opinion of the internists was taken into account, the ICU physicians' estimates did not increase the accuracy in predicting survival.

On the whole, physicians felt rather confident about their survival estimates, ICU physicians more so than internists (in the ICU: mean 4.2 vs. 3.9, on the ward 4.2 vs. 3.8, both $P < 0.001$). Physicians' confidence differed according to the survival probabilities (Additional file 2: Table S2). It was higher for extreme probabilities (i.e., < 10% or > 90%) than for mid-range probabilities.

Discussion

In this study we found that physicians involved in decisions to admit patients to the ICU were able to predict short term survival for admitted and non-admitted patients. The physicians perceived a survival benefit from

Table 3 Estimated gain in survival attributable to intensive care, and observed proportion of patients admitted

Difference in survival categories* between ICU and ward	Intensive care physician		Internist	
	N (%)	Proportion admitted (%)	*N* (%)	Proportion admitted (%)
Loss of 1	5 (2.5)	80.0	–	
Even	58 (28.9)	32.8	24 (11.9)	37.5
Gain of 1	62 (30.8)	79.0	75 (37.3)	61.3
Gain of 2	50 (24.9)	88.0	65 (32.3)	86.2
Gain of 3	22 (10.9)	90.9	29 (14.4)	82.8
Gain of 4	4 (2.0)	100	6 (3.0)	83.3
Test for linear trend		<0.001		<0.001

*Survival was categorized as < 10%, 10–40%, 41–60%, 61–90%, > 90%

Table 4 Patients' observed 28 day survival according to physicians' survival predictions

Predicted survival if care in the ICU	Patients admitted to intensive care ($N=140$)			
	Intensive care physicians		Internists	
	N (column %)	Survived (row %)	*N* (column %)	Survived (row %)
<10%	6 (4.3)	2 (33.3)	2 (1.4)	0 (0)
10–40%	30 (21.4)	18 (60.0)	16 (11.4)	4 (25.0)
41–60%	27 (19.3)	18 (66.7)	28 (20.0)	17 (60.7)
61–90%	42 (30.0)	30 (71.4)	53 (37.9)	40 (75.5)
>90%	35 (25.0)	32 (91.4)	41 (29.3)	39 (95.1)
P for linear trend	$P=0.001$		$P<0.001$	
Area under ROC curve	0.63 (0.53–0.73)		0.76 (0.67–0.84)	
Predicted survival if care on the ward	**Patients NOT admitted to intensive care ($N=61$)**			
	Intensive care physicians		Internists	
	N (column %)	Survived (row %)	*N* (column %)	Survived (row %)
<10%	10 (16.4)	4 (40.0)	12 (19.7)	3 (25.0)
10–40%	11 (18.0)	7 (63.6)	14 (23.0)	11 (78.6)
41–60%	9 (14.8)	7 (77.8)	19 (31.1)	15 (78.9)
61–90%	11 (18.0)	8 (72.7)	13 (21.3)	11 (84.4)
>90%	20 (32.8)	17 (85.0)	3 (4.9)	3 (100)
P for linear trend	$P=0.016$		$P=0.001$	
Area under ROC curve	0.69 (0.54–0.84)		0.74 (0.61–0.89)	

Table 5 Multivariate regression model of survival at 28 days, according to physicians' baseline predictions

Physicians' predictions	Odds ratio*	95% CI	*P* value
	Patients admitted to ICU		
Intensive care physicians	1.32	0.90–1.93	0.15
Internists	3.05	1.87–4.95	<0.001
	Patients on ward		
Intensive care physicians	1.23	0.78–1.96	0.37
Internists	2.23	1.14–4.34	0.019

*The odds ratios are for a 1 category increase on the 5-point survival prediction scale. Predictions made by internists and by ICU physicians are adjusted for each other

an admission to intensive care for a majority of patients. Internists' estimates of survival were higher than ICU physicians', but globally there was a substantial agreement between the 2 groups of physicians. Physicians showed high levels of confidence in their estimates.

The estimated survival benefit was associated with the decision to admit a patient to the ICU: most patients with a high expected benefit were admitted compared to a minority of patients with a low expected benefit. The ICU admission decision was more strongly influenced by the ICU physician's survival prediction than by the internist's. However internists predicted patient survival more accurately than ICU physicians, both for patients admitted to the ICU and for those who remained on the ward.

Our results expand on available data. In a small study based on scenarios, good agreement about ICU survival prediction was also found between internists and ICU physicians, but their prediction accuracy varied [9]. In our study higher accuracy in prediction is likely explained by the fact that physicians estimated survival for patients they had actually assessed. We could not compare physicians' performance with a scoring system as no validated score exists for estimating patient prognosis at the time of triage [10, 11]. However, physicians' clinical judgment has been shown to be at least as accurate as objective risk scores for predicting mortality in patients admitted to the ICU [5] and for predicting medical in-patients' deterioration [12]. Values of the ROC curves in our study were similar to those published for ICU physicians' survival estimates for patients admitted to intensive care. Our findings also show that both internists and ICU physicians are accurate about patient prognosis under different circumstances, i.e., at the time of triage and for continued care on the ward or for care in the ICU.

In keeping with recommendations about ICU admission [1], physicians' predicted gain in survival was associated with admission decisions. Interestingly, some patients with no expected survival benefit were admitted. It suggests that physicians are aware of their limited ability in predicting survival for individuals and prefer to err toward overtriage, an attitude supported by current guidelines [1]. Considerations other than survival may also be deemed important enough for physicians to propose intensive care. Notably, during the updating process of a consensus statement about triage principles, ICU experts could not agree about a survival cutoff precluding ICU admission, not even for a chance of survival of 0.1% or less [13]. Furthermore, ICU physicians seem to use less stringent admission criteria when more ICU beds are available [14–16].

Not surprisingly the ICU physicians' opinions weighed more than the internists' in the decision to admit a patient to the ICU. ICU physicians are considered experts and most capable in estimating the benefit of intensive care for patients. Our findings however challenge this assumption, as internists were more accurate in predicting patient survival for both care on the ward and in the ICU. In this respect, the influence of ICU physicians on the admission decision may not be entirely justified, all the more so that they sometimes assume a dismissive behavior toward requesting physicians and potentially disregard their assessment [8, 17, 18]. Because considerations other than survival benefit influence ICU admission decisions, increased collaborative decision making between ICU physicians and internists seems advisable.

Our study has several limitations. The involved physicians were contacted after they had discussed intensive care for a patient. So their opinions were not independent as they had had the opportunity to come to a shared assessment of the situation. It may partially explain the high level of agreement between the physicians. In some cases, the patient may have died by the time the physicians completed the questionnaire, in which case survival predictions would have been meaningless. However, it would not change the main findings of this study, as it would concern a minority of patients. Moreover, only the physician caring for the patient would know about his death, and for patients assessed during night shifts and week-ends he would not necessarily be the physician in charge at the time of death. Delay between admission decision and completion of the questionnaire may cause an overestimation of physicians' accuracy in prediction, as the physician in charge had the opportunity to observe how the patient's condition evolved. We minimized this risk by contacting physicians twice a day, and by offering them to complete the questionnaire on the phone, thus keeping delays as short as possible. Moreover, on average, the delays were longer for ICU physicians, whose predictions were less accurate than those of the internists. Hence, if delays caused a bias, it should be conservative.

Conclusions

Physicians are able to predict survival probabilities for patients assessed for admission to intensive care, albeit imperfectly. Internists are more accurate than ICU physicians. However, ICU physicians' estimates more strongly influence the admission decision. These results highlight the need for objective risk scores in support to physicians' judgment and for closer collaboration between internists and ICU physicians. Strategies to improve the decision making process should focus on the development of valid triage scoring systems and address potential communication gaps between physicians.

Authors' contributions

Conceived and designed the study: ME, BR, MN, SC, PH, TP. Collected the data: FS. Analyzed the data: ME, BR, MN, TP. Drafted the manuscript: ME. Read and commented the paper: ME, BR, MN, FS, SC, PH, TP. All authors read and approved the final manuscript.

Author details

[1] Pain and Palliative Care Consultation, Division of Clinical Pharmacology and Toxicology, Geneva University Hospitals, Rue Gabrielle-Perret-Gentil 4, 1211 Geneva, Switzerland. [2] Unit of Development and Research in Medical Education, Faculty of Medicine, University of Geneva, Geneva, Switzerland. [3] Division of Intensive Care, Geneva University Hospitals, Geneva, Switzerland. [4] Division of General Internal Medicine, Geneva University Hospitals, Geneva, Switzerland. [5] Division of Primary Care Medicine, Geneva University Hospitals, Geneva, Switzerland. [6] Division of Clinical Epidemiology, Geneva University Hospitals, Geneva, Switzerland.

Competing interests

All the authors declare that they have no conflict of interest.

Funding

This study was funded by the Swiss National Science Foundation, National Research Program "End of Life" (NRP 67), Grant No. 139304. The Swiss National Science Foundation did not contribute to the design of the study, to the collection, analysis, and interpretation of data and to the writing of the manuscript.

References

1. Nates JL, Nunnally M, Kleinpell R, Blosser S, Goldner J, Birriel B, et al. ICU admission, discharge, and triage guidelines: a framework to enhance clinical operations, development of institutional policies, and further research. Crit Care Med. 2016;44:1553–602.
2. Jansen JO, Cuthbertson BH. Detecting critical illness outside the ICU: the role of track and trigger systems. Curr Opin Crit Care. 2010;16:184–90.
3. Vincent J, Moreno R. Scoring systems in the critically ill. Crit Care. 2010;14:207.
4. Christian MD, Fowler R, Muller MP, Gomersall C, Sprung CL, Hupert N, et al. Critical care resource allocation: trying to PREEDICCT outcomes without a crystal ball. Crit Care. 2013;17:107.

5. Sinuff T, Adhikari NK, Cook DJ, Schunemann HJ, Griffith LE, Rocker G, et al. Mortality predictions in the intensive care unit: comparing physicians with scoring systems. Crit Care Med. 2006;34:878–85.
6. Garrouste-Orgeas M, Montuclard L, Timsit JF, Misset B, Christias M, Carlet J. Triaging patients to the ICU: a pilot study of factors influencing admission decisions and patient outcomes. Intensive Care Med. 2003;29:774–81.
7. Boumendil A, Angus DC, Guitonneau AL, Menn AM, Ginsburg C, Takun K, et al. Variability of intensive care admission decisions for the very elderly. PLoS ONE. 2012;7:e34387.
8. Fassier T, Valour E, Colin C, Danet F. Who am I to decide whether this person is to die today? Physicians' life-or-death decisions for elderly critically ill patients at the emergency department-ICU interface: a qualitative study. Ann Emerg Med. 2016;68(28–39):e3.
9. Dahine J, Mardini L, Jayaraman D. The perceived likelihood of outcome of critical care patients and its impact on triage decisions: a case-based survey of intensivists and internists in a Canadian, Quaternary Care Hospital Network. PLoS ONE. 2016;11:e0149196.
10. Sprung CL, Baras M, Iapichino G, Kesecioglu J, Lippert A, Hargreaves C, et al. The Eldicus prospective, observational study of triage decision making in European intensive care units: part I-European Intensive Care Admission Triage Scores. Crit Care Med. 2012;40:125–31.
11. Ramos JG, Perondi B, Dias RD, Miranda LC, Cohen C, Carvalho CR, et al. Development of an algorithm to aid triage decisions for intensive care unit admission: a clinical vignette and retrospective cohort study. Crit Care. 2016;20:81.
12. Patel AR, Zadravecz FJ, Young RS, Williams MV, Churpek MM, Edelson DP. The value of clinical judgment in the detection of clinical deterioration. JAMA Intern Med. 2015;175:456–8.
13. Sprung CL, Danis M, Iapichino G, Artigas A, Kesecioglu J, Moreno R, et al. Triage of intensive care patients: identifying agreement and controversy. Intensive Care Med. 2013;39:1916–24.
14. Sinuff T, Kahnamoui K, Cook DJ, Luce JM, Levy MM, Values E, et al. Rationing critical care beds: a systematic review. Crit Care Med. 2004;32:1588–97.
15. Stelfox HT, Hemmelgarn BR, Bagshaw SM, Gao S, Doig CJ, Nijssen-Jordan C, et al. Intensive care unit bed availability and outcomes for hospitalized patients with sudden clinical deterioration. Arch Intern Med. 2012;172:467–74.
16. Gooch RA, Kahn JM. ICU bed supply, utilization, and health care spending: an example of demand elasticity. JAMA. 2014;311:567–8.
17. Oerlemans AJ, van Sluisveld N, van Leeuwen ES, Wollersheim H, Dekkers WJ, Zegers M. Ethical problems in intensive care unit admission and discharge decisions: a qualitative study among physicians and nurses in the Netherlands. BMC Med Ethics. 2015;16:9.
18. Escher M, Cullati S, Hudelson P, Nendaz M, Ricou B, Perneger T, et al. Admission to intensive care: a qualitative study of triage and its determinants. Health Serv Res. 2018. https://doi.org/10.1111/1475-6773.13076.

19

Targeted temperature management in the ICU: guidelines from a French expert panel

Alain Cariou[1*], Jean-François Payen[2], Karim Asehnoune[14], Gerard Audibert[9], Astrid Botte[15], Olivier Brissaud[16], Guillaume Debaty[13], Sandrine Deltour[19], Nicolas Deye[6], Nicolas Engrand[10], Gilles Francony[1], Stéphane Legriel[7], Bruno Levy[8], Philippe Meyer[17], Jean-Christophe Orban[11], Sylvain Renolleau[18], Bernard Vigue[12], Laure De Saint Blanquat[4], Cyrille Mathien[3], Lionel Velly[5] and for the Société de Réanimation de Langue Française (SRLF) and the Société Française d'Anesthésie et de Réanimation (SFAR) In conjunction with the Association de Neuro Anesthésie Réanimation de Langue Française (ANARLF), the Groupe Francophone de Réanimation et Urgences Pédiatriques (GFRUP), the Société Française de Médecine d'Urgence (SFMU), and the Société Française Neuro-Vasculaire (SFNV)

Abstract

Over the recent period, the use of induced hypothermia has gained an increasing interest for critically ill patients, in particular in brain-injured patients. The term "targeted temperature management" (TTM) has now emerged as the most appropriate when referring to interventions used to reach and maintain a specific level temperature for each individual. TTM may be used to prevent fever, to maintain normothermia, or to lower core temperature. This treatment is widely used in intensive care units, mostly as a primary neuroprotective method. Indications are, however, associated with variable levels of evidence based on inhomogeneous or even contradictory literature. Our aim was to conduct a systematic analysis of the published data in order to provide guidelines. We present herein recommendations for the use of TTM in adult and paediatric critically ill patients developed using the Grading of Recommendations Assessment, Development, and Evaluation (GRADE) method. These guidelines were conducted by a group of experts from the French Intensive Care Society (Société de Réanimation de Langue Française [SRLF]) and the French Society of Anesthesia and Intensive Care Medicine (Société Francaise d'Anesthésie Réanimation [SFAR]) with the participation of the French Emergency Medicine Association (Société Française de Médecine d'Urgence [SFMU]), the French Group for Pediatric Intensive Care and Emergencies (Groupe Francophone de Réanimation et Urgences Pédiatriques [GFRUP]), the French National Association of Neuro-Anesthesiology and Critical Care (Association Nationale de Neuro-Anesthésie Réanimation Française [ANARLF]), and the French Neurovascular Society (Société Française Neurovasculaire [SFNV]). Fifteen experts and two coordinators agreed to consider questions concerning TTM and its practical implementation in five clinical situations: cardiac arrest, traumatic brain injury, stroke, other brain injuries, and shock. This resulted in 30 recommendations: 3 recommendations were strong (Grade 1), 13 were weak (Grade 2), and 14 were experts' opinions. After two rounds of rating and various amendments, a strong agreement from voting participants was obtained for all 30 (100%) recommendations, which are exposed in the present article.

*Correspondence: alain.cariou@aphp.fr
[1] Medical Intensive Care Unit, Cochin University Hospital (APHP) & Paris Descartes University, 27 rue du Faubourg Saint-Jacques, 75014 Paris, France
Full list of author information is available at the end of the article

Introduction

The protective effects of hypothermia were first studied and described in the late 1950s and then seem to have been forgotten for roughly 20 years before intensivists revived interest in this therapeutic method [1, 2]. Experimental data show that the neuroprotective effects of therapeutic hypothermia occur through several mechanisms of action:

- reducing brain metabolism, which restores a favourable balance with cerebral blood flow in injured brain tissue [3, 4];
- lowering the intracranial pressure;
- reducing the initiation of brain cell apoptosis, notably the caspase activation pathway, and of necrosis [5];
- decreasing the local release of lactate and of excitotoxic compounds such as glutamate, that is associated with alteration in calcium homoeostasis during brain ischaemia [6–8];
- reducing brain tissue inflammatory response and systemic inflammatory response syndrome [7, 9];
- decreasing the production of free radicals [7, 10];
- limiting the vascular and cell membrane permeability as seen in brain ischaemia [10].

Accordingly, the use of mild to moderate hypothermia has gained interest for critically ill patients, in particular brain-injured patients in order to limit the extension of initial brain lesions [11]. This can be achieved through various methods and targeted temperatures. The term "targeted temperature management" (TTM) has emerged as the most appropriate referring to interventions used to reach and maintain a specific level temperature for each individual.

The level of targeted temperature may differ according to the situation. TTM may be used to prevent fever, to maintain normothermia, or to lower core temperature. TTM is widely used in intensive care units (ICUs) as a primary neuroprotective method, i.e. in order to protect against neuronal injury or degeneration in the central nervous system. Its indications are, however, associated with variable levels of evidence based on inhomogeneous or even contradictory literature. Our aim was to conduct a systematic analysis of the literature in order to edit national guidelines.

Methods

These guidelines were conducted by a group of experts for the French Intensive Care Society (Société de Réanimation de Langue Française [SRLF]) and the French Society of Anesthesia and Intensive Care Medicine (Société Francaise d'Anesthésie Réanimation [SFAR]). The organization committee defined a list of questions to be addressed and designated experts in charge of each question. The questions were formulated using the PICO (Patient Intervention Comparison Outcome) format (http://www.gradeworkinggroup.org/).

The method used to elaborate these recommendations was the GRADE® method [12]. Following a quantitative literature analysis, this method is used to separately determine the quality of available evidence, i.e. estimation of the confidence needed to analyse the effect of the quantitative intervention, and the level of recommendation. The quality of evidence is rated as follows:

- high-quality evidence: further research is very unlikely to change the confidence in the estimate of the effect;
- moderate-quality evidence: further research is likely to have an impact on the confidence in the estimate of the effect and may change the estimate of the effect itself;
- low-quality evidence: further research is very likely to have an impact on the confidence in the estimate of the effect and is likely to change the estimate of the effect itself;
- very low-quality evidence: any estimate of the effect is very unlikely.

The level of recommendation is binary (either positive or negative) and strong or weak:

- strong recommendation: we recommend (GRADE 1+) or we do not recommend to do (GRADE 1−);
- weak recommendation: we suggest (GRADE 2+) or we do not suggest to do (GRADE 2−).

The strength of the recommendations is determined according to key factors and validated by the experts after a vote, using the Delphi and GRADE Grid method [13] that encompasses the following criteria:

- the estimate of the effect;
- the global level of evidence: the higher the level of evidence, the stronger the recommendation;
- the balance between desirable and undesirable effects: the more favourable the balance, the stronger the recommendation;
- values and preferences: in case of uncertainty or large variability, the level of evidence of the recommendation is probably weak, and values and preferences must be more clearly obtained from the affected persons (patient, physician, and decision-maker);
- cost: the greater the costs or the use of resources, the weaker the recommendation.

The elaboration of a recommendation requires that at least 50% of voting participants have an opinion and that less than 20% of participants vote for the opposite proposition. The elaboration of a strong agreement requires the agreement of at least 70% of voting participants.

Results

Areas of recommendations

Fifteen experts and two coordinators agreed to consider questions concerning TTM and its practical implementation in five clinical situations in the intensive care setting: cardiac arrest (CA), traumatic brain injury (TBI), stroke, other brain injuries, and shock. The PubMed and Cochrane databases were searched for full articles written in English or French published after January 2005 and June 2015. In case of an absence or a very low number of publications during the considered period, the timing of publications could have been extended to 1995. The paediatric literature had a specific analysis.

The experts summarized the work and applied the GRADE® method, resulting in 30 recommendations: 3 recommendations were strong (Grade 1), 13 were weak (Grade 2), and 14 were expert opinions. After two rounds of rating and various amendments, a strong agreement from voting participants was obtained for all 30 (100%) recommendations.

TTM after cardiac arrest

R1.1 We recommend using TTM in order to improve survival with good neurological outcome in patients resuscitated from out-of-hospital cardiac arrest (OHCA) with shockable cardiac rhythm (ventricular fibrillation and pulseless ventricular tachycardia) and who remain comatose after return of spontaneous circulation (ROSC).

(Grade 1+)

Rationale: Seven meta-analyses [14–20] and 4 systematic reviews [13, 21–23] assessed studies on targeted TTM after CA, but none identified separately patients with initial shockable versus non-shockable rhythm. Two studies with patients presenting initial shockable rhythm have been retained in the analysis [24, 25] and were in favour of the TTM use in this population. These trials (one pseudo-randomized [24] and one randomized [25]) found improved neurological outcome for OHCA patients with an initial shockable rhythm. Several studies were not included in the present analysis: (1) the TTM trial [26] because of the absence of a group with no control of body temperature, i.e. the trial compared TTM at 33 °C versus TTM at 36 °C, (2) a trial comparing a combination of hemofiltration with TTM versus hemofiltration alone versus no hemofiltration and no TTM [27], (3) clinical trials that assessed pre-hospital TTM. Observational studies, before–after studies, and matched cohort studies found results in favour of TTM use, despite a low to very low level of evidence [18]. International guidelines using the GRADE method and including Bernard [24] and HACA [25] trials strongly recommended the use of TTM for OHCA patients with an initial shockable rhythm to increase survival with good neurological outcome [13]. A recent meta-analysis also supports the use of TTM in this population [14].

R1.2 We suggest considering TTM in order to improve survival with good neurological outcome in patients resuscitated from OHCA with non-shockable cardiac rhythm (asystole or pulseless electrical activity) and who remain comatose after ROSC.

(Grade 2+)

Rationale: Among 8 meta-analyses [14–20, 28] and 4 reviews [13, 21–23] on TTM after CA, 1 meta-analysis specifically analysed patients with initial non-shockable rhythm [28]. This meta-analysis found decreased hospital mortality in patients with TTM: RR 0.86 (95% CI 0.76–0.99), but there was no difference regarding neurological outcome: RR 0.96 (95% CI 0.90–1.02). One randomized control trial [29] with a limited sample size ($n = 30$) compared patients treated with TTM *versus* no TTM and found no difference between the 2 groups. Most observational studies (low to very low level of evidence) did not observe significant between-groups differences. Although some studies were in favour of TTM use in this population [30–32], a majority of studies did not report a clinical improvement by using TTM [33–38]. Based on the poor prognosis in this population and considering the lack of therapeutic alternatives, the experts considered that TTM could be suggested in this population.

R1.3 We suggest considering TTM in order to increase survival with good neurological outcome in patients resuscitated from in-hospital cardiac arrest (IHCA) who remain comatose after ROSC.

(Expert opinion)

Rationale: There are no published randomized controlled trials with patients presenting in-hospital cardiac arrest (IHCA) patients. From 4 studies having included patients with IHCA or OHCA, it was not possible to separately analyse IHCA patients [37, 39–41]. In the overall population, the results are either in favour of TTM [31, 42] or neutral [34, 37, 39–41].

R1.4 We suggest considering TTM between 32 and 36 °C in order to improve survival with good neurological outcome after CA.

(Grade 2+)

Rationale: Two studies with a high level of evidence and consistent results addressed this question [14, 26]. One randomized controlled trial included 939 patients and found no significant difference in survival and neurological outcome between TTM at 33 °C versus TTM at 36 °C [26]. Similar results were reported in a meta-analysis [14]. This meta-analysis included 6 randomized studies using different degrees of temperature [24–27, 29, 43] and concluded that a TTM strategy using a targeted temperature <34 °C might improve outcome compared to a strategy with no TTM. A randomized controlled trial [43] comparing TTM at 32 versus 34 °C was not included in our analysis because this pilot trial included 36 patients only. A retrospective study, not retained in the analysis, found a better outcome at TTM 32–34 °C versus spontaneous normothermia below 37.5 °C [44]. *Post hoc* study derived from the TTM trial [26] was also not included to avoid duplicate data: it was found a possible worsening in outcome in the TTM 33 °C group for patients with shock at hospital admission [45]. Overall, targeted temperatures in clinical studies can be ranged between 32 and 36 °C, although it is not possible to define the optimal temperature within this range.

R1.5 We do not suggest initiating TTM with infusion of large volumes of cold saline solution during transportation to the hospital after CA.

(Grade 2−)

Rationale: Several randomized studies reported that pre-hospital infusion of cold fluids was not associated with improved outcome, whether this administration was conducted during resuscitation (intra-arrest cooling) or after ROSC [46–50]. In one randomized controlled trial [46], pre-hospital infusion of large volumes of cold saline solution (4 °C) was associated with increased occurrence of re-arrest after ROSC and of pulmonary oedema [46]. Alternative methods of pre-hospital cooling were too limited to assess impact on outcome [24, 51]. The impact of shortening time to reach TTM during the induction phase of TTM is discussed elsewhere (R6.1). Conversely, any onset of hyperthermia after ROSC appears deleterious in terms of outcome [52, 53].

R1.1 Paediatric—In comatose children following resuscitation from OHCA or IHCA with a shockable or a non-shockable cardiac rhythm, we recommend using TTM to maintain normothermia in order to improve neurological outcome.

(Expert opinion)

R1.2 Paediatric—in comatose children following resuscitation from OHCA or IHCA with a shockable or a non-shockable cardiac rhythm, we do not suggest using TTM between 32 and 34 °C to improve survival with good neurological outcome.

(Grade 2−)

Rationale: In a randomized study [54], 270 children (2 days–18 years) with OHCA were compared: 142 children allocated to TTM at 33 °C versus 128 to TTM 36–37.5 °C during 5 days. There was no significant difference between groups in survival rate with good neurological outcome. In this population, hypoxia was the main cause of OHCA (72%), which may explain why these results differed from adults [24, 25]. In a recent study, TTM lower than 32 °C was associated with higher mortality rate [55]. Other retrospective or prospective studies had limited population size, and mixed OHCA and IHCA, cardiac and respiratory causes. Although hypothermia was still recommended in 2010 [56, 57], the latest recommendations by the International Liaison Committee on Resuscitation (ILCOR) endorsed the latest trials and did not recommend any longer using hypothermia in children who remain comatose after resuscitation CA [58].

TTM after traumatic brain injury

R2.1 In patients with severe traumatic brain injury, we suggest considering TTM at 35–37 °C in order to control intracranial pressure.

(Grade 2+)

Rationale: In a case–control series of patients with severe traumatic brain injury (TBI), Puccio et al. [59] showed that patients with TTM maintained at 36–36.5 °C within 72 h of TBI presented a lower averaged intracranial pressure (ICP) and fewer episodes of ICP >25 mmHg as compared with patients who did not receive TTM. Several series of clinical cases [60–62] showed a correlation between core temperature, brain temperature, and ICP. However, there is no randomized controlled study showing that TTM at 35–37 °C in patients with severe TBI was associated with prevention of intracranial hypertension.

R2.2 In patients with severe traumatic brain injury, we suggest considering TTM at 35–37 °C to improve survival with good neurological outcome.

(Grade 2+)

Rationale: In patients with TBI, hyperthermia is associated with higher mortality rates [63, 64], unfavourable neurological outcome [63–66], and prolonged length of stay in the ICU and in the hospital [63, 67, 68]. A cohort of patients with head injury (65% of TBI) did not show improved neurological outcome in patients who received TTM as compared with historical controls with no TTM [69]. There is yet no randomized controlled study showing that TTM in patients with TBI is associated with improved neurological outcome, reduced mortality rate, or length of hospital stay. Despite the low level of evidence, the aggravated outcome associated with hyperthermia supports the recommendation to maintain TTM between 35 and 37 °C.

Several studies with a higher level of evidence [70–74] and meta-analyses [75–77] in adults and children showed no benefit regarding mortality or neurological outcome with the use of therapeutic hypothermia between 32 and 35 °C, compared to normothermia in patients with severe TBI whether they had intracranial hypertension or not.

R2.3 In TBI patients with refractory intracranial hypertension despite medical treatments, we suggest considering TTM at 34–35 °C in order to lower ICP.

(Grade 2+)

Rationale: Several studies showed that TTM at 34–35 °C could lower ICP [70, 75, 78–84], while this effect was not confirmed elsewhere [71, 72], and a raised in ICP was seen during rewarming [69]. Polderman et al. [85] showed in 136 patients (64 patients receiving barbiturates + hypothermia versus 72 patients receiving barbiturates alone) that therapeutic hypothermia was superior to barbiturates alone to treat high ICP and was associated with a reduced mortality rate. In the Eurotherm trial [86], which is the first randomized, multicentre study in a population of TBI patients with ICP above 20 mmHg, 195 patients were treated with TTM (32–35 °C) versus 192 patients treated with normothermia. High ICP was easier to control in patients of the TTM group (barbiturates were used in 41 control patients versus 20 TTM patients). However, several studies found no additional clinical benefit where lowering temperature below 34 °C. In 22 patients with severe head injury, Shiozaki et al. [87] found that intracranial hypertension persisting at 34 °C was not reduced any further by lowering the temperature up to 31 °C. Using multimodal monitoring, hypothermia below 35 °C showed no benefit regarding brain tissue oxygen tension (PtiO2) or biomarkers of brain metabolism [60], and this strategy has a deleterious effect on these parameters [88]. TTM between 32 and 35 °C to treat high ICP can result in side effects, e.g. respiratory infections, that are proportional to the duration and/or depth of hypothermia [75, 76].

The duration of hypothermia should be adapted according to the persistence of intracranial hypertension. In a study of 215 patients with severe TBI, a 5-day duration of hypothermia resulted in better control of ICP and neurological outcome than a 2-day period. In addition, rewarming after 5 days resulted in less rebound effect of ICH than after 2 days [89]. The meta-analysis of McIntyre et al. [90] was in line with these findings.

Sustained elevation of ICP is an independent factor of poor outcome after TBI. Uncontrolled studies indicated that therapeutic hypothermia to treat high ICP could be associated with better outcome [77, 78, 82, 91]. However, the Eurotherm study [86] showed that TTM had a negative effect on neurological outcome at 6 months with an odds ratio of unfavourable outcome after adjustment at 1.53 (1.02–2.30) ($P = 0.04$); favourable outcome (Glasgow Outcome Scale Extended score 5–8) 26% in the TTM 32–35 group versus 37% for patients in the control group ($P = 0.03$). It should be noted that ICP was moderately elevated in that trial, i.e. 20–30 mmHg and of short-term duration (5 min), and that therapeutic hypothermia was initiated with cold saline infusion prior to using treatments for high ICP (osmotic therapy).

R2.1 Paediatric—In children with severe traumatic brain injury, we recommend using TTM at normothermia.

(Expert opinion)

R2.2 Paediatric—In children with severe traumatic brain injury, we do not recommend using TTM at 32–34 °C to improve outcome or control intracranial hypertension.

(Grade 1−)

Rationale: A randomized study including 225 patients [70] and another one with 77 patients, which was terminated prematurely because of futility [73], support the conclusion that moderate hypothermia (32–34 °C) provides no benefit in terms of outcome in severely brain-injured children. A post hoc study by Hutchison et al. [92] showed a higher incidence of low arterial blood pressure and low cerebral perfusion pressure during moderate hypothermia (32–34 °C). A retrospective study in 117 severe TBI children identified early hyperthermia as an independent factor associated with aggravated outcome (OR for lower Glasgow Coma Scale score at PICU discharge: 4.7, CI 1.4–15.6; OR for longer length of stay in PICU: 8.5, CI 2.8–25.6) [93]. TTM may reduce ICP in TBI children as seen in adults.

TTM after stroke, intra-cerebral haemorrhage, and subarachnoid haemorrhage

R3.1 We suggest considering TTM at normothermia during the early phase of severe ischaemic stroke.

(Expert opinion)

Rationale: Hyperthermia or fever is a frequent complication (>50%) in patients at the acute phase of stroke and is correlated with poor functional outcome [63]. However, the efficacy of therapeutic hypothermia has not yet been shown, according to 6 randomized trials that tested hypothermia (33–35 °C) in stroke patients [94–99]. There were few patients and methodological biases were numerous. A single study [99] investigated patients with severe stroke (NIHSS >15). Two randomized studies are ongoing: EuroHYP-1 [100] explores the value of 24 h; 34–35 °C hypothermia following recent stroke, and the recent ICTuS 2/3 trial [101]. In that later study, intravascular therapeutic hypothermia was found safe and feasible in patients treated with recombinant tissue-type plasminogen activator.

Routine use of antipyretics is commonly recommended in patients with hyperthermia, though there is no evidence of their impact on neurological outcome or mortality. The meta-analysis of Ntaios et al. [102] that included 4 major randomized trials [103–106] found no difference in mortality or neurological outcome between hypothermia and hyperthermia (>38 °C).

R3.2 In comatose patients with spontaneous intracerebral haemorrhage, we suggest considering TTM at 35–37 °C to lower intracranial pressure.

(Expert opinion)

Rationale: Observational studies showed that fever is indicative of poor neurological outcome after intra-cerebral haemorrhage [107, 108]. However, most of these studies were observational, with a small number of patients and methodological biases. Two observational studies showed that hypothermia at 35 °C over 8–10 days had a favourable effect on peri-haemorrhagic oedema and ICP, with no benefit on neurological outcome [109, 110]. A case–control study using TTM at 37 °C found no effect on neurological outcome at ICU discharge, while the duration of mechanical ventilation and length of stay in the ICU was prolonged in patients treated with TTM [111]. The effect of hypothermia at 35 °C during 8 days is ongoing in patients with a large intra-cerebral haemorrhage (25–64 mL) (CINCH trial) [112].

R3.3 In comatose patients with aneurysmal subarachnoid haemorrhage, we suggest considering TTM to lower ICP and/or to improve neurological outcome.

(Expert opinion)

Rationale: Observational studies showed that fever is predictive of poor neurological outcome after subarachnoid haemorrhage [113–115]. Most of these studies were observational, with a small number of patients and methodological biases [116–120]. These studies found a decrease in ICP and suggested that the 12-month neurological outcome might be improved with the use of normothermia and hypothermia (32–34 °C) in refractory intracranial hypertension. A randomized controlled study [118] compared normothermia (TTM at 36.5 °C) versus conventional treatment for hyperthermia >37.9 °C: no conclusion could be drawn for the subgroup of patients with subarachnoid haemorrhage.

R.3.1 Paediatric 3.1 Paediatric—In children with subarachnoid haemorrhage, we suggest considering TTM between 36 and 37.5 °C to control intracranial pressure.

(Experts' recommendation)

Rationale: There is no randomized controlled study that explored the use of TTM and therapeutic hypothermia in children with stroke, intra-cerebral haemorrhage, and/or subarachnoid haemorrhage. Reduction of intracranial pressure was reported in one clinical case [121] and in a retrospective study where fever control and therapeutic hypothermia were used [122]. TTM may reduce ICP in children with SAH as seen in adults.

TTM in acute bacterial meningitis and status epilepticus

R4.1 In patients with refractory or super-refractory status epilepticus, we suggest considering TTM at 32–35 °C to control seizure activity.

(Expert opinion)

Rationale: Experimental studies [123–131] showed the anticonvulsant properties of hypothermia that were confirmed in patients with refractory or super-refractory status epilepticus (lasting for more than 24 h) persisting despite maximum treatment. A randomized controlled trial and several reports showed that TTM (32–35 °C) for 24 h was associated with a better control of electrical seizure activity and achievement of burst-suppression pattern [132–134]. In the HYBERNATUS trial, the rate of progression to EEG-confirmed status epilepticus was lower in the hypothermia group than in the control group (11 vs. 22%; odds ratio, 0.40; 95% CI 0.20–0.79; $P = 0.009$) [135].

R4.2 In comatose patients with meningitis or meningoencephalitis, we do not suggest considering TTM when fever is tolerated.

(Expert opinion)

Rationale: No interventional study tested the effect of TTM on outcome of ICU patients with meningitis or meningoencephalitis. Saxena et al. [136] showed that peak temperature in the first 24 h of ICU admission did not increase the hospital mortality rate in patients with infection of the central nervous system (CNS), whereas it was associated with increased mortality rate in patients with stroke and TBI. Other studies did not report consistent results [137, 138]. Interestingly, in the absence of infection, the outcome was better if the temperature over the first 24 h peaked between 37.5 and 37.9 °C, whereas in case of infection the outcome was better if temperature peaked at 38–38.4 °C (UK database) or at 39–39.4 °C (NZ/Australian database) [136]. Fever plays a protective role because it inhibits replication of *N. meningitidis* and *S. pneumoniae* [136] and eases the diagnosis of infection [137]. The use of paracetamol in septic patients can decrease temperature by 0.3 °C, but did not affect mortality or length of ICU stay [139].

R4.3 In comatose patients with bacterial meningitis and no intracranial hypertension, we suggest considering normothermia to improve survival and neurological outcome.

(Expert opinion)
Rationale: In ICU patients with bacterial meningitis, Mourvillier et al. [140] found more deleterious effects in the induced hypothermia group. No other study has been conducted on this topic.

R4.4 In comatose patients with bacterial meningitis and intracranial hypertension, we suggest considering TTM at 34–36 °C to improve survival and neurological outcome.

(Expert opinion)
Rationale: In comatose patients with bacterial meningitis and intracranial hypertension, hypothermia had a favourable effect on non-invasive measurements of ICP [141]. However, the control group was historical and 10 patients from a preliminary study were probably included [142]. In a case report [143], TTM at 35–36 °C controlled refractory intracranial hypertension, in combination with thiopental. In two other studies in patients with severe viral encephalitis and intracranial hypertension, outcome was better in cooled patients [144, 145]. Similar findings were obtained in other case reports [146–151].

R4.1 Paediatric—In children with status epilepticus, we suggest considering TTM (normothermia) to improve outcome.

(Expert opinion)
Rationale: Few clinical cases of refractory or super-refractory status epilepticus [152–154] and encephalitis in children [152, 155] treated with therapeutic hypothermia have been reported. There is a lack of evidence to formalize recommendation. A retrospective study in 43 heterogeneous patients (encephalitis and encephalopathy—viruses, major hyperthermia, shock, status epilepticus) [156] compared 16 patients under normothermia versus 27 patients under therapeutic hypothermia. The cerebral performance category score at 12 months was better in patients under hypothermia. Maintaining normothermia in children with status epilepticus may be appropriate.

TTM after haemodynamic shock

R5.1 We do not suggest considering TTM below 36 °C in patients with cardiogenic shock.

(Grade 2−)
Rationale: There were 4 studies that investigated the effects of moderate hypothermia [157–160]. They were retrospective or uncontrolled, and the number of patients included was low. Therapeutic hypothermia is feasible and not associated with an increased incidence of adverse effects. A prospective study is in progress (clinical trial.gov—NCT01890317).

R5.2 We do not suggest considering TTM below 36 °C in patients with septic shock.

(Grade 2−)
R5.3 We suggest considering TTM at normothermia in patients with septic shock.

(Grade 2)
Rationale: Among five randomized trials [161–164], three were designed to evaluate non-steroidal anti-inflammatory drugs versus placebo with a large proportion of patients without fever in the 2 groups [161, 162, 164]. One study compared acetaminophen versus placebo in patients with fever [139]. These studies showed that antipyretics effectively control temperature with no reported side effects. There was no difference in mortality rate, hemodynamic status, or length of stay in ICU. In one trial that compared TTM versus no TTM, Schortgen et al. [163] found that the vasopressor support (main endpoint) was significantly reduced in the TTM group, as was the duration of shock. However, despite a decreased mortality rate (secondary endpoint) at day 14 observed in the TTM group, there was no difference in mortality rate at both ICU and hospital discharge. TTM improved hemodynamic status in one methodologically well-conducted study [163] in which mortality was a secondary objective. All clinical studies concluded that TTM is feasible in septic shock and is not associated with more frequent side effects.

Implementation and monitoring of TTM

R6.1 We recommend using advanced methods with servo-regulated cooling of central body temperature to optimize TTM.

(Grade 1+)

Rationale: The present recommendation is based on post-cardiac arrest patients. A greater efficacy of advanced methods ("servo-controlled") was constantly found, particularly during the maintenance phase. The benefit of advanced methods during the induction phase of TTM was however variable because it relied upon the initial temperature. The incidence of overcooling/ overshooting was variable between advanced and basic methods. Our analysis included 3 randomized studies [165–167] and uncontrolled studies [168–171]. Regarding the neurological outcome, results were discordant: one study found a trend in favour of advanced methods [165], two studies were either negative [166] or positive (though cerebral performance category score was not reported) [167], and 4 studies gave variable results [168–171]. Overall, these advanced methods might help to optimize TTM, but their effect on survival with good neurological outcome was not established [40].

R6.2 We suggest considering the control of rewarming in patients treated with TTM.

(Expert opinion)

Rationale: After cardiac arrest, it is impossible to distinguish effects associated with the rewarming period from those attributable to induction and maintenance phase. Experts retained 2 randomized trials [165, 166] that found no differences between controlled and passive rewarming. The rate of rewarming and the time to achieve normothermia were found difference between controlled and uncontrolled rewarming in non-randomized studies [178–180]. Rebound or post-rewarming fever was not always suppressed using controlled rewarming [165, 170–172]. Clinical studies found no association between rewarming rate and outcome after adjustment [165, 171–174]. In brain trauma and stroke, a lower rate of rewarming is important in order to prevent rebounds on ICP [89, 173, 174]. However, no randomized trial has specifically addressed this issue other than indirect measurements of ICP [175].

R6.3 We suggest considering measurements of core body temperature in patients treated with TTM.

(Grade 2+)

Rationale: Besides the brain as the most preferable site to measure core body temperature, other sites can be used. Observational studies assessed the agreement between the core body temperature and other sites, i.e. oesophagus, bladder, rectum, nasopharynx, eardrum, and skin [176–180]. Agreement between core body sites of measurement (lungs, oesophagus, bladder, and rectum) was correct. Correlation and agreement were poor for peripheral sites of measurement (skin and tympanic) [176–180]. A study reported a bias of 1 °C between core and tympanic temperature [178].

R6.4 We suggest considering the detection of several complications (sepsis, pneumonia, arrhythmia, hypokalaemia) in patients treated with TTM.

(Grade 2+)

Rationale: The meta-analysis of Xiao et al. [181] found a trend between the use of TTM and the incidence of infectious complications, i.e. sepsis and pneumonia. Not included in this meta-analysis are observational studies performed in large populations [33, 182–184]: they all found an increased incidence of infectious complications in TTM patients.

Hypokalaemia is the most common metabolic derangement reported in TTM studies [26]. Two studies reported an increased occurrence of hypokalaemia (serum potassium <3.5 mmol/L) [37, 185] that was confirmed in the meta-analysis of Xiao et al. [181]. This meta-analysis found higher risk of cardiac arrhythmia in patients treated with TTM [181].

R6.1 Paediatric—We suggest considering methods with servo-regulated cooling of central body temperature in children treated with TTM.

(Expert opinion)

Rationale: One randomized open controlled study showed the superiority of a servo-controlled system in maintaining hypothermia in newborns with perinatal asphyxia managed in the pre-hospital settings with therapeutic hypothermia [186]. Forty-nine infants were allocated to a servo-controlled system, and 51 were cooled according to the unit's usual protocol (passive hypothermia). Newborns cooled with the servo-controlled device were more often close to the target temperature upon arrival at the hospital (median 73% [IQR 17–88] vs. 0% [IQR 0–52] $P < 0.001$). The target temperature was more often reached during transport in the servo-control group (80 vs. 49%, $P < 0.001$) and in a shorter time (44 ± 31 vs. 63 ± 37 min, $P = 0.04$). The number of newborns who reached the target temperature in 1 h was significantly higher in the servo-control group than in the control group (71 vs. 20%, $P < 0.001$).

R6.2 Paediatric—We suggest considering measurements of core body temperature measurement in children treated with TTM.

(Grade 2+)

Rationale: Several studies compared the accuracy of different sites for temperature measurement in children. In a prospective study ($n = 15$), peripheral sites (axillary, tympanic, rectal, oesophageal) were compared to central blood measurements [187]. The best agreement with blood temperature was obtained with oesophageal measurements. Several other studies and meta-analysis confirmed a poor agreement between axillary or tympanic measurements and central blood temperature [188–190].

Authors' contributions

AC and JFP proposed the elaboration of this recommendation and manuscript in agreement with the "Société de Réanimation de Langue Française" and "Société Française d'Anesthésie et de Réanimation"; LSB, CM, and LV wrote the methodology section and gave the final version with the final presentation. ND and GD contributed to elaborate recommendations and write the rationale of question 1 (cardiac arrest). BV, GF, JFP contributed to elaborate recommendations and to write the rationale of question 2 (traumatic brain injury). SD and GA contributed to elaborate recommendations and to write the rationale of question 3 (stroke and subarachnoid haemorrhage). SL and NE contributed to elaborate recommendations and to write the rationale of question 4 (acute bacterial meningitis and status epilepticus). BL and KA contributed to elaborate recommendations and to write the rationale of question 5 (shock). JCO and ND contributed to elaborate recommendations and to write the rationale of question 6 (implementation and monitoring). AB, LSB, PM, and SR contributed to elaborate recommendations and to write the rationale paediatric recommendations. FA and YW provide references. AC, LV, and JFP drafted the manuscript. All authors read and approved the final manuscript.

Author details

[1] Medical Intensive Care Unit, Cochin University Hospital (APHP) & Paris Descartes University, 27 rue du Faubourg Saint-Jacques, 75014 Paris, France. [2] Pôle Anesthésie-Réanimation, Hôpital Michallon, CHU Grenoble Alpes, 38000 Grenoble, France. [3] Service de Réanimation médicale, CH Mulhouse, Mulhouse, France. [4] Hôpital Necker-Enfants Malades, Réanimation Pédiatrique Polyvalente, Assistance Publique - Hôpitaux de Paris, Paris, France. [5] Service d'Anesthésie-Réanimation, Hôpital de la Timone, Assistance Publique-Hôpitaux de Marseille, Marseille, France. [6] Hôpital Lariboisiere, Assistance Publique-Hôpitaux de Paris, Paris, France. [7] Centre Hospitalier de Versailles, Le Chesnay, France. [8] Hôpital Central, CHU de Nancy, Nancy, France. [9] CHU de Nancy, Nancy, France. [10] Fondation Rothschild, Paris, France. [11] Hôpital Pasteur 2, CHU de Nice, Nice, France. [12] Anesthésie-réanimation, Bicêtre, France. [13] CHU de Grenoble, La Tronche, France. [14] Hôpitial Hôtel-Dieu, CHU de Nantes, Nantes, France. [15] Hôpital Jeanne de Flandre, CHRU de Lille, Lille, France. [16] CHU de Bordeaux, Bordeaux, France. [17] Hôpital Necker-Enfants Malades, Assistance Publique-Hôpitaux de Paris, Paris, France. [18] Hôpital Armand-Trousseau, Assistance Publique-Hôpitaux de Paris, Paris, France. [19] Hôpital Pitié-Salpêtrière, Assistance Publique-Hôpitaux de Paris, Paris, France.

Acknowledgements

This article is being published jointly in Anaesthesia Critical Care & Pain Medicine and Annals of Intensive Care. The manuscript validated by the board meeting of SFAR and SRLF (18/02/2016).

Competing interests

Alain Cariou declares speaker fees and transport accommodation from Bard. Nicolas Deye declares speaker fees, transport accommodation, and research grants from BARD and ZOLL. Nicolas Deye was also the primary investigator Francony, Bruno Levy, Cyrille Mathien, Philippe Meyer, Jean-Christophe Orban, Jean-François Payen, Sylvain Renolleau, Laure de Saint Blanquat, Lionel Velly, Bernard Vigue declare no competing interest with this manuscript.

Funding

This work was financially supported by the Société de Réanimation de Langue Française (SRLF) and the Société Française d'Anesthésie et de Réanimation (SFAR).

Guidelines committee (SFAR)

D Fletcher, L Velly, J Amour, S Ausset, G Chanques, V Compere, F Espitalier, M Garnier, E Gayat, JY Lefrant, JM Malinovski, B Rozec, B Tavernier.

Guidelines and evaluation committee (SRLF)

L Donetti, M Alves, T Boulain, Olivier Brissaud, V Das, L De Saint Blanquat, M Guillot, K Kuteifan, C Mathien, V Peigne, F Plouvier, D Schnell, L Vong.

References

1. Benson DW, Williams GR, Spencer FC, Yates AJ. The use of hypothermia after cardiac arrest. Anesth Analg. 1958;38:423–8.
2. Rosomoff HL. Hypothermia in management of cerebrovascular lesions. South Med J. 1961;54:498–505.
3. Lemiale V, Huet O, Vigué B, Mathonnet A, Spaulding C, Mira JP, et al. Changes in cerebral blood flow and oxygen extraction during post-resuscitation syndrome. Resuscitation. 2008;76:17–24.
4. Rosomoff HL, Holaday DA. Cerebral blood flow and cerebral oxygen consumption during hypothermia. Am J Physiol. 1954;179:85–8.
5. Xu L, Yenari MA, Steinberg GK, Giffard RG. Mild hypothermia reduces apoptosis of mouse neurons in vitro early in the cascade. J Cereb Blood Flow Metab. 2002;22:21–8.
6. Busto R, Globus MY, Dietrich WD, Martinez E, Valdés I, Ginsberg MD. Effect of mild hypothermia on ischemia-induced release of neurotransmitters and free fatty acids in rat brain. Stroke. 1989;20:904–10.
7. Polderman KH, Ely EW, Badr AE, Girbes AR. Induced hypothermia in traumatic brain injury: considering the conflicting results of meta-analyses and moving forward. Intensive Care Med. 2004;30:1860–4.
8. Siesjö BK, Bengtsson F, Grampp W, Theander S. Calcium, excitotoxins, and neuronal death in the brain. Ann N Y Acad Sci. 1989;568:234–51.
9. Adrie C, Laurent I, Monchi M, Cariou A, Dhainaut JF, Spaulding C. Postresuscitation disease after cardiac arrest: a sepsis-like syndrome? Curr Opin Crit Care. 2004;10:208–12.
10. Chi OZ, Liu X, Weiss HR. Effects of mild hypothermia on blood-brain barrier disruption during isoflurane or pentobarbital anesthesia. Anesthesiology. 2001;95:933–8.
11. Nunnally ME, Jaeschke R, Bellingan GJ, Lacroix J, Mourvillier B, Rodriguez-Vega GM, et al. Targeted temperature management in critical care: a report and recommendations from five professional societies. Crit Care Med. 2011;39:1113–25.
12. Atkins D, Best D, Briss PA, Eccles M, Falck-Ytter Y, Flottorp S, et al. GRADE Working Group. Grading quality of evidence and strength of recommendations. BMJ. 2004;328:1490.
13. Roche N, Durieux P. Clinical practice guidelines: from methodological to practical issues. Intensive Care Med. 1994;20:593–601.
14. Vargas M, Servillo G, Sutherasan Y, Rodríguez-González R, Brunetti I, Pelosi P. Effects of in-hospital low targeted temperature after out of hospital cardiac arrest: a systematic review with meta-analysis of randomized clinical trials. Resuscitation. 2015;91:8–18.
15. Nielsen N, Friberg H, Gluud C, Herlitz J, Wetterslev J. Hypothermia after cardiac arrest should be further evaluated—a systematic review of randomised trials with meta-analysis and trial sequential analysis. Int J Cardiol. 2011;151:333–41.
16. Wang X, Lin Q, Zhao S, Lin S, Chen F. Therapeutic benefits of mild hypothermia in patients successfully resuscitated from cardiac arrest: a meta-analysis. World J Emerg Med. 2013;4:260.
17. Cheung KW, Green RS, Magee KD. Systematic review of randomized controlled trials of therapeutic hypothermia as a neuroprotectant in post cardiac arrest patients. CJEM. 2006;8:329–37.

18. Arrich J, Holzer M, Havel C, Müllner M, Herkner H. In: Cochrane database of systematic reviews (ed. The Cochrane Collaboration). Wiley. 2012.
19. Arrich J, Holzer M, Herkner H, Müllner M. In: Cochrane database of systematic reviews (ed. The Cochrane Collaboration). Wiley. 2009.
20. Walters JH, Morley PT, Nolan JP. The role of hypothermia in post-cardiac arrest patients with return of spontaneous circulation: a systematic review. Resuscitation. 2011;82:508–16.
21. Polderman KH. Induced hypothermia and fever control for prevention and treatment of neurological injuries. Lancet. 2008;371:1955–69.
22. Sagalyn E, Band RA, Gaieski DF, Abella BS. Therapeutic hypothermia after cardiac arrest in clinical practice: review and compilation of recent experiences. Crit Care Med. 2009;37:S223–6.
23. Maznyczka AM, Gershlick AH. Therapeutic hypothermia in patients with out-of-hospital arrest. Heart. 2015;101:1265–71.
24. Bernard SA, Gray TW, Buist MD, Jones BM, Silvester W, Gutteridge G, Smith K. Treatment of comatose survivors of out-of-hospital cardiac arrest with induced hypothermia. N Engl J Med. 2002;346:557–63.
25. Hypothermia after Cardiac Arrest Study Group. Mild therapeutic hypothermia to improve the neurologic outcome after cardiac arrest. N Engl J Med. 2002;346:549–56.
26. Nielsen N, Wetterslev J, Cronberg T, Erlinge D, Gasche Y, Hassager C, et al. Targeted temperature management at 33 °C versus 36 °C after cardiac arrest. N Engl J Med. 2013;369:2197–206.
27. Laurent I, Adrie C, Vinsonneau C, Cariou A, Chiche JD, Ohanessian A, et al. High-volume hemofiltration after out-of-hospital cardiac arrest: a randomized study. J Am Coll Cardiol. 2005;46:432–7.
28. Kim YM, Yim HW, Jeong SH, Klem ML, Callaway CW. Does therapeutic hypothermia benefit adult cardiac arrest patients presenting with non-shockable initial rhythms? A systematic review and meta-analysis of randomized and non-randomized studies. Resuscitation. 2012;83:188–96.
29. Hachimi-Idrissi S, Corne L, Ebinger G, Michotte Y, Huyghens L. Mild hypothermia induced by a helmet device: a clinical feasibility study. Resuscitation. 2001;51:275–81.
30. Wang CJ, Yang SH, Lee CH, Lin RL, Peng MJ, Wu CL. Therapeutic hypothermia application vs standard support care in post resuscitated out-of-hospital cardiac arrest patients. Am J Emerg Med. 2013;31:319–25.
31. Lundbye JB, Rai M, Ramu B, Hosseini-Khalili A, Li D, Slim HB, et al. Therapeutic hypothermia is associated with improved neurologic outcome and survival in cardiac arrest survivors of non-shockable rhythms. Resuscitation. 2012;83:202–7.
32. Testori C, Sterz F, Behringer W, Haugk M, Uray T, Zeiner A, et al. Mild therapeutic hypothermia is associated with favourable outcome in patients after cardiac arrest with non-shockable rhythms. Resuscitation. 2011;82:1162–7.
33. Vaahersalo J, Hiltunen P, Tiainen M, Oksanen T, Kaukonen KM, Kurola J, et al. FINNRESUSCI Study Group. Therapeutic hypothermia after out-of-hospital cardiac arrest in Finnish intensive care units: the FINNRESUSCI study. Intensive Care Med. 2013;39:826–37.
34. Storm C, Nee J, Roser M, Jorres A, Hasper D. Mild hypothermia treatment in patients resuscitated from non-shockable cardiac arrest. Emerg Med J. 2012;29:100–3.
35. Gräsner JT, Meybohm P, Caliebe A, Böttiger BW, Wnent J, Messelken M, et al. German Resuscitation Registry Study Group. Postresuscitation care with mild therapeutic hypothermia and coronary intervention after out-of-hospital cardiopulmonary resuscitation: a prospective registry analysis. Crit Care. 2011;15:R61.
36. Dumas F, Grimaldi D, Zuber B, Fichet J, Charpentier J, Pène F, et al. Is hypothermia after cardiac arrest effective in both shockable and nonshockable patients? Insights from a large registry. Circulation. 2011;123:877–86.
37. Pfeifer R, Jung C, Purle S, Lauten A, Yilmaz A, Surber R, et al. Survival does not improve when therapeutic hypothermia is added to post-cardiac arrest care. Resuscitation. 2011;82:1168–73.
38. Mader TJ, Nathanson BH, Soares WE 3rd, Coute RA, McNally BF. Comparative effectiveness of therapeutic hypothermia after out-of-hospital cardiac arrest: insight from a large data registry. Ther Hypothermia Temp Manag. 2014;4:21–31.
39. Kory P, Fukunaga M, Mathew JP, Singh B, Szainwald L, Mosak J, et al. Outcomes of mild therapeutic hypothermia after in-hospital cardiac arrest. Neurocrit Care. 2012;16:406–12.
40. Arrich J. Clinical application of mild therapeutic hypothermia after cardiac arrest. Crit Care Med. 2007;35:1041–7.
41. Rittenberger JC, Guyette FX, Tisherman SA, DeVita MA, Alvarez RJ, Callaway CW. Outcomes of a hospital-wide plan to improve care of comatose survivors of cardiac arrest. Resuscitation. 2008;79:198–204.
42. Holzer M, Müllner M, Sterz F, Robak O, Kliegel A, Losert H, et al. Efficacy and safety of endovascular cooling after cardiac arrest: cohort study and Bayesian approach. Stroke. 2006;37:1792–7.
43. Lopez-de-Sa E, Rey JR, Armada E, Salinas P, Viana-Tejedor A, Espinosa-Garcia S, et al. Hypothermia in comatose survivors from out-of-hospital cardiac arrest: pilot trial comparing 2 levels of target temperature. Circulation. 2012;126:2826–33.
44. Hörburger D, Testori C, Sterz F, Herkner H, Krizanac D, Uray T, et al. Mild therapeutic hypothermia improves outcomes compared with normothermia in cardiac-arrest patients—a retrospective chart review. Crit Care Med. 2012;40:2315–9.
45. Annborn M, Bro-Jeppesen J, Nielsen N, Ullén S, Kjaergaard J, Hassager C, et al. TTM-trial investigators. The association of targeted temperature management at 33 and 36 & #xB0;C with outcome in patients with moderate shock on admission after out-of-hospital cardiac arrest: a post hoc analysis of the Target Temperature Management trial. Intensive Care Med. 2014;40:1210–9.
46. Kim F, Nichol G, Maynard C, Hallstrom A, Kudenchuk PJ, Rea T, et al. Effect of prehospital induction of mild hypothermia on survival and neurological status among adults with cardiac arrest: a randomized clinical trial. JAMA. 2014;311:45–52.
47. Debaty G, Maignan M, Savary D, Koch FX, Ruckly S, Durand M, et al. Impact of intra-arrest therapeutic hypothermia in outcomes of prehospital cardiac arrest: a randomized controlled trial. Intensive Care Med. 2014;40:1832–42.
48. Bernard SA, Smith K, Cameron P, Masci K, Taylor DM, Cooper DJ, et al. Rapid Infusion of Cold Hartmanns Investigators. Induction of prehospital therapeutic hypothermia after resuscitation from nonventricular fibrillation cardiac arrest. Crit Care Med. 2012;40:747–53.
49. Bernard SA, Smith K, Cameron P, Masci K, Taylor DM, Cooper DJ, et al. Rapid Infusion of Cold Hartmanns (RICH) Investigators. Induction of therapeutic hypothermia by paramedics after resuscitation from out-of-hospital ventricular fibrillation cardiac arrest: a randomized controlled trial. Circulation. 2010;122:737–42.
50. Kim F, Olsufka M, Longstreth WT Jr, Maynard C, Carlbom D, Deem S, et al. Pilot randomized clinical trial of prehospital induction of mild hypothermia in out-of-hospital cardiac arrest patients with a rapid infusion of 4 C normal saline. Circulation. 2007;115:3064–70.
51. Castrén M, Nordberg P, Svensson L, Taccone F, Vincent JL, Desruelles D, et al. Intra-arrest transnasal evaporative cooling: a randomized, prehospital, multicenter study (PRINCE: pre-ROSC IntraNasal Cooling Effectiveness). Circulation. 2010;122:729–36.
52. Suffoletto B, Peberdy MA, van der Hoek T, Callaway C. Body temperature changes are associated with outcomes following in-hospital cardiac arrest and return of spontaneous circulation. Resuscitation. 2009;80:1365–70.
53. Gebhardt K, Guyette FX, Doshi AA, Callaway CW, Rittenberger JC, Post Cardiac Arrest Service. Prevalence and effect of fever on outcome following resuscitation from cardiac arrest. Resuscitation. 2013;84:1062–7.
54. Moler FW, Silverstein FS, Holubkov R, Slomine BS, Christensen JR, Nadkarni VM, et al. THAPCA Trial Investigators. Therapeutic hypothermia after out-of-hospital cardiac arrest in children. N Engl J Med. 2015;372:1898–908.
55. Fink EL, Clark RS, Kochanek PM, Bell MJ, Watson RS. A tertiary care center's experience with therapeutic hypothermia after pediatric cardiac arrest. Pediatr Crit Care Med. 2010;11:66–74.
56. de Caen AR, Kleinman ME, Chameides L, Atkins DL, Berg RA, Berg MD, Paediatric Basic and Advanced Life Support Chapter Collaborators, et al. Part 10: paediatric basic and advanced life support, international consensus on cardiopulmonary resuscitation and emergency cardiovascular care science with treatment recommendations. Resuscitation. 2010;2010(81):e213–59.
57. American Heart Association. 2005 American Heart Association (AHA) Guidelines for Cardiopulmonary Resuscitation (CPR) and Emergency Cardiovascular Care (ECC) of pediatric and neonatal patients: pediatric basic life support. Pediatrics. 2006;117:e989–1004.
58. Maconochie IK, Bingham R, Eich C, López-Herce J, Rodríguez-Núñez A, Rajka T, et al. Paediatric life support section collaborators. European

Resuscitation Council guidelines for resuscitation 2015. Resuscitation. 2015;95:223–48.
59. Puccio AM, Fischer MR, Jankowitz BT, Yonas H, Darby JM, Okonkwo DO. Induced normothermia attenuates intracranial hypertension and reduces fever burden after severe traumatic brain injury. Neurocrit Care. 2009;11:82–7.
60. Rossi S, Zanier ER, Mauri I, Columbo A, Stocchetti N. Brain temperature, body core temperature, and intracranial pressure in acute cerebral damage. J Neurol Neurosurg Psychiatry. 2001;71:448–54.
61. Tokutomi T, Morimoto K, Miyagi T, Yamaguchi S, Ishikawa K, Shigemori M. Optimal temperature for the management of severe traumatic brain injury: effect of hypothermia on intracranial pressure, systemic and intracranial hemodynamics, and metabolism. Neurosurgery. 2003;52:102–11.
62. Stretti F, Gotti M, Pifferi S, Brandi G, Annoni F, Stocchetti N. Body temperature affects cerebral hemodynamics in acutely brain injured patients: an observational transcranial color-coded duplex sonography study. Crit Care. 2014;18:552.
63. Greer DM, Funk SE, Reaven NL, Ouzounelli M, Uman GC. Impact of fever on outcome in patients with stroke and neurologic injury: a comprehensive meta-analysis. Stroke. 2008;39:3029–35.
64. Li J, Jiang J. Chinese Head Trauma Data Bank. Effect of hyperthermia on the outcome of acute head trauma patients. J Neurotrauma. 2012;29:96–100.
65. Jiang JY, Gao GY, Li WP, Yu MK, Zhu C. Early indicators of prognosis in 846 cases of severe traumatic brain injury. J Neurotrauma. 2002;19:869–74.
66. Bao L, Chen D, Ding L, Ling W, Xu F. Fever burden is an independent predictor for prognosis of traumatic brain injury. PLoS ONE. 2014;9:e90956.
67. Stocchetti N, Rossi S, Zanier ER, Colombo A, Beretta L, Citerio G. Pyrexia in head-injured patients admitted to intensive care. Intensive Care Med. 2002;28:1555–62.
68. Diringer MN, Reaven NL, Funk SE, Uman GC. Elevated body temperature independently contributes to increased length of stay in neurologic intensive care unit patients. Crit Care Med. 2004;32:1489–95.
69. Launey Y, Nesseler N, Le Cousin A, Feuillet F, Garlantezec R, Mallédant Y, Seguin P. Effect of a fever control protocol-based strategy on ventilator-associated pneumonia in severely brain-injured patients. Crit Care. 2014;18:689.
70. Hutchison JS, Ward RE, Lacroix J, Hébert PC, Barnes MA, Bohn DJ, Hypothermia Pediatric Head Injury Trial Investigators and the Canadian Critical Care Trials Group, et al. Hypothermia therapy after traumatic brain injury in children. N Engl J Med. 2008;58:2447–56.
71. Maekawa T, Yamashita S, Nagao S, Hayashi N, Ohashi Y, Brain-Hypothermia Study Group. Prolonged mild therapeutic hypothermia versus fever control with tight hemodynamic monitoring and slow rewarming in patients with severe traumatic brain injury: a randomized controlled trial. J Neurotrauma. 2015;32:422–9.
72. Clifton GL, Valadka A, Zygun D, Coffey CS, Drever P, Fourwinds S, et al. Very early hypothermia induction in patients with severe brain injury (the National Acute Brain Injury Study: hypothermia II): a randomised trial. Lancet Neurol. 2011;10:131–9.
73. Adelson PD, Wisniewski SR, Beca J, Brown SD, Bell M, Muizelaar JP, Paediatric Traumatic Brain Injury Consortium, et al. Comparison of hypothermia and normothermia after severe traumatic brain injury in children (Cool Kids): a phase 3, randomised controlled trial. Lancet Neurol. 2013;12:546–53.
74. Shiozaki T, Hayakata T, Taneda M, Nakajima Y, Hashiguchi N, Fujimi S, et al. A multicenter prospective randomized controlled trial of the efficacy of mild hypothermia for severely head injured patients with low intracranial pressure. Mild Hypothermia Study Group in Japan. J Neurosurg. 2001;94:50–4.
75. Sadaka F, Veremakis C. Therapeutic hypothermia for the management of intracranial hypertension in severe traumatic brain injury: a systematic review. Brain Inj. 2012;26:899–908.
76. Crossley S, Reid J, McLatchie R, Hayton J, Clark C, MacDougall M, Andrews PJ. A systematic review of therapeutic hypothermia for adult patients following traumatic brain injury. Crit Care. 2014;18:R75.
77. Zhang BF, Wang J, Liu ZW, Zhao YL, Li DD, Huang TQ, Gu H, Song JN. Meta-analysis of the efficacy and safety of therapeutic hypothermia in children with acute traumatic brain injury. World Neurosurg. 2015;83:567–73.
78. Jiang J, Yu M, Zhu C. Effect of long-term mild hypothermia therapy in patients with severe traumatic brain injury: 1-year follow-up review of 87 cases. J Neurosurg. 2000;93:546–9.
79. Qiu WS, Liu WG, Shen H, Wang WM, Hang ZL, Zhang Y, et al. Therapeutic effect of mild hypothermia on severe traumatic head injury. Chin J Traumatol. 2005;8:27–32.
80. Qiu W, Shen H, Zhang Y, Wang W, Liu W, Jiang Q, et al. Noninvasive selective brain cooling by head and neck cooling is protective in severe traumatic brain injury. J Clin Neurosci. 2006;13:995–1000.
81. Qiu W, Zhang Y, Sheng H, Zhang J, Wang W, Liu W, et al. Effects of therapeutic mild hypothermia on patients with severe traumatic brain injury after craniotomy. J Crit Care. 2007;22:229–35.
82. Zhao QJ, Zhang XG, Wang LX. Mild hypothermia therapy reduces blood glucose and lactate and improves neurologic outcomes in patients with severe traumatic brain injury. J Crit Care. 2011;26:311–5.
83. Zhi D, Zhang S, Lin X. Study on therapeutic mechanism and clinical effect of mild hypothermia in patients with severe head injury. Surg Neurol. 2003;59:381–5.
84. Shiozaki T, Sugimoto H, Taneda M, Yoshida H, Iwai A, Yoshioka T, et al. Effect of mild hypothermia on uncontrollable intracranial hypertension after severe head injury. J Neurosurg. 1993;79:363–8.
85. Polderman KH, Tjong Tjin Joe R, Peerdeman SM, Vandertop WP, Girbes AR. Effects of therapeutic hypothermia on intracranial pressure and outcome in patients with severe head injury. Intensive Care Med. 2002;28:1563–73.
86. Andrews PJ, Sinclair HL, Rodriguez A, Harris BA, Battison CG, Rhodes JK, Murray GD, Eurotherm3235 Trial Collaborators. Hypothermia for intracranial hypertension after traumatic brain injury. N Engl J Med. 2015;373:2403–12.
87. Shiozaki T, Nakajima Y, Taneda M, Tasaki O, Inoue Y, Ikegawa H, et al. Efficacy of moderate hypothermia in patients with severe head injury and intracranial hypertension refractory to mild hypothermia. J Neurosurg. 2003;99:47–51.
88. Gupta AK, Al-Rawi PG, Hutchinson PJ, Kirkpatrick PJ. Effect of hypothermia on brain tissue oxygenation in patients with severe head injury. Br J Anaesth. 2002;88:188–92.
89. Jiang JY, Xu W, Li WP, Gao GY, Bao YH, Liang YM, Luo QZ. Effect of long-term mild hypothermia or short-term mild hypothermia on outcome of patients with severe traumatic brain injury. J Cereb Blood Flow Metab. 2006;26:771–6.
90. McIntyre LA, Fergusson DA, Hébert PC, Moher D, Hutchison JS. Prolonged therapeutic hypothermia after traumatic brain injury in adults: a systematic review. JAMA. 2003;11(289):2992–9.
91. Liu YH, Shang ZD, Chen C, Lu N, Liu QF, Liu M, Yan J. 'Cool and quiet' therapy for malignant hyperthermia following severe traumatic brain injury: a preliminary clinical approach. Exp Ther Med. 2015;9:464–8.
92. Hutchison JS, Frndova H, Lo TY, Guerguerian AM, Hypothermia Pediatric Head Injury Trial Investigators, Canadian Critical Care Trials Group. Impact of hypotension and low cerebral perfusion pressure on outcomes in children treated with hypothermia therapy following severe traumatic brain injury: a post hoc analysis of the Hypothermia Pediatric Head Injury Trial. Dev Neurosci. 2010;32:406–12.
93. Natale JE, Joseph JG, Helfaer MA, Shaffner DH. Early hyperthermia after traumatic brain injury in children: risk factors, influence on length of stay, and effect on short-term neurologic status. Crit Care Med. 2000;28:2608–15.
94. Piironen K, Tiainen M, Mustanoja S, Kaukonen KM, Meretoja A, Tatlisumak T, Kaste M. Mild hypothermia after intravenous thrombolysis in patients with acute stroke: a randomized controlled trial. Stroke. 2014;45:486–91.
95. Bi M, Ma Q, Zhang S, Li J, Zhang Y, Lin L, et al. Local mild hypothermia with thrombolysis for acute ischemic stroke within a 6-h window. Clin Neurol Neurosurg. 2011;113:768–73.
96. De Georgia MA, Krieger DW, Abou-Chebl A, Devlin TG, Jauss M, Davis SM, et al. Cooling for acute ischemic brain damage (COOL AID): a feasibility trial of endovascular cooling. Neurology. 2004;63:312–7.
97. Hemmen TM, Raman R, Guluma KZ, Meyer BC, Gomes JA, Cruz-Flores S,

ICTuS-L Investigators, et al. Intravenous thrombolysis plus hypothermia for acute treatment of ischemic stroke (ICTuS-L): final results. Stroke. 2010;41:2265–70.
98. Ovesen C, Brizzi M, Pott FC, Thorsen-Meyer HC, Karlsson T, Ersson A, et al. Feasibility of endovascular and surface cooling strategies in acute stroke. Acta Neurol Scand. 2013;127:399–405.
99. Els T, Oehm E, Voigt S, Klisch J, Hetzel A, Kassubek J. Safety and therapeutical benefit of hemicraniectomy combined with mild hypothermia in comparison with hemicraniectomy alone in patients with malignant ischemic stroke. Cerebrovasc Dis. 2006;21:79–85.
100. van der Worp HB, Macleod MR, Bath PM, Demotes J, Durand-Zaleski I, Gebhardt B, EuroHYP-1 investigators, et al. EuroHYP-1: european multicenter, randomized, phase III clinical trial of therapeutic hypothermia plus best medical treatment versus best medical treatment alone for acute ischemic stroke. Int J Stroke. 2014;9:642–5.
101. Lyden P, Hemmen T, Grotta J, Rapp K, Ernstrom K, Rzesiewicz T, Collaborators, et al. Results of the ICTuS 2 Trial (Intravascular Cooling in the Treatment of Stroke 2). Stroke. 2016;47:2888–95.
102. Ntaios G, Dziedzic T, Michel P, Papavasileiou V, Petersson J, Staykov D, Thomas B, Steiner T, European Stroke Organisation. European Stroke Organisation (ESO) guidelines for the management of temperature in patients with acute ischemic stroke. Int J Stroke. 2015;10:941–9.
103. Dippel DW, van Breda EJ, van Gemert HM, van der Worp HB, Meijer RJ, Kappelle LJ, Koudstaal PJ. Effect of paracetamol (acetaminophen) on body temperature in acute ischemic stroke: a double-blind, randomized phase II clinical trial. Stroke. 2001;32:1607–12.
104. Dippel DW, van Breda EJ, van der Worp HB, van Gemert HM, Meijer RJ, Kappelle LJ, Koudstaal PJ, PISA-Investigators. Effect of paracetamol (acetaminophen) and ibuprofen on body temperature in acute ischemic stroke PISA, a phase II double-blind, randomized, placebo-controlled trial [ISRCTN98608690]. BMC Cardiovasc Disord. 2003;3:2.
105. Kasner SE, Wein T, Piriyawat P, Villar-Cordova CE, Chalela JA, et al. Acetaminophen for altering body temperature in acute stroke: a randomized clinical trial. Stroke. 2002;33:130–4.
106. den Hertog HM, van der Worp HB, van Gemert HM, Algra A, Kappelle LJ, van Gijn J, Koudstaal PJ, Dippel DW, PAIS Investigators. The Paracetamol (Acetaminophen) In Stroke (PAIS) trial: a multicentre, randomised, placebo-controlled, phase III trial. Lancet Neurol. 2009;8:434–40.
107. Schwarz S, Häfner K, Aschoff A, Schwab S. Incidence and prognostic significance of fever following intracerebral hemorrhage. Neurology. 2000;54:354–61.
108. Leira R, Dávalos A, Silva Y, Gil-Peralta A, Tejada J, Garcia M, Castillo J, Stroke Project. Early neurologic deterioration in intracerebral hemorrhage: predictors and associated factors. Cerebrovascular Diseases Group of the Spanish Neurological Society. Neurology. 2004;63:461–7.
109. Kollmar R, Staykov D, Dörfler A, Schellinger PD, Schwab S, Bardutzky J. Hypothermia reduces perihemorrhagic edema after intracerebral hemorrhage. Stroke. 2010;41:1684–9.
110. Staykov D, Wagner I, Volbers B, Doerfler A, Schwab S, Kollmar R. Mild prolonged hypothermia for large intracerebral hemorrhage. Neurocrit Care. 2013;18:178–83.
111. Lord AS, Karinja S, Lantigua H, Carpenter A, Schmidt JM, Claassen J, et al. Therapeutic temperature modulation for fever after intracerebral hemorrhage. Neurocrit Care. 2014;21:200–6.
112. Kollmar R, Juettler E, Huttner HB, Dörfler A, Staykov D, Kallmuenzer B, CINCH Investigators, et al. Cooling in intracerebral hemorrhage (CINCH) trial: protocol of a randomized German-Austrian clinical trial. Int J Stroke. 2012;7:168–72.
113. Oliveira-Filho J, Ezzeddine MA, Segal AZ, Buonanno FS, Chang Y, Ogilvy CS, et al. Fever in subarachnoid hemorrhage: relationship to vasospasm and outcome. Neurology. 2001;56:1299–304.
114. Wartenberg KE, Schmidt JM, Claassen J, Temes RE, Frontera JA, Ostapkovich N, Parra A, Connolly ES, Mayer SA. Impact of medical complications on outcome after subarachnoid hemorrhage. Crit Care Med. 2006;34:617–23.
115. Fernandez A, Schmidt JM, Claassen J, Pavlicova M, Huddleston D, Kreiter KT, et al. Fever after subarachnoid hemorrhage: risk factors and impact on outcome. Neurology. 2007;68:1013–9.
116. Gasser S, Khan N, Yonekawa Y, Imhof HG, Keller E. Long-term hypothermia in patients with severe brain edema after poor-grade subarachnoid hemorrhage: feasibility and intensive care complications. J Neurosurg Anesthesiol. 2003;15:240–8.
117. Seule MA, Muroi C, Mink S, Yonekawa Y, Keller E. Therapeutic hypothermia in patients with aneurysmal subarachnoid hemorrhage, refractory intracranial hypertension, or cerebral vasospasm. Neurosurgery. 2009;64:86–92.
118. Broessner G, Beer R, Lackner P, Helbok R, Fischer M, Pfausler B, et al. Prophylactic, endovascularly based, long-term normothermia in ICU patients with severe cerebrovascular disease: bicenter prospective, randomized trial. Stroke. 2009;40:e657–65.
119. Badjatia N, Fernandez L, Schmidt JM, Lee K, Claassen J, Connolly ES, Mayer SA. Impact of induced normothermia on outcome after subarachnoid hemorrhage: a case-control study. Neurosurgery. 2010;66:696–700.
120. Karnatovskaia LV, Lee AS, Festic E, Kramer CL, Freeman WD. Effect of prolonged therapeutic hypothermia on intracranial pressure, organ function, and hospital outcomes among patients with aneurysmal subarachnoid hemorrhage. Neurocrit Care. 2014;21:451–61.
121. Inamasu J, Ichikizaki K, Matsumoto S, Nakamura Y, Saito R, Horiguchi T, Kanai R. Mild hypothermia for hemispheric cerebral infarction after evacuation of an acute subdural hematoma in an infant. Childs Nerv Syst. 2002;18:175–8.
122. Fink EL, Kochanek PM, Clark RS, Bell MJ. Fever control and application of hypothermia using intravenous cold saline. Pediatr Crit Care Med. 2012;13:80–4.
123. Liu Z, Gatt A, Mikati M, Holmes GL. Effect of temperature on kainic acid-induced seizures. Brain Res. 1993;631:51–8.
124. Jiang W, Duong TM, de Lanerolle NC. The neuropathology of hyperthermic seizures in the rat. Epilepsia. 1999;40:5–19.
125. Yu L, Zhou Y, Chen W, Wang Y. Mild hypothermia pretreatment protects against pilocarpine-induced status epilepticus and neuronalapoptosis in immature rats. Neuropathology. 2011;31:144–51.
126. Lundgren J, Smith ML, Blennow G, Siesjö BK. Hyperthermia aggravates and hypothermia ameliorates epileptic brain damage. Exp Brain Res. 1994;99:43–55.
127. Wang Y, Liu PP, Li LY, Zhang HM, Li T. Hypothermia reduces brain edema, spontaneous recurrent seizure attack, and learning memory deficits in the kainic acid treated rats. CNS Neurosci Ther. 2011;17:271–80.
128. Zhou YF, Wang Y, Shao XM, Chen L, Wang Y. Effects of hypothermia on brain injury induced by status epilepticus. Front Biosci (Landmark Ed). 2012;17:1882–90.
129. Maeda T, Hashizume K, Tanaka T. Effect of hypothermia on kainic acid-induced limbic seizures: an electroencephalographic and 14C-deoxyglucose autoradiographic study. Brain Res. 1999;818:228–35.
130. Schmitt FC, Buchheim K, Meierkord H, Holtkamp M. Anticonvulsant properties of hypothermia in experimental status epilepticus. Neurobiol Dis. 2006;23:689–96.
131. Kowski AB, Kanaan H, Schmitt FC, Holtkamp M. Deep hypothermia terminates status epilepticus—an experimental study. Brain Res. 2012;1446:119–26.
132. Corry JJ, Dhar R, Murphy T, Diringer MN. Hypothermia for refractory status epilepticus. Neurocrit Care. 2008;9:189–97.
133. Ren GP, Su YY, Tian F, Zhang YZ, Gao DQ, Liu G, Chen WB. Early hypothermia for refractory status epilepticus. Chin Med J (Engl). 2015;128:1679–82.
134. Bennett AE, Hoesch RE, DeWitt LD, Afra P, Ansari SA. Therapeutic hypothermia for status epilepticus: a report, historical perspective, and review. Clin Neurol Neurosurg. 2014;126:103–9.
135. Legriel S, Lemiale V, Schenck M, Chelly J, Laurent V, Daviaud F, HYBERNATUS Study Group, et al. Hypothermia for Neuroprotection in Convulsive Status Epilepticus. N Engl J Med. 2016;375:2457–67.
136. Saxena M, Young P, Pilcher D, Bailey M, Harrison D, Bellomo R, et al. Early temperature and mortality in critically ill patients with acute neurological diseases: trauma and stroke differ from infection. Intensive Care Med. 2015;41:823–32.
137. Fernandes D, Gonçalves-Pereira J, Janeiro S, Silvestre J, Bento L, Póvoa P. Acute bacterial meningitis in the intensive care unit and risk fac-

tors for adverse clinical outcomes: retrospective study. J Crit Care. 2014;29:347–50.
138. de Jonge RC, van Furth AM, Wassenaar M, Gemke RJ, Terwee CB. Predicting sequelae and death after bacterial meningitis in childhood: a systematic review of prognostic studies. BMC Infect Dis. 2010;10:232.
139. Young P, Saxena M, Bellomo R, Freebairn R, Hammond N, van Haren F, HEAT Investigators, Australian and New Zealand Intensive Care Society Clinical Trials Group. Acetaminophen for fever in critically Ill patients with suspected infection. N Engl J Med. 2015;373:2215–24.
140. Mourvillier B, Tubach F, van de Beek D, Garot D, Pichon N, Georges H, et al. Induced hypothermia in severe bacterial meningitis: a randomized clinical trial. JAMA. 2013;310:2174–83.
141. Kutleša M, Lepur D, Baršić B. Therapeutic hypothermia for adult community-acquired bacterial meningitis-historical control study. Clin Neurol Neurosurg. 2014;123:181–6.
142. Lepur D, Kutleša M, Baršić B. Induced hypothermia in adult community-acquired bacterial meningitis—more than just a possibility? J Infect. 2011;62:172–7.
143. Cuthbertson BH, Dickson R, Mackenzie A. Intracranial pressure measurement, induced hypothermia and barbiturate coma in meningitis associated with intractable raised intracranial pressure. Anaesthesia. 2004;59:908–11.
144. Kutleša M, Baršić B. Therapeutic hypothermia for severe adult Herpes simplex virus encephalitis. Wien Klin Wochenschr. 2012;124:855–8.
145. Kutleša M, Baršić B, Lepur D. Therapeutic hypothermia for adult viral meningoencephalitis. Neurocrit Care. 2011;15:151–5.
146. Wagner I, Staykov D, Volbers B, Kloska S, Dörfler A, Schwab S, Bardutzky J. Therapeutic hypothermia for space-occupying Herpes simplex virus encephalitis. Minerva Anestesiol. 2011;77:371–4.
147. Munakata M, Kato R, Yokoyama H, Haginoya K, Tanaka Y, Kayaba J, et al. Combined therapy with hypothermia and anticytokine agents in influenza A encephalopathy. Brain Dev. 2000;22:373–7.
148. Sakurai T, Kimura A, Tanaka Y, Hozumi I, Ogura S, Inuzuka T. [Case of adult influenza type A virus-associated encephalopathy successfully treated with primary multidisciplinary treatments. Rinsho Shinkeigaku. 2007;47:639–43.
149. Fujita N, Saito H, Sekihara Y, Nagai H. Successful use of mild hypothermia therapy in an adult patient of non-herpetic acute encephalitis with severe intracranial hypertension. No To Shinkei. 2003;55:407–11.
150. Ohtsuki N, Kimura S, Nezu A, Aihara Y. Effects of mild hypothermia and steroid pulse combination therapy on acute encephalopathy associated with influenza virus infection: report of two cases. No To Hattatsu. 2000;32:318–22.
151. Yokota S, Imagawa T, Miyamae T, Ito S, Nakajima S, Nezu A, Mori M. Hypothetical pathophysiology of acute encephalopathy and encephalitis related to influenza virus infection and hypothermia therapy. Pediatr Int. 2000;42:197–203.
152. Guilliams K, Rosen M, Buttram S, Zempel J, Pineda J, Miller B, Shoykhet M. Hypothermia for pediatric refractory status epilepticus. Epilepsia. 2013;54:1586–94.
153. Shein SL, Reynolds TQ, Gedela S, Kochanek PM, Bell MJ. Therapeutic hypothermia for refractory status epilepticus in a child with malignant migrating partial seizures of infancy and SCN1A mutation: a case report. Ther Hypothermia Temp Manag. 2012;2:144–9.
154. Lin JJ, Lin KL, Hsia SH, Wang HS, CHEESE Study Group. Therapeutic hypothermia for febrile infection-related epilepsy syndrome in two patients. Pediatr Neurol. 2012;4:448–50.
155. Vargas WS, Merchant S, Solomon G. Favorable outcomes in acute necrotizing encephalopathy in a child treated with hypothermia. Pediatr Neurol. 2012;46:387–9.
156. Kawano G, Iwata O, Iwata S, Kawano K, Obu K, Kuki I, Research Network for Acute Encephalopathy in Childhood, et al. Determinants of outcomes following acute child encephalopathy and encephalitis: pivotal effect of early and delayed cooling. Arch Dis Child. 2011;96:936–41.
157. Zobel C, Adler C, Kranz A, Seck C, Pfister R, Hellmich M, et al. Mild therapeutic hypothermia in cardiogenic shock syndrome. Crit Care Med. 2012;40:1715–23.
158. Hovdenes J, Laake JH, Aaberge L, Haugaa H, Bugge JF. Therapeutic hypothermia after out-of-hospital cardiac arrest: experiences with patients treated with percutaneous coronary intervention and cardiogenic shock. Acta Anaesthesiol Scand. 2007;51:137–42.
159. Schmidt-Schweda S, Ohler A, Post H, Pieske B. Moderate hypothermia for severe cardiogenic shock (COOL Shock Study I & II). Resuscitation. 2013;84:319–25.
160. Skulec R, Kovarnik T, Dostalova G, Kolar J, Linhart A. Induction of mild hypothermia in cardiac arrest survivors presenting with cardiogenic shock syndrome. Acta Anaesthesiol Scand. 2008;52:188–94.
161. Haupt MT, Jastremski MS, Clemmer TP, Metz CA, Goris GB. Effect of ibuprofen in patients with severe sepsis: a randomized, double-blind, multicenter study. The Ibuprofen Study Group. Crit Care Med. 1991;19:1339–47.
162. Morris PE, Promes JT, Guntupalli KK, Wright PE, Arons MM. A multicenter, randomized, double-blind, parallel, placebo-controlled trial to evaluate the efficacy, safety, and pharmacokinetics of intravenous ibuprofen for the treatment of fever in critically ill and non-critically ill adults. Crit Care. 2010;14:R125.
163. Schortgen F, Clabault K, Katsahian S, Devaquet J, Mercat A, Deye N, et al. Fever control using external cooling in septic shock: a randomized controlled trial. Am J Respir Crit Care Med. 2012;185:1088–95.
164. Bernard GR, Wheeler AP, Russell JA, Schein R, Summer WR, Steinberg KP, et al. The effects of ibuprofen on the physiology and survival of patients with sepsis. The Ibuprofen in Sepsis Study Group. N Engl J Med. 1997;336:912–8.
165. Deye N, Cariou A, Girardie P, Pichon N, Megarbane B, Midez P, et al. Clinical and Economical Impact of Endovascular Cooling in the Management of Cardiac Arrest (ICEREA) Study Group. Endovascular Versus External Targeted Temperature Management for Patients With Out-of-Hospital Cardiac Arrest: a Randomized, Controlled Study. Circulation. 2015;132:182–93.
166. Rana M, Schröder JW, Saygili E, Hameed U, Benke D, Hoffmann R, et al. Comparative evaluation of the usability of 2 different methods to perform mild hypothermia in patients with out-of-hospital cardiac arrest. Int J Cardiol. 2011;152:321–6.
167. Hoedemaekers CW, Ezzahti M, Gerritsen A, van der Hoeven JG. Comparison of cooling methods to induce and maintain normo- and hypothermia in intensive care unit patients: a prospective intervention study. Crit Care. 2007;11:R91.
168. Feuchtl A, Gockel B, Lawrenz T, Bartelsmeier M, Stellbrink C. Endovascular cooling improves neurological short-term outcome after prehospital cardiac arrest. Intensivmed Notfallmedizin. 2007;44:37–42.
169. Flemming K, Simonis G, Ziegs E, Diewok C, Gildemeister R, Wunderlich C, Strasser RH. Comparison of external and intravascular cooling to induce hypothermia in patients after CPR. Ger Med Sci. 2006;4:Doc04.
170. Ferreira I, Schutte M, Oosterloo E, Dekker W, Mooi BW, Dambrink JH, van 't Hof AW. Therapeutic mild hypothermia improves outcome after out-of-hospital cardiac arrest. Neth Heart J. 2009;17:378–84.
171. Gillies MA, Pratt R, Whiteley C, Borg J, Beale RJ, Tibby SM. Therapeutic hypothermia after cardiac arrest: a retrospective comparison of surface and endovascular cooling techniques. Resuscitation. 2010;8:1117–22.
172. Bouwes A, Robillard LB, Binnekade JM, de Pont AC, Wieske L, Hartog AW, et al. The influence of rewarming after therapeutic hypothermia on outcome after cardiac arrest. Resuscitation. 2012;83:996–1000.
173. Schwab S, Georgiadis D, Berrouschot J, Schellinger PD, Graffagnino C, Mayer SA. Feasibility and safety of moderate hypothermia after massive hemispheric infarction. Stroke. 2001;32:2033–5.
174. Povlishock JT, Wei EP. Posthypothermic rewarming considerations following traumatic brain injury. J Neurotrauma. 2009;26:333–40.
175. Lavinio A, Timofeev I, Nortje J, Outtrim J, Smielewski P, Gupta A, et al. Cerebrovascular reactivity during hypothermia and rewarming. Br J Anaesth. 2007;99:237–44.
176. Moran JL, Peter JV, Solomon PJ, Grealy B, Smith T, Ashforth W, et al. Tympanic temperature measurements: are they reliable in the critically ill? A clinical study of measures of agreement. Crit Care Med. 2007;35:155–64.
177. Lefrant JY, Muller L, de La Coussaye JE, Benbabaali M, Lebris C, Zeitoun N, et al. Temperature measurement in intensive care patients: comparison of urinary bladder, oesophageal, rectal, axillary, and inguinal methods versus pulmonary artery core method. Intensive Care Med. 2003;29:414–8.

178. Shin J, Kim J, Song K, Kwak Y. Core temperature measurement in therapeutic hypothermia according to different phases: comparison of bladder, rectal, and tympanic versus pulmonary artery methods. Resuscitation. 2013;84:810–7.
179. Krizanac D, Stratil P, Hoerburger D, Testori C, Wallmueller C, Schober A, et al. Femoro-iliacal artery versus pulmonary artery core temperature measurement during therapeutic hypothermia: an observational study. Resuscitation. 2013;84:805–9.
180. Knapik P, Rychlik W, Duda D, Gołyszny R, Borowik D, Cieśla D. Relationship between blood, nasopharyngeal and urinary bladder temperature during intravascular cooling for therapeutic hypothermia after cardiac arrest. Resuscitation. 2012;83:208–12.
181. Xiao G, Guo Q, Shu M, Xie X, Deng J, Zhu Y, Wan C. Safety profile and outcome of mild therapeutic hypothermia in patients following cardiac arrest: systematic review and meta-analysis. Emerg Med J. 2013;30:91–100.
182. Nielsen N, Hovdenes J, Nilsson F, Rubertsson S, Stammet P, Sunde K, Hypothermia Network, et al. Outcome, timing and adverse events in therapeutic hypothermia after out-of-hospital cardiac arrest. Acta Anaesthesiol Scand. 2009;53:926–34.
183. Mongardon N, Perbet S, Lemiale V, Dumas F, Poupet H, Charpentier J, et al. Infectious complications in out-of-hospital cardiac arrest patients in the therapeutic hypothermia era. Crit Care Med. 2011;39:1359–64.
184. Perbet S, Mongardon N, Dumas F, Bruel C, Lemiale V, Mourvillier B, et al. Early-onset pneumonia after cardiac arrest: characteristics, risk factors and influence on prognosis. Am J Respir Crit Care Med. 2011;184:1048–54.
185. Busch M, Soreide E, Lossius HM, Lexow K, Dickstein K. Rapid implementation of therapeutic hypothermia in comatose out-of-hospital cardiac arrest survivors. Acta Anaesthesiol Scand. 2006;50:1277–83.
186. Akula VP, Joe P, Thusu K, Davis AS, Tamaresis JS, Kim S, et al. A randomized clinical trial of therapeutic hypothermia mode during transport for neonatal encephalopathy. J Pediatr. 2015;166:856–61.
187. Robinson JL, Seal RF, Spady DW, Joffres MR. Comparison of esophageal, rectal, axillary, bladder, tympanic, and pulmonary artery temperatures in children. J Pediatr. 1998;133:553–6.
188. Craig JV, Lancaster GA, Williamson PR, Smyth RL. Temperature measured at the axilla compared with rectum in children and young people: systematic review. BMJ. 2000;320:1174–8.
189. Craig JV, Lancaster GA, Taylor S, Williamson PR, Smyth RL. Infrared ear thermometry compared with rectal thermometry in children: a systematic review. Lancet. 2002;360:603–9.
190. Romano MJ, Fortenberry JD, Autrey E, Harris S, Heyroth T, Parmeter P, Stein F. Infrared tympanic thermometry in the pediatric intensive care unit. Crit Care Med. 1993;21:1181–5.

20

Prognosis of cirrhotic patients admitted to the general ICU

Gaël Piton[1,2*], Claire Chaignat[1], Mikhael Giabicani[3], Jean-Paul Cervoni[4], Fabienne Tamion[3], Emmanuel Weiss[5,6], Catherine Paugam-Burtz[5,6], Gilles Capellier[1,2] and Vincent Di Martino[2,4]

Abstract

Background: The prognosis of cirrhotic patients admitted to the ICU is considered to be poor but has been mainly reported in liver ICU. We aimed to describe the prognosis of cirrhotic patients admitted to a general ICU, to assess the predictors of mortality in this population, and, finally, to identify a subgroup of patients in whom intensive care escalation might be discussed.

Results: We performed a retrospective monocentric study of all cirrhotic patients consecutively admitted between 2002 and 2014 in a general ICU in a regional university hospital. Two hundred and eighteen cirrhotic patients were admitted to the ICU. The 28-day and 6-month mortality rates were 53 and 74 %, respectively. Among the 115 patients who were discharged from ICU, only eight patients underwent liver transplantation, whereas 48 had no clear contraindication. Multivariable analyses on 28-day mortality identified three independent variables, incorporated into a new three-variable prognostic model as follows: SOFA $\geq$ 12 (OR 4.2 [2.2–8.0]; 2 points), INR $\geq$ 2.6 (OR 2.5 [1.3–4.8]; 1 point), and renal replacement therapy (OR 2.3 [1.1–5.1]; 1 point). For a value of the score at 4 (16 % of patients), 28-day and 3-month mortality rates were 91 and 100 %, respectively. An external validation of the score among 149 critically ill cirrhotic patients showed a good accuracy for predicting in-ICU mortality.

Conclusions: Mortality of cirrhotic patients admitted to a general ICU was comparable to that of other studies. A pragmatic score integrating the SOFA score, INR, and the need for extrarenal epuration was strongly associated with mortality. Among the 16 % of patients presenting with score 4 at ICU admission, 100 % died in the 3-month follow-up period. The prognostic evaluation on day 3 remains essential for the majority of patients. However, this score calculable at ICU admission might identify patients in whom the benefit of intensive care escalation should be discussed, in particular when liver transplantation is contraindicated.

Background

The recent developments in the global management of ICU patients and the improved understanding of cirrhosis physiopathology and complications probably account for the better short-term survival of cirrhotic patients reported in the latest studies [1]. Nonetheless, the prognosis of cirrhotic patients admitted to the intensive care unit (ICU) remains poor. Data from the literature of the last decade describe ICU mortality ranging from 36 to 65 % [2–5] and in-hospital mortality varying from 44 to 86 % [6–8], suggesting that despite the initial control of organ failures before release from ICU, 8–21 % of additional patients die in the short term.

An early prognostic assessment is crucial for discriminating the good candidates for ICU from those for whom the situation is hopeless despite strong therapeutic interventions. In this perspective, it has been demonstrated that standard prognostic scores used by hepatologists, such as MELD or Child–Pugh, are insufficient because of focusing on the liver without considering other failures and the hepatic state. The ICU general scores, which reflect the state of the main living functions, are more relevant, particularly in the short term [2, 9–11].

Recently, the literature has underlined the relevance of a prognostic assessment deferred to day 3, which seems

*Correspondence: gpiton@chu-besancon.fr
[1] Intensive Care Unit, Besançon University Hospital, 25030 Besançon, France
Full list of author information is available at the end of the article

more reliable than an assessment on admission [2, 5, 12]. However, the application of such deferred prognostic assessment that can only occur in ICU raises two practical issues: The first is the "permissive" access of cirrhotic patients in ICU and the second is the interruption of organ replacement therapy at day 3 when the situation is deemed hopeless.

The primary objective of our study was to describe the short-term and long-term outcome of cirrhotic patients admitted to a non-specialized general ICU. The secondary objectives were, first, to analyze the performance of prognostic markers to predict 28-day mortality and, second, to develop and evaluate a new prognostic score determined at ICU admission that may identify patients with an extremely poor prognosis in whom intensive care escalation should be discussed, in particular if liver transplantation is contraindicated.

Patients and methods

Population

This is an observational, monocentric cohort study carried out in the medical ICU of the Besancon University Hospital. All cirrhotic patients (cirrhosis either histologically proven or diagnosis made by hepatologists according to clinical, biological, and ultrasonographic criteria) admitted to our medical ICU between 01.01.2002 and 30.05.2014 were included. When a patient had been admitted to ICU more than once, only the first admission was analyzed.

Data collection

For each patient, 170 clinical and paraclinical variables were collected from their medical charts. These parameters were known at ICU admission ($n = 110$) and during ICU stay ($n = 60$). Clinical data included socio-demographic characteristics, comorbidities, cause of admission, history of cirrhosis, baseline clinical conditions, and therapeutics during ICU stay. Biological data included 34 biochemical and bacteriological variables, allowing the calculation of 7 prognostic scores at baseline and day 3. The prognostic scores assessed were the Child–Pugh score, MELD score, D'Amico classification, IGS II score, APACHE II score, SOFA score, and CLIF-SOFA score calculated as global scores.

The main assessment criterion was 28-day mortality. The vital status was confirmed by the review of the computer-based medical record of the hospital which complies information from all units (Axigate database). When a patient released hospital alive, if no data were available after this release, the time was censored at the date of hospital release for statistical analyses.

Statistical analyses

Qualitative variables were expressed by the number and percentages and compared by Fisher's exact tests. Quantitative variables were expressed by the median and interquartile range (IQR) and compared with Wilcoxon's rank test. Survival analyses used the Kaplan–Meier model and log-rank tests. Multivariable analyses of predictors of mortality used a logistic regression model for 28-day mortality. Variables included in the multivariable model were chosen according to univariate analyses, their relevance according to the literature, and the likelihood of collinearity based upon clinical judgment. Indeed, we considered that general ICU scores, all evaluating the risk of mortality and being based upon the sequential assessment of organ failures, would be collinear. Similarly, we considered that validated biological variables of liver failure (i.e., bilirubin, prothrombin rate, and international normalized ratio) would be collinear. A multiple logistic regression model was used for the creation of a new prognostic score, based on 28-day mortality, and taking into account variables collected at the time of ICU admission. This score incorporated among the general ICU scores, the markers of liver failure, and the medical interventions, the one of each which had the best prognostic performance. The local score was externally evaluated in a cohort of 149 cirrhotic patients admitted to the ICU of the Rouen University Hospital. Statistical analyses were performed using SAS 9.3.

Results

Patient baseline characteristics

In the study period, 7427 admissions were recorded, including 258 (3.5 %) admissions for cirrhosis-related complications. Those 258 admissions corresponded to 218 patients. The baseline characteristics of patients are described in Additional file 1: Table S1. Care and outcome in ICU are described in Additional file 2: Table S2. Briefly, the median age was 59 [51–67], there were 165 men (76 %), and alcoholism was the main cause of cirrhosis (85 %). On admission, the medians of the different prognostic scores were as follows: Child–Pugh = 11 [IQR 9–12], MELD = 28 [18–40], SOFA = 12 [9–15], CLIF-SOFA 14 [11–17], and IGS II = 59 [45–72]. The reasons for admission included: hemodynamic failure (53 %), coma (53 %), respiratory failure (36 %), renal failure (25 %), septic shock (17 %), and gastrointestinal bleeding (13 %). One hundred and four patients (48 %) had more than one reason for ICU admission. During ICU stay, 190 patients needed mechanical ventilation (90 %). Of them, 173 (79 %) had been intubated at ICU admission. One hundred and eighty-seven patients (86 %) received catecholamines and 112 (51 %) needed a renal replacement therapy (22 of them (10 %) a MARS).

Outcome events

The median duration stay in ICU was 5 days [IQR 2–12]. The median duration of hospitalization was 13 days [4–36]. In-ICU, 28-day, 3-, 6-month, and 1-year mortality rates were 47 % (103/218), 53 % (116/218), 66 % (139/210), 74 % (145/196), and 77 % (147/190), respectively (Additional file 2: Table S2; Additional file 3: Fig. S1).

The outcome of the 115 ICU survivors is described in Additional file 4: Fig. S2. Forty-eight cirrhotic patients were apparently eligible for liver transplantation according to our retrospective review. Conversely, 67 patients were not good candidates because of old age ($n = 19$), alcohol dependence ($n = 34$), possible advanced hepatocellular carcinoma ($n = 6$), or extrahepatic malignancy ($n = 12$). Finally, only eight (17 %) patients underwent liver transplantation after their ICU stay.

Univariate analysis according to the study period

Renal replacement therapy at ICU admission was performed in 25 and 25 % of the patients before and after 2010 ($p = 1$). Catecholamine use at ICU admission was given in 64 and 77 % of the patients before and after 2010, respectively ($p = 0.04$). Mechanical ventilation was present in 62 and 76 % of the patients before and after 2010, respectively ($p = 0.03$). Liver transplantation during or after ICU stay was performed in five patients in the first study period and in three patients in the second study period. The SOFA score at ICU admission was not significantly different between these two periods (medians of 11 and 12, respectively, $p = 0.25$).

Univariate analysis of factors associated with 28-day mortality

Results of univariate analysis of factors associated with 28-day mortality are given in Table 1. Factors significantly associated with 28-day mortality included low body temperature, low arterial pressure, admission for severe sepsis or septic shock, high INR, high plasma concentrations of creatinine, lactate, and bilirubin, low pH, PaO2/FiO2, platelet count, low albumin, low prothrombin rate, the need of mechanical ventilation, renal replacement therapy, catecholamines, and high levels of all prognostic scores. The period of admission (before or after 2010) did not have significant impact on mortality (log rank $p = 0.45$).

Multivariable analysis of predictors of mortality

We aimed to build a multivariable model including the best general ICU score, the best biological variable of hepatic failure, and the most relevant therapy performed at ICU admission. Among general ICU score (SOFA score, CLIF-SOFA, APACHE II), the SOFA score was the variable which was the most strongly associated with 28-day mortality. Among biological variables of liver failure, INR was the variable which was the most strongly associated with 28-day mortality. Among variables of treatment at the time of ICU admission (i.e., renal replacement therapy, catecholamine use, and mechanical ventilation), RRT was the variable which was the most strongly associated with 28-day mortality. According to these results, we built a multivariable model including the SOFA score, INR, and RRT. For the analysis, the SOFA score and INR were dichotomized at their median value in the cohort, respectively, 12 and 2.6. The results of multiple logistic regressions of variables relating to 28-day mortality are given in Table 2. These three variables were independently associated with 28-day mortality: baseline SOFA score ≥ 12 (OR 4.2 [2.2–8.0]), INR ≥ 2.6 at ICU admission (OR 2.5 [1.3–4.8]), and need for RRT at ICU admission (OR 2.3 [1.1–5.1]).

Creation of a local prognostic score at ICU admission and assessment of its performance

To give to the clinician a pragmatic, powerful, and easy-to-use tool, we created a prognostic score at ICU admission, called "three-variable prognosis score" to predict 28-day mortality. This score incorporated the three independent mortality risk factors identified by multivariable analysis, each variable of the score being weighted by its odds ratio. Baseline SOFA score ≥ 12 was associated with 2 points; INR ≥ 2.6 at ICU admission was associated with 1 point; and need for RRT at ICU admission was associated with 1 point (Table 3). This score varied from 0 to 4 points and was significantly associated with mortality (log rank $p < 0.0001$, Fig. 1). Log-rank test comparing each strata of the score with each other found that the survival probability for score = 3 and score = 4 was different of each other strata (Additional file 5: Table S3; Additional file 6: Fig. S3). AUC of the score for predicting 28-day mortality was 0.79 [0.73–0.84]. This score calculated at ICU admission was able to discriminate survivors and non-survivors at the times of ICU discharge, 28 days, 3, and 6 months (all $p < 0.0001$). Among patients presenting with score at 4 (16 % of patients), 71 % (24/34) died in the first 3 days after ICU admission and 88 % (30/34) died in the first 10 days. For a value of the score at 4, the prediction of 28-day mortality and 3-month mortality was excellent (positive predictive value of 91 and 100 %, respectively).

External validation of the prognostic local score

The prognostic value of the local score was evaluated in a cohort of 149 critically ill cirrhotic patients admitted

Table 1 Predictive factors of 28-day mortality determined by univariate analysis in 218 cirrhotic patients admitted to the ICU

	28-day survivors ($n = 102$)	28-day non-survivors ($n = 116$)	p
Variable			
Age	57 (50–66)	59 (51–68)	0.47
Male sex	75 (74)	90 (78)	0.53
Hepatology transfer	31 (30)	54 (47)	0.02
Diabetes mellitus	36 (35)	24 (21)	0.02
Smoker	88 (86)	89 (77)	0.08
Chronic renal failure	9 (9)	10 (9)	1
Cancer	15 (15)	15 (13)	0.84
Characteristics of cirrhosis			
Alcoholic cause	83 (81)	101 (88)	0.26
Viral cause	14 (14)	18 (16)	0.70
Esophageal varices	72 (71)	86 (75)	0.54
Ascites	63 (62)	86 (74)	0.06
Diagnosis at ICU admission			
Hemodynamic failure	34 (34)	81 (70)	<0.0001
Gastrointestinal bleeding	13 (13)	15 (13)	1
Respiratory failure	43 (42)	36 (31)	0.09
Severe sepsis	18 (18)	42 (36)	0.002
Septic shock	12 (12)	26 (22)	0.048
Renal failure	20 (20)	34 (29)	0.12
Neurological failure	60 (59)	56 (48)	0.14
Cardiorespiratory arrest	2 (2)	16 (14)	0.002
Clinical parameters at ICU admission			
Temperature	37.0 (36.1–37.6)	36.0 (35.0–37.0)	<0.0001
Systolic arterial pressure	110 (100–126)	100 (90–112)	<0.0001
Mean arterial pressure	70 (65–80)	62 (55–68)	<0.0001
Biological parameters at ICU admission			
International normalized ratio	2.1 (1.7–2.8)	3.6 (2.3–6.5)	<0.0001
Blood glucose (mmol/L)	7.4 (6.0–9.5)	6.0 (3.7–8.4)	0.0002
Creatinine (μmol/L)	127 (78–210)	186 (118–293)	0.001
pH	7.37 (7.29–7.44)	7.25 (7.09–7.39)	<0.0001
Lactate (mmol/L)	2.4 (1.7–3.6)	4.7 (2.5–11.3)	<0.0001
PaO_2/FiO_2	290 (190–400)	200 (118–348)	0.003
White blood cells ($\times 10^9$/L)	10.5 (7.4–15.5)	12.5 (8.4–19.0)	0.03
Hemoglobin (g/dL)	9.9 (8.8–11.4)	8.8 (7.4–11.0)	0.005
Platelets ($\times 10^9$/L)	113 (79–172)	90 (62–141)	0.005
Bilirubin (μmol/L)	37 (20–90)	112 (34–248)	<0.0001
Albumin (g/L)	26 (22–30)	22 (18–28)	0.002
Prothrombin rate (%)	43 (33–54)	25 (16–39)	<0.0001
Prognostic scores at ICU admission			
Child–Pugh	10 (8–12)	11 (10–13)	<0.0001
MELD	21 (15–29)	35 (25–45)	<0.0001
IGS II	49 (39–60)	68 (57–81)	<0.0001
APACHE II	23 (18–27)	28 (23–34)	<0.0001
SOFA	10 (7–12)	14 (11–17)	<0.0001
CLIF-SOFA	13 (10–15)	16 (13–19)	<0.0001
Prognostic score after ICU admission			
SOFA at day 3	8 (5–10)	16 (12–19)	<0.0001

Table 1 continued

	28-day survivors ($n = 102$)	28-day non-survivors ($n = 116$)	*p*
Clinical feature during ICU stay			
Mechanical invasive ventilation	76 (75)	106 (91)	0.009
Vasopressor therapy	78 (76)	109 (94)	0.0003
Renal replacement therapy	28 (27)	84 (72)	<0.0001
MARS	8 (8)	14 (12)	0.37
Clinical course in ICU			
Documented infection	76 (75)	94 (81)	0.26
Severe sepsis	56 (55)	88 (76)	0.002
Septic shock	35 (34)	63 (54)	0.004
Gastrointestinal bleeding	30 (29)	39 (34)	0.56
Hepatic encephalopathy	64 (63)	57 (49)	0.06

Numbers are *n* (%), median [interquartile range], *MARS* molecular adsorbent recirculating system

Table 2 Logistic regression analyses of factors associated with 28-day mortality

Variable	Simple logistic regression model		Multiple logistic regression model	
	OR [CI 95 %]	*p*	OR [CI 95 %]	*p*
SOFA score				
<12	1	<0.0001	1	<0.0001
≥12	5.6 [3.1–9.9]		4.2 [2.2–8.0]	
INR				
<2.6	1	<0.0001	1	0.008
≥2.6	4.5 [2.5–8.2]		2.5 [1.3–4.8]	
Renal replacement therapy				
No	1	0.0004	1	0.03
Yes	3.4 [1.7–6.8]		2.3 [1.1–5.1]	

INR international normalized ratio, *SOFA* sequential organ failure assessment score

to the ICU of the Rouen University Hospital (Table 4). These patients had a cirrhosis histologically proven or a diagnosis of cirrhosis made by hepatologists according to clinical, biological, and ultrasonographic criteria. The median age was 56 years (50–62), median INR was 2.2 (1.6–3.0), median SOFA score at ICU admission was 11 [7–14], renal replacement therapy was performed in 22 patients (15 %), and in-ICU mortality was 38 %. In-ICU mortality was 11, 25, 62, 66, and 85 % among patients presenting with local score equal to 0, 1, 2, 3, and 4, respectively (Table 4). In-hospital mortality was 100 % for patients with score equal to 4 at ICU admission. Among the 13 patients classified score 4 (i.e., those having SOFA score ≥ 12 and INR ≥ 2.6 and need for RRT), RRT was indicated but not performed in seven patients despite a deep metabolic acidosis, because of lack of time, because of the death occurring in the first hours after admission, or because the clinician estimated that the patient was moribund and RRT was futile. These seven patients died within 24 h of ICU admission.

Discussion

This monocentric cohort study has evaluated the mortality risk factors in 218 cirrhotic patients consecutively admitted to our general ICU and reports two main results: (1) the prognosis of cirrhotic patients admitted to non-specialized general ICU is comparable to that of other studies, but the long-term prognosis is poor in the absence of liver transplantation; (2) a new prognostic score combining SOFA, INR, and the need for renal replacement therapy improves the prognostic assessment at baseline and could make usefulness the delayed assessment at day 3 in 16 % of patients.

Our study had the merit to collect exhaustive information in a non-selected population from a general ICU in a regional university hospital. Although the proportion of admission for complicated cirrhosis was low during the study period (3.5 %), we were able to report the long-term outcome of almost 200 patients, making our cohort larger than others reported in the majority of published studies on the topic.

In our center, the overall mortality of patients admitted between 2002 and 2014 in our ICU was around 30 %, comparable to that of the literature. In cirrhotic patients, in-ICU mortality was 47 % and was also comparable to that reported in the literature of the last decade, since it ranges from 36 to 65 % [2–5]. Regarding in-ICU and 28-day mortality rates, our data were similar to the 41 % in-ICU and 54 % 28-day mortality rates reported by Das et al. [5], but higher to that reported by Flood et al. [13]. The discrepancies are probably the consequence of the severity of the patients at admission. Interestingly, our results were obtained in a population with a high

Table 3 Prognostic score at ICU admission and its performance

Definition (score calculate at admission)			Points
SOFA score			
<12			0
≥12			2
INR			
<2.6			0
≥2.6			1
Indication of renal replacement therapy			
No			0
Yes			1
Total score			(0–4 points)
Local score	**28-day mortality (*n* = 203)**	**3-month mortality (*n* = 195)**	**6-month mortality (*n* = 181)**
Total			
0 point	14/60 (23)	22/56 (39)	26/47 (55)
1 point	16/33 (48)	19/30 (63)	20/30 (67)
2 points	15/36 (42)	21/35 (60)	21/33 (64)
3 points	31/40 (78)	32/40 (80)	32/37 (86)
4 points	31/34 (91)	34/34 (100)	34/34 (100)

INR international normalized ratio, *SOFA* sequential organ failure assessment score

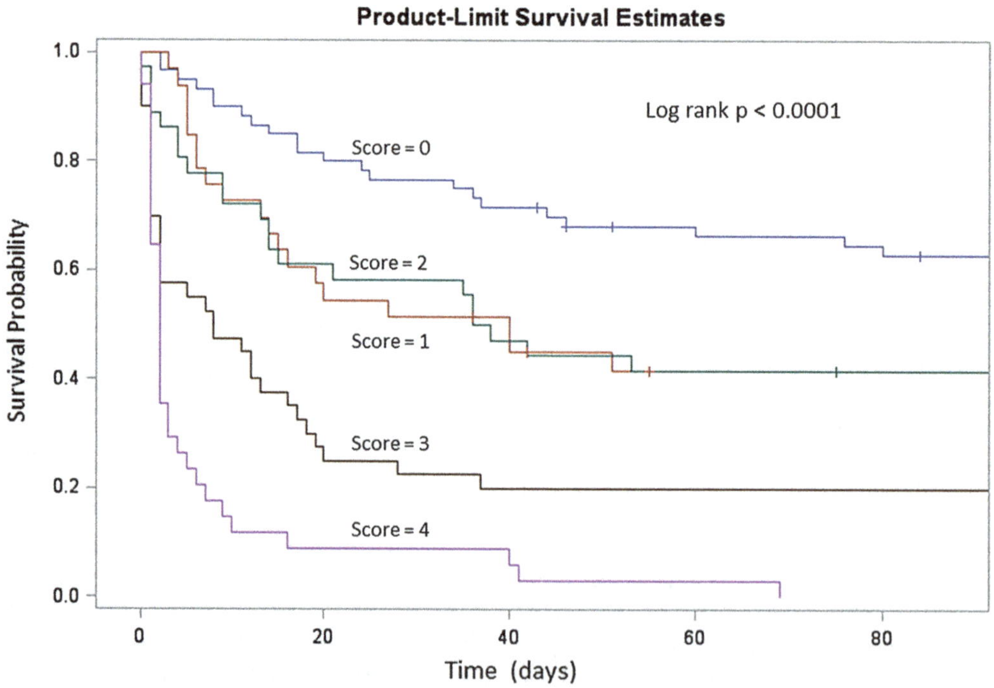

Fig. 1 Survival according to our three-variable prognostic score

proportion of mechanical ventilation (90 %). Regarding long-term mortality, our results were close to the 38 % 6-month survival given by Das [5] and the 31 % one-year survival given by Gildea [6].

The result of initial prognostic assessments was consistent with the literature data. In particular, we found a good performance of organ dysfunction scores: A high SOFA score was particularly a good predictor of in-ICU

Table 4 External validation of the local score in a cohort of 149 cirrhotic patients admitted to the ICU of the Rouen University Hospital

Local score	In-ICU mortality ($n = 149$)
0 point	7/62 (11)
1 point	6/24 (25)
2 points	13/21 (62)
3 points	19/29 (66)
4 points	11/13 (85)

Numbers are n (%)

mortality as reported in the study by Levesque et al. [2]. However, we wanted to improve our initial prognostic assessment as much as possible, and this is why we created a new composite score from this series. The statistical analyses allowed us to identify the best score of organ failures, the best marker of liver failure, and the most relevant organ replacement therapy to predict in-ICU mortality. Thus, the three following variables: SOFA $\geq$ 12, INR $\geq$ 2.6, and need for renal replacement therapy, were selected and incorporated in our new composite score. This score was efficient for the evaluation of short-term and long-term survival.

Recent literature has emphasized the value of a deferred assessment at day 3, justifying in practice a permissive attitude consisting of undertaking intensive support without restriction but with a re-evaluation by SOFA or modified SOFA score after 72 h [5, 11]. In that context, Ginès et al. [14] indicated that therapeutic limitation could be considered if more than 3 organ failures persist at day 3. Such assessment deferred at day 3 is problematic in everyday practice, when considering the financial and human investment it represents, which may appear disproportionated given the suboptimal efficiency of life supports in these patients. In our center, the implementation of therapeutic limitations remains difficult and inconstant. This is why we wanted to optimize and maximize the predictive value of the initial evaluation to establish a thinner selection of cirrhotic candidates for admission in ICU. Our new prognostic score partially solved this issue. A score equal to 4 at ICU admission was associated with a predictive value of 100 % for 3-month mortality. Similarly, in-hospital mortality was 100 % among patients with score equal to 4 in the validation cohort of the Rouen University Hospital.

Further progress concerns the "hepatology" management of these patients. Surprisingly, although priority is given in France to the sickest patients for organ allocation, only 17 % of patients eligible for transplantation actually underwent liver transplantation after their ICU stay in our series. This paradox is not specific to our center and has been clearly highlighted by a meta-analysis dedicated to the prognosis of more than 2600 cirrhotic patients admitted to ICU and included in 13 international studies: Only 3 % of those patients underwent liver transplantation, whereas 55 % survived to ICU stay (Vincent Di Martino, personal communication). We think an ICU stay should be considered as a major event in the natural history of cirrhosis, able to indicate per se a liver transplantation, as well as other events such as a spontaneous bacterial peritonitis.

Our study acknowledges several limitations: (1) This was a retrospective, monocentric, and observational study. However, an external validation of our local score showed a good accuracy for predicting in-ICU mortality in 149 critically ill cirrhotic patients. In this cohort, there was only 9 % patient with a score equal to 4, suggesting that patients considered as moribund may not be systematically admitted to the ICU. (2) The population of cirrhotic patients who have not been admitted to ICU and the reasons why ICU admission did or not occur are not known. This selection of patients undoubtedly influenced our results in "real life." However, this criticism applies to all of the series previously published, because the selection procedures regulating access to ICUs of cirrhotic patients were never described. (3) The inclusion period did not allow us to investigate the prognostic impact of new anti-HCV drugs. (4) As in other studies, our statistical analyses and the determination of our prognostic score presupposed that each relevant variable was not linked to the others. However, it is clear that in those patients, organ failures are intricate and also correlated with the degree of liver failure, the reasons for admission, and the therapeutic interventions. In this context, it is probably unrealistic to argue for the identification of entirely "independent" variables. (5) The long-term analyses were conducted on the entire population, which probably overestimates the impact of initial assessments (especially prognostic scores) because the largest proportion of deaths occurs in ICU. It would have been more appropriate to perform a specific analysis restricted to the 115 patients who survived their ICU stay. However, such analysis would probably have been hampered by a lack of power, making difficult the interpretation of negative results. (6) This study reported critically ill patients admitted to the ICU for medical reasons, and thus, perioperative surgical population was not present in this study. (7) Large prospective validation of this score is necessary before raising definitive conclusions, especially on the possibility to avoid an assessment on day 3 for the most seriously ill patients.

In conclusion, the mortality of cirrhotic patients admitted to a general ICU was comparable to that of other studies. The long-term prognosis of critically ill cirrhotic patients remains poor in the absence of liver transplantation. A pragmatic score calculable at ICU admission might identify patients in whom the benefit of intensive care escalation should be discussed, in particular when liver transplantation is contraindicated.

Additional files

Additional file 1. Table S1 Clinical and laboratory characteristics of 218 cirrhotic patients at ICU admission.

Additional file 2. Table S2 Treatment and prognosis of 218 cirrhotic patients admitted to the ICU.

Additional file 3. Figure S1 Estimated probability of survival of 218 cirrhotic patients admitted to the ICU.

Additional file 4. Figure S2 Outcome of the studied population. Of the 115 patients who survived their ICU stay, 48 were theoritically eligible for liver transplantation, but only 8 underwent liver transplantation.

Additional file 5. Table S3 Survival according to our 3-variables prognostic score comparing score 0, 1 or 2; score 3; and score 4. Log rank test found a significant difference between the three strata of the score.

Additional file 6. Figure S3 Log rank test comparing each strata of the new prognostic score with each other strata.

Abbreviations

ICU: Intensive care unit; MARS: Molecular absorbent recirculating system; INR: International normalized ratio; SOFA: Sequential organ failure assessment score; RRT: Renal replacement therapy.

Authors' contributions

GP, CC, MG, FT, and VDM participated in the design of the study. CC and MG collected data. GP and VDM performed the statistical analysis. GP, CC, and VDM drafted the manuscript. MG, JPC, FT, EW, CPB, and GC have reviewed the manuscript and consistently improved its content. All authors read and approved the final manuscript.

Author details

[1] Intensive Care Unit, Besançon University Hospital, 25030 Besançon, France. [2] Université de Franche Comté, 25000 Besançon, France. [3] Intensive Care Unit, Rouen University Hospital, Rouen, France. [4] Hepatology Unit, Besançon University Hospital, Besançon, France. [5] Intensive Care and Anesthesiology Department, AP-HP, Hôpital Beaujon, Hôpitaux Universitaires Paris Nord Val de Seine, 75018 Paris, France. [6] University Paris Diderot, Sorbonne Paris Cité, 75018 Paris, France.

Competing interests

The authors declare that they have no competing interests.

References

1. Galbois A, Trompette M-L, Das V, Boëlle P-Y, Carbonell N, Thabut D, et al. Improvement in the prognosis of cirrhotic patients admitted to an intensive care unit, a retrospective study. Eur J Gastroenterol Hepatol. 2012;24(8):897–904.
2. Levesque E, Hoti E, Azoulay D, Ichaï P, Habouchi H, Castaing D, et al. Prospective evaluation of the prognostic scores for cirrhotic patients admitted to an intensive care unit. J Hepatol. 2012;56(1):95–102.
3. Jalan R, Saliba F, Pavesi M, Amoros A, Moreau R, Ginès P, et al. Development and validation of a prognostic score to predict mortality in patients with acute-on-chronic liver failure. J Hepatol. 2014;61(5):1038–47.
4. Levesque E, Saliba F, Ichaï P, Samuel D. Outcome of patients with cirrhosis requiring mechanical ventilation in ICU. J Hepatol. 2014;60(3):570–8.
5. Das V, Boelle P-Y, Galbois A, Guidet B, Maury E, Carbonell N, et al. Cirrhotic patients in the medical intensive care unit: early prognosis and long-term survival*. Crit Care Med. 2010;38(11):2108–16.
6. Gildea TR, Cook WC, Nelson DR, Aggarwal A, Carey W, Younossi ZM, et al. Predictors of long-term mortality in patients with cirrhosis of the liver admitted to a medical ICU. Chest. 2004;126(5):1598–603.
7. Cholongitas E, Senzolo M, Patch D, Shaw S, O'Beirne J, Burroughs AK. Cirrhotics admitted to intensive care unit: the impact of acute renal failure on mortality. Eur J Gastroenterol Hepatol. 2009;21(7):744–50.
8. Theocharidou E, Pieri G, Mohammad AO, Cheung M, Cholongitas E, Agarwal B, et al. The Royal Free Hospital score: a calibrated prognostic model for patients with cirrhosis admitted to intensive care unit. Comparison with current models and CLIF-SOFA score. Am J Gastroenterol. 2014;109(4):554–62.
9. Minne L, Abu-Hanna A, de Jonge E. Evaluation of SOFA-based models for predicting mortality in the ICU: a systematic review. Crit Care Lond Engl. 2008;12(6):R161.
10. Pan H-C, Jenq C-C, Tsai M-H, Fan P-C, Chang C-H, Chang M-Y, et al. Risk models and scoring systems for predicting the prognosis in critically ill cirrhotic patients with acute kidney injury: a prospective validation study. PLoS ONE. 2012;7(12):e51094.
11. Cholongitas E, Betrosian A, Senzolo M, Shaw S, Patch D, Manousou P, et al. Prognostic models in cirrhotics admitted to intensive care units better predict outcome when assessed at 48 h after admission. J Gastroenterol Hepatol. 2008;23(8 Pt 1):1223–7.
12. Cholongitas E, Agarwal B, Antoniadis N, Burroughs AK. Patients with cirrhosis admitted to an Intensive Care Unit. J Hepatol. 2012;57(1):230–1.
13. Flood S, Bodenham A, Jackson P. Mortality of patients with alcoholic liver disease admitted to critical care: a systematic review. Available on: http://journal.ics.ac.uk/pdf/1302130.pdf.
14. Ginès P, Fernández J, Durand F, Saliba F. Management of critically-ill cirrhotic patients. J Hepatol. 2012;56(Suppl 1):S13–24.

Daily urinary creatinine predicts the weaning of renal replacement therapy in ICU acute kidney injury patients

Nicolas Viallet[1], Vincent Brunot[1], Nils Kuster[2], Delphine Daubin[1], Noémie Besnard[1], Laura Platon[1], Aurèle Buzançais[1], Romaric Larcher[1], Olivier Jonquet[1] and Kada Klouche[1,3*]

Abstract

Background: In acute kidney injury (AKI), useless continuation of renal replacement therapy (RRT) may delay renal recovery and impair patient's outcome. In this study, we aimed to identify predictive parameters that may help to a successful RRT weaning for AKI patients.

Methods: We studied 54 surviving AKI patients in which a weaning of RRT was attempted. On the day of weaning (D_0) and the following 2 days (D_1 and D_2), SAPS II and SOFA scores, 24-h diuresis, 24-h urinary creatinine and urea (UCr and UUr), creatinine and urea generation rates (CrGR and UrGR) and clearances (CrCl and UrCl) were collected. Patients who remained free of RRT 15 days after its discontinuation were considered as successfully weaned.

Results: Twenty-six RRT weaning attempts succeeded (S_+) and 28 failed (S_-). Age, previous renal function, SAPS II and SOFA scores were comparable between groups. At D_0, 24-h diuresis was 2300 versus 1950 ml in S_+ and S_-, respectively, $p = 0.05$. At D_0, D_1 and D_2, 24-h UUr and UCr levels, UrCl and CrCl, and UUr/UrGR and UCr/CrGR ratios were significantly higher in S_+ group. By multivariate analysis, D_1 24-h UCr was the most powerful parameter that was associated with RRT weaning success with an area under the ROC curve of 0.86 [0.75–0.97] and an odds ratio of 2.01 [1.27–3.18], $p = 0.003$.

Conclusions: In ICU AKI, 24-h UCr appeared as an efficient and independent marker of a successful weaning of RRT. A 24-h UCr $\geq$5.2 mmol was associated with a successful weaning in 84 % of patients.

Keywords: Acute kidney injury, Renal replacement therapy, Weaning, Urine output, Urinary creatinine

Background

Acute kidney injury (AKI) is a common condition in the intensive care unit (ICU). Approximately 5 % of ICU patients suffering from AKI require renal replacement therapy (RRT) [1]. Such patients have a hospital mortality rate of 45–70 % [1–6], and those surviving to hospital discharge continue to carry a high risk for long-term morbidity and mortality [7–10]. Several studies have shown that between 10 and 30 % of patients with AKI who required RRT will remain dialysis dependent at discharge [7–13]. Yet, renal function in AKI surviving patients requiring RRT ultimately recovers in the vast majority of case (more than 90 % of patients) [14]. However, performances of RRT may have untoward effects that contribute to the prolongation of renal failure or impede the ultimate recovery of renal function [15]. Indeed, RRT represents an independent and an added risk factor for mortality [16–18] as it exposes the patient to several complications like catheter-related infections or thrombosis, bleeding favored by anticoagulation, hemodynamic instability. The prolonged continuation of RRT could also be deleterious for renal recovery, particularly in cases of intradialytic hemodynamic instability, inducing renal ischemic lesions [19]. Renal biopsy in patients with prolonged AKI treated by hemodialysis showed regions

*Correspondence: k-klouche@chu-montpellier.fr
[1] Department of Intensive Care Medicine, Lapeyronie University Hospital, 371, Avenue du Doyen G. Giraud, 34295 Montpellier, France
Full list of author information is available at the end of the article

of fresh tubular necrosis days-to-weeks after the initial insult [20]. RRT may also delay renal recovery possibly by purification of mediators and growth factors needful for the tubular repair [21]. Moreover, RRT may remove unpredictable amounts of antibiotics, amino acids and nutrients. Also, RRT represents a significant additional cost in the patient's care. It is therefore a matter of concern to identify which factors present at the time of discontinuation may help physicians in predicting successful cessation of RRT [22]. To the best of our knowledge, a paucity of studies has been reported on RRT weaning during AKI [23–26]. Sepsis-related Organ Failure Assessment (SOFA) score [23, 26] and 2-h creatinine clearance [25] have been reported as a reliable predictive factors, but urine output remains the most consistent parameter significantly associated with the success of weaning [24]. This study was therefore undertaken to investigate and identify parameters, particularly 24-h urinary creatinine, present at the time of RRT weaning that would be associated with successful cessation of RRT during AKI.

Patients and methods

This retrospective study was conducted, from January 2008 to December 2012, in two medical ICUs of the Montpellier University Hospital, France. It was approved by our local institutional review board (Ethic Committee of Montpellier; Comité de protection des personnes: CPP Sud Mediterranée 4) which waived informed consent from the patients or their relatives.

Study population

Patients admitted to the ICU for AKI requiring RRT that survived and in which an attempt of weaning was realized were enrolled in the study. Exclusion criteria included pregnancy, age <18 years old, previous chronic renal failure stage $\geq$4, AKI of obstructive, glomerular or vascular etiology. AKI patients that underwent acute RRT for less than 3 days (no attempt of weaning), and patients without an attempt of weaning RRT or transferred to another unit before an attempt of weaning were also excluded. Decisions regarding the initiation, management and discontinuation of RRT were made by the referring physician according to the guidelines of the intensive care and nephrology societies [22]. The choice of RRT modality was depending on patient hemodynamic stability and was daily re-evaluated. Patients with hemodynamic instability or severe fluid overload were preferentially treated with pre-dilutional continuous venovenous hemodiafiltration (CVVHDF) or on-line sustained low-efficiency daily dialysis-filtration (SLEDD-f), and those with hemodynamic stability were preferentially treated with on-line intermittent hemodiafiltration (IHDF) [27].

Study design

An RRT cessation was considered as an attempt of weaning when referred to a medical decision and if it lasted more than 72 h. Only the first attempt was analyzed for each patient. Current criteria required for weaning attempt were the association of an urine output of at least 20 ml/h without diuretics [24, 28], a restored and stable hemodynamic and respiratory conditions, no new kidney aggression (mainly toxic and predictable), no need to continue RRT for the previously mentioned reasons. A successful weaning was defined as the cessation of RRT for at least 15 days. This endpoint defined two groups of patients: S_+ for the success of the weaning attempt and S_- if it failed.

Data collection

Baseline patient characteristics were recorded, including age, gender, cause of AKI, comorbidities, previous renal function (estimation of glomerular filtration rate—eGFR, by the Chronic Kidney Disease Epidemiology, CKD-epi formula [29]), weight, urine volume. Severity of illness was determined at the inclusion using the simplified acute physiology score II (SAPS II) and the Sequential Organ Failure Assessment (SOFA) score. RRT modalities were collected during treatment.

Day 0 (D_0) was defined as the day of RRT cessation at the weaning attempt, and D_1, D_2 the 2 following days. From D_0 to D_2, we daily collected the following parameters: non-renal SOFA score, patient's weight, 24-h urine output, dose of furosemide, fluid balance (intake output), mean arterial pressure, dose of vasopressors, use of mechanical ventilation, creatinine and urea blood and urine levels. Blood samples were drawn and 24-h urine samples were collected at D_0 and every following day. Creatinine and urea clearance (CrCl and UrCl), diuretic response index and creatinine and urea generation rate (CrGR and UrGR, respectively) were estimated at D_1 and D_2 according to:

- Diuretic response index (ml/mg) = 24-h urine output (ml)/daily dose of furosemide (mg)
- CrGR D_1 (μmol/mn) = [(SCrD_1 − SCrD_0) × 0.6 × weight) + (UCr × urine volume)]/time $D_0 - D_1$
- UrGR D_1 (μmol/mn) = [(SUr D_1 − SUr D_0) × 0.6 × weight) + (UUr × urine volume)]/time $D_0 - D_1$
- CrCl (ml/mn) = (UCr × 24-h urine volume)/(Scr × 1440)
- UrCl (ml/mn) = (UUr × 24-h urine volume)/(Sur × 1440)

where SCr: serum creatinine (μmol/l), UCr: urinary creatinine (mmol/l), SUr: serum urea (mmol/l), UUr: urinary urea (mmol/l), weight (kg), urine volume (l), time (min).

Early re-renal replacement therapy, defined as relapsed need for RRT within 15 days after D_0 was considered as the primary outcome variable. Duration of mechanical ventilation, vasopressor treatment and RRT, hospital and 3-month mortality, and the need of RRT after 3 months were also collected.

Statistical analyses

Statistical analyses were performed using the software R 3.1.0 (R Foundation for Statistical Computing, Vienna, Austria). We first performed a descriptive analysis by computing the frequencies and the percents for categorial data; means or medians, standard deviations, quartiles and extreme values for continuous data. We also checked for the normality of the continuous data distribution using the Shapiro–Wilk tests. The univariate analysis was performed using two-tailed Student's *t* test for continuous variables, Fisher and Chi-square tests for categorial variables or two-tailed Mann–Whitney–Wilcoxon test when appropriate. The areas under the receiver operator characteristic (ROC) curves and their confidence interval (CI) were calculated using the method of DeLong. The optimal threshold value was set for each ROC curve through the Youden index (corresponding to the maximum of the sum sensitivity + specificity). CIs for sensitivity (Se), specificity (Sp), positive predictive value (PPV) and negative predictive value (NPV) were calculated by bootstrap (2000 bootstrap samples). The most relevant variables including urine output, serum creatinine, creatinine clearance, urea and creatinine generation rate and 24-h urinary urea and creatinine obtained by logistic regression were included in multivariate models. The urea and creatinine kinetics in the two groups of patients were modeled using mixed models. A p value less than 0.05 was considered statistically significant.

Results

Population

During the study period, 377 consecutive patients were admitted in ICUs with AKI treated by RRT in which 179 survived (survival rate 47.4 %). After exclusion of 125 patients, 54 were eligible for analysis: 18 females and 36 males (flowchart, Fig. 1). Patient's characteristics, main comorbidities and reasons of ICU admission are summarized in Table 1. The RRT modalities were equally represented in the study population. At D_O, non-renal SOFA score has decreased reaching a median value of 3, and more than half of population was still on mechanical ventilation (Table 2). Median duration of RRT prior to the first attempt of weaning was 11 days.

Factors related to the success of weaning of RRT

Among the 54 patients, 26 attempts of weaning succeeded (S_+ group) while 28 failed (S_- group). Baseline characteristics of the two groups were comparable (Table 1). The proportion of CVVHDF was more important in S_+ group (50 vs 21 %) and conversely for IHDF, but differences were not statistically significant ($p = 0.07$). At the day of RRT cessation, the proportion of patients mechanically ventilated was similar between groups as were non-renal SOFA score and prior duration of RRT. Clinical parameters including mean arterial pressure, dose of vasopressors, mechanical ventilation and fluid balance did not differ between the two groups. However, a higher weight decrease was observed in the success group but without significant differences (Table 2).

At D_0, D_1 and D_2 urea and creatinine blood levels did not differ between the two groups (Table 3). At D_0, 24-h urine output tended to be higher in S_+ group (2300 vs 1950 ml, $p = 0.052$) but most of patients were treated by diuretics in both groups (73 vs 86 %). Diuretic response index was significantly higher in the S_+ group at D_0 with a significant decrease in furosemide dose the following two days as compared to S_- (Table 3). UrCl, CrCl, UUr and UCr levels were significantly higher in group S_+ at D_0, D_1 and D_2. UUr/UrGR and UCr/CrGR ratios were also significantly higher in S_+ group (Table 3). By multivariate analysis, 24-h UCr was the most powerful variable to predict the success of RRT weaning. At D_0, its area under the ROC curve (AUC and 95 % CI) was 0.76 [0.62–0.89] as compared to that of 24-h urine output: 0.66 [0.51–0.80] (Fig. 2). AUC of 24-h urinary creatinine was 0.86 [0.75–0.97] and 0.86 [0.75–0.97] at D_1 and D_2, respectively (Fig. 2). D_1 24-h creatininuria was a strong predictor of successful weaning with an odds ratio at 2.01 [1.27–3.18], $p = 0.003$, independently of age, weight and diuresis and showed Se, Sp, NPV and PPV at 75, 88, 82 and 84 %, respectively, when $\geq$5.2 mmol/24 h [3.1–6.3] (Table 4).

Patients' outcome

A significantly shorter ICU length of stay (13.5 vs 24.5 days) and a shorter duration of RRT (10.5 vs 18 days) were observed in the S_+ group (Table 1). Patients from the S_- group had resumed RRT 4 (3–11) days after the attempt of weaning. Twenty-one of the 28 patients of this group were weaned of RRT after a second attempt, whereas 7 needed more than two attempts (only one patient was re-dialyzed after the seventh day). Hospital survival was at 100 % in both groups, but 3 months later, 4 patients deceased in the S_- group and none in the S_+ group.

Discussion

In this study, we found that almost half of surviving AKI patients treated with RRT had their treatment stopped at the first attempt. We found also that the capability of

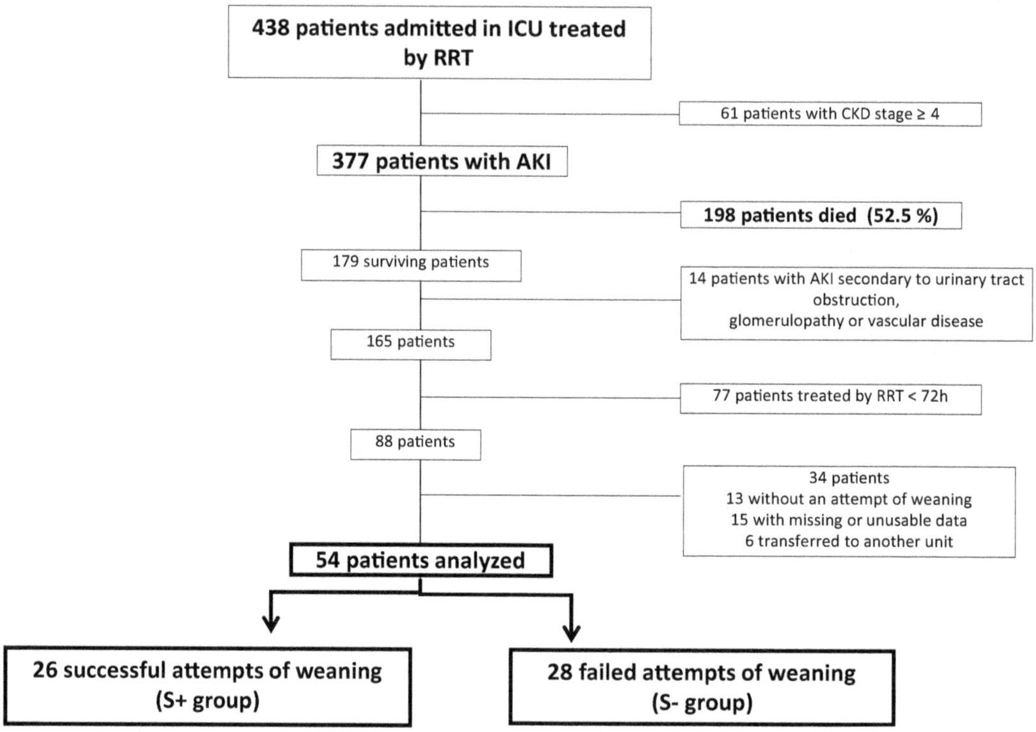

Fig. 1 Flowchart of the study population

24-h urine output to predict RRT weaning was significantly altered by the use of diuretics. In contrast, 24-h urinary creatinine appeared as a powerful marker of successful discontinuation of RRT even if patients received diuretics.

A large majority of ICU patients with AKI may recover sufficient kidney function to be independent of RRT. Indeed, all surviving patients we investigated herein recovered and were weaned from RRT even if several weaning attempts were necessary in some of them. Currently, practices of RRT weaning during AKI depend on every center policy and vary from a "wait and see" and a "go fast" attitudes. The "wait and see" attitude may prolong needlessly RRT and expose the patient to its hazardous effects without any benefits. Conversely a "go fast" attitude may lead to several unsuccessful attempts of weaning with the subsequent requirement of re-institution that is by itself harmful. Appropriate cessation of RRT is obviously critical regarding clinical and economic outcomes. There is, however, a paucity of data about how and when to stop RRT in critically ill patients with AKI, and identification of predictive factors of successful cessation of RRT is scarce. This lack of evidence contrasts with the field of mechanical ventilation, where many studies dealing with the process of weaning have been conducted [30]. We sought therefore to evaluate, in the present study, whether cessation of RRT can be early determined on the basis of clinical and routinely used parameters.

Previous studies have reported the association of the success of an interruption of RRT with age [23], previous renal function [24, 25], the prior length of RRT, the SOFA score at ICU admission [23, 26] and its decrease from admission to the day of attempt [23]. None of these parameters have been found determinant in the success of weaning in our study. Blood parameters including serum urea and creatinine and their kinetic were also helpless to guide the weaning of RRT in our population. Urine output was reported to be the most important predictor of successful discontinuation of RRT. In the trial by Bouman et al. [31], continuous RRT was discontinued when the urine output returned to and was stable at more than 60 ml/h, but there were no data about the optimal rate of urine output predicting the success of weaning. Wu et al. [23] evaluated retrospectively 94 patients weaned from IHDF for 5 or more days, of which 64 were free from RRT for $\geq$30 days. 24-h diuresis was at 1435 $\pm$ 1172 versus 598 $\pm$ 700 ml in the success and the re-dialysis groups, respectively, but diuretics were used in 36 % of patients of both groups. Oliguria (100 ml in 8 h) was independently associated with re-initiation of RRT [23]. The BEST Kidney investigators [24] found that urine

Table 1 Patients characteristics, comorbidities, causes of ICU admission, RRT modalities at initiation of therapy and outcome according to the success or failure of RRT weaning attempt

	All patients ($n = 54$)	S_+ group ($n = 26$)	S_- group ($n = 28$)	p
Age (years)	63.5 [56–72.8]	61.5 [56–71]	67.5 [56.5–75.5]	0.12
Male [n (%)]	36 (67)	20 (77)	16 (51)	0.09
SAPS II	55 [39–69]	54 [39.5–65.8]	56 [40.5–74.5]	0.36
SOFA	11 [8–13]	11 [8.3–13]	11 [8.5–13]	0.51
Previous eGFR (ml/min/1.73 m^2)	70 [45–92]	77 [45–96]	65 [46–89]	0.46
Main comorbidities [n (%)]				
Hypertension	28 (52)	12 (46)	16 (57)	0.16
Diabetes	19 (35)	8 (31)	11 (39)	
Cardiac failure	8 (15)	4 (15)	4 (14)	
Hemopathy	8 (15)	2 (8)	6 (21)	
Main reason for ICU admission [n (%)]				
Septic shock	28 (52)	11 (42)	17 (61)	0.15
Cardiogenic shock/cardiac arrest	10 (19)	5 (19)	5 (18)	
Post-surgical	6 (13)	3 (12)	3 (11)	
Other	10 (13)	5 (19)	5 (18)	
Initial RRT technique [n (%)]				
IHDF	19 (35)	6 (23)	13 (46)	0.07
CVVHDF	19 (35)	13 (50)	6 (21)	
SLEDD-f	16 (30)	7 (27)	9 (32)	
Length of ICU stay (days)	19 [8.3–42]	13.5 [8.3–32.3]	24.5 [17.5–42]	*0.012*
Duration of RRT (days)	15 [5–35]	10.5 [5–14.8]	18 [10–35]	*0.006*
In-hospitality mortality [n (%)]	0 (0)	0 (0)	0 (0)	–
3-month mortality [n (%)]	4 (7.4)	0 (0)	4 (14)	0.11
eGFR at 3 months (ml/min/1.73 m^2)	58 [49–92]	66 [68–92]	55 [49–77]	0.08

Italic values indicate significance of p value ($p < 0.05$)

Results are displayed in median [interquartile range] if quantitative variable; and number and percentage if categorial variable

p: differences between S_+ and S_- groups

SAPS II Simplified Acute Physiology Score, *SOFA* Sequential Organ Failure Assessment, *eGFR* estimated glomerular filtration rate, *IHDF* intermittent hemodiafiltration, *CVVHDF* continuous venovenous hemodiafiltration, *SLEDD-f* sustained low-efficiency daily dialysis-filtration, *RRT* renal replacement therapy

Table 2 Characteristics of the 54 analyzed patients at the first day (D_0) of weaning of RRT

	All patients ($n = 54$)	S_+ group ($n = 26$)	S_- group ($n = 28$)	p
Non-renal SOFA	3 [1–6]	3 [1–5]	3.5 [1–7]	0.21
Mean arterial pressure (mmHg)	83 [77–93]	85 [77–93]	83 [76–94]	0.33
Mechanical ventilation [n (%)]	30 (56 %)	15 (57.7 %)	15 (53.6 %)	0.42
Weight's variation (kg)	−2.5 [− 9.3; −2.3]	−6 [− 11; +1.5]	−1.5 [− 4.9; +4]	0.12
Prior RRT length (days)	11 [5–18]	10.5 [5–14.8]	11 [6.3–24.5]	0.46

Weight's variation means between admission and D0

p: differences between S_+ and S_- groups

SOFA Sequential Organ Failure Assessment

output of >400 ml/day without diuretics had the best operative characteristics with a Se, Sp, PPV and NPV of 0.47, 0.81, 0.81 and 0.77, respectively. However, diuretics administration negatively affected its predictive ability. They concluded that patients with more than 400 ml/day of urine without diuretics or more than 2300 ml/day with diuretics have more than 80 % of chance to successful discontinuation of RRT. Recently, an urine output >8.5 ml/kg/24 h was also found to predict IHDF weaning [32]. In our study, at the day of attempt, 24-h urine output failed to predict the success of weaning (2300 vs 1900 ml/24 h, $p = 0.052$) but a high proportion of our patients, more

Table 3 Serum urea, serum creatinine, 24-h urine output, diuretics, urea and creatinine clearance, 24-h urinary urea and creatinine, urea and creatinine generation rate, urinary urea/urea generation rate and urinary creatinine/creatinine generation rate ratios at the day (D_0) of attempt of weaning and the following two days (D_1, D_2)

	D0			D1			D2		
	S_+	S_-	*p*	S_+	S_-	*p*	S_+	S_-	*p*
S urea (mmol/l)	10 [7.6–13]	7.3 [6.2–12]	0.56	16 [12–24]	17 [14–21]	0.26	22 [15–37]	24 [20–27]	0.54
S creat (µmol/l)	105 [73–170]	83 [64–117]	0.36	177 [136–294]	158 [115–197]	0.15	227 [137–309]	218 [155–314]	0.65
24-h urinary output (l)	2.3 [1.5–3.5]	1.9 [1.0–2.5]	0.05	2.4 [1.8–3.7]	2.6 [1.7–3.3]	0.46	2.7 [2.1–3.4]	2.5 [1.7–3.3]	0.32
Use of furo [*n* (%)]	19 (73)	24 (86)	0.42	15 (59)	25 (89)	*0.009*	9 (35)	21 (75)	*0.005*
Dose of furo (mg/24 h)	470 [215–1000]	1000 [483–1000]	0.06	500 [125–970]	1000 [500–1000]	*0.01*	500 [250–1000]	1000 [500–1000]	*0.01*
Diuretic RI (ml/mg)	6 [2.9–15.4]	2.1 [1.1–6.4]	*0.02*	4.6 [3.6–26.4]	3.2 [1.9–4.3]	0.06	5.8 [2.5–8.2]	3.4 [2.6–5.8]	0.09
UrCl (ml/min)	15 [8–20]	6 [4–12]	*0.008*	12.5 [8–20]	7 [5–9]	*0.001*	13 [9–18]	6 [4–8]	*<0.001*
CrCl (ml/min)	31 [15–41]	18 [7–26]	*0.009*	31 [18–40]	15 [8–21]	*0.002*	31 [16–42]	13 [6–21]	*<0.001*
UUr (mmol/24 h)	187 [72–339]	85.9 [44–157]	*0.031*	357 [195–569]	147 [95–224]	*0.002*	592 [230–672]	236 [113–272]	*0.002*
UCr (mmol/24 h)	4.9 [2.5–6.4]	2.55 [0.7–3.9]	*0.002*	6.65 [5–8.8]	3.5 [1.6–4.4]	*<0.001*	8.1 [6–9.5]	4.4 [2.2–5.2]	*<0.001*
UrGR (µmol/min)				530 [331–722]	318 [254–442]	*0.02*	428 [257–681]	305 [232–393]	0.08
CrGR (µmol/min)				6.8 [5.8–9.9]	4.1 [2.9–5.2]	*<0.001*	6.2 [4.8–7.8]	4 [3.4–4.9]	*0.002*
UUr/UrGR (%)				51 [36–61]	36 [24–48]	*0.03*	71 [62–84]	48 [31–60]	*<0.001*
UCr/CrGR (%)				72 [53–85]	57 [40–67]	*0.047*	94 [77–100]	67 [44–82]	*<0.001*

Italic values indicate significance of *p* value ($p < 0.05$)

Results are displayed in median [interquartile range] if quantitative variable; and number and percentage if categorial variable

p: differences between S_+ and S_- groups

S urea serum urea, *S creat* serum creatinine, *Furo* furosemide, *Diuretic RI* diuretic response index, *Cl* clearance, *UUr* urinary urea, *UCr* urinary creatinine, *UrGR* urea generation rate, *CrGR* creatinine generation rate, *Ur* urea, *Cr* creatinine

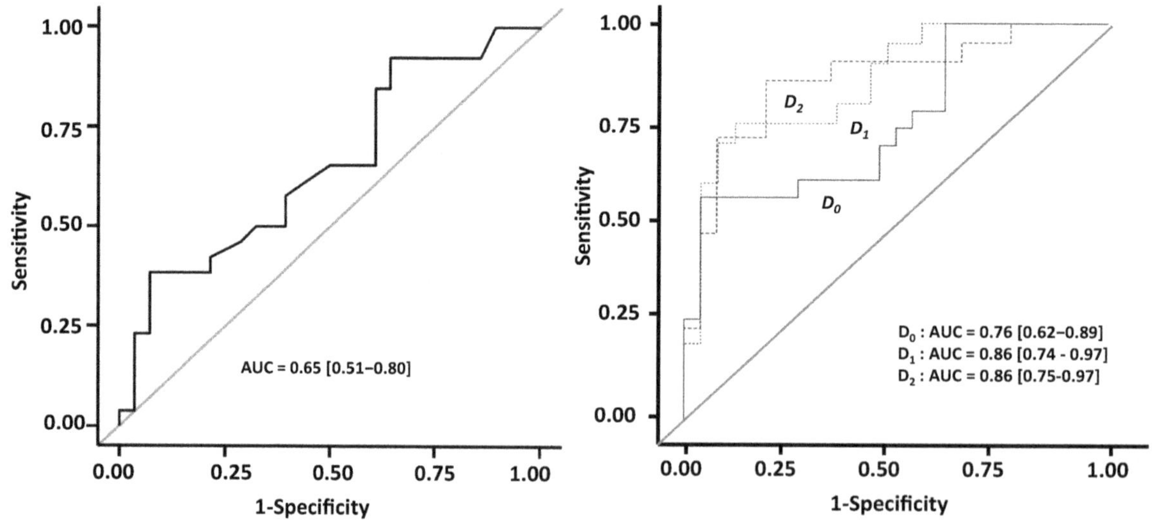

a 24-hour urinary output at D_0 **b** 24-hour urinary Creatinine

Fig. 2 Impact of 24-h urine output (**a**) and 24-h urinary creatinine at Days 0, 1 and 2 (**b**) on predictive ability of successful discontinuation of renal replacement therapy. The area under the receiver operating characteristic curve (AUC) is shown in each graph

than 75 %, received furosemide. We observed, however, that furosemide induced a significantly higher diuresis in the success group. Indeed, recent studies reported a significantly higher urine output in case of successful discontinuation of RRT even if diuretics were used [25, 26]. Nevertheless, the usefulness of diuresis to guide RRT

Table 4 Performances of 24-h urine output, 24-h urinary creatinine and urea to predict the success of an attempt of renal replacement therapy weaning

	Youden index [95 % CI]	Sensitivity % [95 % CI]	Specificity % [95 % CI]	PPV % [95 % CI]	NPV % [95 % CI]
D0 urinary output (ml/24 h)	2575 [1050–3075]	38.5 [19–58]	93 [82–100]	85 [61.5–100]	62 [55–71]
D0 urinary urea (mmol/24 h)	134 [56–322]	65 [48–83]	73 [58–88.5]	68 [53–84]	70 [58–84]
D0 urinary creatinine (mmol/24 h)	4.7 [0.85–5.1]	56.5 [35–74]	96 [88.5–100]	93 [78–100]	71 [62.5–81]
D1 urinary urea (mmol/24 h)	293 [196–363]	70 [50–90]	88 [76–100]	83 [67–100]	79 [68–92]
D1 urinary creatinine (mmol/24 h)	5.15 [3.01–6.3]	75 [55–90]	88 [72–100]	84 [68–100]	82 [70–93]
D2 urinary urea (mmol/24 h)	318 [292–591]	71 [52–90]	85 [69–96]	80 [64–94]	79 [68–92]
D2 urinary creatinine (mmol/24 h)	5.56 [4.67–6.57]	86 [71–100]	81 [65–96]	78 [65–94]	88 [75–100]

PPV positive predictive value, *NPV* negative predictive value, *CI* confidence interval

weaning is clearly reduced since diuretics often may be necessary to correct or avoid a fluid overload [33]. We sought then to determine predictive factors that would be independent of diuretics like urinary creatinine and urea. Urea and creatinine collected in urine during 24-h were significantly higher at the day of attempt of RRT weaning and the following 2 days (with a gradual increase) in the success group. By multivariate analysis, 24-h creatininuria was the most powerful predictor of success of weaning. A level ≥5.2 mmol/24 h had a Sp, Se, NPV and PPV of 75, 88, 82 and 84 %, respectively. Differences of creatinine urinary level observed between the two groups should not be related to muscle mass, as they were independent of patient's age and weight. Also, these differences may not be explained by differences of urea or creatinine generation rate since ratios of urinary levels to generation rates were significantly higher in the success group. Of note, clearance of creatinine (and urea) was significantly higher in the S_+ group, as reported by Fröhlich et al. [25]. In a recent study, Aniort and colleagues [32] sought also to identify predictive factors of intermittent hemodialysis weaning by investigating retrospectively 67 AKI patients. They found that daily urinary urea was the best weaning marker with an optimal threshold >1.35 mmol/kg/24 h (AUC 0.96, 95 % CI 0.93–0.99) as compared to 24-h urine output. In the contrary of our findings, they did not observe any differences in urinary creatinine between weaned and unweaned patients. However, almost 1/3 of their patients (22/67) have a baseline GFR < 30 ml/mn and expectedly 26/67 patients did not recovered renal function. Our population included exclusively patients with a baseline GFR ≥ 60 ml/mn explaining, at least for a part, these discordant results.

RRT modalities (continuous or intermittent) may affect renal recovery and dialysis dependence, but their effects remain a matter of debate. A systematic review of the literature including mainly observational studies concluded that patients who received intermittent RRT had a significant increased risk of dialysis dependency as compared to those who received continuous RRT [34]. We observed indeed a higher proportion of continuous therapies with a higher weight decrease in the success group. However, differences were not significant and our RRT strategy was based on hemodynamic precluding any conclusions from our study. It is noteworthy that two recent studies failed to demonstrate any impact of RRT modalities on renal recovery [35, 36].

Patients who require RRT for AKI have a mortality exceeding 60 %, but most patients that recover function enough to be free from RRT survive to hospital discharge [37]. In the study of BEST Kidney investigators [24], patients whose CRRT was successfully stopped had better outcome than those who needed to be re-treated (mortality: 28.5 vs 42.7 %, p = <0.0001, respectively). In our study, the patients who were weaned from RRT after a second or more attempt had a significantly higher length of RRT and of ICU stay as compared to patients successfully weaned. Moreover, we observed that 4/28 patients of the failed group deceased 3 months later and none in the success group. Whether failure of discontinuation of RRT is just a marker of severity of disease or is harmful by itself remains questioned [38].

This study has several limitations. First, it was a retrospective and bi-center cohort study. Second, the weaning of RRT was not based on standardized criteria but decided by the attending physician who obviously followed general rules. Third, daily urinary creatinine requires 24-h urine collection, a procedure routinely performed with accuracy in ICUs. The measurement of urinary creatinine in a shorter time period or as spot urine concentration would be more easily feasible but may induce less accuracy. Nevertheless, the use of urinary creatinine as a marker of RRT cessation should be internally and externally validated to be used in routine practice. Last, we defined the attempt of weaning as a discontinuation of RRT during 72 h and estimated a success if discontinuation lasted more than 15 days. Various definitions have been used including an interruption of RRT during at least 5 days [23], but we thought that this duration may be too short regarding the severity of our patients. Also, considering RRT weaned after 7 days of interruption, as chosen by others [24, 25] has revealed insufficient. In the BEST Kidney cohort, for example, 15 patients considered as RRT-free were re-treated by CRRT before discharged from the ICU [24]. Indeed, Wu et al. [23] observed that an average of 10.1 ± 6.1 days lasted before re-dialysis if the attempt of weaning RRT failed.

Conclusions

In summary, the usefulness of 24-h urine output to predict the success of RRT weaning in AKI patients treated by diuretics may be significantly altered. Our study showed that 24-h urinary creatinine, in spite of diuretic use, is an independent and performing predictive factor of successful RRT weaning. A 24-h urinary creatinine $\geq$5.2 mmol indicates that RRT will be successfully stopped in 84 % of cases. Larger and prospective studies are needed to confirm our observations and to test a strategy of RRT weaning based on urine output, urinary creatinine and urea, and severity scores.

Abbreviations

AKI: acute kidney injury; AUC: area under the curve; CI: confidence interval; CrCl: creatinine clearance; CrGR: creatinine generation rate; CVVHDF: continuous venovenous hemodiafiltration; D0, D1, D2: day of renal replacement therapy weaning attempt and the following 2 days; eGFR: estimated glomerular filtration rate; ICU: intensive care unit; IHDF: intermittent hemodiafiltration; NPV: negative predictive value; OR: odds ratio; PPV: positive predictive value; ROC: receiver operating characteristic; RRT: renal replacement therapy; SAPS: Simplified Acute Physiology Score; Se: sensitivity; SLEDD-f: sustained low-efficiency daily dialysis-filtration; SOFA: Sequential Organ Failure Assessment; Sp: specificity; UCr: 24-h diuresis urinary creatinine; UrCl: urea clearance; UrGR: urea generation rate; UUr: 24-h diuresis urinary urea.

Authors' contributions

NV, VB and KK designed the study; NK did the statistical analysis; NV, VB and KK interpreted the data and wrote the manuscript; and NK, DD, NB, LP, AB, RL and OJ contributed to interpretation of data. All authors read and approved the final manuscript.

Author details

[1] Department of Intensive Care Medicine, Lapeyronie University Hospital, 371, Avenue du Doyen G. Giraud, 34295 Montpellier, France. [2] Department of Biochemistry, Lapeyronie University Hospital, Montpellier, France. [3] PhyMedExp, INSERM U1046, CNRS UMR 9214, University of Montpellier, Montpellier, France.

Acknowledgements

None.

Competing interests

The authors declare that they have no competing interests.

References

1. Uchino S, Kellum JA, Bellomo R, Doig GS, Morimatsu H, Morgera S, Schetz M, Tan I, Bouman C, Macedo E, Gibney N, Tolwani A, Ronco C. Acute renal failure in critically ill patients: a multinational, multicenter study. JAMA. 2005;294:813–8.
2. Hoste EA, Schurgers M. Epidemiology of acute kidney injury: how big is the problem? Crit Care Med. 2008;36(Suppl 4):146–51.
3. Metnitz PG, Krenn CG, Steltzer H, Lang T, Ploder J, Lenz K, Le Gall JR, Druml W. Effect of acute renal failure requiring renal replacement therapy on outcome in critically ill patients. Crit Care Med. 2002;30:2051–8.
4. Andrikos E, Tseke P, Balafa O, Cruz DN, Tsinta A, Androulaki M, Pappas M, Ronco C. Epidemiology of acute renal failure in ICUs: a multi-center prospective study. Blood Purif. 2009;28:239–44.
5. Mehta RL, Pascual MT, Soroko S, Savage BR, Himmelfarb J, Ikizler TA, Paganini EP, Chertow GM. Spectrum of acute renal failure in the intensive care unit: the PICARD experience. Kidney Int. 2004;66:1613–21.
6. Ympa YP, Sakr Y, Reinhart K, Vincent JL. Has mortality from acute renal failure decreased? A systematic review of the literature. Am J Med. 2005;118:827–32.
7. Coca SG. Long-term outcomes of acute kidney injury. Curr Opin Nephrol Hypertens. 2010;19:266–72.
8. Lafrance JP, Miller DR. Acute kidney injury associates with increased long-term mortality. J Am Soc Nephrol. 2010;21:345–52.
9. Goldberg R, Dennen P. Long-term outcomes of acute kidney injury. Adv Chronic Kidney Dis. 2008;15:297–307.
10. Wald R, Quinn RR, Luo J, Li P, Scales DC, Mamdani MM, Ray JG. Chronic dialysis and death among survivors of acute kidney injury requiring dialysis. JAMA. 2009;302:1179–85.
11. Bagshaw SM, Mortis G, Godinez-Luna T, Doig CJ, Laupland KB. Renal recovery after severe acute renal failure. Int J Artif Organs. 2006;29:1023–30.
12. Uchino S, Bellomo R, Kellum JA, Morimatsu H, Morgera S, Schetz MR, Tan I, Bouman C, Macedo E, Gibney N, Tolwani A, Oudemans-Van Straaten HM, Ronco C. Patient and kidney survival by dialysis modality in critically ill patients with acute kidney injury. Int J Artif Organs. 2007;30:281–92.
13. Van Berendoncks AM, Elseviers MM, Lins RL. Outcome of acute kidney injury with different treatment options: long-term follow-up. Clin J Am Soc Nephrol. 2010;5:1755–62.
14. Delannoy B, Floccard B, Thiolliere F, Kaaki M, Badet M, Rosselli S, Ber CE, Saez A, Flandreau G, Guérin C. Six-month outcome in acute kidney injury requiring renal replacement therapy in the ICU: a multicentre prospective study. Intensive Care Med. 2009;35:1907–15.
15. Palevsky PM, Baldwin I, Davenport A, Goldstein S, Paganini E. Renal replacement therapy and the kidney: minimizing the impact of renal replacement therapy on recovery of acute renal failure. Curr Opin Crit Care. 2005;11:548–54.
16. Elseviers MM, Lins RL, Van der Niepen P, Hoste E, Malbrain ML, Damas P, Devriendt J. Renal replacement therapy is an independent risk factor for mortality in critically ill patients with acute kidney injury. Crit Care. 2010;14:R221.
17. Clec'h C, Darmon M, Lautrette A, Chemouni F, Azoulay E, Schwebel C, Dumenil AS, Garrouste-Orgeas M, Goldgran-Toledano D, Cohen Y, Timsit JF. Efficacy of renal replacement therapy in critically ill patients: a propensity analysis. Crit Care. 2012;16:R236.
18. Bagshaw SM, Uchino S, Kellum JA, Morimatsu H, Morgera S, Schetz M, Tan I, Bouman C, Macedo E, Gibney N, Tolwani A, Oudemans-van Straaten HM, Ronco C, Bellomo R. Association between renal replacement therapy in critically ill patients with severe acute kidney injury and mortality. J Crit Care. 2013;28:1011–8.
19. Schiffl H. Renal recovery after severe acute renal injury. Eur J Med Res. 2008;13:552–6.
20. Solez K, Morel-Maroger L, Sraer JD. The morphology of "acute tubular necrosis" in man: analysis of 57 renal biopsies and a comparison with the glycerol model. Medicine (Baltimore). 1979;58:362–76.
21. Liu KD, Brakeman PR. Renal repair and recovery. Crit Care Med. 2008;36(Suppl 4):187–92.
22. Kidney Disease Improving Global Outcomes: Clinical practice guidelines for acute kidney injury. http://www.kdigo.org/clinical_practice_guidelines/pdf/KDIGO%20AKI%20Guideline.pdf (2012). Accessed 14 April 2016.
23. Wu VC, Ko WJ, Chang HW, Chen YW, Lin YF, Shiao CC, Chen YM, Chen YS, Tsai PR, Hu FC, Wang JY, Lin YH, Wu KD. Risk factors of early redialysis after

weaning from postoperative acute renal replacement therapy. Intensive Care Med. 2008;34:101–8.

24. Uchino S, Bellomo R, Morimatsu H, Morgera S, Schetz M, Tan I, Bouman C, Macedo E, Gibney N, Tolwani A, Straaten HO, Ronco C, Kellum JA. Discontinuation of continuous renal replacement therapy: a post hoc analysis of a prospective multicenter observational study. Crit Care Med. 2009;37:2576–82.
25. Fröhlich S, Donnelly A, Solymos O, Conlon N. Use of 2-hour creatinine clearance to guide cessation of continuous renal replacement therapy. J Crit Care. 2012;27:744.
26. Heise D, Gries D, Moerer O, Bleckmann A, Quintel M. Predicting restoration of kidney function during CRRT-free intervals. J Cardiothorac Surg. 2012;7:6.
27. Klouche K, Amigues L, Serveaux-Delous M, Machado S, Delabre JP, Laydet E, Mauran P, Jonquet O, Canaud B. Implementing on-line hemodiafiltration as a renal replacement therapy for ICU acute renal failure: a single-center report of feasibility, safety and hemodynamic tolerance over a seven-year period. Blood Purif. 2012;34:10–7.
28. VA/NIH Acute Renal Failure Trial Network, Palevsky PM, Zhang JH, O'Connor TZ, Chertow GM, Crowley ST, Choudhury D, Finkel K, Kellum JA, Paganini E, Schein RM, Smith MW, Swanson KM, Thompson BT, Vijayan A, Watnick S, Star RA, Peduzzi P. Intensity of renal support in critically ill patients with acute kidney injury. N Engl J Med. 2008;359:7–20.
29. Levey AS, Stevens LA, Schmid CH, Zhang YL, Castro AF III, Feldman HI, Kusek JW, Eggers P, Van Lente F, Greene T, Coresh J. A new equation to estimate glomerular filtration rate. Ann Intern Med. 2009;150:604–12.
30. Esteban A, Frutos F, Tobin MJ, Alía I, Solsona JF, Valverdú I, Fernández R, de la Cal MA, Benito S, Tomás R, Carriedo D, Macías S, Blanco J, for the Spanish Lung Failure Collaborative Group. A comparison of four methods of weaning patients from mechanical ventilation. N Engl J Med. 1995;332:345–50.
31. Bouman CS, Oudemans-Van Straaten HM, Tijssen JG, Zandstra DF, Kesecioglu J. Effects of early high-volume continuous venovenous hemofiltration on survival and recovery of renal function in intensive care patients with acute renal failure: a prospective, randomized trial. Crit Care Med. 2002;30:2205–11.
32. Aniort J, Ait Hssain A, Pereira B, Coupez E, Pioche PA, Leroy C, Heng AE, Souweine B, Lautrette A. Daily urinary urea excretion to guide intermittent hemodialysis weaning in critically ill patients. Crit Care. 2016;20:43.
33. Bouchard J, Soroko SB, Chertow GM, et al. Fluid accumulation, survival and recovery of kidney function in critically ill patients with acute kidney injury. Kidney Int. 2009;76:422–7.
34. Antoine G, Schneider AG, RinaldoBellomo R, Sean M, Bagshaw SM, Neil J, Glassford NJ, Lo S, Jun M, Cass A, Gallagher M. Choice of renal replacement therapy modality and dialysis dependence after acute kidney injury: a systematic review and meta-analysis. Intensive Care Med. 2013;39:987–97.
35. Truche AS, Darmon M, Bailly S, et al. Continuous renal replacement therapy versus intermittent hemodialysis in intensive care patients: impact on mortality and renal recovery. Intensive Care Med. 2016. doi:10.1007/s00134-016-4404-6.
36. Liang KV, Sileanu FE, Clermont G, Murugan R, Pike F, Palevsky PM, Kellum JA. Modality of RRT and recovery of kidney function after AKI in patients surviving to hospital discharge. Clin J Am Soc Nephrol. 2016;11:30–8.
37. Uchino S. The epidemiology of acute renal failure in the world. Curr Opin Crit Care. 2006;12:538–43.
38. Bell M, Granath F, Schön S, Ekbom A, Martling CR. Continuous renal replacement therapy is associated with less chronic renal failure than intermittent haemodialysis after acute renal failure. Intensive Care Med. 2007;33:773–80.

22

Outcome and features of acute kidney injury complicating hypoxic hepatitis at the medical intensive care unit

Andreas Drolz[1,2*], Thomas Horvatits[1,2], Kevin Roedl[1,2], Karoline Rutter[1,2], Katharina Staufer[1,3], Dominik G. Haider[4,5], Christian Zauner[1], Gottfried Heinz[6], Peter Schellongowski[7], Stefan Kluge[2], Michael Trauner[1] and Valentin Fuhrmann[1,2]

Abstract

Background: Hypoxic hepatitis (HH) is a frequent and potentially life-threatening event typically occurring in critically ill patients as a consequence of hemodynamic impairment. While acute kidney injury (AKI) has been well described in patients with acute liver failure, incidence and outcome of AKI accompanying HH are unclear. The aim of this study was to assess incidence, clinical implications and outcome of AKI and renal replacement therapy (RRT) in critically ill patients with HH.

Methods: A total of 1948 consecutive critically ill admissions were studied at the Medical University of Vienna. Laboratory and clinical parameters as well as the presence of HH and AKI were assessed on a daily basis. Outcome, renal recovery and length of stay were assessed and documented, and patients were followed for 1 year.

Results: A total of 295 admissions (15 %) developed HH. Main precipitators were cardiogenic (44 %) and septic shock (36 %). Occurrence of HH was significantly associated with AKI [OR 4.50 (95 % CI 3.30–6.12)] and necessity of renal replacement therapy [RRT; OR 3.36 (95 % CI 2.58–4.37)], $p < 0.001$ for both. Two hundred forty admissions with HH (81 %) developed AKI, 159 of whom (66 %) had AKI stage 3. Both HH and AKI were significantly linked to mortality. AKI stage 3, international normalized ratio (INR, during HH) and the presence of septic shock were identified as independent predictors of 28-day mortality in admissions with HH, whereas RRT was identified as an independent protective factor. There was a synergistic effect of HH and AKI on length of stay at the ICU. Of all HH survivors treated with RRT, 71 % showed renal recovery during follow-up.

Conclusion: HH is frequently complicated by occurrence of AKI. Severity of HH, AKI stage and the presence of septic shock seem to contribute to poor outcome in these patients. Initiation of RRT in HH with AKI may enable renal recovery and should not be withheld in medical ICU patients.

Keywords: Hypoxic hepatitis, Acute kidney injury, Renal replacement therapy, Mortality

Background

Hypoxic hepatitis (HH) is a life-threatening complication accompanying states of oxygen depletion in critically ill patients at the intensive care unit (ICU) [1–5]. Incidence rates of approximately 10 % have been reported in critically ill patients at the medical ICU [3, 4, 6, 7], and mortality rate in these patients was more than 50 % [1, 4, 5]. Several risk factors for mortality in HH patients have been identified and include the presence of septic shock, sequential organ failure assessment (SOFA) score >10, international normalized ratio (INR) >2, jaundice and necessity of vasopressor therapy [1, 4, 5, 8].

Acute kidney injury (AKI) is a frequent complication in critical illness. As a consequence of various definitions being used over the last decades [9], incidence rates

*Correspondence: a.drolz@uke.de
[2] Department of Intensive Care Medicine, University Medical Center, Hamburg-Eppendorf, Martinistraße 52, 20246 Hamburg, Germany
Full list of author information is available at the end of the article

reported in the literature vary considerably ranging from 13 to 78 % in critically ill patients [10–15].

Yet, little is known about the frequency and features of acute kidney injury (AKI) in HH. Interestingly, some recommendations on the treatment of AKI in critically ill patients suggest not using renal replacement therapy (RRT) in patients with liver failure [9]. These recommendations are based on data obtained from cirrhotic patients with AKI and hepatorenal syndrome, respectively, and are therefore not necessarily applicable to patients with other kinds of liver failure such as HH. In contrast, Kidney Disease: Improving Global Outcomes (KDIGO) recommendations on AKI do not make a statement on patients with liver failure [16]. AKI in acute hepatic injury like HH may differ considerably from kidney injury accompanying chronic hepatic impairment or acute-on-chronic liver failure. This assumption is supported by the gradual recovery of renal function in all patients with AKI following acetaminophen-induced acute liver failure [17], thereby suggesting that renal failure in acute hepatic injury and acute liver failure is frequently reversible. However, to our knowledge, features and outcomes of AKI accompanying HH with respect to RRT have not been studied so far.

The aim of this study was to examine the prevalence, outcomes and renal recovery of AKI in patients with HH, the most frequent cause of severe acute hepatic impairment at the ICU. Furthermore, we aimed to assess the role of RRT in patients with HH and AKI.

Methods

This study is based on a retrospective analysis of prospectively documented data including patient long-term follow-up between January 2005 and December 2011. All patients admitted consecutively to three medical ICUs at the Medical University Vienna were studied. This study was approved by the ethics committee of the Medical University Vienna, which waived the need for informed consent due to the observational character of this study.

On admission, simplified acute physiology score II (SAPS II) [18], SOFA [19], infections, organ dysfunctions (including need for vasopressor support, mechanical ventilation, RRT) and precipitating event for development of HH were documented. Routine laboratory analysis was conducted and documented on a daily basis.

All patients were screened on a daily basis for the presence of AKI defined by urine output and serum creatinine according to the criteria defined below [16], and patients were stratified according to the highest AKI stage observed during the ICU stay. RRT was started in patients with severe metabolic derangement, anuria irresponsive to fluids, hyperkalemia and/or uremic complications, as previously published [20]. In patients requiring RRT, SOFA score was calculated daily for the first 3 days following initiation of RRT. Type, duration and time of initiation of RRT were documented. Additionally, anticoagulation during RRT was documented. Recovery of renal function was assessed during follow-up.

HH was diagnosed according to the following well-established criteria [1, 3]: (a) a sharp but transient elevation of aminotransferase levels to at least 20-fold the upper limit of normal; (b) a setting of cardio-circulatory or respiratory failure; (c) exclusion of other potential causes of liver cell necrosis (viral or drug-induced hepatitis). If these criteria were met, a histologic confirmation was not required for the diagnosis. All patients were screened for the presence of HH by daily laboratory and clinical assessment starting from ICU admission until ICU discharge.

Cardiogenic shock was diagnosed in patients presenting with (a) systolic blood pressure <90 mmHg without the use of inotropes or vasopressors or requirement for vasopressors, (b) signs of decreased cardiac output (low cardiac output measured by any method, low mixed or central venous oxygen saturation), (c) clinical, echocardiographic or radiological signs of pulmonary congestion, (d) absence of hypovolemia and (e) signs of organ malperfusion (e.g., oliguria, cyanosis, lactate, change in mental status) [21, 22]. If available, noninvasive and invasive measurements of hemodynamics were considered for diagnosis, although these methods were not a prerequisite for diagnosis of cardiogenic shock [23, 24].

Septic shock was defined according to the recommendations of the surviving sepsis campaign [25].

Criteria for acute kidney injury were calculated according to the KDIGO clinical practice guideline for acute kidney injury based on serum creatinine and urinary output [16]. The value for baseline creatinine was obtained from the most recently measured creatinine concentration in the year prior to the ICU stay excluding the 7 days directly preceding ICU admission and considered to be representative of the baseline kidney function according to the judgment of the treating physician. If this baseline value was not available, the minimum serum creatinine at the time of admission to the ICU was used as baseline [10, 16, 26]. Renal recovery on hospital discharge was defined as independence from RRT [27].

ICU mortality, 28-day mortality and 1-year mortality were assessed on site or by contacting the patient or attending physician, respectively.

Statistical analysis

SPSS Statistics 20 (IBM, Armonk, NY, USA) was used for statistical analysis. Continuous variables are expressed as median and interquartile range (IQR 25–75 %), binary variables as number (%). Univariate comparisons of continuous variables between groups were carried out using Mann–Whitney U test. Chi-square analysis and Fisher's exact tests, as appropriate, were used to compare categorical variables. Risk factors for AKI in HH were assessed via ordinal logistic regression modeling.

A multivariate Cox regression model was developed in order to assess the impact of AKI and RRT, respectively, on 28-day survival in HH patients after adjustment for predefined confounders. Odds ratios (ORs) and hazard ratios (HRs) are presented with 95 % confidence intervals (95 % CI). A p value of less than 0.5 was considered statistically significant.

Results

Patients' characteristics

A total of 1948 admissions were studied at three medical ICUs. Two hundred ninety-five admissions developed HH (15 %) during their stay at the ICU. In the vast majority ($n = 229$, 78 %), HH occurred within 24 h from ICU admission; 253 (86 %) developed HH within 48 h. Median time from ICU admission to occurrence of HH was 0 (IQR 0–1) days. Main precipitants for occurrence of HH were cardiogenic shock ($n = 130$; 44 %), septic shock ($n = 106$; 36 %), hemorrhagic shock ($n = 8$; 3 %) and mixed cardiogenic/septic shock ($n = 3$; 1 %). A detailed list of underlying conditions associated with occurrence of HH is shown in Additional file 1: Table S1. Two hundred forty-two admissions (12 %) had underlying liver cirrhosis. Clinical and laboratory features of 295 admissions with HH are illustrated in Table 1.

Table 1 Characteristics of 295 admissions with hypoxic hepatitis

Parameter	
Number of patients	295
Admission parameters	
Age (years), median (IQR)	63 (51–72)
Females, *n* (%)	94 (32 %)
SAPS II, median (IQR)	62 (45–79)
SOFA, median (IQR)	11 (8–15)
Heart rate (bpm), median (IQR)	81 (65–104)
MAP (mmHg), median (IQR)	68 (57–82)
Respiratory rate (breaths/min), median (IQR)	20 (16–25)
Body temperature (°C), median (IQR)	36.5 (35.5–37.5)
pH, median (IQR)	7.30 (7.20–7.40)
AST (IU/l), median (IQR)	366 (73–1265)
ALT (IU/l), median (IQR)	139 (39–706)
LDH (IU/l), median (IQR)	599 (360–1523)
INR, median (IQR)	1.4 (1.2–1.9)
Peak values	
AST (IU/l), median (IQR)	2457 (1168–5605)
ALT (IU/l), median (IQR)	1151 (534–2620)
LDH (IU/l), median (IQR)	2439 (1334–4999)
INR, median (IQR)	1.8 (1.4–2.7)
Underlying condition	
Cardiogenic shock, *n* (%)	130 (44 %)
Septic shock, *n* (%)	106 (36 %)
Mixed septic/cardiogenic shock, *n* (%)	3 (1 %)
Hemorrhagic shock, *n* (%)	8 (3 %)
Therapy	
Mechanical ventilation, *n* (%)	225 (76 %)
Vasopressor therapy, *n* (%)	231 (86 %)
Renal replacement therapy, *n* (%)	122 (41 %)
Outcome parameters	
28-day mortality, *n* (%)	170 (58 %)
ICU-LOS (days), median (IQR)	7 (2–14)

SAPS II simplified acute physiology score, *SOFA* sequential organ failure assessment, *MAP* mean arterial pressure, *AST* aspartate aminotransferase, *ALT* alanine aminotransferase, *LDH* lactate dehydrogenase, *ICU-LOS* length of stay at the ICU, *IQR* interquartile range

Acute kidney injury and renal replacement therapy

Of all 1948 admissions studied during the observation period, 55 % (1054 admissions) developed AKI within 48 h after ICU admission. AKI stages 1, 2 and 3 occurred in 128 (7 %), 345 (18 %) and 581 (30 %) admissions to the ICU, respectively. Of those admissions with AKI stage 3, 70 % ($n = 409$) received RRT for a median of 4 (2–10) days. In total, 409 admissions (21 %) underwent RRT during their ICU stay with the median time from admission to initiation of RRT being 1 (IQR 0–3) day. A list of underlying reasons for initiation of RRT stratified according to the presence of HH is shown in Additional file 1: Table S2.

The distribution of AKI stages in admissions with and without HH is illustrated in Fig. 1. HH was significantly associated with AKI and RRT in the univariate analysis [OR 4.50 (95 % CI 3.30–6.12)] and [OR 3.36 (95 % CI 2.58–4.37); $p < 0.0001$ for both]. Two hundred forty admissions with HH (81 %) developed AKI, 159 of whom (66 %) had AKI stage 3. Risk factors for occurrence of AKI in HH are illustrated in Table 2.

In admissions who developed HH, the percentage receiving RRT was significantly higher compared to critically ill admissions without HH (41 vs. 17 %, $p < 0.001$). This relationship is illustrated in a Cox-adjusted hazard plot (Additional file 2: Figure S1; adjusted for age, sex and SOFA score). Of all admissions with HH receiving renal support, 96 (79 %) had continuous RRT, 11 (9 %) underwent intermittent RRT, and 15 (12 %) had both continuous and intermittent types of RRT during their stay at the ICU.

Heparin ($n = 80$, 66 %) and citrate ($n = 26$, 21 %) were the most frequently used substances for anticoagulation. Epoprostenol and danaparoid were used in 5 (4 %) patients and 1 (1 %) patient, respectively. In 10 (8 %)

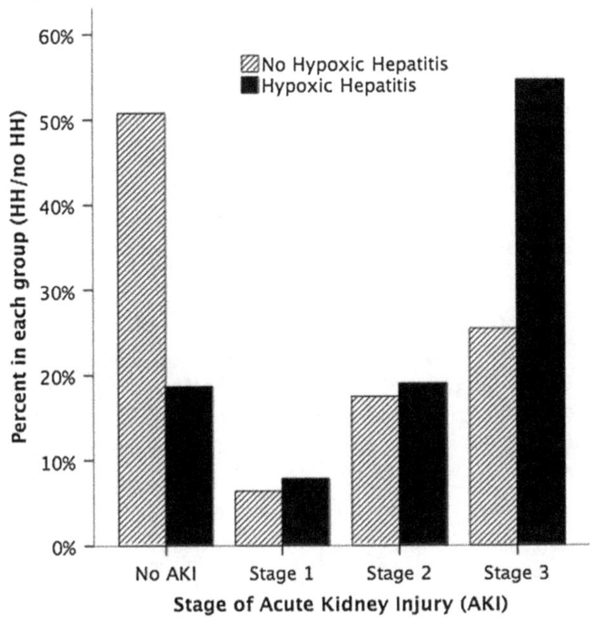

Fig. 1 Distribution of AKI stages (KDIGO) in patients with and without hypoxic hepatitis. *HH* hypoxic hepatitis, *AKI* acute kidney injury—stratified according to the KDIGO criteria [16]

admissions, the substance used for anticoagulation with RRT was changed during the stay at the ICU.

Mortality in HH accompanied by AKI

Both HH and AKI were significantly linked to mortality as illustrated in Cox-adjusted survival curves (Fig. 2, adjusted for age, sex and SOFA score). The worst outcomes, though, were observed in patients with the presence of HH and AKI (28-day mortality 64 %).

AKI stage 3, peak INR (within 48 h after occurrence of HH) and the presence of septic shock were identified as independent predictors of 28-day mortality in admissions with HH by multivariate Cox regression (Table 3). After adjustment for these factors, RRT was identified as an independent protective factor regarding 28-day mortality (Table 3).

In HH patients requiring RRT, SOFA scores and number of organs failing during the first 3 days of RRT were associated with 28-day mortality (Additional file 1: Table S3). Persisting failure of $\geq$5 organs and/or SOFA scores above 20 for more than 48 h despite initiation of RRT was associated with a 100 % mortality rate.

Time from onset of AKI to initiation of RRT did not differ significantly between 28-day survivors and non-survivors [2 (0–7) days vs. 1 (0–3) days, $p = 0.164$]. No difference in 28-day mortality was observed between the two most frequently used methods of anticoagulation [heparin ($n = 64$, 80 %) vs. citrate ($n = 19$, 73 %); $p = 0.457$]. Similarly, incidence of bleeding complications did not differ between HH patients with heparin and citrate anticoagulation [$n = 11$ (14 %) vs. $n = 3$ (12 %), $p = 0.772$].

In the vast majority ($n = 218$, 91 %) of HH patients with AKI, AKI occurred within 48 h prior to or after HH. RRT was initiated after occurrence of HH in 54 patients (44 %), on the same day of HH in 32 patients (26 %), prior to HH in 36 patients (30 %).

Length of stay at the ICU in HH and AKI

Overall length of stay (LOS) at the ICU did not differ significantly between HH admissions with and without AKI [6 (IQR 2–13) days vs. 8 (IQR 3–14) days; $p = 0.295$], which was attributable to the high mortality rate in AKI accompanying HH. However, in ICU survivors, HH and AKI significantly affected ICU-LOS (Additional file 3: Figure S2). Median LOS in ICU survivors was 3 (2–8) days in admissions without HH or AKI, 9 (4–14) days HH without AKI, 5 (2–12) days in AKI without HH and 8 (5–20) days in admissions with both HH and AKI. Additionally, compared to admissions without HH and RRT, respectively, ICU-LOS more than doubled when HH was accompanied by need for RRT [4 (IQR 2–10) days vs. 10 (IQR 3–20) days], $p < 0.0001$.

Renal recovery and long-term outcomes

Twenty-four admissions with HH and RRT survived their stay at the ICU. The ICU survival rate was significantly lower compared to admissions with RRT but without HH (20 % in patients with HH compared to 64 % in non-HH admissions, $p < 0.001$). Seventeen out of the 24 admissions (71 %) showed recovery of renal function at the time of hospital discharge. There was a trend for lower 1-year mortality in HH admissions with RRT and recovery of renal function compared to those without renal recovery [4 (24 %) vs. 4 (57 %), $p = 0.167$].

In admissions requiring RRT who survived the ICU stay ($n = 207$, 51 %), 1-year mortality rate did not differ significantly between those who had and who had not experienced HH [8 (33 %) vs. 68 (37 %), $p = 0.715$].

Discussion

This is the first study that assesses features and outcomes of AKI and RRT in patients with HH compared to a large control group of critically ill patients. Our results demonstrate that HH is frequently accompanied by AKI. Most of the HH patients developed AKI stage 3. Importantly, occurrence of AKI was associated with increased mortality and length of stay in patients with HH.

Our study demonstrates that AKI is a frequent complication in critically ill patients associated with poor outcome [10–14]. In our total cohort, incidence rate of

Table 2 Univariate ordinal logistic regression model linking demographic, physiological and laboratory parameters to AKI in HH

Parameter	Overall	AKI Stage				*p* value*
	n = 295	0 (*n* = 55)	1 (*n* = 23)	2 (*n* = 56)	3 (*n* = 161)	
Baseline characteristics						
Age, years (IQR)	63 (51–72)	60 (45–71)	62 (50–77)	65 (54–71)	63 (52–71)	0.325
Sex (male), *n* (%)	201 (68 %)	31 (56 %)	19 (83 %)	35 (63 %)	116 (72 %)	0.086
SAPS II (IQR)	62 (45–79)	50 (33–68)	52 (37–73)	59 (38–75)	70 (52–86)	<0.001
SOFA (IQR)	11 (8–15)	10 (7–12)	9 (7–12)	10(6–13)	12 (8–16)	<0.001
Respiratory rate, bpm (IQR)	20 (16–25)	18 (15–22)	18 (15–27)	20 (16–25)	21 (17–27)	0.080
Body temperature, C° (IQR)	36.0 (34.8–36.8)	35.5 (33.6–36.5)	35.6 (33.5–36.5)	36.4 (35.2–36.9)	36.1 (35.0–36.8)	0.893
Heart rate, bpm (IQR)	81 (65–104)	79 (61–95)	83 (60–107)	79 (60–98)	83 (66–108)	0.119
Mean arterial pressure, mmHg (IQR)	68 (57–79)	73 (63–83)	72 (58–80)	70 (61–83)	65 (54–76)	<0.01
Preexisting liver cirrhosis, *n* (%)	22 (7 %)	1 (2 %)	0	5 (9 %)	16 (10 %)	<0.05
Cause of HH						
Cardiogenic shock, *n* (%)[a]	133 (45 %)	27 (49 %)	15 (65 %)	28 (50 %)	63 (39 %)	<0.05
Septic shock, *n* (%)[a]	109 (37 %)	12 (22 %)	5 (22 %)	14 (25 %)	78 (48 %)	<0.001
Hemorrhagic shock, *n* (%)	8 (3 %)	0	0	1 (2 %)	7 (4 %)	0.081
Therapy						
Mechanical ventilation, *n* (%)	225 (76 %)	36 (66 %)	19 (83 %)	35 (63 %)	135 (84 %)	<0.01
Vasopressor use, *n* (%)	247 (84 %)	38 (69 %)	18 (78 %)	35 (80 %)	146 (91 %)	<0.001
RRT, *n* (%)	122 (41 %)	0	0	0	122 (76 %)	<0.001
Laboratory parameters on admission						
Arterial lactate, mmol/l (IQR)	3.5 (1.7–8.2)	2.0 (1.2–4.4)	2.7 (1.6–5.7)	3.5 (2.1–6.9)	4.3 (2.1–10.6)	<0.001
Arterial pH (IQR)	7.30 (7.20–7.40)	7.39 (7.30–7.47)	7.32 (7.28–7.39)	7.32 (7.24–7.41)	7.27 (7.15–7.36)	<0.001
Sodium, mmol/l (IQR)	138 (133–142)	138 (133–140)	140 (136–143)	138 (133–141)	138 (133–142)	0.387
Potassium, mmol/l (IQR)	4.5 (3.9–5.2)	4.1 (3.6–4.7)	4.0 (3.7–4.4)	4.5 (4.1–5.1)	4.7 (4.1–5.5)	0.906
Albumin, g/l (IQR)	29.3 (24.1–34.0)	29 (24–32)	30 (26–36)	30 (24–35)	29 (24–34)	0.405
AST, U/l (IQR)	366 (73–1265)	345 (77–781)	474 (85–1341)	699 (108–1599)	248 (57–1475)	0.142
ALT, U/l (IQR)	139 (39–706)	129 (55–639)	219 (54–631)	217 (44–1470)	124 (34–682)	0.731
INR (IQR)	1.4 (1.2–1.9)	1.3 (1.1–1.6)	1.3 (1.1–1.4)	1.4 (1.2–1.9)	1.5 (1.2–2.1)	0.142
Bilirubin, mg/dl (IQR)	1.3 (0.7–2.7)	1.0 (0.6–2.1)	0.9 (0.7–1.6)	1.3 (0.8–3.1)	1.4 (0.7–3.2)	<0.05
Outcome						
28-day mortality, *n* (%)	170 (58 %)	17 (31 %)	6 (26 %)	25 (45 %)	122 (76 %)	<0.001

SAPS II simplified acute physiology score, *SOFA* sequential organ failure assessment, *HH* hypoxic hepatitis, *MCI* myocardial infarction, *RRT* renal replacement therapy, *AST* aspartate aminotransferase, *ALT* alanine aminotransferase, *INR* international normalized ratio, *IQR* interquartile range

* *p* values calculated using univariate ordinal logistic regression modeling with intercept

[a] Three patients had both cardiogenic and septic shock (mixed shock)

AKI was 55 % (and 49 % even in patients without HH), thus considerably higher than recently reported in the FINNAKI study (39 % incidence of AKI) [10]. However, incidence of AKI in our total cohort is comparable to recently published incidence rates according to KDIGO criteria in critically ill patients [26].

AKI was observed in the vast majority of HH patients with only 19 % preserving normal renal function. There was a temporal relationship between HH and AKI, and in most affected patients both events occurred early during the ICU stay. However, the temporal relationship varied between patients. AKI in HH was associated with severity of illness reflected by SAPS and SOFA score, but most importantly with shock, vasopressor use and admission lactate levels. Thus, ischemia and tissue hypoxia seem to play a crucial role in development of AKI in HH.

In accordance with other studies [10, 17], ICU stay was significantly prolonged in patients with AKI; 28-day mortality rate in patients with AKI was 40 % in the total study cohort. In contrast, AKI in HH was associated with significantly higher 28-day mortality rates exceeding 60 % by far. The high mortality rates are in part attributable to the severity of illness reflected by high SAPS and SOFA scores on ICU admission. Yet, AKI, the presence of septic

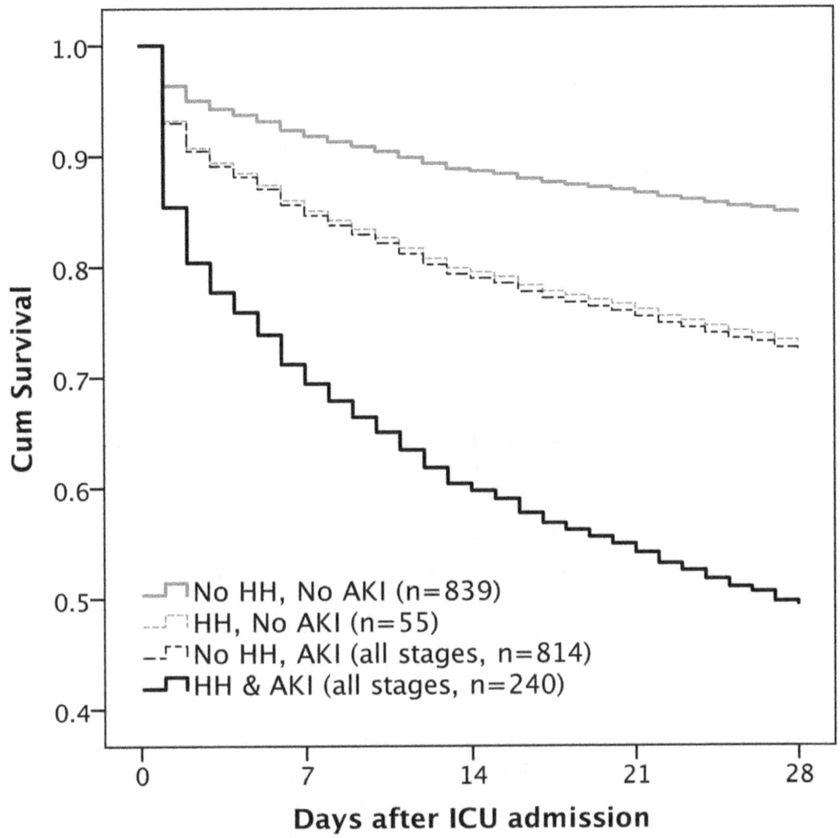

Admissions at risk (n):					
No HH, no AKI	840	784	755	739	727
HH, no AKI	55	46	41	39	38
No HH, AKI (all stages)	814	663	610	578	545
HH & AKI (all stages)	240	142	110	100	87

Fig. 2 Cox-adjusted survival curves illustrating the impact of HH and AKI on survival in critically ill patients. *HH* hypoxic hepatitis, *AKI* acute kidney injury, *ICU* intensive care unit; adjusted for age, sex, sequential organ failure assessment (SOFA) score; significant differences between patients with HH and/or AKI compared to patients without HH or AKI ($p < 0.05$); adjusted hazard ratio (HR) for 28-day mortality in patients with HH and AKI was 4.26 (95 % CI 3.30–5.51), $p < 0.001$

shock and peak INR values during HH were independent predictors of mortality in HH patients. Furthermore, we observed a synergistic effect of HH and AKI resulting in longer stay and increased mortality at the ICU. One reason for that observation may be the described systemic effects of AKI, which may further impair liver function [28].

Initiation of RRT was identified as an independent protective factor regarding survival in patients with HH. While necessity of RRT was significantly associated with increased 28-day mortality in the univariate analysis, this effect was completely abolished after adjustment for demographics, AKI, septic shock, INR and severity of disease. Initiation of RRT may provide beneficial effects in patients with HH. Apart from regulation of fluid balance, metabolic stabilization and removal of water-soluble toxins may contribute to this hypothesis. Best timing for initiation of RRT in critically ill patients is still a matter of debate. A recent large randomized controlled study comparing early versus late initiation of RRT in critically ill patients could not observe a difference in outcome [29]. Yet, future studies are required to assess timing, modality and potential benefits of RRT in patients with HH complicated by AKI.

Renal recovery was observed in the majority (71 %) of ICU survivors with HH and necessity of RRT. This finding is comparable to patients with ALF, where similarly high rates of renal recovery in patients requiring RRT have been described [30].

On the other hand, we observed a 100 % mortality rate in admissions with persisting failure of ≥ 5 organs (or

Table 3 Cox regression model for 28-day mortality in HH

Parameter	Hazard ratio (95% CI)		
	Unadjusted	Adjusted[a]	Adjusted[b]
Age	1.01 (0.99–1.02)	1.01 (0.99–1.02)	1.00 (0.99–1.02)
Gender (male)	1.22 (0.87–1.70)	1.18 (0.83–1.67)	1.26 (0.86–1.84)
Admission SOFA score	1.08 (1.04–1.12)**	1.04 (0.99–1.07)	1.03 (0.99–1.07)
Septic shock	2.07 (1.53–2.80)**	2.15 (1.32–3.50)**	2.37 (1.41–3.97)**
Cardiogenic shock	0.86 (0.64–1.17)	1.62 (0.99–2.63)	1.94 (1.16–3.24)*
INR	1.29 (1.20–1.39)**	1.24 (1.14–1.34)**	1.26 (1.13–1.39)**
Acute kidney injury (AKI)			
AKI 1 vs. no AKI	0.83 (0.33–2.11)	0.77 (0.30–1.95)	0.78 (0.30–2.00)
AKI 2 vs. no AKI	1.69 (0.91–3.12)	1.50 (0.81–2.79)	1.55 (0.81–2.97)
AKI 3 vs. no AKI	3.48 (2.09–5.78)**	3.40 (1.85–6.24)**	3.51 (1.86–6.62)**
Renal replacement therapy	1.86 (1.37–2.51)**	0.64 (0.42–0.97)*	0.62 (0.39–0.97)*

SOFA sequential organ failure assessment, *INR* international normalized ratio, *AKI* acute kidney injury

* p<0.05, ** p<0.01

[a] Patients with chronic liver disease included—adjusted for all variables (total *n*= *295*)

[b] Patients with chronic liver disease excluded—adjusted for all variables (total *n* = *273*)

SOFA scores >20) despite use of RRT for at least 2 days. Thus, our data suggest that continuation of RRT and other therapeutic measures should be repeatedly reevaluated on an individual basis in critically ill HH patients who present with persisting 5- or 6-organ failure despite use of RRT for more than 48 h. Furthermore, future studies are needed to address the question of when to start and to stop RRT in patients with (persisting) multi-organ failure.

Consensus recommendations on prevention and management of AKI in critically ill patients suggest that RRT should not be used in patients with liver failure, who are not candidates for liver transplantation [9]. Yet, the characteristic laboratory pattern of HH presenting with high aminotransferase levels and increased INR frequently fulfills criteria of acute liver failure [2, 7, 31]. Thus, distinguishing HH from other types of acute liver injury is of crucial importance due to its different clinical pattern and therapeutic consequences. It has been suggested that "the ability to manage heart failure or other causes of ischemia successfully will determine outcome for these (HH) patients, and transplantation is seldom indicated" [31]. Given the high incidence rates of HH in critically ill patients [2, 4, 6], HH should be considered as one of the primary differential diagnoses in patients with massive elevation of aminotransferase levels in the setting of critical illness. Our data suggest that, although mortality is still very high, RRT should be initiated in patients with HH developing AKI. Thus, RRT should not be withheld in patients with unclear elevation of aminotransferase levels at the ICU until the etiology has been clarified.

This study has strengths and limitations. This study comprises one of the largest datasets on HH published so far and uncovered for the first time the previously unrecognized association with AKI. Furthermore, the control group (without HH) contains 1653 critically ill medical patients. This sample size enables a good characterization of AKI in HH as compared to AKI in patients without HH. Yet, this study was conducted at three medical ICUs. Thus, our data may not be transferable to surgical ICUs or wards. Residual confounding arising from unmeasured covariates cannot be entirely excluded. Thus, further studies in different samples are required.

Conclusions

In sum, we could demonstrate that AKI frequently occurs in HH and is associated with high mortality and increased length of stay in survivors. Severity of the underlying disease and states of shock seem to contribute to AKI and poor outcome in HH. Initiation of RRT in HH with AKI may enable renal recovery and should not be withheld in medical ICU patients.

Abbreviations
AKI: acute kidney injury; CI: confidence interval; HH: hypoxic hepatitis; HR: hazard ratio; ICU: intensive care unit; INR: international normalized ratio; IQR: interquartile range; KDIGO: Kidney Disease: Improving Global Outcomes; LOS: length of stay; OR: odds ratio; RRT: renal replacement therapy; SAPS: implified acute physiology score; SOFA: sequential organ failure assessment.

Authors' contributions
AD and VF participated in study conception and design. TH, KRo, KRu, KS, CZ, GH, PS, DGH, VF and AD were involved in acquisition of data. AD, VF and TH contributed to analysis and interpretation of data. AD drafted the manuscript. VF, SK and MT were involved in critical revision of the manuscript for important intellectual content. VF and MT participated in supervision. All authors read and approved the final manuscript.

Author details
[1] Division of Gastroenterology and Hepatology, Department of Internal Medicine III, Medical University of Vienna, Vienna, Austria. [2] Department of Intensive Care Medicine, University Medical Center, Hamburg-Eppendorf, Martinistraße 52, 20246 Hamburg, Germany. [3] Division of Transplantation, Department of Surgery, Medical University of Vienna, Vienna, Austria. [4] Division of Nephrology, Department of Internal Medicine III, Medical University of Vienna, Vienna, Austria. [5] Department of Emergency Medicine, Inselspital, University Hospital Bern, Bern, Switzerland. [6] Intensive Care Unit 13H3, Division of Cardiology, Department of Internal Medicine II, Medical University of Vienna, Vienna, Austria. [7] Intensive Care Unit 13I2, Division of Oncology and Infectious Diseases, Department of Internal Medicine I, Medical University of Vienna, Vienna, Austria.

Competing interests
The authors declare that they have no competing interests.

References
1. Henrion J, Schapira M, Luwaert R, Colin L, Delannoy A, Heller FR. Hypoxic hepatitis: clinical and hemodynamic study in 142 consecutive cases. Medicine (Baltimore). 2003;82:392–406.
2. Henrion J. Hypoxic hepatitis. Liver Int. 2012;32:1039–52.
3. Fuhrmann V, Kneidinger N, Herkner H, Heinz G, Nikfardjam M, Bojic A, Schellongowski P, Angermayr B, Kitzberger R, Warszawska J, Holzinger U, Schenk P, Madl C. Hypoxic hepatitis: underlying conditions and risk factors for mortality in critically ill patients. Intensive Care Med. 2009;35:1397–405.
4. Fuhrmann V, Kneidinger N, Herkner H, Heinz G, Nikfardjam M, Bojic A, Schellongowski P, Angermayr B, Schöniger-Hekele M, Madl C, Schenk P. Impact of hypoxic hepatitis on mortality in the intensive care unit. Intensive Care Med. 2011;37:1302–10.
5. Jäger B, Drolz A, Michl B, Schellongowski P, Bojic A, Nikfardjam M, Zauner C, Heinz G, Trauner M, Fuhrmann V. Jaundice increases the rate of complications and 1-year mortality in patients with hypoxic hepatitis. Hepatology. 2012;56:2297–304.
6. Drolz A, Horvatits T, Michl B, Roedl K, Schellongowski P, Holzinger U, Zauner C, Heinz G, Madl C, Trauner M, Fuhrmann V. Statin therapy is associated with reduced incidence of hypoxic hepatitis in critically ill patients. J Hepatol. 2014;60:1187–93.
7. Drolz A, Jäger B, Wewalka M, Saxa R, Horvatits T, Roedl K, Perkmann T, Zauner C, Kramer L, Ferenci P, Fuhrmann V. Clinical impact of arterial ammonia levels in ICU patients with different liver diseases. Intensive Care Med. 2013;39:1227–37.
8. Drolz A, Horvatits T, Roedl K, Fuhrmann V. Shock liver and cholestatic liver in critically ill patients. Med Klin Intensivmed Notfmed. 2014;109:228–34.
9. Brochard L, Abroug F, Brenner M, Broccard AF, Danner RL, Ferrer M, Laghi F, Magder S, Papazian L, Pelosi P, Polderman KH. An official ATS/ERS/ESICM/SCCM/SRLF Statement: Prevention and Management of Acute Renal Failure in the ICU Patient: an international consensus conference in intensive care medicine. In Am J Respir Crit Care Med. 2010;181:1128–55.
10. Nisula S, Kaukonen K-M, Vaara ST, Korhonen A-M, Poukkanen M, Karlsson S, Haapio M, Inkinen O, Parviainen I, Suojaranta-Ylinen R, Laurila JJ, Tenhunen J, Reinikainen M, Ala-Kokko T, Ruokonen E, Kuitunen A, Pettilä V, FINNAKI Study Group. Incidence, risk factors and 90-day mortality of patients with acute kidney injury in Finnish intensive care units: the FINNAKI study. Intensive Care Med. 2013;39:420–8.
11. Medve L, Antek C, Paloczi B, Kocsi S, Gartner B, Marjanek Z, Bencsik G, Kanizsai P, Gondos T. Epidemiology of acute kidney injury in Hungarian intensive care units: a multicenter, prospective, observational study. BMC Nephrol. 2011;12:43.
12. Case J, Khan S, Khalid R, Khan A. Epidemiology of acute kidney injury in the intensive care unit. Crit Care Res Pract. 2013;2013:479730–9.
13. Piccinni P, Cruz DN, Gramaticopolo S, Garzotto F, DalSanto M, Aneloni G, Rocco M, Alessandri E, Giunta F, Michetti V, Iannuzzi M, BelluomoAnello C, Brienza N, Carlini M, Pelaia P, Gabbanelli V, Ronco C. Prospective multicenter study on epidemiology of acute kidney injury in the ICU: a critical care nephrology Italian collaborative effort. Minerva Anestesiol. 2011;77:1072–83.
14. Bagshaw SM, George C, Bellomo R, ANZICS Database Management Committee. Early acute kidney injury and sepsis: a multicentre evaluation. Crit Care. 2008;12:R47.
15. Joannidis M, Metnitz B, Bauer P, Schusterschitz N, Moreno R, Druml W, Metnitz PGH. Acute kidney injury in critically ill patients classified by AKIN versus RIFLE using the SAPS 3 database. Intensive Care Med. 2009;35:1692–702.
16. Kidney Disease Improving Global Outcomes KDIGO Acute Kidney, Injury Work Group. KDIGO clinical practice guideline for acute kidney injury. Kidney Int Suppl. 2012;2012(2):1–138.
17. O'Riordan A, Brummell Z, Sizer E, Auzinger G, Heaton N, O'Grady JG, Bernal W, Hendry BM, Wendon JA. Acute kidney injury in patients admitted to a liver intensive therapy unit with paracetamol-induced hepatotoxicity. Nephrol Dial Transplant. 2011;26:3501–8.
18. Le Gall JR, Lemeshow S, Saulnier F. A new simplified acute physiology score (SAPS II) based on a European/North American multicenter study. JAMA. 1993;270:2957–63.
19. Vincent JL, Moreno R, Takala J, Willatts S, De Mendonça A, Bruining H, Reinhart CK, Suter PM, Thijs LG. The SOFA (Sepsis-related Organ Failure Assessment) score to describe organ dysfunction/failure. On behalf of the working group on sepsis-related problems of the European society of intensive care medicine. Intensive Care Med. 1996;22:707–10.
20. RENAL Replacement Therapy Study Investigators, Bellomo R, Cass A, Cole L, Finfer S, Gallagher M, Lo S, McArthur C, McGuinness S, Myburgh J, Norton R, Scheinkestel C, Su S. Intensity of continuous renal-replacement therapy in critically ill patients. N Engl J Med. 2009;361:1627–38.
21. Goldberg RJ, Samad NA, Yarzebski J, Gurwitz J, Bigelow C, Gore JM. Temporal trends in cardiogenic shock complicating acute myocardial infarction. N Engl J Med. 1999;340:1162–8.
22. Heinz G. Cardiogenic shock–an inflammatory disease. Wien Klin Wochenschr. 2006;118:382–8.
23. Califf RM, Bengtson JR. **Cardiogenic shock**. N Engl J Med. 1994;330:1724–30.
24. Werdan K, Ruß M, Buerke M, Delle-Karth G, Geppert A, Schöndube FA. Cardiogenic shock due to myocardial infarction: diagnosis, monitoring and treatment: a German-Austrian S3 Guideline. Dtsch Arztebl Int. 2012;109(19):343–51.
25. Dellinger RP, Levy MM, Carlet JM, Bion J, Parker MM, Jaeschke R, Reinhart K, Angus DC, Brun-Buisson C, Beale R, Calandra T, Dhainaut J-F, Gerlach H, Harvey M, Marini JJ, Marshall J, Ranieri M, Ramsay G, Sevransky J, Thompson BT, Townsend S, Vender JS, Zimmerman JL, Vincent J-L. Surviving Sepsis Campaign: international guidelines for management of severe sepsis and septic shock: 2008. Intensive Care Med. 2008;34:17–60.
26. Hoste EAJ, Bagshaw SM, Bellomo R, Cely CM, Colman R, Cruz DN, Edipidis K, Forni LG, Gomersall CD, Govil D, Honoré PM, Joannes-Boyau O, Joannidis M, Korhonen A-M, Lavrentieva A, Mehta RL, Palevsky P, Roessler E, Ronco C, Uchino S, Vazquez JA, Vidal Andrade E, Webb S, Kellum JA. Epidemiology of acute kidney injury in critically ill patients: the multinational AKI-EPI study. Intensive Care Med. 2015;41:1411–23.
27. Bagshaw SM, Laupland KB, Doig CJ, Mortis G, Fick GH, Mucenski M, Godinez-Luna T, Svenson LW, Rosenal T. Prognosis for long-term survival

and renal recovery in critically ill patients with severe acute renal failure: a population-based study. Crit Care. 2005;9:R700–9.

28. Singbartl K, Joannidis M. Short-term effects of acute kidney injury. Crit Care Clin. 2015;31:751–62.
29. Gaudry S, Hajage D, Schortgen F, Martin-Lefevre L, Pons B, Boulet E, Boyer A, Chevrel G, Lerolle N, Carpentier D, de Prost N, Lautrette A, Bretagnol A, Mayaux J, Nseir S, Megarbane B, Thirion M, Forel J-M, Maizel J, Yonis H, Markowicz P, Thiery G, Tubach F, Ricard J-D, Dreyfuss D. Initiation Strategies for Renal-Replacement Therapy in the Intensive Care Unit. N Engl J Med. 2016. doi:10.1056/NEJMoa1603017 **(ahead of print)**.
30. Tujios SR, Hynan LS, Vazquez MA, Larson AM, Seremba E, Sanders CM, Lee WM, Acute Liver Failure Study Group. Risk factors and outcomes of acute kidney injury in patients with acute liver failure. Clin Gastroenterol Hepatol. 2015;13:352–9.
31. Polson J, Lee WM. AASLD position paper: the management of acute liver failure. Hepatology. 2005;41:1179–97.

Permissions

All chapters in this book were first published in AIC, by Springer; hereby published with permission under the Creative Commons Attribution License or equivalent. Every chapter published in this book has been scrutinized by our experts. Their significance has been extensively debated. The topics covered herein carry significant findings which will fuel the growth of the discipline. They may even be implemented as practical applications or may be referred to as a beginning point for another development.

The contributors of this book come from diverse backgrounds, making this book a truly international effort. This book will bring forth new frontiers with its revolutionizing research information and detailed analysis of the nascent developments around the world.

We would like to thank all the contributing authors for lending their expertise to make the book truly unique. They have played a crucial role in the development of this book. Without their invaluable contributions this book wouldn't have been possible. They have made vital efforts to compile up to date information on the varied aspects of this subject to make this book a valuable addition to the collection of many professionals and students.

This book was conceptualized with the vision of imparting up-to-date information and advanced data in this field. To ensure the same, a matchless editorial board was set up. Every individual on the board went through rigorous rounds of assessment to prove their worth. After which they invested a large part of their time researching and compiling the most relevant data for our readers.

The editorial board has been involved in producing this book since its inception. They have spent rigorous hours researching and exploring the diverse topics which have resulted in the successful publishing of this book. They have passed on their knowledge of decades through this book. To expedite this challenging task, the publisher supported the team at every step. A small team of assistant editors was also appointed to further simplify the editing procedure and attain best results for the readers.

Apart from the editorial board, the designing team has also invested a significant amount of their time in understanding the subject and creating the most relevant covers. They scrutinized every image to scout for the most suitable representation of the subject and create an appropriate cover for the book.

The publishing team has been an ardent support to the editorial, designing and production team. Their endless efforts to recruit the best for this project, has resulted in the accomplishment of this book. They are a veteran in the field of academics and their pool of knowledge is as vast as their experience in printing. Their expertise and guidance has proved useful at every step. Their uncompromising quality standards have made this book an exceptional effort. Their encouragement from time to time has been an inspiration for everyone.

The publisher and the editorial board hope that this book will prove to be a valuable piece of knowledge for researchers, students, practitioners and scholars across the globe.

List of Contributors

Elie Azoulay, Marine Chaize and Nancy Kentish-Barnes
Medical Intensive Care Unit, Hôpital Saint-Louis, ECSTRA team, Biostatistics and clinical epidemiology, UMR 1153 (Center of Epidemiology and Biostatistic Sorbonne Paris Cité, CRESS), INSERM, Paris Diderot Sorbonne University, Paris, France

Marcelo Park
Intensive Care Unit, Emergency Department, Hospital das Clínicas, University of São Paulo Medical School, Rua Dr. Enéas Carvalho de Aguiar, 255, Room 6040, São Paulo, Brazil

Bruno Adler Maccagnan Pinheiro Besen
Intensive Care Unit, Emergency Department, Hospital das Clínicas, University of São Paulo Medical School, Rua Dr. Enéas Carvalho de Aguiar, 255, Room 6040, São Paulo, Brazil Hospital da Luz, Amil, São Paulo, Brazil

Leandro Utino Taniguchi, Luciano Cesar Pontes Azevedo and Pedro Vitale Mendes
Intensive Care Unit, Emergency Department, Hospital das Clínicas, University of São Paulo Medical School, Rua Dr. Enéas Carvalho de Aguiar, 255, Room 6040, São Paulo ZIP 05403-000, Brazil
Research Institute, Hospital Sírio-Libanês, São Paulo, Brazil

Thiago Gomes Romano
Research Institute, Hospital Sírio-Libanês, São Paulo, Brazil
Nephrology Department, ABC Medical School, Santo Andre, Brazil

Antonio Paulo Nassar Jr.
Intensive Care Unit, Emergency Department, Hospital das Clínicas, University of São Paulo Medical School, Rua Dr. Enéas Carvalho de Aguiar, 255, Room 6040, São Paulo, Brazil A.C. Camargo Cancer Center, São Paulo, Brazil

Fernando Godinho Zampieri
Research Institute, HCor-Hospital do Coração, São Paulo, Brazil
Intensive Care Unit, Hospital Alemão Oswaldo Cruz, São Paulo, Brazil

Christophe E. M. De Block and Luc F. Van Gaal
Department of Endocrinology, Diabetology and Metabolism, Faculty of Medicine, Antwerp University Hospital and University of Antwerp, Wilrijkstraat 10, 2650 Edegem, Belgium

Peter Rogiers
Intensive Care Unit, ZNA, General Hospital Middelheim, Antwerp, Belgium

Philippe G. Jorens and Tom Schepens
Intensive Care Unit, Antwerp University Hospital, University of Antwerp, Edegem, Belgium

Cosimo Scuffi
A. Menarini Diagnostics, Scientific and Technology Affairs, Florence, Italy

Johann Auchabie, François Beloncle and Nicolas Lerolle
Département de Réanimation Médicale et de Médecine Hyperbare, Centre Hospitalier Universitaire, 4 rue Larrey, 49933 Angers Cedex 9, France

Jean-François Augusto
Néphrologie-Dialyse-Transplantation, CHU Angers, 4 rue Larrey, 49933 Angers Cedex 9, France
Service de Néphrologie et Immunologie Clinique, CHRU Tours, Tours, France

Julien Demiselle
Département de Réanimation Médicale et de Médecine Hyperbare, Centre Hospitalier Universitaire, 4 rue Larrey, 49933 Angers Cedex 9, France
Néphrologie-Dialyse-Transplantation, CHU Angers, 4 rue Larrey, 49933 Angers Cedex 9, France

Philippe Gatault
Service de Néphrologie et Immunologie Clinique, CHRU Tours, Tours, France

Steven Grangé
Medical Intensive Care Unit, Rouen University Hospital, Rouen, France

Damien Du Cheyron
Service de Réanimation Médicale, CHU de Caen, Avenue de la Côte de Nacre, CS 30001, 14033 Caen Cedex 9, France

Jean Dellamonica and Sonia Boyer
Medical Intensive Care Unit, Archet 1 University Hospital, Route de St Antoine, CS 23079, 06202 Nice, France

Dimitri Titeca Beauport
Medical Intensive Care Unit, Amiens University Medical Center, 80054 Amiens, Cedex 1, France

Lise Piquilloud
Département de Réanimation Médicale et de Médecine Hyperbare, Centre Hospitalier Universitaire, 4 rue Larrey, 49933 Angers Cedex 9, France
Service de Médecine Intensive Adulte et Centre des Brûlés, Centre Hospitalier Universitaire Vaudois, Lausanne, Switzerland

Julien Letheulle
Service de Réanimation Médicale, Hôpital Pontchaillou, CHU Rennes, 2 rue Henri Le Guilloux, 35033 Rennes Cedex, France

Christophe Guitton
Medical Intensive Care Unit, Hôtel-Dieu, University Hospital of Nantes, 30 bd Jean Monnet, 44093 Nantes, France
UMR 1064, Inserm, 30 bd Jean Monnet, 44093 Nantes, France

Nicolas Chudeau
Service de Reanimation Medico-Chirurgicale, Centre Hospitalier du Mans, 194 Avenue Rubillard, 72037 Le Mans, France

Guillaume Geri
Service de Réanimation Médicale, Hôpital Cochin, Paris, France

François Fourrier
Réanimation, Centre de Réanimation Polyvalente, Hôpital Roger Salengro, CHRU de Lille, Lille, France

René Robert
Service de Réanimation Médicale, CHU de Poitiers, Poitiers, France

Emmanuel Guérot
Service de Réanimation Médicale, Hôpital Européen Georges Pompidou, Paris, France

Julie Boisramé-Helms and Ferhat Meziani
Service de Réanimation Médicale, Nouvel Hôpital Civil, Hôpitaux Universitaires de Strasbourg, Strasbourg, France
EA 7293, Fédération de Médecine Translationnelle de Strasbourg (FMTS), Faculté de Médecine, Université de Strasbourg, Strasbourg, France

Pierre Galichon
APHP, Hôpital Tenon, Urgences Néphrologiques et Transplantation Rénale, Paris, France

Pierre-François Dequin
Service de Réanimation Polyvalente, Hôpital Bretonneau, Tours, France

Alexandre Lautrette
Service de Réanimation Médicale Polyvalente, CHU Gabriel Montpied, 58 rue Montalembert, 63000 Clermont-Ferrand, France

Pierre-Edouard Bollaert
Service de Réanimation Médicale, CHU de Nancy Hôpital Central, 29 Avenue de Lattre de Tassigny, 54035 Nancy Cedex, France

Loïc Guillevin
Département de Médecine Interne, Assistance Public des Hôpitaux de Paris, Hôpital Cochin, Paris, France

Giulliana Martines Moralez
Graduate Program in Translational Medicine, D'Or Institute for Research and Education (IDOR), Rio de Janeiro, Brazil

Ligia Sarmet Cunha Farah Rabello
PPG Internal Medicine, Federal University of Rio de Janeiro, Rio de Janeiro, Brazil
ICU, Hospital Copa D'Or, Rio de Janeiro, Brazil

Thiago Costa Lisboa
Complexo Hospitalar, Santa Casa de Misericórdia de Porto Alegre, Porto Alegre, Brazil

Mariza da Fonte Andrade Lima
ICU, Hospital Esperança Recife, Recife, Brazil

Rodrigo Marques Hatum
ICU, Hospital Total Cor, Rio de Janeiro, Brazil

Fernando Vinicius Cesar De Marco
ICU, Hospital viValle, São José dos Campos, Brazil

Alessandra Alves
ICU, Hospital Rios D'Or, Rio de Janeiro, Brazil

Jorge Eduardo da Silva Soares Pinto
ICU, Hospital Norte D'Or, Rio de Janeiro, Brazil

Hélia Beatriz Nunes de Araújo
Hospital do Coração do Brasil, Brasília, Brazil

Grazielle Viana Ramos and Aline Reis Silva
Department of Critical Care, D'Or Institute for Research and Education (IDOR), Rio de Janeiro, Brazil

Guilherme Côrtes Fernandes
ICU, Santa Casa de Misericórdia de Juiz de Fora, Juiz de Fora, Brazil

Guilherme Brenande Alves Faria
ICU, Hospital Oeste D'Or, Rio de Janeiro, Brazil

Ciro Leite Mendes
ICU, Hospital Universitário Lauro Wanderley, João Pessoa, Brazil

Roberto Álvaro Ramos Filho
ICU, Hospital São Luiz - Unidade Jabaquara, São Paulo, Brazil

Valdênia Pereira de Souza
Complexo Hospitalar de Niterói, Niterói, Brazil

Pedro Emmanuel Alvarenga Americano do Brasil and Fernando Augusto Bozza
Department of Critical Care, D'Or Institute for Research and Education (IDOR), Rio de Janeiro, Brazil
Instituto Nacional de Infectologia Evandro Chagas, Fundação Oswaldo Cruz-Fiocruz, Rio de Janeiro, Brazil

Jorge Ibrain Figueira Salluh
PPG Internal Medicine, Federal University of Rio de Janeiro, Rio de Janeiro, Brazil
Department of Critical Care and Graduate Program in Translational Medicine, D'Or Institute for Research and Education (IDOR), Rio de Janeiro, Brazil

Marcio Soares
PPG Internal Medicine, Federal University of Rio de Janeiro, Rio de Janeiro, Brazil
Department of Critical Care and Graduate Program in Translational Medicine, D'Or Institute for Research and Education (IDOR), Rio de Janeiro, Brazil
Department of Critical Care, D'Or Institute for Research and Education, Rua Diniz Cordeiro, 30. Botafogo, Rio de Janeiro 22281-100, Brazil

Gabor Zilahi
Department of Clinical Medicine, Trinity Centre for Health Sciences, Multidisciplinary
Intensive Care Research Organization (MICRO), Wellcome Trust-HRB Clinical Research, St James's Hospital, St James's University Hospital, Dublin 8, Ireland

Antonio Artigas
Critical Care Center, Parc Taulí Hospital-Sabadell, CIBERes, Parc Tauli s/n., Sabadell, Barcelona, Spain
Centros de Investigación Biomédica en Red (CIBER), Madrid, Spain

Ignacio Martin-Loeches
Department of Clinical Medicine, Trinity Centre for Health Sciences, Multidisciplinary
Intensive Care Research Organization (MICRO), Wellcome Trust-HRB Clinical Research, St James's Hospital, St James's University Hospital, Dublin 8, Ireland
Centros de Investigación Biomédica en Red (CIBER), Madrid, Spain
Wellcome Trust-HRB Clinical Research, Dublin, Ireland
Department of Clinical Medicine, Trinity Centre for Health Sciences, Dublin, Ireland

Xavier Repessé, Margaux Artiguenave, Sophie Paktoris-Papine and, Cyril Charron
Intensive Care Unit, Section Thorax-Vascular Disease-Abdomen-Metabolism, Assistance Publique-Hôpitaux de Paris, University Hospital Ambroise Paré, 9, Avenue Charles-de-Gaulle, 92100 Boulogne-Billancourt, France

Florence Espinasse
Infection Control Unit, Section Biology Pathology and Health Products, Assistance Publique-Hôpitaux de Paris, University Hospital Ambroise Paré, 92100 Boulogne-Billancourt, France

Aurélien Dinh
Infectious Diseases Department, Assistance Publique-Hôpitaux de Paris, University Hospital Ambroise Paré, 92100 Boulogne-Billancourt, France

Faten El Sayed
Microbiology Unit, Section Biology Pathology and Health Products, Assistance Publique-Hôpitaux de Paris, University Hospital Ambroise Paré, 92100 Boulogne-Billancourt, France

Guillaume Geri and Antoine Vieillard-Baron
Intensive Care Unit, Section Thorax-Vascular Disease-Abdomen-Metabolism, Assistance Publique-Hôpitaux de Paris, University Hospital Ambroise Paré, 9, Avenue Charles-de-Gaulle, 92100 Boulogne-Billancourt, France
Faculty of Medicine Paris Ile-de-France Ouest, University of Versailles Saint-Quentin en Yvelines, 78280 Saint-Quentin-en-Yvelines, France
INSERM U-1018, CESP, Team 5 (EpReC, Renal and Cardiovascular Epidemiology), UVSQ, 94807 Villejuif, France

Margareta Ieven, Erlangga Yusuf and Herman Goossens
Department of Microbiology, Antwerp University Hospital (UZA), University of Antwerp, Wilrijkstraat 10, 2650 Edegem, Belgium

Walter Verbrugghe, Philippe G. Jorens and Kristof Bergs
Department of Intensive Care Medicine, Antwerp University Hospital (UZA), University of Antwerp, Wilrijkstraat 10, 2650 Edegem, Belgium

Emiel Goovaerts
Department of Hospital Hygiene and Infection Control, Antwerp University Hospital (UZA), University of Antwerp, Wilrijkstraat 10, 2650 Edegem, Belgium

Kristien Wouters
Department of Biostatistics, Antwerp University Hospital (UZA), University of Antwerp, Wilrijkstraat 10, 2650 Edegem, Belgium

Bruno Van Herendael
Department of Microbiology, Antwerp University Hospital (UZA), University of Antwerp, Wilrijkstraat 10, 2650 Edegem, Belgium
GZA Hospitals, Antwerp, Belgium

Bernard Floccard and Guillaume Marcotte
Department of Anesthesiology and Critical Care Medicine, Edouard Herriot hospital, Hospices Civils de Lyon, Lyon, France

Violette Zorio, Benjamin Delwarde, Julien Textoris and Thomas Rimmelé
Department of Anesthesiology and Critical Care Medicine, Edouard Herriot hospital, Hospices Civils de Lyon, Lyon, France
EA7426 Hospices Civils de Lyon - bioMérieux, University Claude Bernard Lyon 1 "Pathophysiology of Injury Induced Immunosuppression", Lyon, France

Fabienne Venet and Guillaume Monneret
EA7426 Hospices Civils de Lyon - bioMérieux, University Claude Bernard Lyon 1 "Pathophysiology of Injury Induced Immunosuppression", Lyon, France
Cellular Immunology Laboratory, Edouard Herriot hospital, Hospices Civils de Lyon, Lyon, France

Benoit Pilmis
Service de maladies infectieuses et tropicales, Hôpital Necker Enfants malades, Service de maladies infectieuses et tropicales, Université Paris Descartes, Paris, France
Equipe mobile de microbiologie clinique, Groupe Hospitalier Paris Saint-Joseph, Paris, France

Vincent Jullien
Service de Pharmacologie, Hôpital Européen Georges Pompidou, Université Paris Descartes, Paris, France
INSERM U1129, Paris, France

Alexis Tabah
Intensive Care Unit, The Redcliffe Hospital, Brisbane, Australia
Burns, Trauma and Critical Care Research Centre, The University of Queensland, Brisbane, Australia

Jean-Ralph Zahar
Département de Microbiologie Clinique, Unité de Contrôle et de Prévention du risque Infectieux, Groupe Hospitalier Paris Seine Saint-Denis, AP-HP, CHU Avicenne, 125 rue de Stalingrad, 9300 Bobigny, France
Infection Control Unit, IAME, UMR 1137, Université Paris 13, Sorbonne Paris Cité, Paris, France

Christian Brun-Buisson
Réanimation médicale, Hôpital Henri Mondor, Université Paris Est Créteil (UPEC), Créteil, France

Jin-Min Peng, Li Weng, Chun-Yao Wang, Wei Jiang and Bin Du
Medical ICU, Peking Union Medical College Hospital, Peking Union Medical College and Chinese Academy of Medical Sciences, 1 Shuai Fu Yuan, Beijing 100730, People's Republic of China

Hui-Bin Huang
Medical ICU, Peking Union Medical College Hospital, Peking Union Medical College and Chinese Academy of Medical Sciences, 1 Shuai Fu Yuan, Beijing 100730, People's Republic of China
Department of Critical Care Medicine, The First Affiliated Hospital of Fujian Medical University, Fuzhou, China

Océane Garnier, Julie Carr and Albert Prades
Department of Anaesthesia and Critical Care Medicine, University of Montpellier Saint Eloi Hospital, 80, avenue Augustin Fliche, 34295 Montpellier Cedex 5, France

Gérald Chanques, Audrey de Jong and Samir Jaber
Department of Anaesthesia and Critical Care Medicine, University of Montpellier Saint Eloi Hospital, 80, avenue Augustin Fliche, 34295 Montpellier Cedex 5, France
PhyMedExp, INSERM U1046, CNRS, UMR 9214, University of Montpellier, Montpellier, France

Christine M. Rowan
Department of Medicine, Division of Allergy, Pulmonary, and Critical Care Medicine and the Center for Health Services Research, Vanderbilt University School of Medicine, Nashville, TN, USA

E. Wesley Ely
Department of Medicine, Division of Allergy, Pulmonary, and Critical Care Medicine and the Center for Health Services Research, Vanderbilt University School of Medicine, Nashville, TN, USA
Geriatric Research Education Clinical Center (GRECC), Department of Veterans Affairs, Tennessee Valley Healthcare System, Nashville, TN, USA

Fanny Perrigault and Anaïs Eloi
Department of Speech and Language Therapy, School of Medicine, University of Montpellier, Montpellier, France

Sylvie Moritz-Gasser
Department of Speech and Language Therapy, School of Medicine, University of Montpellier, Montpellier, France
Institute of Neurosciences of Montpellier, INSERM U105, University of Montpellier, Montpellier, France

Nicolas Molinari
Department of Statistics, University of Montpellier Hospitals, Montpellier, France

Marie Lecronier
Service de Pneumologie et Réanimation Médicale (Département "R3S"), Groupe Hospitalier Pitié-Salpêtrière Charles Foix, Assistance Publique-Hôpitaux de Paris, 75013 Paris, France

Sandrine Valade and Elie Azoulay
Service de Réanimation médicale, Groupe Hospitalier Saint-Louis - Lariboisière - Fernand-Widal, Assistance Publique- Hôpitaux de Paris, Paris, France

Naike Bigé and Eric Maury
Service de Réanimation médicale, Groupe Hospitalier Est Parisien, Hôpital Saint-Antoine Paris, Assistance Publique- Hôpitaux de Paris, Paris, France

Nicolas de Prost
Service de Réanimation médicale, Groupe Hospitalier Henri Mondor, Assistance Publique-Hôpitaux de Paris, Créteil, France

Damien Roux
Service de Réanimation médico-chirurgicale, Groupe Hospitalier Paris Nord, Hôpital Louis-Mourier, Assistance Publique-Hôpitaux de Paris, Colombes, France

David Lebeaux
Service de Microbiologie, Unité Mobile de Microbiologie Clinique, Hôpital Européen Georges Pompidou, Assistance Publique-Hôpitaux de Paris, Paris, France
Université Paris Descartes, Sorbonne Paris Cité, Paris, France

Alexandre Demoule and Martin Dres
Service de Pneumologie et Réanimation Médicale (Département "R3S"), Groupe Hospitalier Pitié-Salpêtrière Charles Foix, Assistance Publique-Hôpitaux de Paris, 75013 Paris, France
INSERM, UMRS1158 Neurophysiologie respiratoire expérimentale et clinique, Sorbonne Universités, UPMC Univ Paris 06, Paris, France

Fabienne D. Simonis
Department of Intensive Care and Lab. of Experimental Intensive Care and Anesthesiology (L E I C A), Academic Medical Center, Meibergdreef 9, 1105 AZ Amsterdam, The Netherlands

Ary Serpa Neto
Department of Intensive Care and Lab. of Experimental Intensive Care and Anesthesiology (L E I C A), Academic Medical Center, Meibergdreef 9, 1105 AZ Amsterdam, The Netherlands
Department of Intensive Care Medicine, Hospital Israelita Albert Einstein, São Paulo, Brazil

Carmen S. V. Barbas
Department of Intensive Care Medicine, Hospital Israelita Albert Einstein, São Paulo, Brazil
Department of Pulmonology, Faculdade de Medicina da Universidade de São Paulo, São Paulo, Brazil

Antonio Artigas-Raventós
Department of Intensive Care Medicine and CIBER de Enfermedades Respiratorias, Hospital de Sabadell, Corporació Sanitaria I Universitària Parc Taulí, Sabadell, Spain

Jaume Canet
Department of Anesthesiology, Hospital Universitari Germans Trias I Pujol, Barcelona, Spain

Rogier M. Determann
Department of Critical Care, Westfriesgasthuis, Hoorn, The Netherlands

James Anstey and Roger Smith
Department of Intensive Care, St Vincent's Hospital, Melbourne, Australia

Goran Hedenstierna
Department of Medical Sciences, Uppsala University, Uppsala, Sweden

Sabrine N. T. Hemmes and Markus W. Hollmann
Department of Anesthesiology, Academic Medical Center, Amsterdam, The Netherlands

Greet Hermans
Medical Intensive Care Unit, Division of General Internal Medicine, University Hospital Leuven, Louvain, Belgium
Laboratory of Intensive Care Medicine, Department of Cellular and Molecular Medicine, KU Leuven, Louvain, Belgium

Michael Hiesmayr, Werner Schmid and Edda M. Tschernko
Division of Cardiac, Thoracic, and Vascular Anesthesia and Intensive Care, Medical University Vienna, Vienna, Austria

Samir Jaber
Department of Critical Care Medicine and Anesthesiology (SAR B), Saint Eloi University Hospital, Montpellier, France

Ignacio Martin-Loeches
Department of Clinical Medicine, Trinity Centre for Health Sciences, Multidisciplinary Intensive Care Research Organization (MICRO), Welcome Trust, HRB Clinical Research, St James's University Hospital Dublin, Dublin, Ireland
Irish Centre for Vascular Biology, Irish Centre for Vascular Biology (ICVB), Dublin, Ireland

Gary H. Mills
Department of Anaesthesia and Critical Care Medicine, Sheffield Teaching Hospital, Sheffield, UK

Rupert M. Pearse
Barts and the London School of Medicine and Dentistry, Queen Mary University of London, London, UK

Christian Putensen
Department of Anesthesiology and Intensive Care Medicine, University Hospital Bonn, Bonn, Germany

Paolo Severgnini
Department of Biotechnologies and Sciences of Life, Insubria University, Varese, Italy

Tanja A. Treschan
Department of Anaesthesiology, Düsseldorf University Hospital, Düsseldorf, Germany

Marcos F. Vidal Melo
Department of Anesthesia, Critical Care and Pain Medicine, Massachusetts General Hospital, Harvard Medical School, Boston, USA

Hermann Wrigge
Department of Anesthesiology and Intensive Care Medicine, University of Leipzig, Leipzig, Germany

Marcelo Gama de Abreu
Pulmonary Engineering Group, Department of Anesthesiology and Intensive Care Medicine, University Hospital Carl Gustav Carus, Dresden, Germany
Pulmonary Engineering Group, Department of Anesthesiology and Intensive Care Medicine, Technische Universität Dresden, Dresden, Germany

Paolo Pelosi
Department of Surgical Sciences and Integrated Diagnostics, Ospedale Policlinico per la Oncologia, IRCCS per l'Oncologia, University of Genoa, Genoa, Italy

Marcus J. Schultz
Department of Intensive Care and Lab. of Experimental Intensive Care and Anesthesiology (L E I C A), Academic Medical Center, Meibergdreef 9, 1105 AZ Amsterdam, The Netherlands
Mahidol Oxford Research Unit (MORU), Mahidol University, Bangkok, Thailand

José Augusto Santos Pellegrini
Department of Critical Care Medicine, Hospital de Clínicas de Porto Alegre, Universidade Federal do Rio Grande do Sul, Porto Alegre, Brazil

Ricardo Luiz Cordioli
Department of Critical Care Medicine, Hospital Israelita Albert Einstein, São Paulo, Brazil
Department of Critical Care Medicine, Alemão Oswaldo Cruz Hospital, São Paulo, Brazil
Department of Intensive Care Unit, Hospital Israelita Albert Einstein, 627, Albert Einstein St., São Paulo 05652-900, Brazil

Ana Cristina Burigo Grumann
Department of Critical Care Medicine, Nereu Ramos Hospital, Florianópolis, Brazil

Patrícia Klarmann Ziegelmann
Statistics Department and Post-Graduation Program in Epidemiology, Universidade Federal do Rio Grande do Sul, Porto Alegre, Brazil

Leandro Utino Taniguchi
Department of Critical Care Medicine, Hospital das Clínicas de São Paulo, FMUSP, São Paulo, Brazil

Ben de Jong and Arthur R. H. van Zanten
Department of Intensive Care Medicine, Gelderse Vallei Hospital, Willy Brandtlaan 10, 6716 RP Ede, The Netherlands

Anne Sophie Schuppers, Arriette Kruisdijk-Gerritsen and Hubertus Laurentius Antonius van den Oever
Department of Intensive Care Medicine, Deventer Hospital, Nico Bolkesteinlaan 75, 7416 SE Deventer, The Netherlands

Maurits Erwin Leo Arbouw
Department of Clinical Pharmacy, Deventer Hospital, Nico Bolkesteinlaan 75, 7416 SE Deventer, The Netherlands

Fabienne Scherer and Stéphane Cullati
Pain and Palliative Care Consultation, Division of Clinical Pharmacology and Toxicology, Geneva University Hospitals, Rue Gabrielle-Perret-Gentil 4, 1211 Geneva, Switzerland

Monica Escher
Pain and Palliative Care Consultation, Division of Clinical Pharmacology and Toxicology, Geneva University Hospitals, Rue Gabrielle-Perret-Gentil 4, 1211 Geneva, Switzerland
Unit of Development and Research in Medical Education, Faculty of Medicine, University of Geneva, Geneva, Switzerland

Bara Ricou
Division of Intensive Care, Geneva University Hospitals, Geneva, Switzerland

Mathieu Nendaz
Unit of Development and Research in Medical Education, Faculty of Medicine, University of Geneva, Geneva, Switzerland
Division of General Internal Medicine, Geneva University Hospitals, Geneva, Switzerland

Patricia Hudelson
Division of Primary Care Medicine, Geneva University Hospitals, Geneva, Switzerland

Thomas Perneger
Division of Clinical Epidemiology, Geneva University Hospitals, Geneva, Switzerland

Alain Cariou and Gilles Francony
Medical Intensive Care Unit, Cochin University Hospital (APHP) and Paris Descartes University, 27 rue du Faubourg Saint-Jacques, 75014 Paris, France

Jean-François Payen
Pôle Anesthésie-Réanimation, Hôpital Michallon, CHU Grenoble Alpes, 38000 Grenoble, France

Cyrille Mathien
Service de Réanimation médicale, CH Mulhouse, Mulhouse, France

Laure De Saint Blanquat
Hôpital Necker-Enfants Malades, Réanimation Pédiatrique Polyvalente, Assistance Publique-Hôpitaux de Paris, Paris, France

Lionel Velly
Service d'Anesthésie-Réanimation, Hôpital de la Timone, Assistance Publique-Hôpitaux de Marseille, Marseille, France

Nicolas Deye
Hôpital Lariboisiere, Assistance Publique- Hôpitaux de Paris, Paris, France

Stéphane Legriel
Centre Hospitalier de Versailles, Le Chesnay, France

Bruno Levy
Hôpital Central, CHU de Nancy, Nancy, France

Gerard Audibert
CHU de Nancy, Nancy, France

Nicolas Engrand
Fondation Rothschild, Paris, France

Jean-Christophe Orban
Hôpital Pasteur 2, CHU de Nice, Nice, France

Bernard Vigue
Anesthésie-réanimation, Bicêtre, France

Guillaume Debaty
CHU de Grenoble, La Tronche, France

Karim Asehnoune
Hôpitial Hôtel-Dieu, CHU de Nantes, Nantes, France

Astrid Botte
Hôpital Jeanne de Flandre, CHRU de Lille, Lille, France

Olivier Brissaud
CHU de Bordeaux, Bordeaux, France

Philippe Meyer
Hôpital Necker-Enfants Malades, Assistance Publique-Hôpitaux de Paris, Paris, France

Sylvain Renolleau
Hôpital Armand-Trousseau, Assistance Publique-Hôpitaux de Paris, Paris, France

Sandrine Deltour
Hôpital Pitié-Salpêtrière, Assistance Publique-Hôpitaux de Paris, Paris, France

Claire Chaignat
Intensive Care Unit, Besançon University Hospital, 25030 Besançon, France

Gaël Piton and Gilles Capellier
Intensive Care Unit, Besançon University Hospital, 25030 Besançon, France
Université de Franche Comté, 25000 Besançon, France

Mikhael Giabicani and Fabienne Tamion
Intensive Care Unit, Rouen University Hospital, Rouen, France

Vincent Di Martino
Université de Franche Comté, 25000 Besançon, France
Hepatology Unit, Besançon University Hospital, Besançon, France

Jean-Paul Cervoni
Hepatology Unit, Besançon University Hospital, Besançon, France

Emmanuel Weiss and Catherine Paugam-Burtz
Intensive Care and Anesthesiology Department, AP-HP, Hôpital Beaujon, Hôpitaux Universitaires Paris Nord Val de Seine, 75018 Paris, France
University Paris Diderot, Sorbonne Paris Cité, 75018 Paris, France

Nicolas Viallet, Vincent Brunot, Delphine Daubin, Noémie Besnard, Laura Platon, Aurèle Buzançais, Romaric Larcher and Olivier Jonquet
Department of Intensive Care Medicine, Lapeyronie University Hospital, 371, Avenue du Doyen G. Giraud, 34295 Montpellier, France

Nils Kuster
Department of Biochemistry, Lapeyronie University Hospital, Montpellier, France

Kada Klouche
Department of Intensive Care Medicine, Lapeyronie University Hospital, 371, Avenue du Doyen G. Giraud, 34295 Montpellier, France
PhyMedExp, INSERM U1046, CNRS UMR 9214, University of Montpellier, Montpellier, France

Christian Zauner and Michael Trauner
Division of Gastroenterology and Hepatology, Department of Internal Medicine III, Medical University of Vienna, Vienna, Austria

Andreas Drolz, Thomas Horvatits, Kevin Roedl, Karoline Rutter and Valentin Fuhrmann
Division of Gastroenterology and Hepatology, Department of Internal Medicine III, Medical University of Vienna, Vienna, Austria
Department of Intensive Care Medicine, University Medical Center, Hamburg-Eppendorf, Martinistraße 52, 20246 Hamburg, Germany

Stefan Kluge
Department of Intensive Care Medicine, University Medical Center, Hamburg-Eppendorf, Martinistraße 52, 20246 Hamburg, Germany

Katharina Staufer
Division of Gastroenterology and Hepatology, Department of Internal Medicine III, Medical University of Vienna, Vienna, Austria
Division of Transplantation, Department of Surgery, Medical University of Vienna, Vienna, Austria

Dominik G. Haider
Division of Nephrology, Department of Internal Medicine III, Medical University of Vienna, Vienna, Austria
Department of Emergency Medicine, Inselspital, University Hospital Bern, Bern, Switzerland

Gottfried Heinz
Intensive Care Unit 13H3, Division of Cardiology, Department of Internal Medicine II, Medical University of Vienna, Vienna, Austria

Peter Schellongowski
Intensive Care Unit 13I2, Division of Oncology and Infectious Diseases, Department of Internal Medicine I, Medical University of Vienna, Vienna, Austria

Index

www.ingramcontent.com/pod-product-compliance
Lightning Source LLC
LaVergne TN
LVHW080727210926
848485LV00003B/531